Laboratory Animal Science and Medicine

Volume 3

Series Editors
Aurora Brønstad, Laboratory Animal Science, University of Bergen, Bergen, Norway

José Sanchez Morgado, Bioresearch and Veterinary Services, The University of Edinburgh, Edinburgh, UK

This book series aims at providing an easily accessible and complete toolbox for researchers, Veterinarians and technicians who design animal studies or/ and work with research animals. The series equips the readers with the theoretical and practical knowledge to successfully run an animal facility, to monitor and maintain animal health and wellbeing in compliance with international ethical guidelines, to proof the genetic status of laboratory rodents and furthermore it profoundly introduces on how to design reproducible animal experiments. In a unique way, each volume focuses on a distinct topic which is always explored in a comprehensive manner.

This series is endorsed by the European Society for Laboratory Animal Veterinarians (ESLAV). As a leading voice in European Laboratory Animal Medicine, ESLAV's objectives are to promote and disseminate expert veterinary knowledge within the field of laboratory animal science, with a special focus on advancing skills in subjects connected with the breeding, health, welfare and use of laboratory animals.

Javier Guillén • Viola Galligioni
Editors

Practical Management of Research Animal Care and Use Programs

Questions and Answers

Springer

Editors
Javier Guillén
AAALAC International
Pamplona, Navarra, Spain

Viola Galligioni
Netherlands Institute for Neuroscience,
Royal Netherlands Academy of Arts
and Sciences
Amsterdam, The Netherlands

ISSN 2730-7859 ISSN 2730-7867 (electronic)
Laboratory Animal Science and Medicine
ISBN 978-3-031-65416-9 ISBN 978-3-031-65414-5 (eBook)
https://doi.org/10.1007/978-3-031-65414-5

UK Research and Innovation
This work was supported by UK Research and Innovation - Medical Research Council.

This Springer imprint is published by the registered company Springer Nature Switzerland AG
The registered company address is: Gewerbestrasse 11, 6330 Cham, Switzerland

Preface

Animal facility managers and other professionals involved in the care and use of animals used for research purposes face a cascade of challenges on a daily basis. Between planning a new animal facility and completing research projects, there are numerous aspects to be considered, many of them repeated every day to support the development of each new project while addressing animal welfare issues. Management of animal care and use programs is performed by a variety of professionals, including not only veterinarians but also animal technologists, biologists, researchers, and others. Regardless of the background of the ultimate responsible person, management of an animal care and use program is always a collective and multidisciplinary effort, where the knowledge and input of diverse personnel are needed.

There are not so many postgraduate courses addressing all the topics involved in such business that ranges from animal welfare to legislative requirements, to engineering needs, to personnel and users management, to financial administration, to health and safety and communication. Facility managers entering the job most of the time learn from personal experiences and the knowledge gained through their network.

This book, part of the book series promoted and endorsed by the European Society of Laboratory Animal Veterinarians (ESLAV), aims to become a reference in management of the daily challenges of the business. It discusses in detail the aspects to be considered for the implementation and management of a successful animal care and use program. The target audience is anybody involved at different levels in the management of animal care and use programs. The main objective is to present information in a very practical way for those responsible to address all needs, especially for those starting out in this business. For this purpose, the chapters are presented in a question and answer (Q&A) format, to give response to the potential questions of interest in each particular program area. We understand that in our profession, we typically simplify using the term "facility" to refer not only to the physical facility but to all the events happening in it on a daily basis. Therefore, except in the chapter focusing on the physical facility, the reader may assume that the term "facility" may be interchangeable with the concept of "animal care and use program" in most cases.

The order of the chapters considers a theoretical sequence of the areas to be addressed during the hypothetical planning and implementation of a program. However, each chapter stands on its own, and its Q&A can be used independently as a source of information for each addressed program area.

Because this book belongs to the ESLAV book series, a large proportion of authors are based in European animal care and use programs. Also, some of the contents may have a particular focus on the European environment, but since we believe that the main concepts and principles of laboratory animal science are shared by all professionals across the world, we think that the book can be useful for professionals in all geographical areas.

We believe that all professionals involved in the animal care and use program can benefit from the practical Q&A presented in this book.

Pamplona, Spain — Javier Guillén
Amsterdam, The Netherlands — Viola Galligioni

Contents

About the Editors and Contributors

About the Editors

Javier Guillén, D.V.M., is the AAALAC International Senior Director for Europe and Latin America. He is also responsible for the AAALAC activities in Africa and the Middle East. Previously, he was for 17 years Director of the Laboratory Animal Services at the University of Navarra in Pamplona, Spain.

He is a member of the Council of Management of Laboratory Animals Ltd., which publishes the journal *Laboratory Animals*, and of the Board of Management of the European Animal Research Association (EARA), an association that promotes openness/transparency through the establishment of national agreements. He is one of the promoters of the Spanish Transparency Agreement launched in 2016.

He is former President of the Federation of European Laboratory Animal Science Associations (FELASA) and of the Spanish Association for Laboratory Animal Science (SECAL), and he was also a member of the Governing Board of the International Council for Laboratory Animal Science (ICLAS) for eight years. He is currently a member of the ICLAS European Regional Committee.

He has published many articles/chapters on several topics relating to the care and use of animals in research, education, and testing, with special emphasis on legislation, ethics, and quality, including two editions of the book *Laboratory Animals: Regulations and Recommendations for the Care and Use of Animals in Research.*

He participated in several Expert Working Groups by the European Commission for the implementation of European Directive 2010/63/EU.

Viola Galligioni, D.V.M., PhD, is the Head of the Animal Facilities at the Netherlands Institute for Neuroscience, Royal Netherlands Academy of Arts and Science, the Netherlands. She has been involved in facility management in different European countries, Italy, Czech Republic, Ireland, and the Netherlands. Her experience spans across a variety of species (rodents, sheep, pigs, zebrafish, *Xenopus*, rabbits, cephalopods, and NHPs).

At the time of publication, she is President-elect of the European Society of Laboratory Animal Veterinarians (ESLAV) and Board member of the

Italian Association for Laboratory Animal Sciences (AISAL). She is also AAALAC International ad hoc consultant.

She has published scientific articles and chapters on the implementation of the 3Rs, animal welfare, and cephalopods. She believes in education and training of future facility managers and veterinarians, and therefore, she has been involved in the organization of multiple ESLAV-ECLAM Summer schools.

Contributors

Xavier Abad IRTA-CReSA, Bellaterra, Spain

Marion Berard Institut Pasteur, Université Paris Cité, Paris, France

Alessandra Bergadano University of Bern, Bern, Switzerland

Thomas Bertelsen Novo Nordisk, Maaloev, Denmark

Delphine Bouard Vetsalius, Lyon, France

Elodie Boucheaux Sanofi, Vitry-sur-Seine, France

Dorte Bratbo Sørensen University of Copenhagen, Copenhagen, Denmark

Tina Brønnum Pedersen H. Lundbeck A/S, Valby, Denmark

Aurora Brønstad University of Bergen, Bergen, Norway

James Bussell University of Oxford, Oxford, UK

Guillermo Cantero IRTA-CReSA, Bellaterra, Spain

Sabine Chourbaji University of Heidelberg, Heidelberg, Germany

Joachim Coenen Merck KGaA, Darmstadt, Germany

Thierry Decelle DCL Solutions, Paris, France

Delphine Denais-Lalieve IRSN, Fontenay-aux-Roses, France

Nicolas Dudoignon Sanofi, Gentilly, France

Alberto Elmi University of Pisa, Pisa, Italy

Paul Finnemore AstraZeneca, Cambridge, UK

Paul A. Flecknell Newcastle University and Flaire Consultants Ltd., Newcastle, UK

Rafael Frías Karolinska University Hospital, Solna, Sweden
Karolinska Institutet, Huddinge, Sweden

Viola Galligioni Netherlands Institute for Neuroscience, Amsterdam, The Netherlands

Mark Gardiner Mary Lyon Centre, MRC Harwell, Didcot, UK

Javier Guillén AAALAC International, Pamplona, Spain

Stefanie Hansborg Kolstrup University of Southern Denmark, Odense, Denmark

Patrick Hardy Centre Lago, Vonnas, France

Jann Hau University of Copenhagen, Copenhagen, Denmark

Gabi Itter Sanofi-Aventis, Frankfurt, Germany

Rony Kalman The Hebrew University of Jerusalem, Jerusalem, Israel

William W. King University of Michigan, Ann Arbor, USA

Axel Kornerup Hansen University of Copenhagen, Copenhagen, Denmark

Jan A. M. Langermans Biomedical Primate Research Centre, Rijswijk, The Netherlands

Kirk Leech European Animal Research Association, London, UK

Annet L. Louwerse Biomedical Primate Research Centre, Rijswijk, The Netherlands

Bertrand Luissier Université de Montréal, St-Hyacinthe, Québec, Canada

James D. Macy Yale University, New Haven, CT, USA

Jean-Philippe Mocho Joint Production System Ltd, Potters Bar, UK

Helena Paradell Zoetis Manufacturing & Research Spain, Vall de Bianya, Spain

Jan Parker-Thornburg MD Anderson Cancer Center, Houston, TX, USA

Belén Pintado CNB-CBMSO, CSIC, Madrid, Spain

Patricia Preisig Yale University, New Haven, CT, USA

Yannick Raeves Janssen Pharmaceutica NV, Beerse, Belgium

Thomas Steckler Janssen Pharmaceutica NV, Beerse, Belgium

Martina Stocker Biomedical Primate Research Centre, Rijswijk, The Netherlands

Susanne Rensing AbbVie Deutschland GmbH & Co KG, Ludwigshafen, Germany

Tanusha Singh University of Johannesburg, Johannesburg, South Africa

David Solanes Zoetis Manufacturing & Research Spain, Vall de Bianya, Spain

Bob Tolliday European Animal Research Association, London, UK

Eric Troncy Université de Montréal, St-Hyacinthe, Québec, Canada

Pascalle L. P. Van Loo Animal Welfare Body Utrecht, Utrecht, The Netherlands

Nicola Watts Laboratory Animal Science, London, UK

Sara Wells Mary Lyon Centre, MRC Harwell, Didcot, UK

Sarah Wolfensohn University of Surrey, Surrey, UK

Hanno Würbel University of Bern, Bern, Switzerland

The Ethical and Legal Framework

1

Javier Guillén, Paul Finnemore, and Hanno Würbel

Abstract

The management of an animal care and use program implies compliance with the legal requirements and observation of the societal and professional ethical concerns, both in constant evolution. This chapter answers in a practical and orderly way many questions relating to ethical and legal matters that should be considered first when setting up the program, second when attending research activities and operating the program, and third when dealing with aspects arising after animal use. Whereas the ethical aspects in this area of work are common in all continents, the practical aspects of legal compliance vary according to different supranational, national, and local legislation. This chapter focuses mainly on the legal framework of the European Union, but also offers multiple examples concerning the United Kingdom and the United States.

J. Guillén (✉)
AAALAC International, Pamplona, Spain
e-mail: jguillen@aaalac.org

P. Finnemore
Global Ethics and Compliance, AstraZeneca, Cambridge, UK
e-mail: paul.finnemore@astrazeneca.com

H. Würbel
Vetsuisse Faculty, Division of Animal Welfare, Veterinary Public Health Institute, University of Bern, Bern, Switzerland
e-mail: hanno.wuerbel@unibe.ch

Keywords

Ethics · Legislation · Research · Animal use

1.1 Where Are We on Legal and Ethical Grounds on Animal Use? (How Are We Allowed to Use Animals in Research)

The use of animals in research is regulated by a complex and dynamic set of laws, ordinances, policies, guidelines, and procedures that may differ across jurisdictions. Despite these differences, however, the legal and ethical conditions for using animals in research are largely similar around the world [1]. First, they all rest on the fundamental assumption that (some) animals are sentient and may thus experience negative affective states such as pain and other forms of suffering. And second, they are based on the principle of proportionality, which implies that any use of animals for scientific procedures must promote relevant societal interests (knowledge gain, human and animal health and well-being, and environmental protection), without imposing unnecessary harm on animals. The ultimate decision as to whether a particular study or research program is legitimate is, therefore, taken by a harm–benefit analysis [2]. A harm–benefit analysis is explicitly required by the European Union

J. Guillén, V. Galligioni (eds.), *Practical Management of Research Animal Care and Use Programs*, Laboratory Animal Science and Medicine 3, https://doi.org/10.1007/978-3-031-65414-5_1

(EU) Directive 2010/63 [3], but is also implied in the US Guide for the Care and Use of Laboratory Animals [4] and emphasized in the Terrestrial Animal Health Code by the World Organization for Animal Health [5] and the updated Principles of the Council for International Organizations of Medical Sciences (CIOMS) and the International Council for Laboratory Animal Science (ICLAS) [6]. The principle and procedure of harm–benefit analysis in animal research are further explained in Question 1.7.

Adherence to the principle of proportionality is further supported by various complementary legal and ethical conditions governing the use of animals in research. Thus, all staff interacting with, or taking responsibility for using, animals in research need to be adequately educated, trained, and competent or must be supervised until they have obtained and demonstrated the requisite competence. Animal facilities must provide the legal minimal requirements (e.g., space, environmental enrichment) for the housing of research animals, as well as adequate veterinary care by responsible staff for all animals in their establishments. Certain procedures are deemed inhumane a priori and are therefore prohibited, and humane endpoints must be used whenever possible (further discussed in Question 2.4). Also, adherence to a good research practice is required to guarantee reliable, robust, and reproducible results in view of maximizing the epistemic benefit, and the 3Rs principle (replace, reduce, and refine; further explained in Questions 1.7 and 2.1) must be applied to minimize the use of animals for research and the harm imposed on them [7]. Finally, institutions using animals in research should have an animal welfare body in place to offer advice on animal welfare issues, and the monitoring of compliance with the legal and ethical conditions should be facilitated by record keeping on all procedures and by regular inspections (both internal by the animal welfare body, and external by the competent authority).

1.2 Setting Up the Program

1.2.1 What Legislation Applies to an Animal Care and Use Program?

The most important is the legislation on the protection of animals bred for or used in research. In the EU, this is represented by Directive 2010/63/EU on the protection of animals used for scientific purposes [3], which every EU Member State has transposed into their national legislation. In the United Kingdom (UK), the Animals (Scientific Procedures) Act 1986 applies [8]. In the United States (US), there are two sources of legislation, the Animal Welfare Act and subsequent amendments and related Regulations [9], but which do not cover rats, mice, and some birds; and the Public Health Service Policy on humane care and use of laboratory animals [10] with requirements for each institution receiving Public Health Service funds for research involving animals. This policy requires compliance with the Guide for the Care and Use of Laboratory Animals [4], which is not a piece of legislation per se but is also followed in other areas of the world.

This type of legislation normally defines the scope, species covered, and the mechanisms to ensure the welfare of animals from the acquisition of the animals to the end of the experiments. Different laws protecting animals in research share common ethical principles (i.e., the 3Rs), though may differ in practical aspects. For example, all agree on the ethical evaluation of research projects using animals, but they may require different ways to implement the ethical review process.

In addition to legislation, there are a number of international documents that promote the same principles, which serve as guidance especially in countries where legislation has not been implemented. The most widely recognized are Chapter 7.8. of the Terrestrial Animal Health Code [5] and the International Guiding Principles for Biomedical Research Involving Animals [6].

However, there are other legislative areas applying to an animal care and use program that have to be considered for the program management, and that have to be identified in the respective geographical area. These include legislation pertaining to specific requirements on:

- Personnel training/competence
- Occupational health and safety of personnel
- Biosafety
- Use of genetically modified organisms
- Animal transportation
- Drug management
- Waste disposal

These areas are described in their respective chapters in this book.

Extensive descriptions of worldwide legislation on the protection of animals bred for or used in research in all areas of the world, and references to other applicable legislation can be found elsewhere [11].

1.2.2 What Is the Body to Ensure Evaluation and Oversight of the Animal Care and Use Program?

There may be one or more oversight bodies (OBs). They can be institutional or government, and in some cases external, independent of institution and government. In most cases of countries with specific legislation, the evaluation and oversight processes are performed through a combination of institutional and government OBs.

The institutional OB can be in the form of Ethics Committee (EC), Animal Welfare Body (AWB, as in the EU), Animal Welfare and Ethical Review Body (AWERB, as in the UK), Institutional Animal Care and Use Committee (IACUC, as in the US), or other denominations. Differences about these institutional OBs do not only apply to the denomination, but rather may relate to the functions they are assigned to perform (see Sect. 1.2.4).

When there are government OBs, they can be at regional and/or national level.

In some countries (e.g., Spain, the Netherlands) the government may delegate some functions (e.g., project evaluation) to external OBs if they demonstrate expertise, competence, and impartiality [12].

1.2.3 What Roles and Representation Are Required/Appropriate for an Oversight Body?

An "Oversight Body" (OB) is a committee or body tasked with overseeing and evaluating an animal care and use program at an establishment. It is a collective term comprising bodies established under different international guidelines or regulations, but which have similar functions. Examples include the Animal Welfare Body (AWB) and Ethics Committee in the European Union, the Animal Welfare and Ethical Review Body (AWERB) in the United Kingdom, and the Institutional Animal Care and Use Committee (IACUC) in many other parts of the world, particularly North America and the Asia-Pacific region.

The composition of the AWB is set out in Article 26 of the European Directive 2010/63/EU (European Parliament and the Council of the European Union 2010). It specifies the minimum membership as being the person or persons responsible for the welfare and care of the animals and, in the case of establishments where scientific procedures are carried out, a scientific member. The Designated Veterinarian (DV) is required to provide input to the AWB but is not needed to be a formal member.

The Animals (Scientific Procedures) Act 1986 defines minimum AWERB membership as broadly similar to the AWB, with the exception that the Named Veterinary Surgeon is a full member rather than providing input. In addition, guidance accompanying the Act [13] sets out expectations for a wider membership still, to include persons who hold no responsibilities themselves under the Act (sometimes called the "lay member"), as well as persons who are independent of the establishment.

IACUC composition is described in the Guide to the Care and Use of Laboratory Animals [4] and is quite similar to the AWERB so far as veterinarians and scientists are concerned. A Chair role is also required, and the additional roles are somewhat more specifically defined compared to the AWERB. For instance, the equivalent to the lay member is required to come from a non-scientific background, and the "community member" is defined as someone from outside the establishment who can represent community interests in animal care and use.

Regardless of legal requirements, composition and competence of OBs can be enhanced with the addition of professionals such as bioethicists, biostatisticians, representatives of the competent authorities, etc. Ideally, institutions should go beyond legal requirements to establish an efficient OB according to the complexity of the animal care and use program.

1.2.4 What Are the Principal Tasks and Responsibilities of an Oversight Body?

Article 27 of the European Directive 2010/63/EU [3] sets out the minimum suite of tasks expected of an "Animal Welfare Body" (AWB). There are three principal elements: the provision of advice to staff at the establishment on matters such as the application of and development in the 3Rs, care and accommodation of animals, and rehoming of animals; the development and review of operational processes for overseeing the welfare of animals at the establishment; and a duty to follow the progress and outcomes of projects at the establishment with a view to further application of the 3Rs. In many EU Member States, the competent authorities also delegate the project evaluation to an institutional OB, which can be organized either by adding this function to the legally defined AWB tasks, or using other institutional OBs such as an ethics committee.

The Guide to the Care and Use of Laboratory Animals [4] sets out a more expansive set of responsibilities for the Institutional Animal Care and Use Committee (IACUC). In addition to responsibilities similar to those of an AWB, IACUCs are explicitly tasked with the prospective review and approval of projects involving animals ("Protocol Review"), a formalized and ongoing review process for approved projects ("Post-Approval Monitoring" or "PAM"), and regular inspection of the facilities where animals are kept and used along with the supporting infrastructure ("semi-annual facility inspection"). In a further contrast to AWBs, IACUCs are made responsible for the entire animal care and use program as defined by the Guide, including broader components such as occupational health and safety.

In practice, many "Oversight Bodies" (OBs) recognize the value in taking on accountabilities beyond the minimum expectations defined in guidelines or statute. An example in relation to Animal Welfare and Ethical Review Bodies (AWERBs) can be found in Guiding Principles on Good Practice for Animal Welfare and Ethical Review Bodies [14], which both deepens the core functions of AWERBs and further introduces concepts such as establishing a "culture of care" and providing a "forum for discussion" as good practice accountabilities. AWBs, AWERBs, and IACUCs are increasingly embracing openness and transparency as a core part of their role, both within their own institutions and externally with local communities and society at large (see for example, the University of Washington https://oaw.uw.edu/iacuc/) ([15]-UnivWash).

1.2.5 How Are Project Proposals Evaluated and Authorized?

Methods and processes for project evaluation and authorization vary widely around the world, similarly use of the terms "project" versus "protocol." Even within the European Union where EU Directive 2010/63/EU applies [3], there remains latitude for individual Member States to take different approaches to how and where project evaluation and authorization takes place. For these reasons, work involving animals should never start until the specific regulations that apply in that location have been confirmed.

"Project" most commonly means a program of work conducted for a specific scientific purpose, comprising one or more procedures involving animals. This is the definition found in EU Directive 2010/63/EU, and implicit within this definition is a harm–benefit review where the "harms" caused to animals in terms of their number, species, and procedures which they undergo are weighed against the scientific "benefits" likely to accrue from the work. "Protocol" in the IACUC context is more of a descriptive specification of an animal experiment, and although usually it provides a rationale for the use of animals, a formal harm–benefit assessment is not a part of the process. Evaluation and approval of protocols sits exclusively with the IACUC.

Guillén et al. [12] compared 5 (at the time) EU Member States and their approach to project evaluation and authorization. A general theme is that accountability for project authorization tends to be retained by, or very close to, the Competent Authority itself, whereas project evaluation is often delegated to regional or even institutional bodies.

An assessment of the degree to which the 3Rs have been applied, including the specification of scientific and humane endpoints, use of analgesics and anesthetics to minimize suffering, and the justification for specific procedures are common features of protocol and project evaluation. Consideration of the ethical case for the use of animals at all and the scientific merits on which the arguments are based are further characteristics of project evaluation. Protocols or projects that are found not to satisfy the various evaluations are returned to the applicant for revision and resubmission, or denied outright. Satisfactory evaluations lead to the authorization of animal use for the specific case or cases presented, often with an accompanying time limit for that authorization.

1.2.6 What Are the Available Sources to Identify Alternatives to Animal Use?

By "alternatives" to animal use, we refer to the 3Rs (Replacement, Reduction, Refinement), originally developed by Russell and Burch [16]. We thus consider here any change in the practice of animal use that leads to the replacement, reduction, or refinement of animal use. This includes methods that directly replace or avoid the use of animals where they would normally be used (replacement), methods that either reduce the number of animals per project or increase the amount of information gained per animal (reduction), as well as methods that reduce any form of harm to animals or otherwise improve their welfare (refinement).

There are increasingly many good open access sources available on the Internet to identify alternatives to animal use. In particular, most national 3Rs organizations host websites with information on alternatives to animal use and links to other sources of alternatives. Among those organizations providing the most extensive libraries of 3R resources and link lists are the UK's National Centre for the Replacement, Refinement & Reduction of Animals in Research (NC3Rs, https://www.nc3rs.org.uk/3rs-resources), the North American 3Rs Collaborative (https://www.na3rsc.org/resources/), Norway's National Consensus Platform for the Replacement, Reduction and Refinement of animal experiments (Norecopa, https://norecopa.no/alternatives), the Johns Hopkins Center for Alternatives to Animal Testing (CAAT, https://caat.jhsph.edu/), and the European Union Reference Laboratory for alternatives to animal testing (EURL ECVAM, https://ec.europa.eu/jrc/en/eurl/ecvam). In addition, conventional biomedical databases such as PubMed (https://pubmed.ncbi.nlm.nih.gov/) and Embase (https://www.embase.com/) can be searched with the use of appropriate terms. Leenaars et al. [17] detail a systematic approach to query such databases for all entries relevant to any particular animal model.

1.2.7 What Is the Harm/Benefit Analysis and Why It Is So Important?

Research on animals is regulated on the explicit understanding that it will provide important new knowledge to promote scientific discovery, to advance human or animal health, or to facilitate nature conservation, without causing unnecessary harm to animals. Both maximizing epistemic benefit and minimizing harm to animals are therefore necessary conditions for legitimate animal research [18]. The harm–benefit analysis (HBA) is the common tool employed in project evaluation to decide whether study protocols meet these expectations [2, 7].

Minimizing harm to animals is achieved by implementing the 3Rs: replace, reduce, and refine [16]. Thus, the use of animals in research can be legitimate only if such use is *necessary* for achieving the study goals, that is, if the study goals cannot be achieved without using (sentient) animals (replace) or by using fewer animals (reduce) or less harmful procedures (refine). Good program management can contribute substantially to the reduction of animal numbers by optimizing breeding programs, and to the refinement of animal experiments by improving housing and care of animals.

However, unless a study yields scientifically valid and reproducible results, animals may be used unnecessarily for inconclusive research, regardless of how little harm is imposed on them [19]. Thus, prior to assessing implementation of the 3Rs, study protocols should be reviewed for whether they are *suitable* for achieving the study goals in the first place. Similar to the 3Rs for minimizing harm to animals, the 3Vs offer a guiding principle for maximizing epistemic benefit, whereby the 3Vs represent the three key aspects of scientific validity in animal research: construct validity, internal validity, and external validity [7, 18]. Construct validity refers to the validity of an animal model of a disease (e.g., stroke) or of an outcome variable for measuring a property of interest (e.g., anxiety). Internal validity refers to the study design (e.g., use of proper control groups) and the use of measures against risks of bias (e.g., randomization, blinding, sample size calculation). Finally, external validity refers to the generalizability of the results to other study populations and conditions, which also determines the reproducibility and translatability of study findings [20]. However, even if a study protocol is perfectly suitable and the harm to animals is necessary for achieving the study's goals, whether the study protocol is also deemed *reasonable* depends on ethical deliberation, that is, whether the study's benefit to society is considered to "outweigh" the harm to animals.

A formal harm–benefit analysis (HBA) thus proceeds in logical order along three steps, thereby systematically assessing whether a study protocol is [1] *suitable*, [2] *necessary*, and [3] *reasonable* for achieving its goals. HBA follows the principle of proportionality, which is used to settle conflicts between different legal rights—for example, the freedom of research and the protection of animal welfare. Taken together, a formal HBA offers a coherent framework for a logically structured evaluation procedure to decide about the legitimacy of animal research projects.

1.2.8 What Is To Be Considered in Terms of Openness/ Transparency, Such as Non-technical Summaries in the European Union?

In recent years, the scientific community is responding to the societal concerns on the use of animals through openness/transparency activities, to allow the public have a more informed opinion on why, when, and how animals are used for research purposes. Hundreds of institutions in several countries have voluntarily joined openness/ transparency agreements and participated in other initiatives such as the Biomedical Research Awareness Day (BRAD) or the Global Openness/ Transparency Day. Some regulators have also incorporated this concept in the legislation. For example, one of the three main reasons to update EU legislation with Directive 2010/63/EU [3] was to enhance openness/transparency. In addition to the requirements on statistical reporting (see Question 3.2), non-technical summaries (NTS) have to be part of the documentation submitted to the Competent Authorities as part of the application for project authorization. The NTS must include in an anonymous manner (a) information on the objectives of the project, including the predicted harm and benefits and the number and types of animals to be used; and (b) a demonstration of compliance with the requirement of replacement, reduction, and refinement. The EU Member States (MS) may require NTS to specify whether a project is to undergo a retrospective assessment, and they must make NTS available to the public.

A consensus guiding document on NTS was initially published by the European Commission in 2013 [21], which, after implementation of Regulation (EU) 2019/1010 [22], was replaced by a Working Document in 2021 [23]. The Regulation established timelines for updating NTS after retrospective assessment (6 months), for publication of NTS (at the latest within 6 months of authorization), and required the European Commission to establish a common NTS format and an open access database. The 2021 Working Document provides the required template for the NTS, and guidance on the content to be included in it.

Since the objective of the NTS is to inform the public, only language and terminology which will be easily understood by the public should be used. The institutional Animal Welfare Body may be helpful in assisting on content and accuracy, and it is the responsibility of the competent authority to authorize projects only when they include a satisfactory NTS.

Information to be part of an NTS includes the title and duration of the project; keywords; purpose, objectives, and predicted benefits of the project; predicted harms; and application of the Three Rs (Replacement, Reduction, and Refinement).

1.2.9 What Individual Roles/Positions Are Required to Be Appointed in the Program?

There are several individual key roles/positions that have to be officially appointed as having some kind of responsibility for the program. First, someone with the authority and legal responsibility on the entire program. In the Directive 2010/63/EU [3], this is named as "the person responsible for ensuring compliance with the provisions of this Directive …," while it is called the "Institutional Official" in the US, or "Establishment Licence Holder" in the UK and other countries. A second key role is that of the veterinarian, named as "Designated veterinarian" in the EU Directive, "Attending Veterinarian" in the US framework, or "Named Veterinary Surgeon" in the UK. The third one is relating to the person having overall responsibility on animal welfare. In the EU, this is called the person "responsible for overseeing the welfare and care of the animals in the establishment," with the UK equivalent being the "Named Animal Care and Welfare Officer." In general, it is known internationally as the "Animal Welfare Officer." This third position is not defined as such in the US environment, since welfare responsibilities fall on the Attending Veterinarian. A Designated Veterinarian can also occupy the role of Animal Welfare Officer in the EU.

In addition to these three common international roles/positions, the EU Directive also requires one or several persons on site to "ensure that the staff dealing with animals have access to information specific to the species housed in the establishment" and "be responsible for ensuring that the staff are adequately educated, competent and continuously trained and that they are supervised until they have demonstrated the requisite competence."

There is no impediment for one single person to hold more than one responsibility. However, attention should be paid to avoiding conflicts of interest that could negatively impact decisions on animal welfare (e.g., same person as Institutional Official and Attending Veterinarian).

1.2.10 What Are the Legal Requirements on Training and Competence?

Most existing legislation include requirements on training and continuous professional development of personnel relating to the care and use of animals in research. They refer to the different types of personnel and functions/activities performed, such as:

- Basic animal care personnel (husbandry activities)
- Specialized animal care personnel (animal welfare responsibilities)
- Veterinarians (veterinary care)
- Researchers (experimental design and procedures)
- Oversight body members (ethical review process and oversight)

Some functions/activities may be common to different types of personnel (e.g., euthanasia). Nowadays it is not just a matter to complete the required training programs, but also to demonstrate the competence to perform the functions/activities, and in the species used. Modern frameworks (e.g., based on European Union guidance for Member States) [24] establish and define specific syllabus in training modules, learning outcomes for the modules, assessment criteria, a supervision period before being able to perform the function, and a continuous professional development program. In the European case, Member States have established particular duration of training modules and validity periods for the achieved training and competence, which have to be renewed periodically.

The chapter on Training and Competence in this book describes in detail the current systems in place.

1.2.11 Are There Different Requirements for Field or Agricultural Studies Compared to Those for Laboratory Studies?

Scientific procedures are most commonly carried out on laboratory animals within dedicated facilities. However, there are two key circumstances where institutions need to be aware of animal procedures going on outside the usual bounds of their establishment.

The first of these cases is where procedures that form an integral part of research projects at the establishment must by necessity be conducted at a place away from the establishment itself. This might, for instance, be the case where the studies involve animals on working farms, or where wild animals are being studied in their natural habitat. In these cases, the work remains fully within the remit of the Oversight Body (OB) as for any other project. Agricultural studies are often conducted with food and production animals, where the work by necessity must take place where the animals are normally kept. The Guide for the Care and Use of Agricultural Animals in Research and Teaching [25] is a comprehensive resource which may assist OBs with their responsibilities for such work. Studies with wild animals are usually undertaken for conservation or ecological purposes. Article 9 of European Directive 2010/63/EU [3] mandates specific conditions for work with animals taken from the wild, but most jurisdictions will have additional regulations that apply to trapping and working with wild animals; care should be taken to establish what rules are in effect, particularly where protected or endangered species are involved.

The second case is where the institution is more distantly associated with animal studies outside of their own establishment (see Chap. 19). This may be because the work is a scientific collaboration where a second institute has the formal accountability for the work, despite the involvement of the first. Alternatively, the work may be being conducted overseas or in another jurisdiction, as is often the case with wildlife and conservation studies. Finally, the animal work could be covered by different regulations to those for scientific research, as might be the case for veterinary clinical trials. In these situations, the establishment and their OB may not have a legal or formal duty towards the studies, but they should nevertheless remain aware of the public perception of such work. A common expectation is that the same standards of care and oversight should be applied to all work involving animals, regardless of whether it meets the specific requirements for OB responsibility. It is a good practice for an OB to at least maintain an awareness of, and interest in, such work.

1.3 Attending Research Activities/Operating the Program

1.3.1 How Can We Help Promoting 3Rs in the Research Activities?

The animal care and use program is key to the promotion and implementation of 3Rs in the research activities. Researchers are experts in their specific fields of research and know the scientific requirements of their research projects. Sometimes, however, they have limited knowledge of the best practice in terms of the 3Rs, and little reward and motivation for developing specific 3Rs alternatives to their procedures. It is, therefore, of utmost importance to establish such expertise within the program and to build sufficient capacity to be able to support researchers and study directors in the implementation of the 3Rs. To this end, the personnel of the program (veterinarians, animal care staff, technicians) need to be trained and supported in searching for and implementing 3Rs alternatives, and in communicating with the researchers and study directors. Ideally, researchers are invited to explain their research projects, their needs in terms of animal care, and the scientific requirements of their projects. This in turn gives the program personnel the opportunity to explain to the researchers any challenges associated with the planned research. The better the program staff understands the scientific requirements of a research project, the better they will be able to propose adequate solutions (e.g., in terms of the animal breeding program, environmental enrichment, non-aversive handling, pain management, monitoring of humane endpoints, and humane killing), and the better these solutions will be accepted by the researchers. It may also be helpful to produce standard operating procedures (SOPs) describing best practices and agree on all specific procedures, e.g. using a checklist or a contract between researchers and the program. The institutional ethics committee/animal welfare body or equivalent may also be the tool to facilitate the input of the animal care program personnel to promote the 3Rs in the research activities where direct communication with researchers is not fluid.

1.3.2 How Can We Ensure There Is Oversight of the Entire Animal Care and Use Program?

There are several persons/bodies and roles that are expected or required by legislation to be appointed/performed in the program (see Question 1.9). However, not all guidance/legislation describes in detail how to implement a comprehensive oversight process of the entire program. European Directive 2010/63/EU [3] in Art. 27 assigns several tasks to the Animal Welfare Body (e.g., review internal operational processes; follow the development of projects) that can be considered as oversight activities. The Guide for the Care and Use of Laboratory Animals [4] may be the guidance document that more specifically addresses this, considering the IACUC "responsible for oversight and evaluation of the entire Program and its components ..." and assigning oversight functions including "review and approval of proposed animal use (protocol review) and of proposed significant changes to animal use; regular inspection of facilities and animal use areas; regular review of the Program; ongoing assessment of animal care and use; and establishment of a mechanism for receipt and review of concerns involving the care and use of animals at the institution."

Regardless of the applicable legal requirements, the oversight of the entire program is to be efficiently organized, and the best way to do it is to assign the responsibility to the institutional Oversight Body, in which the key personnel are represented and coordination can be ensured. The most important point is that oversight activities should not be restricted to protocol/project review, but should include processes for protocol/project post-approval monitoring, regular review of the animal program, and visits to the animal facilities to evaluate the program performance. A report of each of these processes, including observations and proposed corrective actions, should be submitted to the responsible person at the institution, who will provide the authority and resources to implement these actions.

1.3.3 What Is the Main Documentation that May Be Necessary for Record Keeping Within the Program?

Documentation and record keeping is an important part of the program, for reasons including operational planning and delivery, ensuring quality and compliance, and achieving continuous improvement of the program itself. Some records and documents are mandated by the regulations which apply to the work; these will vary across jurisdictions so care should be taken to understand the specific requirements in effect. The broad categories of records which might be kept include:

- Animal source, use, and disposal records: Accurate records of how many animals have been obtained and used, where they came from, and what was their ultimate fate is a cornerstone requirement of the program. The data contained is vitally important for demonstrating compliance, as well as tracking performance trends relating to animal care and use.
- Project and procedure records: The scientific use of animals should be documented in order to track progress against approved purposes and to verify that procedures were carried out in accordance with authorizations.
- Oversight Body (OB) deliberations, advice, and reporting: The OB should maintain records of its advice and decisions in order to demonstrate it is fulfilling its obligations. Such advice is not limited to protocol and project decisions, but also to the overall running of the program and management of the establishment.
- Training, competence, and supervision records: A primary accountability for the care and welfare of animals rests with the person who applies procedures to them. Being able to demonstrate suitable training and supervision is essential for compliance and animal welfare, both for in vivo researchers and animal care staff.
- Occupational health and safety records: The safety and well-being of personnel involved in the program is effectively monitored and protected through records such as health surveillance, vaccination and preventative medicine, and accident and injury reporting.
- Environmental and facility data: The environment and the quality of the facility can have profound effect on the health and well-being of the animals, and in the turn the data they produce. Environmental records are necessary to ensure conditions are optimally maintained, along with records relating to routine husbandry and sanitation procedures at the establishment.
- Veterinary records: The Designated or Attending Veterinarian will provide advice on the care and welfare of animals at the establishment, as well as supervising health records for animals and colonies under their care. Veterinarians may also be accountable for the safe storage, prescribing and disposal of prescription medicines and controlled drugs, for which accurate record keeping is vital.

1.3.4 What Are Humane Endpoints and How Are They Used with Severity Assessments?

A considerable amount has been written about "humane endpoints" and the term is used widely with subtly different meanings according to circumstance. Wallace [26] offers a succinct and inclusive definition contextualizing humane endpoints with scientific (experimental) endpoints; "*Scientific endpoints are criteria that determine the outcome of an experiment. Humane endpoints are finite, compassionate limits placed on the amount of pain or distress any experimental animal will be allowed to experience.*" The limits imposed by a humane endpoint are often achieved by humane killing, though severity can also be limited by the timely application of interventions such as analgesia, anesthesia, dosing breaks, etc. This is made more explicit in the definition by Hendriksen, Morton, and Cussler [27], which additionally introduces an upper limit on morally justifiable severity; "*The earliest indicator in an animal experiment of (potential) pain and/or dis-*

tress that, within its scientific context and moral acceptability, can be used to avoid or limit adverse effects by taking actions such as humane killing, terminating the study or alleviating the pain and distress." Therefore, in practice, humane endpoints are applied:

- At a level of severity that never exceeds that of the scientific endpoint
- As soon as the scientific objective can be achieved or can no longer be achieved
- At a set limit of severity regardless of whether the scientific objective has been achieved

The successful implementation of humane endpoints requires that they are defined in advance, during the planning phase of the study, collaboratively between investigators, veterinarians, and Oversight Bodies. The factors that must be determined are:

- What will be measured or observed? Potential indicators include general signs such as spontaneous and provoked behavior, posture, bodyweight or condition, and common physiological measures. Biochemical, preclinical, or technological markers might be available which are more specific to particular models.
- How do the selected variables relate to severity? Measures must have a validated link to severity if they are to be useful. Where such evidence is not available, pilot studies may be needed.
- What interventions are available? Suitable interventions will be effective at limiting or terminating the adverse effects experienced by the animal, while not confounding the scientific objectives.
- What training of personnel and validation of observations are necessary to recognize and apply effective humane endpoints in practice?

Score sheets and welfare assessment schemes offer a formalized way of defining and refining humane endpoints. Wolfensohn and Lloyd [28] present an accessible review including the concepts of lifetime experience and cumulative suffering.

As a means to minimize severity, humane endpoints are principally a tool of refinement. Recital 14 of the European Directive 2010/63/EU [3] explicitly refers to the use of humane endpoints to "*avoid, so far as possible, death as an endpoint.*" The Guide to the Care and Use of Laboratory Animals [4] states "*The use of humane endpoints contributes to refinement by providing an alternative to experimental endpoints that result in unrelieved or severe animal pain and distress, including death.*" Humane endpoints are vitally important to Oversight Bodies and regulators as prospective indicators of likely severity, one side of the harm–benefit analysis. Similar they provide an opportunity for challenge and review, to ensure the ongoing application of refinement in practice.

1.3.5 How Can an Effective Procedure to Report Animal Welfare Concerns Be Implemented?

Whereas most animal care and use is performed according to ethical and legal principles, there may be situations where individuals feel concerned about the care and welfare of animals in the institution. The reasons for concern may be diverse, such as the application of humane endpoints, adequacy of analgesia, conduct of experimental procedures, or potential mistreatment of animals. To manage these potential situations, institutions should implement a way for concerned employees to report it in an effective way, what is usually called "whistle blower policy." The procedure should be defined at institutional level, and everyone associated with the animal care and use program should be aware of it through training. It is an ethical (and in some cases legal) responsibility to report these concerns. Key elements for an effective procedure are:

- A mechanism to allow reporting in an anonymous manner should be considered. This can be done, for example, via letterboxes in several places.

- As a reminder, signage on this procedure should be posted in prominent locations in the animal facility and institutional website.
- There should be several potential recipients of the report to ensure effective processing. These may include senior management, the Oversight Body Chair, the responsible veterinarian, or the manager of the facility.
- Each report should be investigated, and the findings communicated to the concerned employee(s) unless reported anonymously.
- There should be a guarantee that, when not reported anonymously, there is no reprisal against the concerned employee(s).

These basic elements are described in the Guide for the Care and Use of Laboratory Animals [4], which indicates it as a mandatory procedure for institutions (in the United States, responsibility for review and investigation of these concerns rests with the Institutional Official and the IACUC), and summarized in an AAALAC International FAQ (https://www.aaalac.org/accreditation-program/faqs/#B7):

1.3.6 What Is Meant by Non-compliance and How Should We Respond to Different Types of Event?

Non-compliance means the failure to obey or abide by the terms of a rule that applies to an action being carried out. Implicit within this definition is an expectation on the part of those setting the rule that it will be followed, and the acceptance of responsibility by those carrying out the action in question to do so in accordance with the rule. Consequently, there are different types of non-compliance which can be categorized according to the nature of the rule and the degree to which it was not met.

King et al. [29] describe a hierarchy of rules in order of level of obligation. At the highest level and extrinsic to an establishment are legislative controls applied by Governments as laws or regulations, sometimes supplemented by guidelines containing additional details. At an intermediate level are publications and industry standards, which may be seen as expressions of contemporary good practice and may sometimes be recommended or required by regulations. The most local levels of control are those that are intrinsic to the establishment, such as institutional policies and standard operating procedures. It is at this level where quality systems play an important role in addressing non-compliance. A Quality System (QS) is a collection of organizational processes defined in policies, standard operational procedures, work instructions, protocols, guidelines, or other documents (see Chap. 18).

Within each of these levels, the scale of non-compliance can also vary from minor technical or administrative errors, to major breaches or deviations from authorized practice. The combination of these factors generally determines the appropriate speed and intensity of response by an establishment to non-compliance, as well as the need to inform or involve outside agencies. Regardless of the scale or nature of non-compliance, it is a good practice always to try to identify the root causes of the non-compliance in order to rectify any process or procedural shortcomings and so reduce the likelihood of future recurrence. Formalized approaches such as Root Cause Analysis (RCA) and the use of documented Corrective and Preventative Actions (CAPA) are effective ways of ensuring remediation and maximized learning from non-compliance events. The Oversight Body (OB) should play a key role in directing and reviewing investigations into non-compliance, as part of its duty to oversee and evaluate the animal care and use program.

1.3.7 How Are Project Amendments Processed?

During the lifetime of a project, it is not uncommon that either the initial considerations and objectives of the project change, or so might the procedures and associated controls used to achieve them. Where either or both of these situations arise, amendment of a project may be necessary to ensure that the authorized project continues to describe fully the work intended to be carried out.

Much like the processes for initially evaluating projects (see Question 1.2.5), processes for amending an existing project vary across different institutions and jurisdictions. In general, amendment of an active project is a less intensive process than initial evaluation of a new one, although very large or complex amendments can require almost as much scrutiny as new proposals. A minor administrative amendment that does not materially affect the procedures applied to animals might merit a simplified fast-track approach, whereas more substantive amendments that introduce new procedures or changes to severity might require the entire harm–benefit assessment to be reconsidered.

In the European Union, Directive 2010/63/EU [3] grants to Member States the responsibility to publish conditions for the amendment of project authorizations, though the Directive itself refers to formal evaluation being required only where amendments "*may have a negative effect on animal welfare*." Similarly, in the USA, the Public Health Service Policy on Humane Care and Use of Laboratory Animals [10] and the Animal Welfare Act and Regulations [9] require review and approval of "*significant*" changes to IACUC protocols (refs). "Significant" is generally taken to mean only those changes that have a material impact on the welfare of animals, but individual institutions are encouraged to draw up their own lists of types of amendments the IACUC would wish to review, which may well be broader. For these reasons, precisely as for initial authorization of new projects, it is vitally important to establish the specific rules and regulations that apply to amendment of authorities wherever the work is being carried out.

1.3.8 How Can Program Operations Help Improve Good Science?

The scientific quality of animal research depends in many ways on the quality of the animal care and use program. There are three interconnected elements that may have a positive impact on the quality of science: animal welfare, risk of bias, and communication within the program.

First, good welfare is key to good science [30]. Pain, distress, and other forms of impaired welfare can impact scientific results in unpredictable ways. They have thus to be considered as confounding factors.

Second, the validity and reproducibility of results from animal experiments depends on scientific rigor, that is, adherence to the principles of a good research practice. This includes all kinds of measures to minimize risks of biases, such as randomization, blinding, a priori definition of inclusion and exclusion criteria, as well as measures taken to guarantee stable conditions and equal treatment of all animals. Many of these aspects depend on adequate program operations, including stable conditions of the macroenvironment (e.g., temperature, humidity, and noise), consistency in inspections and handling of animals (e.g., order of cage checking and cage changes counterbalanced across treatment groups), and reliable criteria for interventions (e.g., separation of animals in case of aggression, treatment of wounded or sick animals, exclusion criteria, and humane endpoints). All of these operations should be optimized in view of both maximal animal welfare and minimal risks of bias in experimental results. Ideally, not only the researchers but personnel interacting with animals should be blind to treatment.

Finally, all of this requires an effective interface between the researchers and the program staff to facilitate the implementation of optimal program operations. As with the promotion of the 3Rs, promotion of scientific validity and reproducibility by program operations depends on adequate training of personnel (e.g. on measures to avoid risks of bias). However, because risks of bias may be highly study-specific, it also depends on good communication between the researchers and the program staff. Direct communication will help to identify and eliminate potential conflicts between program operations and study protocols and will help with appropriate reporting of animal studies.

1.4 Compliance After Animal Use

1.4.1 How Is Animal Reuse to Be Legally and Ethically Implemented?

Researchers and members of ethical review bodies are sometimes faced with the difficult task of deciding between the use of fewer animals or a reduction of the burden per animal, for example, when deciding between cross-sectional or longitudinal studies or between reusing animals for further experiments or using new animals. Most regulations leave it to the researchers and ethical review bodies to take these decisions on a case-by-case basis. A recent online survey of animal facilities involved in preclinical studies suggested that reuse of animals in multiple independent studies is a common practice [31]. According to the Guide for the Care and Use of Laboratory Animals [4], refinement and reduction goals should be balanced on a case-by-case basis, principal investigators are strongly discouraged from advocating animal reuse as a reduction strategy, and reduction should not be a rationale for reusing an animal or animals that have already undergone experimental procedures especially if the well-being of the animals would be compromised.

Because animal welfare is ultimately about the well-being of individual animals, one might argue—from an ethical point of view—that the reuse of animals should only be considered in cases where the previous use did not have a lasting effect on the animals' well-being. In that case, the effect of reuse on overall animal welfare would be equal to the effect of using new animals, in which case reuse should be preferred to reduce animal numbers without increasing the harm on animals. However, procedures rarely leave no lasting traces and often may even sensitize animals to perceive the same or similar procedures more harmful. Therefore, reuse of animals should only be considered for animals exposed to mild or moderate procedures at maximum. For instance, Article 16 of European Directive 2010/63/EU [3] only allows reuse when the previous procedure was mild or moderate and the further procedure is classified as mild, moderate, or non-recovery. Similarly, in Switzerland, reuse is permitted only for animals exposed to procedures of no to low severity [32].

1.4.2 How Can Statistical Reports Be Produced Effectively?

Countries may have different legal requirements on reporting animal use, with the purpose of increasing transparency and public awareness, and also responding to societal concerns on the use of animals. In the European Union, Directive 2010/637EU [3] requires Member States, on an annual basis, to collect, publish, and submit to the European Commission statistical information on the use of animals in procedures, including information on the actual severity of the procedures and on the origin and species of non-human primates used in procedures (the same systems are also established in the UK). The Directive also mandated to establish a common format for the submission of this information, which has been recently revised [33]. The European Commission has also established the "ALURES Statistical EU Database," where all the statistical information collected from Member States and Norway are made available to the public (https://ec.europa.eu/environment/chemicals/lab_animals/alures_en.htm).

The main categories of information, in addition to basic items such as species, numbers, or origin, refer to the reason for use (e.g., specific research area, type of testing), and the severity (mild, moderate, severe) actually experienced by each animal. Effectively collecting these details, especially at big institutions, is a challenge. Whereas the reasons for animal use are easy, as they can be prospectively obtained from the reviewed and authorized projects, collecting the actual severity for each animal use is a more difficult task.

To effectively produce accurate statistical data, the collaboration between animal care personnel, the Oversight Body (Animal Welfare Body, Ethics Committee), and the researchers is necessary. Traditionally the animal facility managers, with the help from the Oversight Body, have collected the statistics, but in many instances, it is the research team who has the information on the actual severity. Therefore, a reporting system between researchers and the responsible person(s) in the animal program to collect the information is needed, with the collaboration of the Oversight Body to provide retrospective data of the projects when needed. This may be implemented through manual reporting systems after completion of experimental procedures, or through animal facility management software available in the market, which are being continuously adapted to facilitate these aspects of legal compliance. Because the statistical reports focus on animal uses rather than just animal numbers, and have to be submitted on an annual basis, the system should facilitate the continuous reporting during the project development, without waiting for its completion. Knowledge of these legal requirements by the institutional management will help to get the necessary support and authority to ensure collaboration of all involved parties.

1.4.3 What Is "Retrospective Severity Assessment," and How Can It Be Applied in Practice?

In jurisdictions where prior authorization of animal studies depends on a favorable harm/benefit analysis, a forward-looking or "prospective" estimate of likely severity must be made as part of that analysis. For example, Article 15 of the EU Directive 2010/63/EU [3] requires an assessment and categorization of the likely severity of each procedure. Under this system, projects are also prospectively assigned an overall severity rating, which is determined by the highest level of severity expected to be experienced by any individual animal. Alongside the anticipated numbers and species of animals to be used, the aggregated assessment of likely severity completes the "harm" side of the equation. Prospective severity assessment can only ever be an estimate however, based on the best knowledge available at the time of how the specific procedures are likely to affect the animals being used. In practice, the harms may vary quite widely from the prior assessment, either due to unexpected effects and outcomes or simple limitations of the original estimate.

"Retrospective" severity assessment is the practice of looking back and quantifying the actual harms that were experienced by individual animals. Article 54 of the EU Directive [3] requires reporting of the actual severity experienced by the animals, in order to provide statistical information. At face value, retrospective severity assessment therefore serves a purpose around openness and transparency, by detailing what actually happened during procedures as opposed to what may have been anticipated. Perhaps more important is that the existence of this data enables retrospective assessment of entire projects (see Question 3.4), allowing the original assumptions, estimates, and harm–benefit analysis itself to be reviewed in light of the facts. By closing the loop and learning from actual outcomes, future prior authorizations can be made more robust and better apply all three of the Rs.

A number of frameworks exist that can be applied to assess and report retrospective severity. An early resource is the report published by a working group co-sponsored by the UK Animal Procedures Committee (APC) and Laboratory Animal Science Association (LASA) [34] illustrating a number of possible approaches, as well as recommending the adoption of retrospective severity reporting in European legislation. A consensus document from a European Commission Expert Working Group published in 2012 [35] offers more specific advice on meeting the current requirements of the European Directive. A supplement to the consensus document [36] offers a series of worked examples. Smith et al. [37] provide detailed guidance and examples on both prospective and retrospective reporting of severity.

1.4.4 What Are the Requirements for Retrospective Assessment of Projects?

Retrospective assessment of a project is the process of systematically evaluating a project in order to test the assumptions on which the original evaluation was made and to learn any lessons of relevance to the authorization or conduct of future projects. Retrospective assessment can only be conducted after an appreciable amount is known about project outcomes, which requires that the project itself has at least reached as far as some interim milestones. More commonly retrospective assessments are carried out after projects have been fully completed, and in some cases long after completion where there is a delay before final results are known. Although retrospective assessment of projects is mandated only by a limited number of legislative frameworks, it may be a valuable exercise for any kind of institution in any part of the world on ethical grounds.

Article 38 of European Directive 2010/63/EU [3] makes consideration of the need for, and timing of, retrospective assessment of a project part of the initial evaluation and authorization of that project. Article 39 requires that all projects using non-human primates or projects involving "severe" procedures are mandated for retrospective assessment. Member States can, through Article 39, define other categories of project to be assessed, whereas Article 40 allows for limited exemption from the requirement for assessment where the project involves only "mild" or "non-recovery" procedures.

The key elements of a retrospective assessment are:

- A consideration of whether and to what extent the project achieved its original objectives. The prospectively authorized objectives determine the benefits likely to accrue from the project, so retrospective assessment is intended to test whether these benefits were in fact realized.
- An evaluation of the harms caused to animals, both in severity and in number. While these are by necessity estimated in advance, it is only through the practice of retrospective severity assessment (see Question 3.4) that the actual harms can be quantified, to enable the original harm–benefit assessment to be tested.
- Identification of findings or elements that may improve the future implementation of the 3Rs, not just in the conduct of projects but also in their initial evaluation and authorization.

A European Commission-sponsored Expert Working Group published guidance which includes advice on the purpose and practice of retrospective assessment [35, 36]. Smith et al. [37] and RSPCA guidance from 2016 offers further practical advice, including a worked example [38].

1.4.5 What Can Be Done with Animals at the End of the Experiments?

There are several choices for what to do with animals at the end of experimental procedures:

- Many animals have to be killed to obtain scientific information post-mortem. In these cases, killing must follow accepted methods (see Chap. 12). But when killing is not necessary, there are other options:
- The animals can be reused, if ethical and legal requirements are met (see question on reuse in this chapter).
- The animals can be rehomed (see question on rehoming considerations in this chapter).
- The animals can be maintained on site without further use, if none of the previous options are possible and the animal is in good health status:
- According to some legislation such as European Union, Directive 2010/63/EU [3], a decision to keep an animal alive at the end of a procedure shall be taken by a veterinarian or by another competent person and the animal shall be killed when it is likely to remain in moderate or severe pain, suffering, distress, or lasting harm.

Animals that have been killed, which do not pose any kind of risk and there is no need to obtain further scientific information relating to the project, can be potentially used for other purposes after death. For example, organs and tissues can be shared (https://www.animatch.eu/), carcasses can be used for training handling or experimental techniques, or used for feeding other animals.

1.4.6 What Considerations Should Be Made Around Rehoming Programs?

Rehoming is one of the choices for disposition of animals at the end of experimental procedures subject to certain conditions being met. It may happen that these conditions are defined in legislation, for example in European Directive 2010/63/EU [3], the conditions are that: the state of health of the animal allows it; there is no danger to public health, animal health, or the environment; and appropriate measures have been taken to safeguard the well-being of the animal. Whereas most rehoming cases concern larger species such as dogs (for adoption) or non-human primates (sanctuaries as destination), it can be applied for any species as far as the established conditions are met.

Rehoming should follow a defined institutional procedure which in general, and regardless of legislation, should include aspects regarding the suitability of both the animal (taking into account its life experience) and the new owner (or host). Concerning the animal, aspects to consider may include:

- Veterinary input to determine if the animal is in good health and not likely to pose a risk to human and animal health and the environment.
- The behavioral records (if existing), including housing conditions and socialization with other animals and humans.
- The age of the animal, the time it has spent in the facility, and the procedures it has been subjected to.

Concerning the new owner or host:

- The knowledge of the animal research environment. Quite often in adoption programs, institutional staff are the first choice when possible, but this may not necessarily be a condition.
- Experience with the species.
- Commitment to ensure the well-being of the animals. This can be formalized through a signed document where the new owner/host commits to maintain the animal under certain conditions (e.g., ensuring veterinary care when needed, etc.), and not to use the animal for certain activities (e.g., work-related).

It will also be interesting to take into consideration published guidelines on adoption of certain species [39], or institutions may work with external agencies that are set up on either voluntary or statutory basis to support them with rehoming projects and assessing the suitability of new homes. Useful international guidance on rehoming has been recently published [40].

1.4.7 What Rules or Guidelines Apply to the Disposal of Animal Tissues and Carcasses?

Great care is required to ensure that all waste arising from the use of animals in research, including animal tissues and carcasses, is disposed of safely and in accordance with all relevant local and national regulations. Inappropriate disposal of such waste might expose humans, animals, or the environment generally to risk. Laboratory animal wastes present particular hazards because of the procedures in which the animals were used. This might, for instance, include the animals having been exposed to infectious organisms, dosed with radionuclides, or administered toxic substances. Such hazards might remain present in waste derived from the animals, and in the tissues and carcasses of the animals themselves. In most circumstances, these waste materials are at the least treated as infectious or clinical waste, typically disposed of by incineration at regulated facilities. Stricter controls might apply where radionuclide activity exists beyond certain thresholds, where microorganisms of higher hazard groups are involved, or where genetically modified organisms have been used. Legislation varies widely by geography and the nature of the potential hazards, so institutions must ensure that they have conducted proper risk assessments and identified the specific regulations that apply. Institutions often rely on authorized waste contractors to manage their waste materials, but even so the institution still has a duty to make such contractors aware of the specific risks they are handling.

Carcasses and tissues can be useful resources for other researchers or serve other purposes.

References

1. Guillén J, Vergara P. Global guiding principles: a tool for harmonization. Laboratory animals: regulations and recommendations for the care and use of animals in research. 2nd ed. Cambridge: Academic; 2018.
2. Brønstad A, Newcomer CE, Decelle T, Everitt JI, Guillen J, Laber K. Current concepts of harm–benefit analysis of animal experiments – report from the AALAS–FELASA working group on harm–benefit analysis – part 1. Lab Anim. 2016;50(1_suppl):1–20. https://doi.org/10.1177/0023677216642398.
3. The European Parliament and the Council of the European Union, Directive 2010/63/EU of the European Parliament and of the Council of 22 September 2010 on the protection of animals used for scientific purposes. Off J Eur Union. 2010;L276:33–79.
4. National Research Council, National Academy of Sciences. Guide for the care and use of laboratory animals. Washington: National Academy Press; 2011.
5. World Health Organization. Terrestrial Animal Health Code 2012. Available at: http://www. oie.int/international-standard-setting/terrestrial-code/access-online/
6. Council for International Organizations for Medical Sciences; and International Council for Laboratory Animal Science 2012. International Guiding Principles for Biomedical Research Involving Animals. Available at: www.iclas.org.
7. Würbel H. More than 3Rs: the importance of scientific validity for harm–benefit analysis of animal research. Lab Anim. 2017;46:164–6.
8. United Kingdom Home Office. Animals (Scientific Procedures) Act 1986, c.14. Available at https://www.legislation.gov.uk/ukpga/1986/14/contents (Accessed: 19 January 2021).
9. US Department of Agriculture, 1966. Animal Welfare Act of 1966 (Pub. L. 89-544) and subsequent amendments. U.S. Code. Vol. 7, Secs. 2131-2157 et seq. Available at: https://www.nal.usda.gov/awic/animal-welfare-act
10. US Public Health Service. Public health service policy on humane care and use of laboratory animals. Office of Laboratory Animal Welfare, National Institutes of Health, Public Health Service; 2015. Available at: https://olaw.nih.gov/policies-laws/phs-policy.htm
11. Guillén J. Laboratory animals: regulations and recommendations for the care and use of animals in research. 2nd ed. Cambridge: Academic Press; 2018.
12. Guillén J, Robinson S, Decelle T, Exner C, Fentener Van Vlissingen M. Approaches to animal research project evaluation in Europe after implementation of Directive 2010/63/EU. Lab Anim Europe. 2015;44(1):23–31.
13. Her Majesty's Stationery Office (2014). Guidance on the operation of the animals (Scientific procedures) Act 1986. Available at https://assets.publishing.service.gov.uk/government/uploads/system/uploads/attachment_data/file/662364/Guidance_on_the_Operation_of_ASPA.pdf (Accessed: 19 January 2021)
14. RSPCA and LASA, 2015. Guiding principles on good practice for animal welfare and ethical review bodies. A report by the RSPCA Research Animals Department and LASA Education, Training and Ethics Section. Editor: M. Jennings.
15. University of Washington, Office of Animal Welfare. Available at https://oaw.uw.edu/iacuc/ (Accessed: 24 February 2021)
16. Russell WMS, Burch RL. The principles of humane experimental technique. Potters Bar: Special edition. Universities Federation for Animal Welfare; 1959.
17. Leenaars M, Hooijmans CR, van Veggel N, ter Riet G, Leeflang M, Hooft L, van der Wilt GJ, Tillema A, Ritskes-Hoitinga M. A step-by-step guide to systematically identify all relevant animal studies. Lab Anim. 2012;46(1):24–31. https://doi.org/10.1258/la.2011.011087.
18. Eggel M, Würbel H. Internal consistency and compatibility of the 3Rs and 3Vs principles for project evaluation of animal research. Lab Anim. 2021;55(3):233–43.
19. Bailoo JD, Reichlin TS, Würbel H. Refinement of experimental design and conduct in laboratory animal research. ILAR J. 2014;55(3):383–91.
20. Voelkl B, Altman NS, Forsman A, Forstmeier W, Gurevitch J, Jaric I, Karp NA, Kas MJ, Schielzeth H, Van de Casteele T, Würbel H. Reproducibility of animal research in light of biological variation. Nat Rev Neurosci. 2020;21:384–93. https://doi.org/10.1038/s41583-020-0313-3.
21. National Competent Authorities for the implementation of Directive 2010/63/EU on the protection of animals used for scientific purposes Working document on Non-Technical Project summaries Brussels, 23-24 January 2013. https://ec.europa.eu/environment/chemicals/lab_animals/pdf/Recommendations%20for%20NTS.pdf

22. European Parliament and the Council of the European Union (2019) Regulation (EU) 2019/1010 of The European Parliament and of The Council of 5 June 2019 on the alignment of reporting obligations in the field of legislation related to the environment, and amending Regulations (EC) No 166/2006 and (EU) No 995/2010 of the European Parliament and of the Council, Directives 2002/49/EC, 2004/35/EC, 2007/2/EC, 2009/147/EC and 2010/63/EU of the European Parliament and of the Council, Council Regulations (EC) No 338/97 and (EC) No 2173/2005, and Council Directive 86/278/EEC https://eur-lex.europa.eu/legal-content/EN/TXT/PDF/?uri=CELEX:32019R1010&from=EN
23. National Competent Authorities for the implementation of Directive 2010/63/EU on the protection of animals used for scientific purposes (2021). Working document on Non-technical Project Summaries. Brussels, XX-XX XXXX 2021, replacing consensus document of 23–24 January 2013. https://environnement.brussels/sites/default/files/user_files/draft_nts_guidance_document_for_users.pdf
24. National Competent Authorities for the implementation of Directive 2010/63/EU on the protection of animals used for scientific purposes 2014. A working document on the development of a common education and training framework to fulfil the requirements under the Directive. Replacing consensus document of 18–19 September 2013. https://ec.europa.eu/environment/chemicals/lab_animals/pdf/Endorsed_E-T.pdf
25. American Dairy Science Association®, the American Society of Animal Science, and the Poultry Science Association 2020. Guide for the Care and Use of Agricultural Animals in Research and Teaching, 4th Edition. Illinois, 2020. Available at: https://www.asas.org/docs/default-source/default-document-library/agguide_4th.pdf
26. Wallace J. Humane endpoints and cancer research. ILAR J. 2000;41(2):87–93.
27. Hendriksen C, Morton D, Cussler K. Use of humane endpoints to minimise suffering. In: Howard B, Nevalainen T, Perretta G, editors. The COST manual of laboratory animal care and use: refinement, reduction and research. CRC Press; 2010.
28. Wolfensohn S, Lloyd M. Handbook of laboratory animal management and welfare. 4th ed. Wiley-Blackwell; 2013.
29. King WW, Paramastri YA, Guillen J. Compliance and regulatory programs. In: Weichbrod RH, Thompson GAH, Norton JN, editors. Management of animal care and use programs in research, education, and testing. Chapter 7. 2nd ed. Boca Raton, FL: CRC Press/Taylor & Francis; 2018.
30. Poole T. Happy animals make good science. Lab Anim. 1997;31:116–24.
31. Kovalcsik R, Devlin T, Loux S, Martinek M, May J, Pickering T, Tapp R, Wilson S, Serota D. Animal reuse: balancing scientific integrity and animal welfare. Lab Anim (NY). 2006;35(9):49–53. https://doi.org/10.1038/laban1006-49.
32. Swiss Federal Department of Home Affairs, Federal Food Safety and Veterinary Office. French version: 455.1 Ordonnance sur la protection des animaux (OPAn) du 23 avril 2008 (Etat le 1er décembre 2015). German version: 455.1 Tierschutzverordnung (TschV) vom 23. April 2008 (Stand am 1. Dezember 2015).
33. European Commission, 2020. COMMISSION IMPLEMENTING DECISION (EU) 2020/569 of 16 April 2020 establishing a common format and information content for the submission of the information to be reported by Member States pursuant to Directive 2010/63/EU of the European Parliament and of the Council on the protection of animals used for scientific purposes and repealing Commission Implementing Decision 2012/707/EU.
34. LASA/APC Working Group, 2008. Final report of a LASA/APC Working Group to examine the feasibility of reporting data on the severity of scientific procedures on animals. Available at: http://www.lasa.co.uk/PDF/LASA_APC_severity_project.pdf
35. National Competent Authorities for the implementation of Directive 2010/63/EU on the protection of animals used for scientific purposes. 2012. Working document on a severity assessment framework. https://ec.europa.eu/environment/chemicals/lab_animals/pdf/Endorsed_Severity_Assessment.pdf
36. National Competent Authorities for the implementation of Directive 2010/63/EU on the protection of animals used for scientific purposes. 2013. Examples to illustrate the process of severity classification, day-to-day assessment and actual severity assessment. https://ec.europa.eu/environment/chemicals/lab_animals/pdf/examples.pdf
37. Smith D, Anderson D, Degryse AD, Bol C, Criado A, Ferrara A, Franco NH, Gyertyan I, Orellana JM, Ostergaard G, Varga O, Voipio HM. Classification and reporting of severity experienced by animals used in scientific procedures: FELASA/ECLAM/ESLAV Working Group report. Lab Anim. 2018;52(1_suppl):5–57.
38. RSPCA, 2016. Road Map Resource Pack, Focus on Severe Suffering, Part 4: Retrospective Review. Available at: https://science.rspca.org.uk/documents/1494935/9042554/Road+map+resource+pack+4+After+a+project+has+finished+%28retrospective+assessment%29+%28PDF+1.58+MB%29.pdf/e328d546-3f22-4e64-a0df-e9111e32a411?t=1553008407422
39. RSPCA, 2018. Guidance on the rehoming of laboratory dogs. https://www.lasa.co.uk/wp-content/uploads/2018/05/LASA-Guidance-on-the-Rehoming-of-Laboratory-Dogs.pdf
40. FELASA, 2023. FELASA recommendations for the rehoming of animals used for scientific and educational purposes. Ecuer E, Boxall J, Louwerse AL, Mikkelsen LF, Moons CP, Roth M, Spiri AM. Lab Anim. 2023. doi: https://doi.org/10.1177/00236772231158863

2 Management: Governance—Finances—Human Resources

Patricia Preisig, James D. Macy, and Jann Hau

Abstract

The focus of this chapter is the internal operation of an animal program. The first part deals with organization structure, including the components of an animal program, the reporting structure, checks and balances that ensure compliance with all relevant regulations, and financial sustainability. The second part delves into the services associated with an animal program, including research cores, research and development activities, and the outsourcing of services. The third section focuses on the finances of an animal program, including income and expenses, the resulting net cash flow, and how a deficit is handled, should the program have an operational deficit. This section also touches on cost accounting methodologies. The last section focuses on staffing, including operational structure of staff and metrics used to determine staffing requirements. The chapter ends with a brief discussion about the best approach for programs to benchmark themselves against their peers. The take-home message is that there is more than one way to have a robust, compliant, and financially sustainable program. The key to having such a program is to involve the expertise of staff at every level in decision-making, emphasizing the need for more "performance-based standards," i.e., standards that meet regulatory requirements while being both practical and feasible for the program to achieve, than "engineering standards," i.e., prescriptive ways to achieve the standards needed to meet regulatory requirements.

Keywords

Program · Governance · Structure · Finances · Staffing

2.1 Part 1: Animal Program Governance

1. **What are the Advantages and Disadvantages of Centralization of the Animal Care and Use Program**?

   Understanding a centralized organizational structure requires an understanding of the opposite structure: a decentralized organizational structure. The dictionary definitions are

   - Centralized: Decision-making and power are in the hands of few
   - Decentralized: Decision-making and power are spread among several participants

P. Preisig · J. D. Macy
Yale University, New Haven, CT, USA

J. Hau (✉)
University of Copenhagen, Copenhagen, Denmark
e-mail: jhau@sund.ku.dk

J. Guillén, V. Galligioni (eds.), *Practical Management of Research Animal Care and Use Programs*, Laboratory Animal Science and Medicine 3, https://doi.org/10.1007/978-3-031-65414-5_2

By the above definitions the advantages and disadvantages of a centralized structure are:

- Advantages
  - Clear leadership and responsibilities
  - Faster progress and uniform implementation of changes—few voices involved
  - More efficient workflow—policies and Standard Operating Procedures (SOPs) are developed by few
  - More flexibility—consensus is not a requirement
- In summary: A few individuals, typically at the top, are "running the show."
- Disadvantages
  - Assumption is that those "at the top" are fully informed and have experience with the "world" of those "at the bottom"
  - Assumption is that the leadership is trustworthy and trusted
  - Greater risk of rogue behavior
  - Little transparency required
  - Lack of checks and balances
  - Heterogeneity and compliance with policies, rules, and regulations at risk

Logically, then, the advantages and disadvantages of a decentralized program would effectively be reversed. For example, the inherent heterogeneity of a decentralized program enables geographic and programmatic catering to specific investigator needs, but comes at the expense of consistency and efficiency across the program.

In the European Union (EU), each institution's animal unit must comply with the EU Directive [1] and National laws and regulations, and each country is required to have a National Committee that advises the National authorities responsible for issuing licenses in compliance with the Directive. The Directive's compliance requirements include approval of the facilities, having an animal welfare body, ensuring competence of staff, etc. This is obviously an incentive to have some central control over the management and operations of the animal programs throughout the EU and within each country. Similarly, in the United States (US), the Animal Welfare Act [2], US Federal Regulatory bodies, i.e., the Office of Laboratory Animal Welfare (OLAW) [3], and the National Academies of Science [4] provide "central" oversight that delegates, using internal checks and balances, the requirements for an animal program to meet the highest-level requirements. Neither of these organizational structures, however, are a "centralized" program by the definition above.

2. **What are the Operational Units Within an EU or US Animal Program that Accomplish the Required Tasks?**
   - A unit that scrutinizes and approves the use of live animals in each proposed experiment (Approval Unit; IACUC or equivalent unit)
     - Approval Unit should have the following expertise within its organizational structure:

       Members with broad competence and experience with research that uses live animals as research subjects

       Investigators experienced in the research use of all of the animal species on census in the program

       Members not involved in research that uses live animals as research subjects, the so-called community member who represents the voice of the public

       Members licensed in veterinary medical care
   - A unit responsible for the husbandry and medical care of all animals on census (Animal Resource Center; ARC)
     - An Animal Resource Center should have the following expertise:

       A veterinarian that oversees all aspects of the animal care, i.e., Attending or Designated Veterinarian (AV), that is licensed and certified in the subdiscipline of laboratory animal veterinarian. This individual may also serve as the Director of the Animal Resource Center, but in some programs the AV and Director may be different individuals

Veterinarians with laboratory animal training and experience with each animal species on census in the program

Veterinarians with field research experience, if field research is conducted by the institution's investigators

Veterinarians with laboratory animal infectious disease experience

Depending on the size of the program, the veterinary staff may be supported by veterinary technicians with expertise in the medical care of each animal species on census

Staff trained and with experience in all aspects of animal care, i.e. husbandry, euthanasia, sanitation, intra-institution transportation, inter-institution transportation (import/export). Depending on the size of the program, staff may be organized in a hierarchical system with a director, manager, supervisor, unit leaders, etc.

Staff responsible for training new staff. These individuals need to be experienced in the skills they are teaching

Staff responsible for developing SOPs and policies that govern the responsibilities of the veterinary and animal care staff. These individuals need to be versed in all relevant regulations

- A unit with the ultimate authority for the compliance and financial sustainability of the program [Institutional Official (US term) or Governing Body (EU term)]
  - The IO/Governing Body is responsible for ensuring

    That the program is compliant with all relevant supranational, federal, state/regional/local, and institutional requirements

    Reportable non-compliance is accurately reported to the relevant body in a timely manner

    Mandatory reports to higher regulatory agencies are complete, accurate, and submitted by the deadline

    Financial sustainability of the program

    Approval Unit and ARC have the resources needed to meet all relevant regulations

    That the focus of research that uses live animals as research subjects is consistent with the mission of the institution

In both the US and EU, several of the functions described above are legal requirements, such as the EU Directive [1] and the US regulatory/guidance documents [2–4].

3. **Are Checks and Balances Needed?**
   - As mentioned above, at a minimum an animal program must have the units focused on and with the expertise to complete their dictated responsibilities—typically the three types of units described above. In the US, checks and balances are built into the regulatory documents such that each of the units ("arms" of the program) "keeps an eye" on the other two arms and have a responsibility for ensuring that the three "arms" can work together. Examples include:
     - The Governing Body/IO cannot require an activity that the other unit(s) have decided should not occur. For example, the Governing Body/IO (a) could disapprove the use of an animal that the Approval Unit approved, but it cannot approve the use of an animal that the Approval Unit did not approve and (b) cannot approve the care of an animal that does not meet the standards of the Animal Resource Center but could raise the standard of care
     - Veterinarians and the Governing Body/IO have input into animal use approved by the Approval Unit
     - Approval Unit and Governing Body have input into the standards set by the Animal Resource Center/IO

- Approval Unit and Animal Resource Center have authority to restrict the Governing Body/IO

4. **How Should an Animal Care and Use Program Be Organized?**
   - In most US programs and about half of the EU programs that participated in the League of European Research Universities (LERU) pilot study "ultimate accountability" resides with the Institution's leadership, i.e., Governing Body, with a "local" level of accountability residing at the operational/administrative "location," e.g. School, Department, Section, Division [5].
   - While such an organizational structure has a defined leader, giving the appearance of a centralized structure, the authorities and accountability given to the "local" levels capitalize on the expertise of the involved individuals at each level, which has advantages over a true centralized pyramid structure in which decisions are made by the few at the top. However, this model requires that clear expectations and responsibilities exist to avoid misunderstandings and different priorities between involved parties within the institution.
   - In the EU it is common for larger institutions (one Governing Body) to oversee more than one ARC—a decentralized model by the "animal program world" definition. In most of these situations, the Governing Body manages the capital budget, designated veterinarian, other veterinarians and veterinary staff, husbandry and sanitation staff, occupational safety and health program, and transport services as if the individual ARCs were one ARC. But all Governing Bodies manage the operating budget and regulatory compliance as if the ARCs were one ARC. In smaller universities, there will be variations with respect to the operational organization of their animal facilities, but most Governing Bodies are unlikely to oversee more than one ARC.
   - Advantages and disadvantages of the different animal program structures under one Governing Body:
     - Advantages: Whether a one ARC structure or centralized structure at the level of the Governing Body (multiple ARCs), advantages include:
       Economies of scale for fixed expenses
       Lack of need to duplicate resources
       Easier insurance of consistent standards, policies, and SOPs within operational units, e.g. rodent versus non-human primate (NHP) vivaria
       In the "multiple ARCs under one Governing Body" model, allowing individual ARCs to establish performance-based standards that are feasible and practical for their situation, while being in compliance with the animal program as a whole
       More efficient self-assessment programs
       Creates a critical mass of investigators needed to support a specialized research service
     - Disadvantage of the "multiple ARCs under one Governing Body" model is that it is more difficult for ARCs and investigators to access specialized resources if the resource is not housed at their ARC location, e.g. genome editing, cryopreservation

5. **How Should Compliance with Legislation and Relevant Guidelines Be Organized Effectively?**

   This book contains a chapter on ethical and legal compliance. Readers are referred to it for a more detailed information on legal compliance.

   In brief:

   In the US, the animal programs must follow the requirements and guidance of the regulatory documents [2–4], which dictates that

- each of the three entities of the animal program (IO, Approval Unit, Animal Resource Center) should ensure that its membership has the qualifications and experience to perform the unit's responsibilities
- each of the three entities should have an internal assessment program to evaluate its own performance
- the "checks and balances" listed above provide oversight of each unit by the other two units
- besides approving the use of an animal for a research study, Approval Units are typically responsible for leading their and the ARC's self-assessment activities, the outcome of which is reported to the Governing Body
- reportable non-compliance is led by the Governing Body
- third-party review, i.e., AAALAC International, provides an assessment by individuals not responsible for the tasks of each unit and not biased by their perception of their own program

In the EU

- The European Directive [1] ensures compliance by mandating that member states' national authorities issue licenses for institutions and scientists, and audit/inspect facilities, programs, and experiments to ensure compliance with national legislation and the Directive.

6. **What Should the Reporting Structure Be?**
   In the EU there is a legal requirement for annual reporting to the National Authorities for all license holders, and the information provided is organized in the ALURES statistical database (https://environment.ec.europa.eu/topics/chemicals/animals-science/statistics-and-non-technical-project-summaries_en#statistical-database), which consists of three sections.

- Section 1 gives the numbers of animals (conventional and genetically altered) that are used for the first time for research, testing, routine production, and for education and training.
- Section 2 gives numbers of all uses (first use and subsequent reuses) of animals for research, testing, routine production and for education and training. It also gives the reason for use (e.g., specific research area, type of testing), the actual severity (mild, moderate, severe) experienced by animals, the animal's genetic status, and the use of animals to meet legislative requirements.
- Section 3 gives the numbers of genetically altered animals to support scientific research. These animals were used for the creation of new lines or for the maintenance of existing colonies. Section 3 provides the actual numbers of animals used for the first time and details of all uses, and the type of research for which new genetically altered lines have been created. In addition to the EU's requirement for annual reports, there may be National requirements for regular reporting as well as institutional requirements.

In the US, all animal programs that receive Public Health government funding must report annually to the Office of Laboratory Animal Research (OLAW) and those programs with US Department of Agriculture (USDA) species on census must report annually to the USDA. OLAW and the USDA reports are required to provide the specific information required by each entity. Additionally, AAALAC accredited facilities are required to report annually.

The above describes the reporting structure to external regulatory bodies. Internally the reporting structure within each unit of the animal program should be based on the organization of that unit. In smaller programs, the organizational structure may be a single person or only two levels deep, while in larger programs the organizational structure may be multiple layered. Within the institution, the reporting structure may involve a number of designated leadership positions, such as the IO, AV, facility manager, and/or the program oversight body.

For multi-ARC programs, the organizational structure may need both an internal reporting structure and a secondary reporting structure to the overall leadership of the animal program (Governing Body).

By design the organizational structure of multiple units working together for the betterment of the animal program makes for a matrix working relationship that minimizes the chance for rogue behavior by any one arm, i.e. ARC, IO/Governing Body, IACUC.

This design is neither a centralized nor decentralized organizational structure by the definitions at the beginning of this section but capitalizes on the positives and shortcomings of each. For example, decisions are not made by just a few at the top (positive) but operational processes may take longer to implement and be less efficient (negative). However, given what is at stake, i.e., animal welfare, public opinion, advancement of knowledge, financial support for research, etc., the positives outweigh the negatives.

7. **What is the Role of an IACUC in the Animal Care and Use Program and How Does It Differ from the Role of the EU's Animal Welfare Body?**

This book contains a chapter on ethical and legal compliance. Readers are referred to it for a more detailed information on oversight bodies and IACUCs.

In brief, the IACUC has several responsibilities, including

- Reviewing and approving an initial proposal and require modifications or withhold approval to conduct *in vivo* research. The proposed use of a live animal must demonstrate
  - Justification to conducting the study, specifically addressing its value to society and the advancement of knowledge, and confirming that it does not unnecessarily duplicate already published work
  - That the 3Rs have been met
  - That the appropriate species is being used
  - That the minimal number of animals will be used
  - All involved personnel are appropriately trained
  - Animals will be appropriately monitored, pain and distress managed in compliance with American Veterinary Medical Association (AVMA) standards, and criteria stated for euthanizing an animal using an AVMA-approved method prior to the study endpoint for humane reasons
- Reviewing every 6 months the institutions program for humane care and use
- Inspecting every 6 months facilities and non-vivarium spaces where live animals are taken, including labs
- Preparing results from above and submit to the Institutional official which must include reasons for any departures and/or deficiencies, and a plan for correction
- Reviewing concerns involving animal care and use
- Making recommendations for program improvements and/or compliance resolutions regarding any aspect of the institution's animal program, facilities, or personnel training
- Suspending any non-compliance activities involving live animals

In contrast, the EU's Animal Welfare Body is primarily an advisory body, and the "advice" is directed by the European Directive document. Advice is focused on the following topics:

- Matters related to the welfare of animals, in relation to their acquisition, accommodation, care, and use
- Application of the requirement of replacement, reduction, and refinement, and keep the Animal Welfare Body informed of technical and scientific developments con-

cerning the application of that requirement

- Establishing and reviewing internal operational processes as regards monitoring, reporting, and follow-up in relation to the welfare of animals housed or used in the establishment
- Development and outcome of projects, taking into account the effect on the animals used, and identify and advise as regards elements that further contribute to replacement, reduction, and refinement
- Rehoming schemes, including the appropriate socialization of the animals to be rehomed

Unlike the IACUC, the EU Animal Welfare Body (AWB) does not "issue" approval for investigators to conduct the proposed experiments. Although AWB normally performs an initial evaluation and helps improve the project, official authorization is granted by the competent authorities of the member states, who are responsible for the ethical cost–benefit analysis of the experiment and implementation of the 3Rs, sometimes referred to as "Ethics Committees." The number of such committees varies between countries from one to several (at regional level).

8. **What are the Advantages of Accreditation by Third Parties like AAALAC International**?

- "Arm's length" set of eyes on the program, which supplement the animal program's self-assessment program
- Ensures compliance and a consistent standard for animal use and care across animal programs—within and between states and countries
- Provides assurance to funding agencies that use of their support meets regulatory requirements
- Provides assurance to the public that the animals are not being abused and public funds are not supporting animal abuse

Summary

In some ways the EU, made up of individual countries, is similar to the US, made up of individual states. In both, standards and regulatory requirements come from the "top," i.e. the EU Commission or the US Government. At the highest level the animal program operation must have the same/very similar components, i.e., separate units that approve the use of each live animal, provide husbandry and medical care of the animals, ensure financial sustainability, ensure compliance with all relevant regulations, and has an individual/body with ultimate responsibility for the animal program.

Neither in the EU nor US can animal programs be classified as "centralized" or "decentralized" by the dictionary definition at the beginning of this section. In no EU or US program is all decision-making and power in the hands of a few at the top. Rather decision-making and authorities are delegated or granted to those with expertise in the aspect of the animal program in which they are involved. The value of this model, which has the potential of meeting some of the dictionary characteristics of a decentralized structure and was established by the regulatory agencies, is that it better ensures both proper care of the animals and research of the highest quality. However, the regulatory agencies also recognized the shortfalls of such a model, so established an internal "checks and balances" system, which got embedded in the regulatory documents, and is supplemented by third-party entities that review animal programs, which in the EU are National regulatory authorities.

Thus, the model set up by the regulatory agencies avoided the potential "negative" aspects of either a pure centralized or decentralized organization structure and capitalized on the potential "positive" aspects.

2.2 Part 2: Animal Program Services and Operation

1. **Which Services Should Be Included in an Animal Care and Use Program?**

Depends entirely on the type of institution (university, biotech company, contract house, etc.) and could vary from only providing basic husbandry and care of the animals to providing everything, i.e., care, experimental procedures, molecular and genetic manipulation, breeding, testing, licenses and experimental design, imaging, pathology, statistics, etc., so the scientist never needs to leave her or his office but just write the report or publication based on the information and data provided by the Program. Services included in a Program may involve insurance of compliance and state-of-the-art husbandry and care, and where relevant behavioral management including training of animals. Other services often offered by the Program are teaching and training such as mandatory courses for license applicants, as well as anesthesia and aseptical surgical procedures.

In a recent survey of university Programs in the US and the EU [5, 6], breeding was reported to be the responsibility of all participating EU Programs This contrasts with US Programs, where ~40% of rodent breeding is managed by researchers. However, the US Programs that participated in the survey were responsible for all animal purchasing and per diem and fee-for-service billing. There were several services for which >50% of participating EU and US Programs were responsible, including veterinary clinical services, import/export, billing, euthanasia, transportation, technical services, animal purchasing, and serology/virology/molecular diagnostics.

2. **Should Relevant "Hands on" Training and Didactic Teaching, Such as Mandatory Courses in Laboratory Animal Science, Be a Component of the Program?**

For investigators, the short answer is yes. The veterinary and academic staff of the centralized program would in general be the institutions' experts in laboratory animal science. Thus, for an institution to maintain the highest possible standards for the animal-based research, it is logical to place responsibility for compliance and relevant teaching and training to these experts. In some EU countries, e.g., Ireland, Netherlands, and the UK (not a member of the EU) there is a designated Training Officer, who is responsible for training and competence assessment.

For ARC staff, some European countries, e.g., Scandinavia, have specific college education for laboratory animal technicians/caretakers, and only staff with this education are allowed responsibility for the husbandry of laboratory animals. In other countries, it is mandatory for technicians to follow specific educational programs at vocational schools.

3. **How Should Core Facilities Offering Special Animal-Based Services Interact with the Animal Care and Use Program?**

The complexity of specialized equipment and technologies that are invaluable to advancing animal-based research is ever increasing and are frequently not technologies that are practical for an individual research lab to set up. Consequently, many institutions have established core facilities offering specialized services to the Institution's scientific community, e.g., fish and rodent transgenics, imaging, phenotyping assays/procedures, sequencing, etc. These core facilities are typically operated on a fee-for-service basis where the revenue covers the costs of consumable supplies, labor, equipment maintenance, and service contracts, and ultimately replacement costs. The cores that offer the above type of services are most often operated outside the umbrella of the ARC. The research support services typically operated by the ARC are services such as diagnostic and comparative pathology, molecular and serological diagnostics, and technical, e.g., procedure and surgical support, services that the ARC needs itself for regulatory and QA processes. However, some ARCs also oversee cores that are animal related, e.g., gene editing, phenotyping, and have the advantage of centralization of animal services which aids in compliance and provides "one stop shopping" for animal-related services.

4. **What are Satellite Facilities and How do They Differ From Core Facilities?**

   Satellite facilities is a term used to describe animal facilities located outside the boundaries of the main facilities. This location may be due to space constraints in the main facility or because the satellite facilities need to be close to specialized equipment located outside the main animal facilities. Operationally, a satellite facility may be managed by the centralized animal care and use program, or it may be operated by local research staff. Either way it is recommended that satellites have the same oversight stringency and adhere to the standard operating procedures that are in use in the main facilities, such as husbandry practices, veterinary care, experimental procedures, documentation, training, and sanitation practices, for overall institutional program consistency. Satellite facilities often serve one or a few research groups and the facilities are thus not available to the wider scientific community and—contrary to a core facility—a satellite facility does not provide services to scientists who are not members of the local research group.

5. **Should an Animal Care and Use Program Include Research and Development?**

   Yes, laboratory animal science is a complex and constantly evolving field, so if an institution aims to operate a first-class animal care and use program, it is important to allocate resources to in-house research and development activities. This will also help to attract and retain competent staff, ensure an effective animal care and use program with focus on animal welfare and the 3Rs, facilitate effective implementation of refinement initiatives, and collaboration and interaction with the wider scientific community of the institution. Additionally, development of emerging technologies and new animal-based services requires competent veterinary and academic expertise often in collaboration with the institution's scientific and managerial staff.

6. **What are the Advantages and Disadvantages of Outsourcing Activities, Such as Sanitation and Health Monitoring?**

   The advantages of outsourcing activities include lower labor costs, and minimizing investments in equipment and expert staff, allowing ARC staff to focus on more "attractive" job responsibilities. The decision to outsource a task needs to be balanced by the potential disadvantages, which could include the lack of in-house control and competence, lack of a critical mass to perform expert judgment on the quality of services bought in, leading to reliance on a potentially limited number of outside vendor, beholden to market pricing, and the cultural impact if staff numbers are, consequently, reduced.

   When services are outsourced, ARCs need to ensure that all relevant health and safety practices are followed, and the delivered service(s) are compliant with all relevant regulatory requirements and have appropriate quality control.

7. **What are the Major Cost-saving Possibilities in Programs?**

   From surveys of programs in the EU and the US [4, 6], opportunities for increased automation provide the major cost-saving potential. Process improvement approaches such as Lean Six Sigma can improve animal resource performance by reducing operational waste and limiting process variation (see, e.g., https://leansixsigmainstitute.org). In particular, process re-engineering combined with automation of environmental monitoring, colony management, sanitation and husbandry are prevalent areas for automation and cost savings.

2.3 Part 3: Animal Program Costs and Income

1. **What are Direct and Indirect Costs?**

   Animal Facilities/Program: The components of direct and indirect operational costs are often customized for the animal facility for costing purposes. The US NIH Cost Analysis and Rate Setting Manual for Animal Facilities [7] provides a representative framework for determining direct and indirect costs specific to allocating animal care costs. The manual provides guidance on expenses that are considered "direct costs," such as consumable expenses incurred for animal husbandry, labor, and veterinary care that can be costed and specifically allocated to a species and/or service level. "Indirect costs" are expenses that are incurred by all species. These aggregated expenses are proportionally distributed across all species and can include expenses such as program leadership, business office expenses, and cage wash.

Institutional Level: The definition and components of indirect cost vary by funding source. Further, not all funding sources allow financial support for indirect costs. The NIH costing manual also provides categories and definitions of institutional indirect costs. The manual refers to these "indirect" costs as Facilities and Administrative costs and includes:

- Space costs that include building and equipment depreciation or use allowances, interest expenses associated with the construction or renovation of facilities or the acquisition of equipment, and operation and maintenance of physical plant (e.g., utilities, repairs and maintenance, security, pest control).
- Institutional general administration and general expenses that include the central university administration, general accounting, purchasing, and similar administrative costs.
- Regulatory compliance costs that include activities that are necessary for the conduct of research but are not directly attributable to individual research projects. These activities are typically mandated as an institutional responsibility and include review of protocols for proposed research involving laboratory animals; monitoring of approved protocols; development, provision, and certification of training to qualify individuals to perform certain types of animal procedures; employee occupational health costs; oversight of animal study areas; and advice and consultation on reduction of animal numbers, refinement of research techniques, and alternatives to animal use [3]

2. **What are Full Costs?**

The definition of full costs is highly variable as is the cost basis for setting per diem rates. The costs of labor, food, bedding, medications, detergents/chemicals, and general supplies associated with husbandry, sanitation, and veterinary care are almost always included in full costs. However, the components of full costs vary significantly when other costs associated with the animal facility operation and maintenance are considered. What is considered full costs is also influenced by costs that are "allowable" costs by funding agencies. Thus, the animal facility budget—what the animal facility often defines as full costs—may only include allowable costs to ensure unallowable costs are not inadvertently incorporated into per diem rates and charged to funding agencies. Thus, the unallowable costs may be "lumped" into another budget at the institution and not fully known by the animal facility but are part of the full costs. In surveys in both the US and EU the inclusion of costs such as building depreciation, rent, major maintenance, IT, university administrative services, and legal services is variability as to whether these costs are incorporated into a "full cost" analysis [6]. Of those programs that do include such costs in their calculation almost 50% indicated that the Institution covers these costs [6]. Such data illustrate the lack of a universal definition of "full cost" and, thus, a lack of consistency in the approach to subsidies to animal programs. It is tempting to speculate that institutions with lower per diem rates have lower costs and, hence, are more efficient (or vice versa), but with no consistent approach to determining full costs, such assumptions can be significantly inaccurate.

3. **How Should Costs Associated with the Program Be Calculated?**

The goal of cost accounting is to ensure costing for each species and/or service level represents its specific cost, and that one species/service level does not cross-subsidize another. A cost accounting methodology should be used to calculate the per diem rate and other services expenses offered by the animal facility. This includes allocation of direct and indirect animal facility costs to each species and level of service. For example, mice may have more than one service level, so cost allocation should take into consideration the service level. Since labor represents the largest expense of an animal program's operation, appropriately allocating labor costs is among the most important factors for accurately costing species and/or services. The allowable indirect costs should be allocated to the direct cost center using an approach that proportionally spreads indirect costs to direct cost center that uses the service, e.g. care days, species, space, service level, etc. The approach should be consistent, defensible, and as objective as possible to ensure each species and service accrues appropriate expenses.

The US NIH Cost Analysis and Rate Setting Manual for Animal Facilities [7] outlines the basic steps to animal facility cost accounting:

- List all the internal costs of the animal program
- Identify the direct cost centers of the animal program, such as daily care of a category of laboratory animals, and the internal support cost centers, such as ARC administration
- Assign the internal animal program costs to the appropriate direct and support cost centers
- Allocate to appropriate cost centers those institutional Facilities and Administrative (indirect) costs that are eligible to be assigned to the animal program
- Allocate the costs of the internal support cost centers to the direct cost centers
- Calculate unit costs by dividing the total allocated costs of each direct cost center by the units of service provided

4. **How Should the Program's Research and Development Be Funded?**

Animal program research and development is vital to advancing program enhancements. These activities also provide opportunities for animal care and veterinary personnel to engage in research that directly benefits animal care and use, thereby providing an incentive to attract and retain exceptional personnel. Ideally, program research and development would be funded by external grants, but few mechanisms exist to fund program enhancements. Thus, funding for program enhancements and refinements relies on institutional support. The funding source for these activities should not come from per diem rates for the following reasons:

- To ensure the per diem income from one species does not "cross-subsidize" the research and development benefiting another species
- Because program development such as developing/adding new services, acquiring new techniques, caring for new species, refinements in animal care and use often reflects institutional research priorities and not the priorities of the grants used to pay the per diems
- Development of animal care and use refinements that benefits the animals is an institutional responsibility. Once the outcome of the research and development process has demonstrated a benefit to the animal care and use programs, processes, and/or activities, the implementation and ongoing cost to maintain these new initiatives can be allocated to appropriate costs centers and included in relevant per diem rates

5. **What is the Range of the Percent of Per Diem Income to Total Income in Animal Care and Use Programs?**

   In general, animal programs have two mechanisms to generate income: per diems and fee-for-service activities. In both US and EU programs, per diem income is ~70–80% of the Animal Programs' income, with the remaining coming from non-subsidy sources, such as transportation and fee-for-service work, e.g. technical services [6].

6. **Which Factors are Important to Consider When Setting Per Diem Rates?**

   The charging of a per diem unit can be for individual animals or for cages/tanks or per day or per week. For countries in which many of the rodent and fish species do not require a precise census, per diem charge unit, e.g., per animal or per cage/tank, typically reflects how the animals are housed. For example, mice and rats per diem rates are typically per cage, fish per tank, and larger species, e.g., pigs, NHPs, sheep, dogs, per animal. The above describes the approach typically used by academic institutions for species in which the census can be estimated, independent of their "public" versus "private" status. For-profit companies use a variety of mechanisms to account for their animal costs and may not be based on a "per diem unit."

   In academia, per diem charges are paid mostly from investigators' research budgets. This results in needing an "affordable" per diem rate for investigators, which then impacts the need for the Animal Program to cover its operating expenses. The most influential factor in establishing academic per diem rates is cost accounting [6]. However, three other factors, institution acceptance of a deficit, having competitive rates with peer institutions, and percent increase from prior years, challenge charging the fully costed per diem rate, often leaving the animal program "caught in the middle" with an operational deficit. The institutional cost factors (cost accounting, deficit acceptance) and two more investigator-focused factors (competitive rates with peer institutions and percent increase from prior years) underscore the competitive dynamics among rate-setting factors and highlight the growing financial sustainability issues emerging among institutions that conduct animal-based research.

7. **Which Costs Can Be Included in Per Diem Rates and Which Cannot?**

   The costs that can be included in the per diem rate are determined by the funding bodies and hence vary. Again, the NIH Cost Analysis and Rate Setting Manual [7] provides guidance about allowable and unallowable costs that can be included in the per diem rate. Many of the unallowable costs, appropriately, should not be included in the per diem cost base because these expenses are already accounted for in the institution's facilities and administration [Facilities and Administration (F&A) "indirect"] rate. The F&A portion of an award is provided to the institution to ensure investigators have the appropriate infrastructure to conduct the research set forth in the award. Examples of F&A expenses typically included in the institution's negotiated F&A indirect rate are:

   - Space expenses: Building and equipment acquisition and depreciation, the interest on construction and renovation projects, physical plant maintenance.
   - Institutional administration expenses: President's office, general accounting, purchasing, etc.
   - Regulatory compliance expenses: Federally mandated institutional responsibilities, IACUC protocol development and review, animal program self-assessment, monitoring of approved protocols, development, provision, and certification of training for animal procedures, employee occupational health costs, oversight of study areas, advice/consultation on the reduction of animal numbers, refinement of procedures and alternatives to animal use [3]. This guidance provides a common framework for US academic programs to establish the cost base for setting animal per diem rates.

Animal programs in the EU do not have a uniform set of costing guidelines used by all programs, resulting in a variety of approaches to establishing the cost base for per diem rates and potentially leading to more variability in the expenses included in the cost base. In addition, many LERU institutions are struggling with funding bodies' reluctance to accept realistic indirect costs (overhead) when awarding grants, which may result in some institutions including costs in the per diem rates that would be considered "indirect" and not allowable in the US. Nevertheless, while the approach is likely more consistent in the US, it clearly does not allow inclusion of all operational expenses.

8. **Which Costs Will Funding Bodies Accept To Be Included in Per Diem Rates?**

   As noted above, allowable expenses to be included in the per diem rate depend on the funding body. In general, the direct animal care costs are usually funded with little questioning. However, it is less clear when a portion of the Institutions indirect costs is included in the per diem rate to cover a portion of the Institutional "overhead" costs, e.g., building utilities, maintenance, and operation, general administration, purchasing, libraries, etc. This is further complicated because most institutions also have an indirect rate which is negotiated with the funding bodies. Thus, those portions of the "overhead" expenses in the institutional indirect rate and those that are in the per diem rate often require clarification. Some funding bodies, e.g., smaller foundations, may not fund the institutional indirect rate at all. In some cases, the institution may have one per diem rate for funding bodies that pay the full institutional indirect rate and a separate (higher) rate for those that do not provide funds (or insufficient funds) to fund the indirect rate. In such cases where per diem rates may vary by funding sources, an administrative mechanism is needed to ensure financial compliance, i.e., the correct per diem rate is charged to the funding source, especially if an investigator has multiple funding sources.

9. **How Should Per Diems for External Users of the Program's Services Be Calculated?**

   The per diem rate should include the total cost to care for the species. In many cases, this includes the internal per diem rate, the indirect rate, any deficits, including those arising from direct animal care and/or under recovery from the indirect rate, space costs, and the administrative costs to administer services to external investigators. The appropriateness of charging more than it costs to deliver a service, i.e., making a profit, should be reviewed with the institutions' administrative leadership to ensure it does not infringe on institutional or other broader policies governing institutional financial compliance.

10. **Is the NIH Cost Accounting Manual Relevant for Setting Per Diem Rates in Animal Care and Use Programs Outside the US?**

    Yes, it provides a framework for developing a cost accounting approach. This guidance provides a common framework for animal programs to establish the cost base for setting per diem rates and can be customized to meet specific institutional and funding bodies' needs.

11. **How Does Net Cash Flow Vary Between Programs?**

    The net cash flow is dependent on which costs are included in the animal facility budget and whether an institutional subsidy or deficit coverage is considered "income" when the balance is calculated. As noted above, there is wide variability in the specific costs included in the animal program budget and this variability is further confounded by differences in how institutions cover these costs. Similar to the "full cost" issue there is not a universal approach to calculating operational balances or the definition of a "balanced budget" and highlights the pitfalls when comparing operational balances among different animal programs.

12. **How are Deficits Handled?**

    The definition of a "deficit" is also not universal. For example, a program that balances its budget based on a pre-defined institutional financial supplement may report that it "broke even," whereas other animal programs would consider the institutional financial support required to balance the budget a deficit. Likewise, the definition of "subsidy" is also not universal either as a program may report no subsidy because no institutional financial support was provided for the budget, yet the deficit is covered by the institution. However, the reconciliation of similar income and expense categories exposes the financial result with deficits being a frequent reality. A notable difference between the net cash flow in US and EU programs is the larger frequency and magnitude of the deficit in US programs. Thus, an overarching factor in an animal program's financial sustainability is how the deficit is managed. In both EU and US programs, deficits are mostly funded by the institution but other options include allowing the deficit to accumulate, use of reserve funds (if available) and loans to the animal program. It is not surprising that that there is much higher institutional debt "forgiveness" in US programs where there is more debt as it represents an essential approach to financial sustainability among US animal programs [6].

    Summary: There is no standard nomenclature or practices for reporting animal program financial data, and costing can be customized. Staffing is highly dependent on infrastructure, species, and services. Thus, comparisons between or among animal programs require a detailed analysis of each program to ensure comparisons are "apples to apples." Without such analysis, animal program comparisons have the potential to be "apples to oranges."

2.4 Part 4: Animal Program Staffing

1. **What Factors Affect Staffing Levels?**

    There are many factors that affect staffing. The degree to which each factor contributes to staffing levels is dependent on local animal program infrastructure, services offered, species and census, operating processes, and the staff themselves.

    Infrastructure issues that drive staffing levels include:

    - The facility layout, degree of decentralization
    - Cage type, e.g. IVC vs static caging for rodents, disposable caging
    - Water sources, e.g. bottles/water pouches vs. automatic watering
    - Washer center automation
    - Software applications for animal program management, e.g. census and billing, environmental monitoring, staff assignments, veterinary care

Services offered that could impact needed staffing levels include:

- Biohazard housing
- Gnotobiotics
- Technical services
- Outsourcing services and activities

Processes that can affect needed staffing numbers include:

- Regulatory requirements for cage sanitation, cage components, and cage contents
- The degree to which such processes have been evaluated and optimized for maximal efficiency
- Onboarding new species
- Breeding and colony management services

Species-specific factors that can impact staffing needs, include:

- The species diversity, census, and turnover
- Very low numbers of one species can erode economies of scale, whereas high census numbers can promote economies of scale, unless high census levels exceed the infrastructure's capacity

Staffing-specific issues that affect needed staff number, include:

- Staff training, including time "away" from normal assignment for cross training and staff onboarding
- Work rules, e.g. benefit time, work schedule flexibility options
- Staffing redundancy to account for staff benefit time, unexpected staff absences and unplanned operational challenges (especially given the long training period required for new staff)

2. **What are the Typical Staffing Categories for Animal Programs?**

   Position description and categories are often institution specific in order to conform to categorical job descriptions within the institution's human resource framework, which might be influenced by the size and complexity of the program.

   Typical examples of staffing categories are:

- Program Leadership (Program Director, Attending or Designated Veterinarian, Associate Director, Assistant Director)
- Veterinary Services (Chief/Head of Veterinary Service, Clinical Veterinarian, Veterinary technician)
- Operations Managerial/Supervisory Positions (Head of Husbandry or Daily Operations, Unit Operations Manager, Unit Staff Supervisor)
- Facility Infrastructure Manager
- Technical/Special Service Manager
- Diagnostic Pathology Chief/Manager and staff
- Virology Chief/Manager and staff
- Administrative Manager
- Financial Manager
- Trainer(s) for investigators and/or staff
- Technical Staff

In many programs, particularly smaller ones, not all of the above positions may exist, and in fact, some positions may be combined or an individual may have multiple roles and responsibilities, depending on the size and complexity of the program.

3. **How Should Animal Staffing Levels Be Determined?**

   Labor is the largest proportion of direct costs making staffing levels an important cost factor. The method that is used should be as objective as possible, equitable, and defensible. Since species come and go, census fluctuates, service requests are not always constant, and absenteeism is not linear, establishing metrics for adequate staffing levels is extraordinarily challenging. Ensuring staff assignments are equitable and minimizing "burn out" are important staff scheduling and retention considerations as high staff turnover drives both costs and quality of service. Time motion studies and establishing labor metrics for various tasks is one approach.

   Although establishing labor metrics is very time consuming and, therefore, costly, it may be the most accurate way to both determine appropriate staffing levels, ensure equitable job responsibilities, and project staffing levels based on changes in census and/or species. Establishing such metrics can be done by manually having an individual follow an individual(s) in a category of job for a predefined number of days, recording the time it takes to do each task within that job description. The data are then compiled to establish a metric for each activity/task and utilized to build an assignment and/or schedule for each staff member based on what activities/tasks need to be accomplished on that day/week/

month, etc. For example, a metric established for single cage change for the specific species, service level, caging type, etc., is then calculated to assign the number of cages that require changing by an individual. Conversely, all of the activities/tasks that are required over a specified period of time can be used to quantify overall staffing levels. Thus, while time consuming, metrics provides an objective, defensible approach to immediate staffing level needs and for projecting future needs that predictably track with demand.

Another approach which would not require the resources described above is to use a budgetary approach, e.g., income, of the unit to assign staffing levels.

Regardless of the method used, the use of scheduling software driven by the above collected data can aid in scheduling and refining staffing levels to achieve better equity between jobs categories and obtain more accurate labor allocation for cost accounting purposes.

2.5 Part 5: Animal Program Comparisons

1. **How Should Cost Among Animal Programs Be Compared?**

   The ideal way is to have a database that collects the same information from many animal programs, including demographic information that could impact program expenses.

   In the US, Yale University has been conducting a "Yale Animal Resource Cost and Benchmarking" survey© (Yale survey) every two to three years since the mid-1990s. While the survey items have changed and improved over the years, there are themes that can be trended over time and participants can benchmark themselves against their peers in any given survey. In 2018, the Yale survey was revised to reflect terminology and infrastructure of EU animal programs with the goal of collecting similar information about the operation and finances of EU programs. Fourteen members of the LERU participated in a pilot study [4, 6]. Data were compared between the LERU database and the 2016 and 2019 Yale surveys, which bracket the LERU survey. While there were many similarities identified, there were many differences found in organizational structure, operations, and management of finances between the EU and US programs.

   Over the years, the Yale survey has improved in its ability to be used by individual participants to benchmark their program against that of their peers. Some of the key improvements included:

   - Clarification as to exactly what piece of information each survey item is requesting.
   - Have the survey calculate key pieces of data. For example, when asked if a program is subsidized the definition of "subsidized" must be clear. Some programs have a revenue line item in their budget that comes from the institution, which coincidentally is the exact amount needed for net cash flow to be $0.00. Many of these institutions do not consider this revenue a subsidy because it is a fixed line item in their proposed budget for the fiscal year. Thus, these programs never have an internal operational deficit, which is not really correct.
   - So, in the survey the participant is asked for their revenue, which is mostly per diems and fee-for-service work, and their expenses, which are lumped together by major categories. The survey then calculates the net cash flow, thereby determining if the program has an operating deficit. This approach allows peer institutions to compare revenue types and amounts, expenses, and the net cash flow outcome.
   - Demographics: The survey should provide an analysis in multiple ways, looking at the impact of demographics so that one can benchmark themselves against a "similar" program. Demographics that have been shown to have an impact include:

- Physical location or region
- Public or private institution
- Workers unionized or not
- Size of the animal program, both in terms of the number of species and the total number of animals
- Species on census
- Automation priorities

AAALAC program accreditation is not likely to impact cost benchmarking mostly because many programs have some sort of accreditation and if they do not, the animal program operation still must comply with the same relevant federal, state/regional, local, and institutions requirements.

The industry does have optional program certifications, such as GLP, GMP, and ISO, that allow the program to provide specialized services which do have specific infrastructure and operational requirements. These certifications can be helpful when benchmarking against peer institutions because they signify that the program has additional infrastructure, resources, and costs embedded in their operation.

In both the US and EU, the value of cost comparisons between programs is totally dependent on the quality of the data being used for comparisons—as the saying goes "Garbage in, Garbage out." Hopefully, the LERU survey will grow in the number of participating institutions to the point where trends within its domain can be evaluated and a more robust comparison can be done "across the pond" between US and EU animal programs, which will be of value to all programs. What was shown with just a simple comparison between the US surveys and the LERU pilot survey is that "one size does not fit all, i.e., the best practice/approach of one institution may not be the appropriate practice/approach of another, but there is clearly something to be learned from one's peers" [6].

2. **Can Per Diem Rates Be Used as Surrogate for Costs and/or Efficiency?**

   Not at face value for a couple of reasons.

   - Unless the cost accounting is fully transparent showing that all expenses related to animal care have been included. In the surveys described above, there is significant variability between animal programs in the EU and the US in the expenses considered when calculating the "full cost of the animal program" [6]. For example, about 50% of the institutions that participated in the LERU pilot study or in the last Yale Animal Resource Cost and Benchmarking survey© do not include any of the following in the full cost of the animal program: building depreciation, building rent, major maintenance expenses, University administrative assistance, IT services, human resource services, or legal services, whereas the other 50% of participating programs include such expenses to a variable extent. In the US, government grants and some other sponsored awards provide funds that partially cover infrastructure expenses ("indirect rate"). About 30% of programs do not consider the portion of the expenses not covered by the indirect rate as animal program expenses.

     Thus, while one can benchmark their per diem rates against their peers, one cannot assume that your peers have the same or different costs or operational efficiencies without knowing the true full cost of running their animal program.
   - Not unless the difference between the cost-accounted per diem expenses is compared to the per diem rate charged to investigators. Some programs have sources of revenue, e.g., subsidies, that allow their per diem rate to be less than that of their cost-accounted rate to deliver a unit of service.

     Thus, the rate charged to investigators may or may not reflect the full cost of the animal care and, thus, not reflect the operational efficiency of the program.

3. **Are There Key Performance Indicators Allowing Benchmarking Programs Between Institutions?**

   As mentioned above, it is paramount that the survey items are stated in such a way that the piece of information being requested is interpreted the same by all participants. To allow for a comprehensive comparison data from all aspects of the animal program must be collected, including operational expenses, regulatory expenses, labor costs, veterinary care, administrative costs, etc. Because of the differences in care costs between species, it is difficult to collect metrics data about staffing numbers, workload, etc. However, when the above-described surveys attempted to collect such pieces of data, it has been limited to mice because that is the species that all programs have on census in large enough numbers for cost accounting to have some degree of accuracy.

References

1. Directive 2010/63/EU of the European Parliament and of the Council of 22 September 2010 on the protection of animals used for scientific purposes
2. Animal Welfare Act and Animal Welfare Regulations. United States Department of Agriculture. November, 2013
3. Office of Laboratory Animal Welfare. The Public Health Service Policy on Humane Care and Use of Laboratory Animals. NIH Publication No 15-8013, revised 2015. Based on the Heath Research Extension Act of 1985; Public Law 99–158, November 20, 1985. https://olaw.nih.gov
4. National Research Council of the National Academies. Guide for the care and use of laboratory animals. 8th ed. Washington, DC: The National Academies Press; 2011.
5. Preisig P, Macy JD, Hau J. Comparing United States and European Union academic animal programs: organization, operation, and services offered. Lab Anim. 2024;58(2):149–59.
6. Preisig P, Macy JD, Hau J. Comparing United States and European Union academic animal programs: finances. Lab Anim. 2024; 58(2):138–48.
7. Cost Analysis and Rate Setting Manual for Animal Research Facilities. National Center for Research Resources (U.S.) Bethesda, MD: U.S. Dept. of Health and Human Services, National Institutes of Health, National Center for Research Resources; 2000.

3 Facility Planning

Nicola Watts and Sarah Wolfensohn

Abstract

Whilst the use of animals continues to be a key requirement in the progression of biomedical research, there is a need to house them in appropriate accommodation for both breeding and experimental purposes. The physical environment that the animals are kept in plays a critical part in the quality of science generated by an institution and the welfare of those animals. The planning, design and building or refurbishment of laboratory animal facilities is a complex and lengthy process, requiring diverse expert input via carefully managed specialist teams to optimise success. This chapter provides an overview of these aspects, which will be discussed in greater detail elsewhere.

Keywords

Facility planning, design and build · Animal welfare · Scientific integrity

N. Watts (✉)
London, UK

S. Wolfensohn
Present Address: University of Surrey, Guildford, UK
e-mail: s.wolfensohn@surrey.ac.uk

3.1 Introduction

An appropriate physical environment for laboratory animals is fundamental to a strong animal care and use programme. It is recognised that quality of scientific output is linked with good animal welfare [1]. The five domains concept of animal welfare [2] sets out internationally accepted standards of animal care that safeguard an animal's access to basic needs. It includes five interacting physical/functional domains: (1) Nutrition, (2) Environment, (3) Health, (4) Behaviour and (5) Mental state, seeking to assess the impact of the physical and social environment on the affective state of an animal. The Five Domains may be used as an evaluation tool for 'particular physical/functional disruptions and imbalances, as well as restrictions on behavioural expression, and then to identify the specific negative affects each disruption, imbalance or restriction would be likely to generate' [2].

Moreover, the 3Rs (replacement, reduction, and refinement) developed in the 1950s by Russell and Burch [3] is used throughout the world as an ethical framework for improving laboratory animal welfare and there is an expectation set by legislation, e.g., the European Directive [4] and international organisations, such as AAALAC International, for the application of these principles, which can also be found in the ICLAS-CIOMS principles [5] and OIE Terrestrial code [6]. Even when the 3Rs are

J. Guillén, V. Galligioni (eds.), *Practical Management of Research Animal Care and Use Programs*, Laboratory Animal Science and Medicine 3, https://doi.org/10.1007/978-3-031-65414-5_3

applied and less animals are used and the use of in vitro research using cells increases, these tissues still come from animals which need to be bred and raised in a controlled lab environment. Therefore, it is clear that the physical environment that the animals are kept in plays a critical part in the quality of science generated by an institution and the welfare of those animals.

1. What May Be the Drivers for a New Facility?

The building of a new animal facility is a complex, expensive and time-consuming project which, if not designed carefully, can end in a building that is not fit for the purpose intended, may struggle to gain approval by local authorities or at the very least be very difficult to 'make work' on a day-to-day basis for both animals and staff. This chapter will focus on aspects to consider with respect to experimental rather than breeding facilities.

The usual driver for a new facility is the deterioration of old buildings, the need to consolidate or an entirely new venture. When there are old facilities already on site, consideration is often given to the refurbishment of the existing buildings rather than starting afresh. This strategy may appear a cheaper option, but it rarely is and may meet challenges with unexpected issues in the original infrastructure, which could hinder progress or even invalidate the original plan. Using specialist laboratory animal facility expertise can be invaluable in the development of an initial brief. Without initial appropriate expert input and the involvement of a wide range of stakeholders, the building may not fit the needs of the animals, researchers or technical staff and may not function as required (e.g. if noisy physical plant is located too close to procedure rooms).

2. What Considerations Should Be Taken into Account When Planning a New Facility?

- Legal compliance
- Type and volume of research; current and future
- Animal species required and their specific requirement
- Working environment for the staff
- Level of biosecurity required
- Location
- Access to the facility including large trucks delivering supplies and animals
- Security
- IT support
- Layout and space
- Budget

By the very nature of the laboratory animal facilities, they are a costly investment and extensive value engineering rarely results in a fit for the future build. Cost comes from the requirement for an extensive physical plant (which can be up to 40–50% of the gross space) to maintain temperature, ventilation and humidity; biosecurity, specialist cleaning equipment; bespoke enclosures for animals to meet species-specific behavioural needs; specialist procedural areas; health & safety and staff considerations, to name but a few. Space is at a premium and every effort must be made to be as economical as possible to avoid suboptimal late-stage changes. Insufficient storage can result in expensive animal holding and animal procedure areas being used instead.

Depending on the siting of the proposed facility and the external scientific environment, a centre of excellence focussing on key research strengths could be considered instead of a more general multi-user facility but there may be concern over the potential of this business model to stifle diversity of research and innovation.

3. What Are the Principal Phases of a Facility Design Project?

Initial Design Phase

(i) Programming and feasibility including goals of the project, feasibility study, space planning, flows and barriers, all applicable regulations and site suitability. This phase includes the expression and formalisation of user requirements specifications (URS).

(ii) Schematic design of the facility including named functional layout of the building with areas and room allocation, physical flows, equipment to be integrated in the construction.
(iii) Budget, design, timeline are finalised and resources defined for construction; contractual documents are issued including final drawings and specifications, as well as documents used for tender.

Procurement phase: Orders, purchases, rental of materials, tools and services necessary to complete the project.

Construction phase: Involving mainly the project manager, design and engineering teams as well as the contractor and subcontractors.

Post-construction/close-out phase: To detect tasks that are not correctly completed and specifications that are not respected before reception of the building.

4. **Who are the Key Players Involved to Create an Effective Team Approach?**

It may take some years to reach full realisation of a new build concept so ensuring sign off of the project and initial budget approval by appropriate senior leader(s) of the institution is key in order to avoid any misunderstandings at a later stage. Any new build project should be achievable and justifiable. To ensure a team approach, with clear lines of communication throughout the project and robust budgetary control, a suitable governance structure including Board oversight and robust project teams are required with a clear remit, milestones and appropriate membership. Stakeholder management must be a priority. Laboratory animal facility experts may be able to offer a rough estimate of likely cost based on the size of facility required. Benchmarking of other newly built facilities at an early stage can aid stakeholders in their vision and prevent errors later in the process. A feasibility study to test scope and location can be undertaken, followed by a more detailed costing with architects experienced in the design of laboratory animal facilities. Coming to the table with an unrealistically low budget could impact the likelihood of a successful outcome. On the other hand, in a shrinking economic environment, pragmatism is paramount and 'must haves' will need to be separated and prioritised above 'nice to haves'. The inclusion of 'lean' methodology in the planning of a new build will be discussed later.

To clarify the scope of the project and URS, initial consultation with animal experts and researchers is strongly recommended, combined with floor planning exercises and a review of key risks. From there a series of potential options can be drawn up for consideration. Institutional research strategy as well as individual research plans for expansion or reduction of work will heavily influence the type of animal facility required. Meticulous note taking, official minutes and robust version control of documentation are important to avoid confusion and poor decision-making as well as the potential to make a fundamental mistake with a design element of the build. A real size 'mock up' room, appropriately equipped for stakeholders to assess can be invaluable to avoid costly mistakes in the actual build (e.g. door/ corridor/ceiling configuration such that trolleys or animal housing units cannot fit around or through into the required rooms).

5. **What are the Legal Issues to Be Considered? (See Chap. 1 on Legal Questions)**

Depending on the country where the institution is sited, there may be particular legal frameworks which must be complied with regarding the physical finish and function of laboratory animal facilities in order to safeguard the welfare of the animals to be housed there. There may be legal statutes, recommended guidance or the reliance on a third party such as AAALAC International to assess performance outcomes. There must also be compliance with legislation relating to health and safety, biosafety and release of genetically modified organisms. It is likely that commissioning data and/or inspections as well as decontamination are required before animals are imported into the new facility and the lead-in for these tasks should be carefully integrated into project timelines to avoid unexpected delays to research activities.

6. **What Aspects Should Be Considered Regarding Selection of the Best Location?**

There are many aspects that influence the location of a new facility including:

- Cost of the land
- Secure location
- Terrain and space
- Flood risk
- Adjacency to existing research laboratories
- Accessibility to internal/external visiting researchers
- Accessibility to road, rail and airports for animal deliveries

Once there is a clear understanding of the type of research to be carried out, the siting of a new animal facility is a major decision. The most economical, quickest to build and most efficient facilities to operate are ones located on a flat site. Adjacency to researchers and wet labs (if not contained within the animal facility itself) must also be taken into account, as well as the ability to keep the facility secure, yet also accessible to users and deliveries including appropriate space for large trucks to turn as well as potential for an integrated lobby area.

7. **What Factors Should Be Considered for the Building Structure?**

The type of build depends on the budget, location and scope of research it is intended for. Institutional strategy may dictate a brick build with specific sized rooms or greater flexibility may be achieved through the use of modular, prefabricated builds or those with the ability to vary the internal layout or repurpose, depending on changing need. It must be recognised, however, that the species to be housed must be carefully considered before approving building plans, and animal welfare staff are critical to the decision-making.

Multi-floored facilities can be very difficult to manage if there are biosecurity issues to be considered and if animals need transferring between floors. A multi-storey facility is inherently more expensive because a large proportion of each floor is taken up by lifts and stairwells and biosecurity/flow of animals across the floors becomes difficult to manage. Lifts need to be large enough to accommodate caging racks and other large pieces of equipment.

Historically, many rodent facilities consisted of multiple small rooms; however, with the increasing recognition of laboratory animal allergens, the advent of large biosecure ‘sealed’ caging solutions, e.g., individually ventilated cages and robotic cage cleaners, has driven more open plan building designs in recent years, since these are more space-efficient in terms of housing capacity. Farm animals and equines have a different set of needs to more typical laboratory species, such as ventilation, drainage or grazing. When incorporating a fish facility, the load bearing strength of facility flooring must be considered (to take account of the weight of the water) and if not on the ground floor, consideration of any particular rooms on lower floors that could be impacted by flooding. The strength of flooring in a multi-storey build is, in general, critical because of the weight of equipment and feed, etc., which may be stored on each floor. Potential for noise and vibration must be avoided or mitigated in the design. For example, disturbance from lifts or cage wash adjacent to rodent rooms can cause significant behavioural impact. This is important for all animal research activities but particularly mammalian behavioural studies or for aquatics because of the potential impact on animal welfare and therefore the science.

Historically, laboratory animal facilities were built in the basement and therefore without windows, for security. However, more recently, there has been a move to incorporating as much natural as light as possible to improve the wellbeing of both the staff and animals. In some situations, this has included external access for some animal species, e.g. dog, farm. The provision of windows for natural light must be caveated against security requirements and also the type of research being carried out which may require the addition of window/door coverings to control photoperiod within animal holding rooms, reducing environmental variables that may impact scientific integrity. In addition, external blinds and reflective glazing can be installed depending on the perceived security risk of the site.

Weather also has an influence in that very sunny climates may require the addition of brise soleil, an architectural feature of a building that reduces heat gain within that building by deflecting sunlight. Such a system allows low-level sun to enter a building in the mornings, evenings and during winter but cuts out direct light during summer. Alternatively, the number of windows can be reduced in order to maintain constant temperatures within for animals' and staff health, as well as for preservation of feed supplies, etc.

The physical plant requires not only considerable space but careful positioning in relation to the animal facility to allow accessibility for maintenance. Accessing the plant from within the animal facility is to be avoided due to the complexities of importing contractor equipment through a clean animal facility as well as the potential of wild rodent ingress to animal holding areas if accessing the plant via a ceiling void, etc.

8. **How Can the Biosecurity Level Impact the Design?**

The level of biosecurity required in a laboratory animal facility is a fundamental consideration in the planning stages of build design. Historically, the quality of scientific data has relied heavily upon the minimisation of experimental variables. Within a laboratory animal facility setting this has been delivered via ultra clean barriered facilities and the supply of purpose bred, disease free animals. Some institutions require staff to shower-in and wear full personal protective equipment (PPE) and all items being imported whether husbandry or research are 'sterilised' before entry. In general, animal facilities remain barriered (albeit at different levels) to protect animal health and safeguard against highly significant disease outbreaks. The importance of the mammalian microbiome and its potential to influence some research is an increasingly hot topic. The housing of gnotobiotic animals is discussed in the next chapter.

Thus, the type of research carried out in an institution heavily influences the strength of biosecurity required (and associated build design) and may have legal implications. For example, regulatory work must meet Good Laboratory Practice (GLP) requirements; cancer and immunology work must avoid infection of immune deficient animals; breeding establishments must avoid the supply of animals with subclinical disease. Infectious disease research requires a physical environment that acts to keep the infectious agents contained which is dependent on the defined Biosafety level at which that agent must be handled. These all require consideration of 'flow' within an animal facility from clean to dirty if required, air flow and room pressures, careful design of loading bay areas and specialist staff change facilities with wet or air showers. There may also be requirement for animal quarantine areas, interlocks to animal areas, specially designed animal holding areas and a facility built to allow appropriate process, storage and removal of waste materials including carcases.

Understanding and complying with genetically modified organism (GMO) legislation is becoming more important with the increasing use of genetically altered rodents and fish in biomedical research. There are strict requirements regarding the containment of these animals and facility design must reflect this, for example in the avoidance of floor drains in rodent holding areas/addition of drain traps and rodent barriers. Precision breeding technologies, such as gene editing, are aimed at developing new traits more precisely and more efficiently than traditional breeding techniques. Larger species such as pigs are used in this research and while such technologies have the potential to improve the health and welfare of the animals and improve the sustainability of farming systems, the design of the research facility must be appropriate.

9. **How Does Biosafety Impact the Design?** (See also Chap. 15 on Biosafety)

Zoonotic disease and potential for human cross infection and ensuring that infectious agents are not inadvertently released will also require detailed consideration when designing new facilities depending on the species and the infectious agents as well as the potential routes of transmission. Wild rodents pose a significant threat to the health status of laboratory rats and mice, so every effort must be made in the design of the facility to mitigate this. Ceiling voids, lift shafts, access lobbies, diet stores, etc., are all vulnerable and require consideration to safeguard the physical integrity of the facility, together with the systems for access and use of humane pest control where appropriate.

10. What are the Health and Safety Aspects to Consider?

Health and safety is governed by increasingly robust legislation across many countries. This is particularly true of laboratory animal allergen and manual handling risks associated with staff working in a laboratory animal environment. The former has been one of the drivers for barriered facilities and associated engineering standards such as ventilated type caging systems, specialist machinery in cage cleaning areas and specialist ventilated cabinets for animal procedures. Mitigating risk of manual handling injury requires specialist machinery such as robotics to reduce lifting, twisting or repetitive strain. All these require careful facility design to ensure appropriate space planning but also budget for expensive equipment. Ignoring the risk could significantly impact staff health and become costly if a breach of legislative compliance is proven.

Bespoke imaging facilities and radiation protective functions/equipment must be considered for a new build design, especially considering the potential use of radioactive material in research and imaging as well as a veterinary requirement for imaging on welfare/treatment grounds. Due consideration must also be given to the handling and access of hazardous materials, drugs and anaesthetic exhaust, and needles, sharps, waste all of which pose a health risk to staff and will require a degree of engineering design. Health and safety legislative requirements for the construction of high biosafety level (BSL) rooms are complex, require specialist advice and will not be covered in this chapter.

11. Which and How Staff Needs Should Be Addressed?

Historically, animal facilities were built in basement areas for security and those working within these areas had a very poor working environment. This has improved with time and more recently, new builds have incorporated natural light for the staff, at least in break out areas as well as providing for dedicated comfortable office space to support the increasing administrative burden on animal staff; toilets and change areas must meet gender, religious and disabled needs; facility parking and 24/7 access must be provided for animal care staff. Within animal areas, appropriate health and safety equipment is required to safeguard staff from repetitive manual tasks and laboratory animal allergens.

12. What are the Security Elements to Consider?

Laboratory animal facility security always has been and remains a priority in the feasibility assessment of a new build. The needs for a facility in the country or city may differ; however, the concepts will remain aligned. The facility perimeter must be contained, especially if some animals have access to outdoor areas and the wider issue of wild animal ingress may be important depending on the laboratory species housed on site. If laboratory animals have outside access, vocalisation from inside the site such as dogs barking could also create a security challenge. Access for animal, diet and bedding deliveries via loading bays, etc., must be secure and monitored on a day-to-day basis. Staff entry must be secured, something that can be difficult if 24-hour access is required for research purposes; the ubiquitous carrying of mobile cell phones has challenged traditional methods of security and priority is now best placed on the smooth delivery of a robust ethical care and use programme in case of animal rights infiltration. The code to keypads needs to be updated regularly so in practical terms, biometrics are better placed at facility entry points although if there is an IT issue there must be back up access through master keys or some such like. Visual access may also be required depending on the proposed Biosafety Level. CCTV could be installed in general, across the facility but data protection would need appropriate management.

The increasing use of natural light has already been discussed from a wellbeing perspective; however, the security element of windows into animal research areas can be challenging depending on the location. Reflective glass can be installed but beware that this will fail if room lights are switched on in the evening in which case additional automatic blinds may be required. Dawn and dusk lighting are necessary for some species and for some research purposes reverse lighting may be required. From a disposal perspective, secure removal of waste must also be a consideration, including confidential waste.

13. **What are the IT Aspects to Consider?**

Due to the location and physical build of animal facilities, Internet and phone signals can be a challenge. Input from IT at the design phase is key to ensure all rooms have Wi-Fi and data transfer cabling is included for research purposes, especially when imaging data is concerned. In addition, in recent years, telemetry studies have increased as well as cage side remote monitoring, all of which require proactive involvement of the IT for an optimal solution.

14. **What are the Sustainability Considerations?**

Eco-friendly building design solutions are becoming increasingly important in the face of climate change and carbon reduction, particularly as animal facilities can be energy consumption intensive and sometime wasteful. Potential considerations include:

- Build materials
- Demand based ventilation control to allow reduction in room air changes when stocking density is low or the room is empty
- Ventilated caging which can reduce cage changes and therefore bedding waste
- Bedding waste may be sent for composting instead of for incineration
- Recycling of plastics such as caging

15. **What are the Specific Species-related Considerations?** (See also Chap. 7 on Housing)

The design of an animal facility depends on the species housed within it. The species housed depend on the type of research activities carried out. Thus, an initial strategic review of the institution's future research goals prior to agreeing the design of any new animal facility is key. Although many laboratory animal species were historically housed individually, in small bare cages, the negative impact on scientific outcomes through stressed animals is now recognised. To promote animal wellbeing, they need a range of different environments to support the expression of 'normal' species-specific behaviour. Please see the following for some examples not already covered:

Non-Human Primates (NHPs): Old World

These are extremely intelligent, gregarious animals that often experience some of the most severe research procedures over time because of their similarities to man and that they are usually not used unless there is no alternative. Providing the appropriate environmental enrichment to reduce their stress as much as possible is critical both from a welfare perspective but also scientific integrity. Most reputable institutions now aim to house their NHPs in social groups with tall ceilings or even multi-floored accommodation to better reflect the species' natural environment, need for sufficient space to support hierarchical groups and tendency to seek elevated positions for safety. Toxicology research often uses juvenile animals which are easier to group house. Where sexually mature animals are required, social housing is still possible but their sex, size, strength and temperament must be taken into consideration. The type of study may also dictate whether animals can only be socially housed whilst they are stock animals. Even if single housing can be justified for primates for a particular procedure, they can usually be allowed visual, auditory and even tactile contact with conspecifics if the housing facilities are well designed. All these aspects influence the design of the building, the caging and the procedural areas.

Health and safety of those staff interacting with the animals should be considered both from a physical perspective and also possible disease transmission—both from primate to human and from the human to the primate. Key considerations include:

1. Provision of quarantine facilities for recently imported animals
2. Size and height of caging, avoiding animals being maintained in cramped accommodation close to the ground
3. Decision on the ability to provide natural light (scientific/security issues)
4. Orientation of bars to avoid trapping extremities or negatively impacting visual acuity
5. Sufficient distance between cage tops and ceiling tiles to avoid damage to the room from curious animals reaching through bars
6. Appropriate drainage for cleaning and swimming pools for enrichment
7. Extremely robust physical finishes to allow for rigorous, routine cleaning
8. Appropriate design features for waste management including shavings
9. Moveable partitions to allow transfer of animals to different cage areas during cleaning
10. Solid flooring to allow foraging
11. Space for, and provision of, suitable enrichment items that can be rotated
12. Appropriate features to allow for positive reinforcement training, non-stressful capture, restraint for simple interventions such as blood sampling or injections +/− transfer of animals to procedural areas
13. Design features to take into account the enrichment requirements of singly housed animals, e.g. within sight and smell of conspecifics; provision of TVs to reduce boredom, etc., ability to climb and perform 3-dimensional activities
14. Large enough procedural areas to accommodate multiple NHP restraint devices for dosing
15. Provision of bespoke veterinary rooms for treatment, isolation and imaging
16. Provision of large enough high spec surgical theatres with pre- and post-operative areas, anaesthetic scavaging, piped gases
17. Consideration of the type of imaging modalities required and behavioural suites
18. Provision of a postmortem facility with biological safety cabinets

Non-Human Primates (NHP): New World

New World monkeys originate from tropical rain forests in Central and South America, where they are exclusively arboreal. They climb well and if startled they flee upwards, not along the ground, so cages for these species should be taller to reflect this. The stocking density within the room must be kept low, since high stocking densities and overcrowding are associated with increased levels of disease. Marmosets are usually housed in family groups composed of an adult pair and offspring. They are agile and like to climb, and so benefit from branches or other suitable perches within the cage. They will walk along branches on all four feet and use their tails to balance. New World monkeys may thrive in one captive environment but exhibit poor reproductive capacity or ill health in another very similar environment, or even if moved to a different position in the same room. Social and environmental enrichment appear to play a particularly important role in maintaining the health of these small primates.

Farm Animals:

Successful animal facilities used for housing farm species reflect the concepts implemented for agricultural buildings—grass, grazing, browsing, natural light, good ventilation, temperature control, robust physical finish, nonslip flooring, sloping floors with drainage and appropriate width of entrances to allow movement of farm machinery. Social housing should be the default. These species have different requirements to dogs and so facility design may need to cater for both. Having said that, there is an increased use of the mini pig which does seem to adapt to dog enclosures with minimal repurposing. Farm species can be used as specialised surgical models, and surgical theatres must balance the need for stringent aseptic conditions, transfer of extremely large animals through the building (with automatic doors, hoists and appropriate bump rails) and hygiene considerations There are some species-specific considerations and requirements that will need appropriate planning such as: fleece clipping for sheep; outdoors rooting, mud wallowing and preventing of tail docking for pigs foot trimming, dehorning, provision of an appropriate comfortable laying area for cattle. Also, for these larger species, there must be well designed areas for killing, with facilities for stunning, hauling up for exsanguination and post-mortem examination.

Dog:

Increased knowledge about dog behaviour has aided in the design of dog facilities in recent years. Dogs are now generally group housed, on solid floors with inter-pen partitions for flexibility. Alternative facility designs to the traditional narrow gangway pens seem to have improved the animals' awareness of the environment around them and led to quieter, calmer dogs including increased use of transparent barriers and appropriate orientation of bars for improved visual acuity and multiple height benching. Outdoor space remains a contentious issue but is one worth discussing in the design phase in case it can be justified for the benefit of the dogs' welfare. If outdoor space is inappropriate, suitable internal play areas should be provided as well as veterinary and imaging facilities for sick animals and preventative care. Data capture technology for telemetered animals has advanced significantly in recent years and it is now possible to monitor individual animals within social groups. This requires specialist advice in the design phase of a new build. With the introduction of solid floors for animal welfare and shavings to absorb urine, there can be challenges with vacuum systems and drains clogging, so these require careful thought.

Cat:

The use of cats in research has declined in recent years. They have complex behavioural needs and require quiet facilities away from noisy areas and animals such as barking dogs which is a stressor to them as a prey species. For colonies, ensure there is suitable well designed space for co-existence including multiple, multilevel protected sleeping areas and perches to help to meet their behavioural needs as well as separate feeding stations, litter areas and scratching posts.

Rabbit, Guinea Pig and Ferret:

The physical facilities are often similar for these species, but they have different temperature requirements. Sufficient space should be provided for social groups, in floor pens where possible, pending study or gender need.

Rabbits are social animals, which are able to utilise a complex, three-dimensional environment. If given sufficient space, laboratory rabbits will exhibit the full range of behaviours seen in their wild ancestors, including standing on their hind legs, climbing up to a good vantage point, exploratory and tunnelling behaviour, and social activity. It is essential to provide sufficient space for the animals to perform these behaviours, to prevent boredom and skeletal problems. Cages should allow the rabbit to stretch out in at least one direction and be tall enough for the animal to stand and include a box or shelf they can sit on. Environmental enrichment can be provided by giving hay, chew sticks or cardboard boxes to play with. Rabbits should always be housed where they can see other rabbits. Solid floors with bedding are preferred: if grid floors are used, these should be carefully designed to allow urine and faeces to drain without predisposing to sore hocks. Trays beneath the grid should be lined with an absorbent pad, or high ammonia levels can trigger the development of respiratory disease. Low-intensity light should be provided for albino animals. Rabbits are sensitive to high pitched sounds, so care should be taken not to expose them to excessive ultrasound. Background noise can help to prevent the animals from being startled by sudden noises. Ventilation is particularly important for rabbits. Poor ventilation, allowing a build-up of ammonia, or low relative humidity levels predispose to respiratory diseases.

Ferrets spend up to 75% of the day asleep, but the remainder of the time will be very active. They are agile and like to explore and burrow, and they will make good use of three-dimensional environments containing playthings and multi-level perches. Housing for ferrets needs to be particularly secure. Their slender bodies and extreme flexibility allow them to exploit the smallest gaps, and they are notorious escapers which may have tragic consequences for both the ferret and any rodents or birds housed in adjacent areas. Ferrets like to sleep in dark, enclosed areas, need an area for food storage, and a latrine area within the enclosure so they can keep the rest of the cage clean, and they can be trained to use a litter box. Ferrets prefer solid floors with bedding such as sawdust or shavings rather than grid floors. Photoperiod can be important for ferrets, and installation of appropriate light monitoring systems could be important for assurance of correct photoperiod delivery.

Fish:

The major requirement for husbandry of aquatic species is keeping the water clean and aerated; otherwise animals are exposed to toxins from their own excreta. To achieve this, they should be either kept in static water systems at low stocking density and the water changed regularly or kept in circulating systems with biological filters to remove toxins. The water treatment systems required to maintain fish welfare can be very complex depending on species requirements. Salt and/or fresh water as well as cold water and tropical species may all be maintained in the same facility if supported by a centralised bespoke electronic water monitoring system which requires highly specialist input for successful facility design. Noise and vibration from the water system plant can be significant and must be located away from fish holding and experimental rooms to reduce impact on the animals and therefore quality of the science. Rooms for fish need a high-quality water source, a sink, a floor drain, a power supply, and must be able to support the weight of the tanks. All fittings need to be able to withstand high humidity and exposure to water. If circulating systems are used, back up pumps are advised in case of equipment failure. Tanks can be made from glass or plastic (latter may become scratched). Tanks should be kept on a dark surface away from light, and tubing carrying fresh and wastewater should be non-transparent, to minimise algal growth. Breeding of fish is often manipulated through the local light regime and monitoring/control features should be incorporated to the design of the plant to ensure the correct photoperiod is delivered. Many fishes are sensitive to visual stimuli, especially light, so handling in a dimly lit area may help lessen handling stress. Fish do well in dim light, and bright light encourages algal growth. The use of zebrafish is a growing research sector and contingency space planning for future growth of the unit may hold merit, including the capacity of water delivery system, tank washing and procedural areas.

Birds:

Birds constitute a very diverse group of animals and different species of birds have different requirements with regard to housing, husbandry and care. In general terms, housing for birds should be secure to prevent escapes or ingress of predators and must be large enough to allow the bird to stretch its wings fully and to exercise and fly. Some species like to rest on perches rather than the floor, so several perches at different heights can provide a suitable environment. The type of flooring used depends on the species and the need for hygiene. Dirt or gravel floors may allow birds to forage but solid floors may be more hygienic. Sloping floors may be a consideration for ease of cleaning in the case of long-term studies with relatively high stocking densities. Food can be scattered through bedding to allow birds to perform natural foraging behaviour. A secluded area in the cage gives the birds somewhere in which to feel safe. Some like to bathe in water, others in dust baths. The requirement and siting of nest boxes depends on the species. The light cycle is important since it can influence breeding performance and behaviour. Birds produce a lot of dust and dander, so good ventilation is vital to keep dust levels to a minimum.

16. What Has to Be Considered for the Refurbishment of an Older Facility?

Refurbishment of one older animal facility or consolidation of several facilities into one older existing facility can be successful but the following should be considered:

1. Reconfiguring an existing space can be expensive and may not deliver the agreed scope and constrain future research strategy.
2. Reconfiguring an existing space may not meet biosecurity or biosafety needs; the health status of the new facility will probably reflect historical health status which may or may not impact future scientific initiatives; the risk of laboratory animal allergy may increase through increased movement of animals out of contained areas or inability to fit appropriate protective equipment into the existing rooms.
3. Refurbishment may negatively impact the welfare of animals by the noise and vibration of building works if they remain nearby.
4. The cost and impact of the refurbishment works should be balanced against the extra longevity achieved and whether this meets the aims and scope of the original project.
5. A refurbishment of an ageing facility embedded in a larger building could be problematic if both areas share the same utilities. The failure of those utilities in the larger building could put animal welfare at risk.
6. Without a dedicated generator, a refurbished facility within a larger building is vulnerable to power outages elsewhere with significant risk to animal welfare.
7. Repairing some existing components of an animal facility instead of replacing with new could lead to subsequent failures once animals have re-populated the area, this could be very complicated to resolve due to biosecurity, contractor noise and dirt/dust.
8. Refurbishing an existing facility usually requires all animal work to cease or to be transferred elsewhere. Proposals to continue animal research during a building project is likely to impact scientific quality for all the reasons discussed previously. However, ceasing studies could impact research grants and researcher employment in some institutions; relocating work carries many of the complexities related to a new build unless there are pre-existing animal facilities elsewhere that could be brought up to required specification promptly to meet the criteria previously discussed, or, purpose built temporary accommodation can be imported in a timely fashion and sited in an appropriated location for research work to continue in a meaningful way (something which can be very costly and should be incorporated into the scope of the project if refurbishment is the main focus).

Surveying an old building before committing to a refurbishment programme provides a foundation on which to base the level of refurbishment required and balance the cost of this with the research need and the benefits of maintaining the existing location of the facility.

Stakeholder management is particularly crucial when refurbishing an existing multi-user facility due to the complexities of matching a programme of building works against the backdrop of ongoing animal research carried out by multiple different research groups, all needing different start/stop dates. If facilities are to be completely emptied for refurbishment, an achievable programme of building works and a clear re-opening date is paramount for research planning. This can create tension and impact not only research delivery, but animal wastage if unexpected building issues slip the completion date.

17. **Should Outsourcing the Animal Research Work Be Considered as an Alternative to a New or Refurbished Facility?**

An alternative option to self-investment is to close the animal facilities, repurpose them and outsource the animal work to a third party. This may have financial, compliance, risk and governance benefits for the institution but there may be other criteria to consider before making such a decision including:

- Impact on Institutional reputation depending on where the animal work is outsourced to
- Maintaining appropriate oversight of research activities and therefore scientific integrity

- Maintaining appropriate oversight of the welfare of the animals being used at a third party and the ethical implications
- Physical location and access for researchers, or clarity on the competency of those undertaking work on behalf of the original researchers and how this would be assured.

If, after all options have been exhausted, a decision may be made to postpone any animal facility changes and retain status quo. Although this may seem like a cheaper option, the exponential increase in cost of buildings maintenance of an ageing estate could outstrip the initial investment of any new build. Moreover, ongoing existing facilities need to be able to support changes in future scientific direction as technology evolves and older facility layouts may struggle to support this effectively. This may include:

- Fit for purpose holding and procedural areas including novel surgical areas required by changing research strategy
- Ability to accommodate new imaging modalities
- Ability to support increasingly genetically modified work
- Ability to support future work at different Biosafety containment levels
- Whether the existing facility is connected to another failing building which may need extensive work, the noise and vibration of which could negatively impact animal welfare and scientific delivery

If a buildings survey and risk review has not already been completed, this can be highly informative in identifying key areas that might need some focussed, prioritised work to ensure ongoing compliance and a facility capable of supporting a meaningful animal care and use programme.

18. How Can 'Lean' Thinking Be Introduced to an Existing or New Animal Facility?

'Lean' is a management methodology, first developed by Toyota in the 1940s to analyse and improve processes; to reduce operational waste and increase efficiencies. Lean is seen as a process improvement toolkit consisting of 5 phases: Define, Measure, Analyse, Improve and Control which is not dissimilar to other project management tools. Utilising Lean methodology in the animal research sector has the potential to lower operating costs, improve sustainability, increase capacity, and lower space requirements. Embracing Lean early in new animal facility discussions and applying it to existing facilities could help identify efficiencies that may influence programme requirements and decisions about whether to build new or refurbish animal facilities. In some cases, changing operational process may be sufficient.

A process-driven facility design overlaying the layout can show the distance people travel when performing tasks and reveal ways to minimise the time and motion required to complete the task [7]. More organised and productive workspaces can be created using Lean 5S methods to reduce 'waste', e.g. careful location of key pieces of equipment to reduce footfall, the removal of obsolete/unnecessary pieces of equipment to maximise space, the standardisation of equipment and processes to reduce cycle time. Using 'just in time 'thinking for food and consumables versus bulk delivery reduces storage space required for these supplies although careful consideration must be given to the minimal level of stockpiling required to safeguard the welfare of the animals in case of unexpected delivery failure. Cage processing can also utilise 'just in time' so that clean cages are prepared on demand instead of blocking expensive storage space to store clean cages for unnecessary periods of time.

Carrying out time and motion studies up front to identify key processes and ways to improve efficiency, e.g., appropriate space in cage washing areas either for robotics or for multiple technicians to reduce number of steps and therefore turnaround time. The evolution of Artificial Intelligence technology may play an important part in the design in animal facilities in the future, from flagging caging that requires cleaning or topping up of feed, managing inventory, optimising space utilisation and monitoring animal welfare. This has the potential to redirect staff resource to other key activities. However, the argument can be made that AI may struggle to replace the complex welfare assessment of an animal by expert technicians observing and handling their animals [8].

19. **What are the Basic Architectural Elements to Be Considered for the Build Design?**

Having discussed key concepts in any animal facility new build or refurbishment, here is a summary list of practical architectural elements;

1. Maintain a functional barrier:

    - Biosafety levels 1,2,3,4 as required.
    - Staff changing areas with appropriate shower facilities and PPE
    - Pass-throughs for incoming small supplies
    - Vaporised hydrogen peroxide (VHP) and autoclave for incoming equipment
    - Pressure gradients between rooms and corridors to protect either the animals or the staff.

2. Appropriate internal spaces:

    - Entry
    - Corridors
    - Quarantine
    - Cage wash
    - Appropriate ratio of holding and procedural areas
    - Euthanasia and necropsy
    - Laboratories/imaging, storage, etc.
    - Staff accommodation

3. Environmental parameters with appropriate monitoring, emergency alerts and back up mechanisms in case of failure:

    - Temperature
    - Humidity
    - Ventilation (mechanical air changes)
    - Lighting of sufficient lux within rooms to see but not negatively impact albino animals
    - Systems to provide different photoperiods plus/minus dawn and dusk
    - Reverse lit rooms with 'animal' appropriate red light, for staff
    - Noise levels
    - Generator back up with regular black starts to ensure functionality

4. Cage processing to protect staff health and safety and improve efficiency:

    - Robotic cage dumping and bedding up
    - Walk in cage/rack washers
    - Walk in autoclave
    - Automated bottle processing

5. Feed and bedding supply, efficient storage and waste removal including automation such as industrial vacuum systems, wild rodent control
6. Staff accommodation including workstations, toilets and rest areas
7. Security:

    - Location
    - Access
    - External barriers
    - IT system
    - Phone use
    - CCTV
    - Alarm systems

References

1. NC3Rs. Improving quality of science through better animal welfare: the NC3Rs strategy. Lab Anim. 2017;46(4):152–6. https://doi.org/10.1038/laban.1217.
2. Mellor DJ. Updating Animal Welfare Thinking: Moving beyond the "Five Freedoms" towards "A Life Worth Living". Animals. 2016;6(3):21. https://doi.org/10.3390/ani6030021.
3. Russell WMS, Burch RL (1959) The principles of humane experimental technique. Special Edition UFAW 1992.
4. Directive 2010/63/EU of the European Parliament and of the Council of 22 September 2010 on the protection of animals used for scientific purposes. Official Journal of the European Union, 276/33-276/79

5. CIOMS-ICLAS (2012) International guiding principles for biomedical research involving animals. https://iclas.org/cioms-iclas-international-guiding-principles-for-biomedical-research-involving-animals/
6. OIE - Terrestrial Animal Health Code Twenty-eighth edition, 2012 ISBN 978-92-95108-85-1 csat-vol 1.book (woah.org)
7. Lean Principles at Houston University, USA. https://www.tradelineinc.com/reports/2019-3/lean-principles-transform-design-and-operation-animal-research-facilities#:~:text=The%20University%20of%20Houston%20used,and%20leverage%20employees'%20full%20potential
8. Vivarium operational excellence network. https://www.voenetwork.com

Animal Facility Equipment

4

Patrick Hardy

Abstract

Laboratory animal facility equipment went through multiple and impressive technological and design evolutions marked by the availability of a larger range of options responding not only to animal welfare and 3Rs obligations, but also to the evolution of experimental needs and possibilities. Equipment selection and acquisition is obviously a major component of all animal facility projects and operational management, contributing in a major way both to better care and better science.

In addition to these core issues, any progress in the field must also address more recent requirements such as their multi-component environmental impact (linked to environmental and societal responsibility) and the ever-growing increase of related costs (capital and operational expenditures), which require a close attention to cost management and operational efficiency.

Finally, the quality system(s) of the institution (e.g.: GLP, AAALAC International, ISO), the research environment, and occupational health and safety requirements are also to be taken into consideration to ensure the adequate level of overall compliance.

This chapter reviews what categories and type of equipment should be considered for acquisition and use in an animal facility, not only for housing but also, more widely, for the overall management of the facility and the conduct of research projects. The purpose is not to get into details as species or research specificities are addressed in other chapters, but to share more general issues dealing with facility and equipment decision-making, project management as well as systems and equipment acquisition, installation, and use. These elements aim at providing support to facility design, renovation, and compliance (to regulations, quality standards, and applicable guidelines).

A more detailed attention is paid to topics which are not addressed in other chapters, such as safety-related issues and protective equipment, or validation/qualification processes applicable to animal facility equipment.

Keywords

Animal research · Caging & housing · Research equipment · Safety & containment · Washing & sanitization

P. Hardy (✉)
Veterinary Support Services, Finilios SAS, Paris, France

J. Guillén, V. Galligioni (eds.), *Practical Management of Research Animal Care and Use Programs*, Laboratory Animal Science and Medicine 3, https://doi.org/10.1007/978-3-031-65414-5_4

Acronyms

AAALAC	Association for the Assessment and Accreditation of Laboratory Animal Care
ABSL	Animal Biosafety Level
AK-KAB	Arbeitskreis Käfigaufbereitung—Working Group for Cage Processing
ANSI	American National Standards Institute (see NSF)
ASD	Airborne Surface Disinfection
ATP	Adenosine triphosphate
BMBL	Biosafety in Microbiological and Biomedical Laboratories
BMS	Building Management System
BSC	Biosafety Cabinet
BSL	Biosafety level
CDC	Center for Disease Control (USA)
CFU	Colony Forming Unit
CMR	Carcinogenic, Mutagenic and Reprotoxic agents
COVID-19	Coronavirus Disease 2019
DPTE	Double Porte pour Transfert Etanche (See RTP)
DQ	Design Qualification
EEC	European Economic Community
EMS	Environment Monitoring System
EN	European Norm
ETS	European Treaty Series
EU	European Union
GLP	Good Laboratory Practices
GMM	Genetically Modified Microorganism
GMO	Genetically Modified Organism
HEPA	High Efficiency Particulate Air [filter]
HVAC	Heating, ventilation, and air conditioning
ICH	International Committee for Harmonization
IQ	Installation Qualification
IVC	Individually Ventilated Cage
ISO	International Organization for Standardization
MQ	Maintenance Qualification
MRI	Magnetic Resonance Imaging
NF	Norme Française
NIH	National Institute for Health (USA)
NMR	Nuclear Magnetic Resonance
NRC	National Research Council (USA)
NSF/ANSI	National Sanitation Foundation/American National Standards Institute
OECD	Organization for Economic Co-operation and Development
OHS	Occupational Health and Safety
OQ	Operational Qualification
PAPR	Powered Air Purifying Respirator
PET	Positron Emission Tomography
PPE	Personnel Protective Equipment
PQ	Performance Qualification
qPCR	Quantitative Polymerase Chain Reaction
RFID	Radio-Frequency Identification
RLU	Relative Light Unit
RTP	Rapid Transfer Port (see DPTE)
SPECT	Single Photon Emission Computed Tomography
SPF	Specific Pathogen Free
SOPF	Specific and Opportunistic Pathogen Free
TOC	Total Organic Carbon
URS	User Requirement Specifications
UV	Ultraviolet
VHP	Vaporized Hydrogen Peroxide
VP	Validation Plan
WHO	World Health Organization

4.1 Definition and Scope of Animal Facility Project with Regard to Equipment

4.1.1 What Kind of Animal Facility Projects Are Concerned?

All animal facilities, whatever the scope of activity: model creation, breeding, housing, all research, or other scientific uses, as well as the overall technical requirements and management resources. Several regulations, guidance, and reference document are applicable in research animal facilities. Ensuring a strict implementation of animal protection and welfare is one of the several critical requirements [1–4].

4.1.2 What Are the Categories of Equipment to Be Considered?

Any equipment or material resource that might be useful to consider ensuring the success of a project, for housing, care, and use of animals as well as for all support areas and activities.

4.1.3 How and When Should the Equipment Requirements Be Addressed?

As early as possible, from the initiation of the project, when the project group is appointed, when the equipment to be used is defined, especially if it requires specific and sometimes demanding installation fittings.

4.1.4 For a New Building or a Building Renovation, What Are the Key Players in Equipment-Related Project Management?

It is important to benefit from the contribution of a team representing all competences: project management, building construction/renovation, future users from research teams and animal facility key persons. The list includes the project sponsor, the contract administrator, the project manager, the future facility manager, the construction superintendent, the architect, contractors and subcontractors, specialized engineers in all relevant fields, the health and safety manager (and/or any other institutional officer appointed to deal with specific risks), experienced user representatives from the research and animal facility teams and if necessary external consultant(s).

Material and equipment key suppliers may also be invited to participate. All these stakeholders are involved as needed, depending on the project meeting nature and agenda.

Regulations related to occupational health and safety are another set of references which must be strictly implemented, both for general requirements [5–7] and for specific risks and work environment [8–14].

In GLP-compliant facilities, the Quality Assurance department must also be represented to ensure the implementation of Quality regulatory standards, such as Good Laboratory Practice [15–17].

4.1.5 Are Recent Evolutions Worth to Be Mentioned in Animal Facility Project Management, and in Equipment Selection?

Due to societal pressure, sensitive evolutions emerged about sustainability in European Union legislation (Directive 2014/25/EU) [18] and in societal pressure towards sustainable procurement, including the requirement to assess the whole life cycle of equipment, from manufacturing to disposal through running impacts on environment. Some administrations already included this requirement in their bidding process. Furthermore, there is a strong synergy between environmental impact and running cost, especially the ever-growing cost of energy and greenhouse effect of gas emissions (calculation of CO_2 equivalence). A very clear example is the use of an autoclave, an equipment originally designed for sterilization, for routine caging equipment disinfection, requiring a very high level of energy (for steam production) and volume of water (for steam production and for chamber cooling).

In a similar way to 3Rs implementation for animal use in research, biomedical R&D community is expected to assess the harm/benefit of research projects vs their environmental impact: can we justify the environmental impact of a project with regard to its cost in human or animal life or suffering and provide evidence that a research program on a disease is not more detrimental than the disease?

In the field of sustainability, FELASA issued a communication *"Reduce–Reuse–Recycle"* [19] addressing the intensive use of plastic sent for recycling after a single experiment. Other examples/issues mentioned are the use of deep freezers (−80 °C) when warmer temperatures could be used (−60 °C to −70 °C), saving a third of energy consumption, or the high greenhouse effect of anesthetics. Accreditation schemes and policies were set up to reduce environmental impact. Designing a new facility and deciding on solutions for heating, ventilation, and air conditioning (HVAC), disinfection and sterilization, energy and water use reduction became major issues.

4.1.6 What Does "URS" Mean and Why Is It So Important Before Equipment Acquisition?

"URS" stands for "User Requirements Specifications". It includes the technical requirements describing the operational needs, drafted by end-users in collaboration with occupational health and safety (OHS) and Quality Assurance representatives. URS allow completing regulatory and safety requirements and are usually used for later steps such as Installation Qualification (IQ), Operational Qualification (OQ), and Performance Qualification (PQ), or User Acceptance Testing. They can be combined with functional requirements and include commercial terms including shipping, installation, and commissioning.

Properly written URS help the suppliers to fully understand the final user's requirements and to design equipment or systems that entirely fulfill user needs and expectations. The absence of URS can lead to miscommunication or create confusion between parties, resulting in wasting time and resources. URS are also used to initiate the tender process to purchase new equipment and should mention what is mandatory *vs*. "nice to have".

4.2 Quality Processes Applicable to Installations and Equipment

4.2.1 What Is the Difference Between Validation and Qualification?

Validation and qualification are essential components of the same concept, with a common objective, i.e. demonstrating through documentary evidence that a procedure, a process, or an activity achieves and maintains the desired level of compliance and quality at all stages.

The term qualification is normally used for equipment, utilities, and systems, and the term validation is rather used for processes. In this sense, qualification is part of validation.

4.2.2 About Validation, What Are the Key Components of the Quality Process When Dealing with Installations or Equipment?

In Quality management, the concept of Validation Plans (VP) defines the scope and goals of a validation project for a single project or a piece of equipment. It is sometimes written concurrently with the URS and includes the deliverables to be generated during the validation process, the acceptance criteria demonstrating that the system or equipment meets all defined and compliance requirements. Validation plans are the rule in GLP-compliant and biocontainment facilities but are recommended for any animal facility project relying on critical equipment use, e.g., to ensure adequate cleaning, disinfection, or sterilization related to autoclaves, washers, washer-disinfectors, airborne surface disinfection devices, etc. As an example, AAALAC International recommends a regular evaluation of equipment, which is applicable to washer. Good practices in the field include examination of key mechanical components to ensure that they are functioning appropriately, and that the equipment is exposed to the desired conditions (e.g., temperature level and plateau, product concentration, pressure).

4.2.3 What Is an Equipment Validation Plan (VP) and What Is the Process?

A Validation Plan includes Design Qualification (DQ), Installation Qualification (IQ), Operational

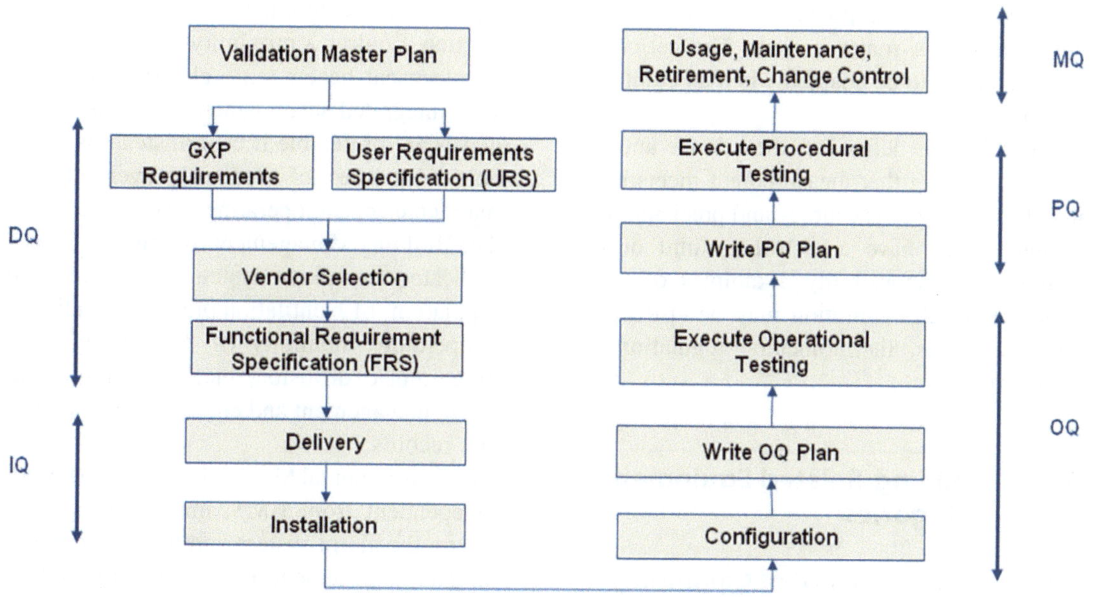

Fig. 4.1 Steps usually included in a comprehensive Validation Plan—Design Qualification (DQ), Installation Qualification (IQ), Operational Qualification (OQ), Performance Qualification (PQ), and Maintenance Qualification (MQ)

Qualification (OQ), Performance Qualification (PQ), and Maintenance Qualification (MQ) (Fig. 4.1).

- DQ verifies that the design deliverables are consistent with the URS and the expected use and performance of the equipment.
- IQ verifies that it has been installed and configured (installation checklist).
- OQ verifies, through a series of tests the proper functioning, as defined in the Functional Requirements Specification.
- IQ and OQ are generally conducted by the equipment supplier.
- PQ is the final step of qualifying equipment, generally conducted by the end user (or a subcontractor). It aims at verifying, through appropriate testing and the use of adequate indicators, that the equipment achieves all performance requirements for functionality and safety and that procedures are effective and reproducible, as defined in the URS.
- PQ generally relies on the use of appropriate indicators, allowing to objectively demonstrate the efficacy of the process, e.g. chemical indicators, thermal indicators, and biological indicators. To illustrate the selection and use of indicators, a publication listed in references describes the PQ of a washer-disinfector in a research animal facility.
- MQ reviews the adequacy of the maintenance process to ensure the system/equipment integrity, with no adverse effect on safety and performance, and allowing to maintain a validated state.

4.2.4 What Is Meant by Calibration of an Instrument and By Metrology?

Instrument calibration is one of the primary processes used to verify and maintain measuring instrument accuracy through testing and/or restoring its accuracy by comparing it with an established standard, with the aim to ensure that it is operating safely and efficiently.

Calibration schedule/periodicity is based on the application and manufacturer's recommendations and is generally anticipated when an equipment experiences a potentially harmful event, before and after major project. The periodicity may also have to be adapted when an equipment gets older.

Metrology is defined as the science and process of ensuring that measurement meets specified degrees of both accuracy and precision. GLP establishments have a metrology unit or outsource that responsibility. Examples of equipment for which calibration may be critical are: pipettes, scales, thermometers, regulation and alarm probes.

4.3 Building-Related Equipment Categories

4.3.1 What Is the List of Commonly Used Heavy, Fixed, or Building Integrated Equipment?

4.3.1.1 At Site and/or Facility Level

- At barrier level specific equipment could be required, such as air showers, air locks, chemical locks, interlocked pass-box(es), autoclaves …, allowing the transfer in/out of various small items (laboratory supplies, test compounds, documents, biological samples …).
- Chemicals locks are generally used with an ASD (airborne surface disinfection) system, which may by fixed/integrated or mobile.
- The HVAC system also includes air filtration (for supply and exhaust) at the appropriate level (HEPA or at least opacimetric filtration) and is associated with supply and exhaust air ducts, and all regulating valves (rooms, corridors, and airlocks), including local redundancies options in case of power or ventilator outage.
- Water heaters: Sometimes hot or warm water must be produced for the animal facility use (heating or pre-heating), relying on gas (from a tank or city gas) or electricity.
- If required, a central site steam production unit and network may have to be used for autoclave/washer steam supply, water, and/or HVAC heating (utility steam or clean steam depending on the application). With some equipment, the absence of central steam production requires a proximity production with an electrical heater (e.g., electric autoclaves with integrated steam generator). Steam autoclaves are preferable if central steam is available, because of reduced cycle times, maintenance, and operating costs.
- The Building Management System (BMS) is a dedicated computer system controlling the regulation of ventilation/pressure gradients, temperature, humidity (if regulated), lightning, music diffusion, etc., with integrated alarm management and environmental parameter records.
- An Environmental Monitoring System (EMS), independent from BMS, may be needed to secure the alarm system and the environmental data management. Further to alarm redundancy, it allows maintaining the permanent qualification status of EMS, with the purpose to ensure GLP compliance (a BMS system undergoes too frequent interventions to maintain a permanent validated status).
- An emergency power supply station (shared on-site or animal facility dedicated) ensuring permanent power supply, at least to listed critical equipment.
- Internal communication and computer systems: Wired, Wi-Fi, and Bluetooth local networks for all required applications and connections within the animal facility: e-mails, equipment alarm reporting, lone-worker alarm, laboratory animal management system, experimental data acquisition system(s), access control, and security system.
- Electricity supply, with all suitable voltages.
- Water treatment and distribution for all required uses, with suitable treatment and quality: Drinking water, steam production/autoclave, washing equipment, laboratory devices, i.e. demineralized, deionized, pre-filtered, micro or ultra-filtrated, UV-treated, reverse osmosis …

4.3.1.2 For Agriculture Species

- Agriculture species with conventional health status in standard conditions are commonly housed in enclosures with at least a limited surface percentage of slatted flooring, built over a manure pit system. As an alternative, ruminant facilities may have to be equipped with a manure scraping system. Both scraping and manure pit systems require highly specific indoor and outdoor building design and fittings.

- For pig breeding, maternity rooms require special temperatures, relying either on heating ground areas, pads, or lamps.
- Avian facilities with breeding activities may require installing incubators, hatchers, and post-hatching brooders or rooms/caging systems with heating lamps.

4.3.1.3 For Aquatic Species

- Most fish water systems used in biomedical research are recirculating-type, adapted to high-density fish tanks capacity. Tank water biofiltration, treatment, and quality monitoring require a dedicated room and equipment, allowing to produce the suitable water quality to supply fish tanks (temperature, pH, alkalinity, removal of fish waste products, hardness, UV disinfection, salinity if required, etc.).
- An upstream water treatment may be required depending on the origin of the water and the need to process, e.g., by reverse osmosis.
- The aquatic breeding of research area must be fitted with water piping system (in and out flow) allowing to connect all fish tanks and rack to the water treatment and monitoring system.
- A washing room should be dedicated to the fish area, with all adequate fittings and tank washing equipment, e.g. a dedicated washer.

4.3.1.4 Other General Technical Equipment

- Fire detection system and sprinkling system if required.
- Storage and distribution of CO_2, liquid nitrogen, and other gases.
- Storage of hazardous supplies (infectious material, inflammable, toxic or volatile chemicals, radioactive reagents …) is submitted to specific regulations that include adequate equipment (fire-proof of ventilated cabinets, spill containment tanks, restricted access room, defined room or cabinet ventilation …), all decided in close collaboration with the OHS department.
- Central vacuum pump and lines with connections available at required locations.
- Laboratory grade air compressor may be required: either a large/centralized unit (with pipes and point of use accessories) or small/mobile air compressor(s). In animal facilities, this equipment should be silent, contaminant free and vibration free.
- Central automatic watering station, with selected options for filtration, water treatment, capacity, distribution.
- Heavy load handling equipment in logistic and storage area: e.g., big-bag handling, with railing system, forklift.

4.3.1.5 Washing Area

- Washing equipment must cover qualitative and quantitative needs for rack-washing, cage and bottle washing.
- Bottle and cage parts washing may be fully automated, semi-automated, or manual, depending on the size of the operation.
- Robots can be selected and programmed for caging components handling, at one or several steps, from dirty bedding collection to cage filling with clean bedding.
- Soiled bedding can be eliminated through a central vacuum or augur system from dirty washing area to external container(s).
- A central system can be installed for clean bedding handling and distribution (from storage area to washing area), with the addition of a cage filling unit.

4.3.1.6 Waste Management

- Waste management requires to define specific flows according to the nature and level of risk, as well as suitable storage conditions before collection by dedicated service companies.
- Special equipment or room conditions may be required (infectious material containers, radioactivity decay room, inflammable or toxic chemicals or fumes, fire-proof of ventilated cabinets, spill containment tanks, suitable room or cabinet ventilation, etc.) in close collaboration with the OHS department.

- Depending on the size of the operation, an effluent treatment plant (generally managed at site level) may be required before release in the sewer system.
- Large volumes of effluents, even with a site waste station, may require concluding an agreement with the local sewer treatment plant.

4.3.1.7 What Kind of Building/Technical Requirements Are Prerequisites to Equipment Acquisition, Installation, Especially If Heavy or Bulky?

- Access (to site and building) for delivery may require the access and circulation of heavy trucks and lifting cranes/equipment, with sufficient maneuvering area.
- Large doors or dismountable panel(s) in wall opening(s), allowing the introduction/replacement of bulky/heavy equipment or parts, to/from their installation place.
- At sensitive locations such as barriers for SPF areas or biosafety level (BSL)-3 units, possibility to mount an airtight partition after installing the "barrier" equipment (e.g., in BSL-3 units, the sealing of double-door/pass-through autoclaves allowing airtight separation between the hazardous and safe sides at secondary containment level). Partition sealing relies on a flexible component designed to maintain barrier integrity with pressure differential and temperature variations.
- For washers, autoclaves, chemical locks, airlocks ..., equipment size/capacity is determined based on throughput prevision prevision, considering factors such as load capacity and cycle duration.
- Redundancy could be a critical operational issue with washers or autoclaves to allow maintaining operations during periodic maintenance and other outage situation.
- Some equipment such as large autoclaves may be both very bulky and heavy. Further to identifying path dimensions for installation/replacement from the loading dock to the final location, weight should also be taken into consideration, both for the final location and the installation/replacement path, considering that units may have to undergo periodic hydrostatic testing, with the chamber filled with water. They may also require specific floor depth considerations.
- Adequate access and space must be provided for service activities/maintenance tasks on large pieces of equipment, with access outside of the SPF barrier area or the BSL-3 secondary containment.

4.4 Rooms and Equipment Non-related to Housing/Caging

4.4.1 What Are Examples of Common Laboratory and Support Room Equipment?

- Refrigerators/cold rooms (from 1 to 10 °C), freezers/deep freezers (below −18 °C, as low as −40 °C), ultra-low temperature deep freezers (−60 to −86 °C), cryo-freezing tanks (with cryogenic liquids, e.g. liquid nitrogen at −196 °C), for various purposes and all suitable volume storage (including for animal carcasses storage before elimination). Depending on the use and context of use, some of these units may have to be connected for temperature monitoring and alarm reporting.
- Laboratory ovens or Incubators dedicated to various purposes (research, health monitoring bacteriology, water and environment monitoring bacteriology, process qualification…), refrigerators and freezers (at different ranges of temperature).
- Centrifuges (low or high speed, floor standing or benchtop).
- Scales/balances of different types for specific purposes (weighing small and larger animals, measuring feed consumption, analytical balances to prepare substances to be administered, balancing the weight of centrifuge tube holders/buckets), all with the suitable weight range and accuracy level. Some may have to be periodically calibrated.

4.4.1.1 What Is Required for Surgery?

- Surgical procedures are very common in research facilities, ranging from minor or superficial acts (subcutaneous implants, osmotic pumps, catheters …) to invasive surgery (such as thoracic, abdominal, orthopedic, brain surgery).
- The surgery suite ventilation should benefit from HEPA filtrated air, with a sufficient level of air changes per hour to control air particle level and an adequate room temperature control. It should be easy to clean and disinfect and have a specific personnel access control.
- Availability of a dedicated washer and a sterilization autoclave is a must, each with a capacity adapted to the nature and the level of activities.
- Other pieces of equipment may be required, such as cold sterilization systems for temperature sensitive equipment (e.g., endoscopes).
- In the surgery room, the usual equipment for superficial surgery includes at least species-adapted tables (with warming system), room and surgical table lights, instrument trolleys, and volatile anesthesia equipment. For more invasive procedures and depending to the type of surgery, the list of equipment may also include cardiac and respiratory monitoring, patient temperature monitoring, radioscopic equipment, blood gas analysis, micro-surgery equipment, etc.
- Suitable trolleys could be necessary for animal transfers, for pre-surgery operations (hairs' clipping, skin preparation).

4.4.1.2 What Are Examples of Imaging Technology Usable in Research Animal Facilities?

- Several types of imaging technology can be used in research animal facilities. Some require complying with safety/OHS regulation, e.g. those relying on the use of radioactive tracers or ionizing radiations.
- Examples are:
- Magnetic resonance imaging (MRI) is based on the principles of nuclear magnetic resonance (NMR), MRI scanners use strong magnetic fields and radio waves to generate images of the organs in the body, especially of soft tissues. It does not involve X-rays or the use of ionizing radiation.
- Positron Emission Tomography scan (PET-scan) is an imaging technology revealing metabolic or biochemical function of tissues and organs, using positron emitting radioactive tracers (a micro-PET technology is usable with rodents).
- Scintigraphy or Single Photon Emission Computed Tomography (SPECT) uses radionucleotides tracers emitting gamma-ray detected by a dedicated camera.
- X-ray imaging (radiography and radioscopy with or without contrast agent use,) in 2 or 3 dimension (X-scanner/microcomputed tomography).
- Ultrasound echography, with or without Doppler.
- Bioluminescence (luciferase-based) uses photon detection by a dedicated camera in a black chamber.

4.4.1.3 What Are Other Equipment Categories Common in Research Animal Facilities?

- Telemetry equipment for rodents or larger species, with standard implants or "jacketed external telemetry" through Bluetooth communication and dedicated software.
- X-ray irradiator (generally self-shielded, benchtop, or a free-standing unit), for small rodent irradiation (creation of immune-compromised models).
- Neurosciences studies require highly specific equipment, such as behavioral mazes and video tracking cameras with dedicated software, that need to be implanted in a very quiet and standardized room macro-environment, avoiding nonsuitable external stimuli (sound, ultrasounds, vibrations, odors, light/vision …).

4.5 Equipment Categories Related to Housing/Caging

4.5.1 What Are the Main Categories of Housing and Caging Equipment for Small Rodents, and Their Gross Features?

- The selection of caging systems (for breeding, maintenance and during use) depends on several factors such as the species, the health standard, the nature of the animal model and its use …
- Cage categories are standard (open) cages, filter-top cages (with static ventilation), standard individually ventilated caging (IVC) systems (used in negative or positive pressure mode), negative or positive pressure sealed IVC systems (used, respectively, for biocontainment or gnotobiology).
- Open cages can be placed on racks and exposed to the room macro-environment or kept in a bioexclusion device such as isolators, with HEPA-filtered air in positive or negative pressure.
- Positive pressure isolators (with sealed chamber and HEPA filter air supply, built with flexible film or rigid or semi-rigid chamber) are used to keep and use SPF, SOPF or even gnotobiotic rodent models in stricter bioexclusion conditions. They also allow conducting aseptic hysterectomies, maintaining high values animal colonies, such as foundation colonies … The gnotobiology section addresses the use of positive pressure/bioexclusion isolators in a more detailed way.
- Negative pressure isolators (flexible film maintained by a frame, semi-rigid or rigids) are mainly used for quarantine use, e.g., to maintain rodents with an unknown, poorly specified or suspect health standard while implementing a suitable health screening program. The biohazard section also addresses the use of negative pressure/biocontainment isolators.
- For many years, ventilated cabinets are not used anymore for basic housing, but are sometimes still used to maintain a specific environment such as temperature for rodent post-surgery recovery, or reverse/special lighting conditions.
- The use of standard IVC systems is now a very common practice, for many reasons. They allow maintaining in the same secondary enclosure (a room or a set of rooms) multiple animal models used by different research groups, with different health standards (SPF or SOPF exclusion lists), benefiting from a double bioexclusion barrier (at the facility and at the cage level) against external sources of contamination. Their correct use slows down the spreading of a contamination before it is detected. They create a barrier between personnel and rodents allowing to exclude not only pathogens or undesirable agents potentially carried by personnel but also human commensal opportunistic agents. Further to the health management benefit, IVC systems reduce personnel exposure to allergen and dust, decrease the impact of macro-environmental interfering factor such as sound, ultrasound and, in some cases odors from neighbor cages (see sections on "facility-integrated ventilation" and "thimble use"). They also allow decreasing the bedding change, commonly from every week to every second week.
- Standard IVC systems versatility rely on a double ventilation (supply and exhaust, both with prefiltration and HEPA filtration) that allows using a rack either in positive pressure mode, or in negative pressure mode, depending on the rack ventilation option selected.
- The IVC rack double ventilation and air filtration units (supply and exhaust) are available at rack level (installed on rack top), as an independent mobile unit (on wheels) allowing the connection of a few racks, as a fixed unit (wall or ceiling mounted), also allowing the connection of a few racks. Another option, which must be anticipated at building design and construction phase, is to create a "facility integrated ventilation and filtration" with high-performance units, installed at an interstitial building level above the housing rooms.

- Whatever the ventilation option, air used to ventilate the IVC systems is always taken at room level (benefiting from macro-environment settings and monitoring).
- With rack or room mounted ventilation and filtration systems, exhaust air is rejected into the room. With a "facility integrated ventilation and filtration" or with a "thimble connection" system, exhaust air is collected directly in a building exhaust air duct, allowing to reduce cage originating odors, which presents a double benefit: working conditions for personnel and control of odor/pheromones interferences with rodents. Again, these options need to be discussed very early in the building design and construction process.
- Standard IVC caging system is available with various cage capacity, with single or double face racks.
- Some IVC systems can be used either with reusable or disposable cages (see the "disposable IVC cage section").
- Multiple other options are also available to meet user needs, related to: drinking water (automatic watering, water bottles, or water bags), cage top options (with bottle inside or outside the IVC cage), rack integrated health monitoring (particle collection system at rack exhaust for qPCR periodic screening, avoiding or minimizing the need for sentinel animals, and other operational drawbacks associated with other sampling methods for health monitoring), remote ventilation, temperature monitoring and alarm system.
- More common options also include RFID-based systems (Radio-Frequency Identification) using electromagnetic fields to automatically identify and track tags attached to cages, developed for rapid and reliable cage identification, location, and census.
- Other, more recent options were also developed, such as mouse intra-cage monitoring system, combining electronic sensors and a software to collect cage information such as animal activity or water leak detection.
- Some racks can also be adapted to use video camera monitoring systems.

4.5.2 What Are the Main Ventilation and Filtration-Related Differences Between Standard and Sealed IVC Systems?

- Standard IVC systems use a double ventilation, supply, and exhaust, each with a HEPA filtration. The control unit allows balancing the blower airflows to maintain the rack cages either in positive or negative pressure. For safety reasons and to maintain a high-pressure differential, sealed IVC system works either with supply blowing (for positive pressure mode) or exhaust blowing (for negative pressure mode) ventilation. Each blower unit consists of two parallel-mounted ventilators ensuring redundancy, benefits from battery power back-up. Of course, both supply and exhaust rack ventilation are fitted with prefiltration and HEPA filtration.
- Standard IVC systems are not fitted with sealed connections at cage and rack docking level, and their cage cover includes a static filter (ensuring a minimum cage passive ventilation in case of power failure or when a cage is undocked from the rack for long time). When a standard IVC cage is undocked from its rack, air movements from rack inlet and outlet continue from and to room air.
- Further to the HEPA air filtration at rack level, cages of sealed IVC systems are fitted with an intra-cage HEPA cartridge, placed either at cage air-supply (for positive pressure models, used for gnotobiology) or air-exhaust level (for negative pressure models, used for biocontainment). Some models can be fitted with a HEPA cartridge placed both at cage air-supply and air-exhaust levels. Such small HEPA filters are made of a PTFE (polytetrafluoroethylene, Teflon) filter, i.e. a thin media layer but with high capture efficacy surface filtration.
- In addition, on standard IVCs, when the water bottle is placed on the external face of the cage top, an opening allows the introduction of the sipper tube in the cage cover (standard IVC systems are available with different watering

solutions: bottles, pouches, or automatic watering), which is never the case with sealed IVC system. The cage airtightness is even reinforced between cage bottom and top parts (type of gasket and locking system).

- The rack and cage connections of sealed IVC systems are fitted with double gasket self-closing valves, cages are not fitted with a static filter and are fully airtight to maintain the intra-cage positive or negative pressure even when undocked from the rack.
- With these sealed systems, cages are not ventilated at all when undocked: working practices must be designed to include that critical constraint (maximum time of disconnection before reconnection or opening).

4.5.3 What Are the Equipment Options for Cage and Animal Handling with IVC Systems?

- With standard IVC systems, a few users consider that, with swift and cautious cage and animal handling and if room air quality is adequate, the cage change operations can be conducted on a simple clean table. Such a practice cannot be recommended, as it obviously represents a breach in the overall bioexclusion or biocontainment process.
- The most common way to open the cage, to handle its content and the animals is to use a "change" or "transfer" station, which is a workstation specifically designed for that purpose, with easy access and ergonomic handling under the protection of a vertical flow of HEPA-filtered air (matching ISO class 3 air quality), either for one single operator or for two face-to-face operators. Such workstations ensure animal and cage content protection as well as operator protection (against airborne particles, allergens …).
- Another option (mandatory for biocontainment and for gnotobiology) is to work in a BSC-II, which is designed and certified for primary biocontainment (standards NSF/ANSI 49, USA or EN 12469, Europe). When selecting a BSC-II for use with rodent caging and procedures, it is critical to pay attention at least to two important features: (i) the front opening should be high enough to allow easy cage introduction and cage/animal handling (see BSC-II section) and (ii) the dimensions of the work surface should be sufficient to allow separating the clean, working, and contaminated areas, especially for use in gnotobiology or biocontainment. The BSC-II option provides the most reliable combined protection of the operator and the cage/animals.

4.5.4 What Are Disposable Rodent Cages and What Are Examples of Uses?

- Disposable IVC cages, developed for use in IVC racks are made of recyclable plastic such as PET and, for some parts, polypropylene. Metallic parts, e.g., in aluminum or, reusable, in stainless steel can also be used. Cages are using disposable water bottles that may be bought loaded pre-filled (micro-filtrated water, use of reverse osmosis …)
- Cages preloaded with bedding can be disinfected by radiation and bought ready to use.
- Before the COVID-19 pandemic, some facility managers decided to use exclusively disposable cages, to avoid capital and operational expenditures related to washing and disinfection and claiming the environmental benefit of this option. Most had to change their mind due to supplier stock shortage and sky-rocketing costs, as well as cost related to waste management.
- Examples of rational use of disposable IVC cages are for rodent quarantine units, allowing to avoid any cross-contamination risk at washing area level, for studies with radionuclide marked compounds, making it possible sending cages to decay storage and destruction, or in ABSL-2 units with limited autoclave capacity …

4.5.5 What Kind of Housing and Caging Equipment Can Be Used for Guinea Pigs, Rabbits, and Ferrets?

- These species can be maintained either on bedding or perforated floors (with holes diameter adapted to the species and animal size). Some recently available slatted plastic floors are particularly well designed and finished and may also be a good option when operational constraints support this option (bedding use is always the best options for animal welfare, but for large facilities, sanitation issues may become dominant).
- As a key rule, any housing option and equipment should be comprehensively tested over a sufficient time and in real conditions before purchase.
- For rabbits and guinea pigs, pen group housing on bedding is promoted as the best animal welfare option. However, rabbit adult behavioral characteristics must be considered, mainly but not exclusively for males. Consequently, structural enrichment is a very important component of pen group housing.
- When pens cannot be used for a valid and documented reason, group or pair caging may be an alternative addressing behavior or scientific use issues, after review and approval of the Animal Welfare Body.
- Usually, perforated or suitable slatted plastic floor cages are positioned on racks over individual cage trays allowing to collect feces and urine manually.
- For large rabbit units, such as breeding colonies, the cages can be fitted on racks equipped with a single waste tray with automatic scrapers, a slope, and a water flush system, pushing urine and feces towards a collector and a drain. This option requires a suitable building design.
- Provision of drinking water is either with water bottles or with an automatic watering system, requesting central water treatment and circulation, a facility water duct system, peripheral flow control and, at room level, a flushing device, as well as equipment of all racks with water distribution and water.
- Ferret is not a widely used species in research. For this reason, if pens are not used, ferret caging systems are often created using rabbit housing systems as a basis, then adding various fittings to adapt them to use with ferrets (structural enrichment, feed and water distribution, cage locking system …).

4.5.6 What Kind of Housing and Caging Equipment Can Be Used for Larger Animals?

- Frequently, for several reasons (including regulatory housing standards and health management issues), agriculture equipment is not appropriate in research facilities, and tailored solutions must be used.
- As for rabbits and guinea pigs, a gold rule is that any new housing option, equipment, fittings, and accessories should be comprehensively tested over a sufficient time and in real conditions before purchase.
- Some enclosure systems are designed to provide a maximum versatility and modularity, e.g. allowing to house two species (such as mini-pigs or dogs, pigs or small ruminants) and/or different size/weight ranges. This objective requires special attention to ensure meeting not only surface requirements through adequate pen modularity and partition design, but also suitable species-specific solutions for feeder, watering system, pen cleaning, rest areas, structural enrichment, etc.
- Also see the section addressing "building design" for agriculture species.
- Examples of common materials used for larger animal enclosures construction are:
  - Stainless steel (widely used to build enclosures structures as well as for drinking water piping and nipples, bowls, for feeders, or other parts, screws …). For animal housing or caging, grade 304 is used as the minimum standard and grade 316 is often preferred because of its much higher resistance to corrosion.

- High-Pressure compact Laminate (HPL) panels, are made in a material resistant to shocks, gnawing, humidity, not only usable for animal enclosures but also for showers, lockers, wall cladding, bench tops …
- Polypropylene panels, a cost-effective, highly durable, water resistant, and flexible material, widely used for its ability to resist impacts and corrosive chemicals, for its versatility in a variety of applications, as well as its resistance to acids and other chemicals.
- Tempered glass panels, made of a type of safety glass with increased strength. If broken, it shatters into small granular chunks, less likely to cause injury.

4.5.7 What Kind of Housing and Caging Equipment Can Be Used for Fishes (Zebrafish) or Amphibians?

- See "heavy, fixed or building integrated equipment" section for area design and equipment.
- This section purposefully mentions only zebrafish and Xenopus, but other fish or amphibian species are used in research, such as the medaka and the killifish, but also larger species such as the rainbow trout, which requests a specific and very different vivarium facility.
- Complete zebrafish tank sets are commercially available for housing or breeding: single- or double-sided racks with shelves dimensioned for various tank capacities, with a housing capacity and configuration adapted to requirements.
- Tank sets, shelves, and accessories are also available for Xenopus housing.
- Central recirculating water treatment, filtration, UV disinfection, water quality monitoring and alarm notification systems, supplying multiple racks also commercially available and are mainly used.
- For small capacity research projects or for educational use, a stand-alone zebrafish housing rack could be the best option, when compared with the implantation of a central water treatment station.

4.6 Safety-Related Equipment

4.6.1 What Are the Different Hazard Categories Requiring Dedicated Units and Special Equipment for Animal Housing and/or Use, in Compliance with Applicable Needs, Regulations, and Guidelines?

4.6.1.1 Biological Hazards: Use of GMO, GMM, and Infectious Agents

European/national regulations and guidance for biosafety, related to the use of infectious agents and GMO/GMM require, all depending on a site- and protocol-specific risk analysis, the following:

- Implementing suitable biocontainment at primary level ("at the source," critical for protection of personnel with infectious hazard) and secondary level (protection of the environment), both with adequate physical barriers and associated practices.
- Requirements vary according to the class of risk (1–4), the nature of the agent and its expected use. They include waste management.
- With small animals (e.g., rodents, birds, ferrets), primary containment is easier to implement and relies on the use of biosafety cabinets (BSC) such as BSC-II and BSC-III and, for rodents, IVC caging systems (always in negative pressure, standard or sealed system depending on the risk analysis outcome). Class 2 agents might be used with standard IVC in negative pressure. The choice is based on regulatory requirements and the outcome of the risk assessment.
- Larger species require tailor-made isolators or other biocontainment caging systems. In BSL-3, EU directive 2000/54/EC (on the protection of workers from risks related to exposure to biological agents at work) [7] requires that infected material including any animal is to be handled in a registered safety cabinet or in other suitable primary containment systems. A risk assessment should determine the appro-

priate type of personal protective equipment to be utilized and a qualification process should demonstrate that it achieves the expected protection level.

- With very large species, such as ruminants, horses, adult pigs, usual primary containment equipment is not usable. The alternative is to rely on the use of high-level PPE's selected according to the outcome of a risk analysis by the biosafety committee according to applicable biosafety guidance. Examples are full protective gowning with garments, helmets, gloves, footwear, goggles, face protection devices, hooded coveralls, half-suit hood or full facepiece particulate respirator (PAPR for Powered Air Purifying Respirator, with HEPA filters) combined with a disposable hood, etc.
- As an example of solutions applicable for primary containment, two approaches are used in BSL-4 units, depending on the outcome of the risk analysis, addressing the species, the nature of biological hazard, and the conditions of use: either full manipulation of agents in BSC-III, or work in a "suit unit" where personnel permanently wear a positive pressure supplied air protective suit.
- When quarantine of animals received from a facility with non-reliable health standards is judged necessary, a biocontainment system is also used. Quarantine may be infrequent in some research facilities and outsourced or, e.g., in breeding facilities, routinely practiced. To minimize the risk of cross-contamination, a quarantine unit should be fully independent of the breeding and use barrier units, with separated flows, dedicated equipment and located as far as possible. The infectious agents motivating a quarantine may be considered or not as a biohazard for humans and other animal species and may not require working in compliance with biosafety regulations. If compliance is applicable, implementation of ABSL-2 or even ABSL-3 requirements will be necessary (e.g., with exotic wild animals or from unreliable origin, which are potential carriers of zoonotic agents).

4.6.1.2 Radiation Hazards (Sealed and Non-sealed Sources)

- Radioactive sealed sources or unsealed radioisotopes must be used in premises and working conditions compliant with applicable regulations and guidelines (including for waste storage and management), except for self-contained (i.e., fully self-shielded) X-ray equipment used with small animals.
- Otherwise, X-ray equipment is installed in a dedicated room with shielded walls, equipped with glass control window and shielded door(s).
- A dedicated working environment is also required with non-sealed sources such as radionuclides, frequently used with imaging techniques and radiolabeled compounds for drug metabolism and pharmacokinetic studies.
- Caging systems designed specifically for studies with radionuclides allow a suitable containment level and an easy pre-washing decontamination process. With rodents, single-use IVC caging systems are a very interesting option, as they simplify and secure the cleaning and sanitization operations.

4.6.1.3 Chemical Hazards

- Several categories of chemical hazards are commonly used in research animal facilities, with a potential impact on personnel and the environment. The first action is to list and document all hazardous chemicals expected to be used, before conducting a risk analysis for each type of use, allowing to define and implement prevention measures including the safety equipment needed.
- Solvents and flammable chemicals require appropriate storage cabinets in dedicated storage area, with suitable ventilation.
- Biocides, detergents, acids are kept over retention tanks of suitable capacity.
- Anoxic gases (carbon dioxide, nitrogen) are stored and used in sufficiently ventilated rooms, with leak detectors connected to an alarm system prohibiting access to the room at risk.

- Further to managing the risk of anoxia, cryogenic solids (dry-ice) or liquids (liquid nitrogen) required specific cryo-tanks or insulated containers, with appropriate handing.
- Regulations include specific provisions for carcinogenic, mutagenic, and reprotoxic agents (CMR) that require very strict conditions of use in studies. Such test substances (with the addition of "high pharmacological activity" compounds) are received, stored in locked cabinets, and used in laboratory equipped for chemical hazard handling, with chemical hood(s) or cytotoxic safety cabinet connected to air exhaust (hard-duct connection). When a double protection is required (not only personnel, but also the product sterility), a cytotoxic safety cabinet, with a design similar to BSC-II (see that section) can be used, with an "indirect" connection to air exhaust ("thimble" connection).
- Formalin (used as tissue fixative in histology) storage and use may require a ventilated chemical hood (for large volume distribution in smaller containers) and dedicated ventilated benches during necropsies and organ collection.
- Volatile anesthetics are expected to be used as far as possible in close circuit. Further to sufficient room ventilation, additional ventilation should be provided for all systems at bench level, either through a table purposefully designed with integrated air extraction, or through a fume extraction arm allowing a safe capture as close as possible to the source.

4.6.2 For Use of Biological Hazards, What Are the Equipment-Related Facility Requirements?

Depending on their biological hazard group (1–4) and their conditions of use (risk assessment), infectious agents must be used at the appropriate biocontainment level, BSL-1 to 4 for laboratories and BSL-1 to 4 for animal facilities.

- BSL-3 biocontainment level requires equipment and waste decontamination at secondary containment barrier level. At this level, thermal decontamination is the most reliable solution, when compared with chemical processes (which may be suitable for BSL-2 or ABSL-2). For solid waste removal, a double-door autoclave is required, with a suitable capacity and programs duly qualified (PQ: see validation and qualification section) with defined loads and in worst-case conditions (use of the "overkill" approach). For biologically contaminated liquids and effluents, small volume can be absorbed by solid waste (e.g., dirty bedding) but larger volumes generally require a pre-decontamination collection/storage followed by high-temperature decontamination, either with a batch or a continuous-flow technology. After thermal decontamination, effluents must generally be cooled down before release into a sewer system.
- In BSL-3 units, the double-door autoclave must be designed for decontamination. A standard or walk-in model can be selected depending on the operation. It must be adapted to the type of biological solid waste or equipment to be processed and to the type and volume of waste generated. In BSL-2 units, a decontamination autoclave must be available in the building. For walk-in equipment, safety of operators is also an important aspect. For example, AAALAC International has a very strict policy to ensure the safety of personnel entering "walk-in"/floor-level autoclaves or rack washers.
- Steam autoclaves and some washers use a central steam source; electric autoclaves and most washers produce steam with an integrated steam generator. Steam autoclaves are recommended to reduce cycle times, maintenance, and operating cost. Clean steam is generally not required.
- The washing area should be located outside the BSL unit, to allow processing decontaminated equipment and sharing it with non-contained areas.
- Chemical lock(s) must be available to introduce equipment and supplies. After any transfer into the secondary containment area, the empty lock(s) is disinfected with a validated process and qualified equipment of airborne surface disinfection, before reopening to the non-contaminated area.

4.6.3 What Are the Different Classes of Biosafety Cabinets (BSC) Usable for Animal Handling and Use? What Are Their Main Features?

4.6.3.1 Class I BSC (BSC-I)

The use of this BSC class is very limited as most have been replaced with BSC-II. A BSC-I provides personnel and environmental protection, but no "product" protection. BSC-I air movement is similar to a chemical fume hood, with the addition of a HEPA filter in the exhaust system to protect the room environment from bioaerosols. Unfiltered room air is drawn across the work surface, the inward airflow ensuring personnel protection by its air velocity level through the front opening. As with BSC-II, appropriate work practices are critical.

BSC-I are named "hard-ducted" when they are fitted with a direct and airtight connection the building exhaust system, which provides the negative pressure necessary to draw room air into the cabinet.

4.6.3.2 Class II BSC (BSC-II)

- BSC-II are widely used, as they provide personnel, environment, and "product" protection. There are different types (A1, A2, B1, B2, and C1), all with airflow drawn into the front grille of the cabinet, providing personnel protection. In addition, a downward laminar flow of HEPA-filtered air in the cabinet chamber provides product protection, by minimizing the chance of cross-contamination across the work surface. As BSC-II rely on laminar air movement to provide containment, personnel training is a critical requirement to avoid disruption of the air curtain by the operator while working.
- With types A1 and A2, cabinet exhaust air passes through a HEPA filtration, allowing air recirculation into the laboratory or to be discharged into a room exhaust duct via a canopy or "thimble" connection. It is also possible to exhaust the air from a Type A1 or A2 cabinet outside of the building. It must be done without altering the balance of the cabinet exhaust system.
- With types B1 and B2, air must be discharged to the outdoors via the room air exhaust duct, through a hard connection.
- With hard-ducted types B1 and B2, and with thimble-connected types A1 and A2, as air is directly exhausted and not recirculated, small quantities of volatile chemicals may be worked with in, after qualification of the installation. See the "thimble" section for more information.
- For all BSC-II types, an internal blower draws sufficient room air through the front grille to maintain a minimum required inflow velocity at the face opening of the cabinet. Air flows through a HEPA filter and supplies a particulate-free, laminar, unidirectional, airflow to the work area.

4.6.3.3 Class II BSC Type C1 (BSC-IIC)

- This C1 type is designed to have airflow characteristics of both type A2 and type B2 BSC-II.
- Depending on safety requirements, it may or may be hard-ducted or not to laboratory exhaust and may allow or not working with chemical hazards such as cytotoxic compounds, gas, hazardous particles, chemical vapors, or radionuclides. A risk analysis is required to identify the appropriate cabinet design to be used, based on the nature of the chemical compound and on the type of handling.
- It has two blowers, one for supply positioned above the supply HEPA filter (for the recirculation of air from the front grille and sides of the work area), and one for exhaust, located before the exhaust HEPA filter, drawing air from the center of the work area, and pushing it through the filter, discharging HEPA-filtered air either back into the laboratory, or into the room air exhaust system, or through a "thimble" or canopy connection.

4.6.3.4 Class III BSC (BSC-III)

- BSC-III design allows working with highly infectious microbiological agents and risky use conditions. It provides maximum protection for the environment and the worker and is particularly appropriate for BSL-4 biocontainment or BSL-3 work with highly resistant and/or airborne transmitted agents.

- It is an airtight enclosure with transparent walls or viewing windows. Flows are managed through double-door pass-through chamber(s) for decontamination. Both supply and exhaust air are HEPA filtered (two for exhaust air). They can also be fitted with a fully qualified RTP/DPTE transfer system (Rapid Transfer Port/Double Porte pour Transfert Etanche). Handling is exclusively allowed with arm-length gloves, attached in a gas-tight manner to glove ports with O-ring.

4.6.4 What Are Other Example of Small/Portable Equipment?

Some pieces of equipment have a double utility in environmental monitoring, to control both personnel work environment and animal housing conditions.

- Audiometer (measuring sound intensity in dB)
- Portable room gas/vapor detector used to measure hydrogen peroxide residues, level of CO_2, NH_3, and other gas/vapor to be monitored on site
- Lux light meter

4.7 Additional Information on Laminar Flow and Biosafety Cabinets

4.7.1 What Are Laminar Flow "Clean Benches" and Other Equipment Used with IVC Systems When Compared with BSC-I or BSC-II?

- Laboratory laminar flow clean benches are not biological safety cabinets. They exist in two varieties, with horizontal or vertical unidirectional HEPA-filtered air flow and discharge air across the work surface and towards the room and the user. They only provide product protection and no user protection for allergens, chemicals, biologicals. They should never be used (especially horizontal flow cabinets) when handling cell culture materials, drug formulations, potentially allergenic or infectious materials, as the worker will be exposed to the materials being manipulated on the clean bench.
- They can be used for certain clean activities, such as the dust-free assembly or packaging of sterile equipment or supplies.
- In rodent IVC caging rooms, "change" or "transfer" stations, with an ISO Class 3 vertical air flow, are widely used. They are specifically designed for cage and animal handling, when standard (not sealed) IVC cages are opened. They aim at providing a large work surface area with maximum allergen protection for personnel, with ergonomic working conditions while maintaining the animal health status (SPF or SOPF). Their double face opening also allows the collaboration of two operators, standing face to face. Their lighter weight allows moving them around IVC caging rooms. Some models benefit from an additional "outside of sash" air curtain for increased protection.
- Soiled bedding dump stations (working as a chemical hood, to capture soiled and allergenic particles) when emptying cages, and clean bedding dispensers (delivering a calibrated bedding volume) are other very common pieces of equipment used in rodent facilities.
- It is important to stress again on the fact that, even if the quality of design and performance of this IVC associated equipment allow protecting personnel and animals, they are not registered BSC-I or BSC-II cabinets.

4.7.2 What Are the Specificities of BSC-II and Laminar Clean Benches Designed for Cage and Animal Handling?

- A BSC-II can be built and certified NSF49 with two usual dimensions of frontal opening, either 254 mm H (standard BSC-II laboratory model) or 305 mm H (for use in animal facility, allowing comfortable introduction and handling of cages and animals, without disrupting the cabinet air flow). This higher opening dimension requires a variable speed blower, adjusted not only to increasing HEPA filter load but also to allow maintaining the required air output level and velocity. It is important to pay attention to the difference before ordering any BSC-II for use in an animal facility.

4.7.3 What Is a Thimble Connection (Usable with IVC Systems and BSC's)?

- A "thimble" connection is used with BSC-II type A1 or A2, or with an IVC rack that is ducted to the outside. It is located on an exhaust air duct, at room ceiling level, over the cabinet or IVC rack, allowing to collect and suck the air expelled from the cabinet or IVC rack into a duct that leads outside. A small opening must be maintained between the "thimble" and the cabinet's exhaust to enable room air to be drawn into the exhaust ducting system. The capacity of the exhaust system must be sufficient to capture both room air and the cabinet or IVC exhaust. The objective is to avoid affecting the performance of a thimble-connected BSC or IVC rack by fluctuations in the room airflow.
- A "thimble" connection should not need any room ventilation adjustments and the pressure in the room should remain nearly constant. To keep a controlled, constant, lowered pressure within the containment room, a damper control for the exhaust system is usually needed to enable the air flow through the thimble to be balanced with the exhaust capacity of the extractor fan placed at the end of the ducting.
- NSF/ANSI 49 Standard requires BSC-II types A1 or A2 cabinets with a canopy or "thimble" connection to be fitted with an audible and visible exhaust alarm to indicate when air flow is being returned to the room rather than being exhausted out. Annual certification of cabinets with these "thimble connections" must include alarm function certification.

4.7.4 What Are the Differences Between the European and the American Standards for BSC's?

The two standards, the European [11] and the American [12] are available. For BSC-II, they are basically identical: they both provide protection for the product, the operator, and the laboratory environment and they operate with the same principles, which include HEPA-filtered vertical down-flow and exhaust, inward airflow at the front opening, etc.

- The American standard describes different BSC-II designs (Class II type A1, A2, B1, and B2), while the European defines only general requirements for Class II cabinets.
- Despite some minor differences, BSC-II available on the European market conforming to the EU standard are virtually identical in terms of construction principles to American standard. Both standards provide an identical level of quality and safety, when they are used by trained personnel and operated according to manufacturer instructions.

4.8 Equipment for Gnotobiology Housing and Research

4.8.1 What Are the Different Model Categories Uses in Gnotobiology and What Kind of Environment and Facility Equipment Is Required?

- Gnotobiology is a scientific discipline that includes the creation, breeding, maintenance, and use of gnotoxenic animal models, i.e., characterized by a fully defined microbiota (at least for all known and detectable microorganisms) in order to study the multiple interactions between host organisms and their microbiota.

- Gnotoxenic animals, mainly but not exclusively rodent models, must be maintained in a strict bioexclusion system allowing to maintain the microbiota over the required time.
- The different categories of gnotoxenic microbiota are axenic/germ-free (the starting point also used to create all other categories), oligoxenic (a few bacteria), predefined/standard microbiota (10–12 bacteria, in "isobiotic" breeding colonies), extended microbiota (e.g., to study "bacterial cooperation"), and very complex microbiota (from animal or human donors by fecal microbiota transplantation, to study pathology interactions).
- It is important to keep in mind that gnotobiology requires access to a neighbor microbiology resources to create the microbiota to be used in research protocols and for regularly monitoring of the animal microbiota in breeding and experimental groups.
- Depending on the model category used, access to services of a specialized molecular technology laboratory may also be required. Complex microbiota analysis and comparisons require large memory and high-performance computing resources, which may be difficult to access.
- Whatever the bioexclusion system, it is highly recommended to dedicate room(s) to gnotobiology activities, with a restricted access and a very clean environment.
- For access and flow control reasons, some gnotobiology units are fully independent, i.e., benefit from their own washing room and equipment, and independent logistics.
- A gnotobiology unit cannot work without a sterilization autoclave of suitable capacity. Equipment and supplies are sterilized in transfer cylinder allowing steam penetration or in autoclave bag or wrapping. Note that the cages of the "sealed IVC systems" (see below) can also be autoclaved when docked to dedicated autoclave rack, which require a suitable autoclave chamber dimension. See the "biosafety" section for technical requirement" related to autoclaves.

4.8.2 What Kind of Equipment Is Available for Gnotobiotic Animal Housing and Handling?

- High-performance bioexclusion isolators, maintained in positive pressure with HEPA filtration (supply and exhaust) are the original equipment used to house animals while maintaining their defined microbiota. Flexible-film isolators are commonly used for rodents, but semi-rigid and rigid isolators are also used. Cages and animals can be handled with the isolator gloves, and the various transfers are managed through ports with aseptic procedures relying on autoclaved feed, water, caging/equipment, and supplies.
- "Cold sterilants" (commonly based on peracetic acid and/or hydrogen peroxide) are routinely used for chemical sterilization during transfers, which require to be validated in worst-case conditions.
- Different isolator designs can be used for housing, animal procedures, transfer and cold sterilization management, sterile storage, animal transfer and shipment …
- An alternative to isolators is the use "sealed IVC system" (operated only in positive pressure), specifically designed for gnotobiology. Many facilities use both systems in parallel. Sealed IVC system requires less room surface and allows managing several microbiotas in parallel, decreasing constraints related to the cage capacity of isolators and to study design. Animal procedures are also more easily conducted in a BSC-II that with isolator gloves.
- The conditions of use of "sealed IVC" are very different from isolators as the sealed cages must be opened in a sterile environment, without losing time during transfer (while disconnected from the rack, cages are not ventilated). The recommended solution is to use a BSC-II installed in the same room. Some use two of them, one for cage changes and another one for procedures. The BSC-II can be equipped with various lateral fittings such as a

RPT/DPTE door, a standard port connection and/or a transfer chamber for cage processing cages and supplies with cold sterilant.
- Dedicated containers are used for autoclaving supplies and equipment before introduction into isolators, or for transfers
- Isolators can be fitted with "standard ports" (cylinders with openings closed by airtight plastic caps or doors) of with a RTP/DPTE transfer system (Rapid Transfer Port/Double Porte pour Transfert Etanche). This type of transfer system is expensive, but allows major time saving.
- Isolator can be ventilated with their own ventilators or with a central system. In both cases, alarm and redundancies are critical.
- Cold sterilants can be used either by manual spraying (operator dependent) or with a dedicated automated vaporizing unit. Both options can be used in parallel, e.g. spraying for small volumes (isolator port) and use of an automated vaporizer for larger volumes (isolator, sealed IVC system …)
- Different transfer/shipping containers or systems can be used for animal transfer between isolators on site or between sites, depending on the distance and the duration of shipment: autonomous (battery powered) racks (for sealed IVC systems) or isolators, static ventilation isolators or containers … The selection of an option should be submitted to a risk analysis by the Animal Welfare Body.

4.9 Equipment for Washing and Support Areas

4.9.1 What Are the Most Common Types of Equipment Associated to Enclosures and Pen Sanitation?

- Animal facilities housing exclusively large species do not need large cage and rack washer capacity, but may use a washer for smaller items (feeders and feed preparation items, water bottles or bowls, enrichment, toys …).
- Fixed enclosures are sanitized manually with high and/or low-pressure equipment (mobile or centrally installed). High-pressure washing is effective with heavy soiling whereas low pressure may be required for less resistant surfaces, and when dosing and applying detergent foam or disinfectant with a foam lance. The same lance is used for rinsing.
- Depending on the nature and volume of equipment, washing areas of rodent and aquatic facilities are equipped with one or several washers, to ensure a washing capacity adapted to the weekly volume of cages or tank components, racks and other items.

4.9.2 Are Some Reference Documents Available in the Field of Equipment Processing (Washing, Disinfection …), Applicable to Animal Facilities?

Most reference documents have a general or different scope, such as those applicable to airborne disinfection [20] or washer-disinfectors [21]. Some are very specific to use in research animal facilities and address process efficacy [22, 23].

4.9.3 What Are the Washing Efficiency Parameters and the Different Types of Washers Usable with Rodent Caging Equipment?

Washing efficiency is the result of the combination of a chemical effect (detergent), a physical effect (water pressure), a temperature effect (high temperature), time of exposure of all these parameters, plus the quality/homogeneity of the load coverage during washing.

4.9.3.1 Rack Washers

- Rack washers are designed to wash a wide range of equipment of various sizes, including cage racks. Cage parts and other small items must be placed in specifically designed holding supports or baskets, allowing a suitable and homogenous exposure to washing.

- Rack washers are fitted with a single door or with interlocked double doors. They can be used with different programs.
- As they allow rolling-in large equipment, they require a floor pit for installation.
- Their large chamber capacity also allows high throughput for small items washing.
- Some models are designed and equipped for airborne disinfection with hydrogen peroxide (after chamber cooling) and/or thermal disinfection.
- Steam or electric water heating options are generally available.
- As for rolling-in/floor-level chamber autoclaves, rack washers require to be installed in a floor pit adjusted to suitable dimensions.

4.9.3.2 Cabinet Washers

- Their smaller chamber dimensions allow washing various sizes and types of caging, bottles, and miscellaneous small equipment but not racks. Their technical features and washing efficacy vary according to the model: cage capacity, number of tanks for washing/rinsing, washing temperature, water pressure, load coverage, chamber volume and loading versatility, equipment throughput level, loading ergonomics, washing and rinse programming possibilities …. Some have a high efficacy thermal disinfection option.
- They are available with single door or interlocked double doors, and either with steam or electric water heating.

4.9.3.3 Aquatic Cabinet Washers

- Their design is similar to rodent cage cabinet washers, but they are generally exclusively dedicated to aquatic equipment washing, with suitable technical features and programs, which allows avoiding any risk of chemical residues and removing algae and biofilm without any manual scrubbing or chemical pretreatment. Programs generally include multiple rinses, and a final one with reverse osmosis water.

4.9.3.4 Tunnel Washers

- They are generally custom-designed and built with dimensions adapted to the type and dimensions of equipment to wash (e.g., adjusting conveyer belt width and design, chamber height), to allow processing a wide variety of equipment types (e.g., caging parts, bottles, feeders, trays, nest boxes, enrichment items) with suitable programs.
- Design options also include different modules (tunnel sections): loading, pre-wash, wash, pre-rinse, rinse, drying (heated air), and unloading. Window and access doors on wash and rinse modules allow visual inspection and access by operators (with adequate safety fittings).
- Due to their level of output, they are generally used in facilities requiring high washing capacity needs. Water heating is also available with steam or electricity.

4.9.3.5 Bottle Washers

- They are available with single or double door (pass-through), or with a hood system, with variable technical features and washing efficacy, such as chamber capacity, washing temperature, water pressure, load coverage, and rinsing quality.
- Some sophisticated models are automated and able to manage bottle decapping and emptying, washing, rinsing, bottle refilling and recapping.

4.9.4 What Is a Washer-Disinfector? What Are Their Specific Features When Compared with Washers? What Means "A0"?

- Thermal disinfection with high-temperature water is an option available in some high-range washer models, particularly cabinet washers (due to the technical challenge related to rack washers chamber volume). It is based on the A0 concept (cf. EN ISO 15883-1), which was originally developed for disinfection of medical devices in hospitals. A0 is similar to the F0 concept used with autoclaves. It represents the number of seconds of exposure at 80 °C.

- Microorganisms inactivation performance is directly related to the A0 value. A0 = 600 can be reached with 660 s at 80 °C or 150 s at 84 °C. When exposing equipment 300 s at 85 °C, a A0 = 1500 is reached.
- Washer-disinfectors use thermal disinfection programs set in accordance with a time and temperature combination having a proven and suitable biocidal activity. As an example, an A0 value of 600 is specified for disinfection processes deployed against bacteria, including mycobacteria, fungi, and heat-sensitive viruses.
- With a cabinet washer-disinfector, thermal disinfection with high-temperature water is achieved after the washing phase and before the rinsing phase of the program. The process can be validated using temperature data loggers and biological indicators for the performance qualification. A performing washer-disinfector cabinet should be able to manage a disinfection phase with water temperature plateau around 85 °C for 300 s, allowing to each a A0 of 1500. To reach this performance level with rodent cages, a first water tank is dedicated to washing and fitted with a high-power pump, and the dosage of an appropriate detergent (e.g., a neutral pH detergent with rats and mouse caging), at a water temperature of 60–65°. A second water tank is hence dedicated to thermal disinfection. No detergent is used, and a lower pressure pump can be used if a homogeneous load water coverage is reached. The tank water heating system should allow reaching about 85 °C in a few minutes at load level. The time at the plateau temperature is the main contribution to the disinfection efficacy level. A third water tank must be exclusively used for rinsing. By contrast with the other higher volume washing and disinfection tanks, to avoid chemical residues, rinsing water is not recycled by returning to the tank, but is eliminated and renewed after each use. It is also heated at 81–85 °C. The rinsing time (around one minute) allows increasing the duration of the temperature plateau and increasing the overall A0 value of the program.

4.9.5 What Are the Different Uses and Types of Autoclaves? What Means "F0"?

- Steam sterilization or bio-decontamination in animal facilities and laboratories responds to defined specifications and requirements, depending on their intended use, which includes sterilization (of surgical instruments, glassware, culture media, caging, drinking water, porous loads as feed pellets and bedding …), thermal disinfection (of caging components, bedding and feed …), barrier decontamination (of equipment and waste leaving a biocontainment unit).
- The term "F0" is defined as the number of equivalent minutes of steam sterilization at 121 °C, recorded at load core level. For example, an autoclave cycle with a F0 value of 12 has a sterilization efficacy equal to 12 minutes at 121 °C, whatever the process temperature and the cycle time used in the program used.
- Sterilization requires specific packing or containers (cylinders) allowing steam penetration, both aiming at preserving sterility after autoclave opening and unloading.
- Sterilization and decontamination autoclaves do not have the same design as they must comply with specific efficacy requirements. Their performance qualification processes are different.
- BSL-3 barrier autoclaves must be fitted with interlocked double-door for pass-through use and installed with an airtight partition at barrier level.
- All types are available with various chamber and overall sizes, from benchtop small autoclaves, e.g., used for sterilization of surgical instruments, to large capacity units with single or double pass-through interlocked doors, roll-in/floor-level loading, as well as inter-

mediate capacity models with standard chambers ... Depending on the load and its heat resistance, different programs are required to allow adjusting temperature between 105 and 135 °C. In addition to temperature fixed probes of the chamber, it is also important to place probe(s) in the load core (e.g., with liquids, animal carcasses, large porous masses ...).

- Autoclaves, especially with large chamber dimensions, are very expensive to buy and to operate (heating for steam production) and use a lot of water (for steam production and chamber cooling). It is both important to ensure a sufficient autoclaving capacity and to avoid oversizing the capacity. In that context for equipment disinfection purposes, when feasible, using a washer-disinfector could be an interesting alternative. Similarly, a small dry-heat sterilizer may be sufficient for sterilization of a limited quantity of small heat resistant surgical instruments.
- The location and access to autoclave service cubicle by technical personnel is also important to define.
- Finally, both use for sterilization and for biohazard decontamination purposes require a robust performance qualification as well as inspectable records of use and maintenance, even if the performance qualification is different.

4.9.6 What Are the Available Robotic Solutions in Washing Area and the Operations Potentially Benefiting from Such Equipment?

- In facilities processing many items, robotic equipment can be used for IVC cage parts handling, allowing to benefit from an interesting throughput and manpower-related return on investment, as well as for ergonomics and work conditions (avoiding repetitive lifting and handling, tedious and repetitive work and, with soiled equipment, reducing exposure to allergens and other particles). The relevance of investing in robotic equipment requires site-specific studies based on multiple parameters.
- Robotic equipment can be pre-programmed for use with different caging items. Some large-scale facilities automated all repetitive material handling processes, at dirty and clean sides of the washing area (from cage soiled bedding emptying to cage stacking after clean bedding filling, through loading and loading washers).
- Each robot requires a defined floor surface, which includes its maneuvering area. For personnel safety reasons, that area must be delimited by a fence or a transparent panel prohibiting access during robot operation.

4.9.7 What Are the Available Options for Disinfection Locks/Chambers? What Kind of Airborne Surface Disinfection Equipment Can Be Used in Animal Facilities for Room and Enclosure Disinfection?

- Chemicals locks category includes various capacity chambers, used for high-efficiency airborne surface disinfection. The disinfectant used is generally hydrogen peroxide (high and wide range efficacy, leaving no residue), with two main diffusion system option (either integrated or independent). Two technologies are mainly used: VHP systems, which vaporize hydrogen peroxide (30–35% concentration), and dry-fogging systems, which generate micro-droplets (ca. 7.5% concentration) with different diffusion technical solutions.
- VHP and dry-fogging systems are also widely used for room and fixed enclosure disinfection.
- Different models are available, depending on the context the intended use and the volume to be disinfected. Whatever their use, all systems are supported by a process control and must be performance qualified for each type of application, in real and worst-case conditions, which require appropriate indicators (usually bacterial spore indicators, with an objective of 5 to 6 log reduction).

4.9.8 What Are Other Transfer Systems that Are Worth to Be Mentioned?

4.9.8.1 Small Volume Pass-Through Boxes

- This equipment category is used for small items transfers into or from a barrier area, often in "non-regulated situations," i.e., with no mandatory demonstration of disinfection or decontamination efficacy.
- They are available either for floor or wall installation.
- Depending on the design, they work as a passive/static chamber, or they may be designed to provide dynamic airflow.
- Some models can be equipped with UV lights or used with disinfectant spraying.
- All models should be equipped with an interlocking door system to avoid simultaneous door opening (and turning out UV lights before opening).
- It is advised to design and to use such small volume pass-through boxes according to the criticality of the transfer, and to set an expected performance level, and to assess it accordingly through a performance qualification. Homogenous UV light disinfection is practically difficult to achieve and to control as it depends on surface exposure time.

4.9.9 What Are the Main Types of "Indicators" Usable for Performance Qualification of Sterilization or Disinfection?

Amongst a wide choice of different indicators or data loggers' categories and models, three types are mainly used in animal research facility environment [23].

4.9.9.1 Chemical Indicators

They have two common applications:

(i) For autoclave sterilization, chemical indicator tape is fixed on each packing unit or each cylinder. A color change does not prove that the item is sterile but is useful to visualize that an item was were actually exposed to heat autoclave heat. It says nothing about what temperature was achieved internally, particularly a load core level.

(ii) For airborne surface disinfection with hydrogen peroxide, color strip indicators allow visualizing easily the homogenous vapor or mist diffusion in the volume to disinfect, including on remote spots. It does not mean that disinfection was achieved, but it is a very useful preliminary test.

4.9.9.2 Electronic Temperature Data Loggers

- They allow recording a temperature curve over a defined time. Using several of them, it is possible to establish a cold or warm chamber cartography or to record the temperature curves at multiple points in a load placed in an autoclave or in a washer-disinfector, and to collect data over the entire program duration [23].

4.9.9.3 Biological Indicators

- Various models are also available, allowing to demonstrate the impact of a sterilization or disinfection process on highly resistant or target microorganisms. They should always be used as the final demonstration of efficacy to validate a process or conduct a performance qualification. A common biological indicator is made of three stainless steel disks, inoculated each with a defined spore load of *Geobacillus stearothermophilus* (10^4, 10^5, and 10^6). The three disks are sealed in a Tyvek porous envelope. It is a very convenient indicator for exposure to a steam sterilization or a hydrogen peroxide vapor disinfection process. Each disk is then incubated in a culture media under defined growth conditions, to determine whether any spores survived the process. During a process validation or an equipment performance qualification, such indicators can be easily placed in different locations (in a room, in a chemical lock or autoclave or chemical chamber load …), always using the "worst case" approach.

4.9.10 What Are Examples of "Indicators" Usable for Performance Qualification of a Washer?

4.9.10.1 Washing Indicators

- The first solution is a comparative macroscopic examination before and after washing, taking pictures as records.
- It is also possible to use commercial "soil test" strips with different standard loads of a chemical mimicking different soil levels or to apply a "soil test solution" at different place of the equipment items.
- Another option is the use of contact Petri dishes before and after washing, to compare the number of CFU's (Colony Forming Units) after incubation, using media valid for environmental bacteria and yeast.
- An ATP (adenosine triphosphate) surface test measures the level of ATP on a surface, thus its cleanliness level as ATP is a molecule found in all living cells for transferring and storing energy. The presence of ATP on a surface indicates improper cleaning and the presence of organic soil (microorganisms, biofilm, food residues, and other biological residues). After surface swabbing, the swab from the test-kit is transferred into a solution where ATP reacts with luciferin and luciferase to produce a green-yellow light, measured by a portable luminometer in Relative Light Units (RLU). The higher the RLU number, the more contaminated the sample. RLU values can be calibrated with viable plate counts expressed in Colony Forming Units (CFU) per area of surface tested. After calibration a RLU value can be immediately converted into CFU, allowing a rapid cleanliness assessment.

4.9.10.2 Rinsing Indicators

The absence of residue after rinsing can be detected by mass spectrometry (if equipment available on site), total organic carbon (TOC) test, or (with alkaline and acid detergents) pH indicator strips for pH measurement of a volume of water used to rinse items, after the end of the washing process.

References

1. Directive 2010/63/EU on the protection of animals used for scientific purposes
2. European Convention ETS 123 for the Protection of Vertebrate Animals Used for Experimental and Other Scientific Purposes (Council of Europe" (ETS 123)" and its Appendix A (revised 2006) "guidelines for the accommodation and care of animals"
3. The Guide for the Care and Use of Laboratory Animals, NRC, 8th edition, 2011 (principal AAALAC accreditation standard)
4. The Guide for the Care and Use of Agricultural Animals in Research and Teaching, American Dairy Science Association, American Society of Animal Science, and Poultry Science Association, 4th edition, 2020
5. Council Directive 89/391/EEC of 12 June 1989 on the introduction of measures to encourage improvements in the safety and health of workers at work
6. Occupational Health and Safety in the Care and Use of Research Animals (NRC, 1997)
7. EU directive 2000/54/EC on the protection of workers from risks related to exposure to biological agents at work
8. WHO Laboratory Biosafety Manual, 4th edition (2020)
9. Biosafety in Microbiological and Biomedical Laboratories (BMBL), 6th edition, CDC, NIH (2020)
10. Canadian Biosafety Standards/Lignes Directrices Canadiennes sur la Biosécurité, 3rd edition, Public Health Agency of Canada/Agence de la Santé publique du Canada (2022)
11. European Standard EN 12469:2000 '- Biotechnology - Performance criteria for microbiological safety cabinets
12. American National Standard NSF/ANSI 49 - 2008 - Biosafety Cabinetry: Design, Construction, Performance, and Field Certification
13. Directive 2013/59/Euratom laying down basic safety standards for protection against the dangers arising from exposure to ionizing radiation
14. European regulation 528/2012 concerning the making available on the market and use of biocidal products
15. Directive 2004/10/EC of the European Parliament and of the Council of 11 February 2004 on the harmonization of laws, regulations and administrative provisions relating to the application of the principles of good laboratory practice and the verification of their applications for tests on chemical substances
16. OECD series on principles of Good Laboratory Practice and compliance monitoring, number 1 (revised 1997)
17. ICH (International Council for Harmonization of Technical Requirements for Pharmaceuticals for Human Use), ICH safety guidelines
18. Directive 2014/25/EU on procurement by entities operating in the water, energy, transport and postal services sectors

19. https://felasa.eu/about-us/library/3rs-reduce-reuse-recycle
20. NFT 72281 and EN 17272:2020 standards - Chemical disinfectants and antiseptics - Methods of airborne room disinfection by automated process - Determination of bactericidal, mycobactericidal, sporicidal, fungicidal, yeasticidal, virucidal and phagocidal activities
21. EN ISO 15883-1 - Washer-disinfectors – Part 1: General requirements, definitions and tests
22. AK-KAB (Working Group for Cage Processing), Cage Processing in Animal Facilities, 5th issue, 2016 / AK-KAB (Working Group for Cage Processing), Fisk Tank Processing in Animal Facilities, 1st issue, 2020
23. Mocho JP, et al. Assessment of microbial reduction by cage washing and thermal disinfection using quantitative biologic indicators for spores, viruses and vegetative bacteria. J Am Assoc Lab Anim Sci. 2021;60(5):529–38.

5 Animal Procurement and Transport: Connecting the Dots

Nicolas Dudoignon

Abstract

Transportation is a typically stressful experience for animals. Whether it is primarily between their breeding place and the facility they will be used at, or in the scope of an inter-institutional collaboration (see Chap. 19), or after being used in laboratories in order to reach a rehoming place, every animal used for scientific purpose is subject to transport in a way or another during its life. As the way animals are transported is often—not to say always—transparent for the researchers, this step may not be given the attention it deserves. However, transport, with all different aspects and the complexity in it, shall not be neglected as it does directly impact animals, from a welfare standpoint, and their ability to meet the standards required for scientific purposes, and humans, from a health and safety perspective. Addressing different considerations, this chapter seeks to illustrate that every transport may have a diversity of impacts on animals, that must all be anticipated and addressed to ensure animals will go through the journey in the best possible manner and remain fit for scientific purpose.

N. Dudoignon (✉)
Sanofi, Corporate Social Responsibility, Gentilly, France
e-mail: nicolas.dudoignon@sanofi.com

Keywords

Transport · Health and welfare · Safety · Security · Roles and responsibilities · Planning

5.1 What Are the Regulations and Standards on the Health and Welfare of Animals During Transport?

5.1.1 Are There Specific and Overarching Regulations that Apply to the Transport of Research Animals?

Given the high standards for the breeding and the use of animals for scientific purposes (aka, research animals) in all related regulatory pieces, it would seem obvious that these same texts would include a substantial section on the appropriate conditions for transporting these animals. This is not the case.

For instance, in Directive 2010/63/EU [1], Member States are required to ensure "animals are transported under appropriate conditions" as part of the general considerations on animal care and accommodation (Article 33), without any further details or specific requirements. The only other mention of "Transport" in Directive 2010/63/UE is about the capture and transport of

J. Guillén, V. Galligioni (eds.), *Practical Management of Research Animal Care and Use Programs*, Laboratory Animal Science and Medicine 3, https://doi.org/10.1007/978-3-031-65414-5_5

animals taken from the wild (Section A: General section/3. Care of animals/3.2. Animals taken from the wild/(a)). In this regard, Appendix A of European Treaty Series No. 123 [2] is a bit more descriptive with a paragraph on packing and transport conditions (4.3) and one on acclimatisation (4.4.2), followed by species-specific provisions. So does USDA Animal Welfare Regulations, with transportation standards by species categories in "Part 3—Standards" [3].

Nevertheless, although not specific to research animals, a wide range of regulations and standards are relevant to animal transport. They primarily apply to livestock animals, which represent the main category of animals transported worldwide. Adding diversity and complexity in when and where these regulations apply does not make things easy to manage end-to-end international journeys. However, general provisions apply to all species, particularly vertebrates, and regulations also include specific considerations based on individual species needs. But being species-specific does not necessarily mean being fully relevant in terms of welfare or health status in a context of animals bred and used as research models. For such reason, additional guidelines are available for animal species used for scientific purposes. In addition to such guidelines published by the laboratory animal science community, there is a push from animal welfare NGOs to include specific provisions in the regulation [4].

5.1.2 What Are the Key References on the Welfare of Animals During Transport?

Although subject to change as part of the revision of the European Union legislation on animal welfare [5], the most detailed and relevant regulation one should refer to is European Council Regulation (EC) No. 1/2005 of 22 Dec 2004 on the protection of animals during transport and related operations [6]. After European Convention for the Protection of Animals during International Transport (aka European Treaty Series—No. 193) [7], seeking to harmonise standards for all live vertebrate animals transported within the European Union (EU), and based on the understanding that poor animal welfare is often due to a lack of education, the Regulation imposes rules to Member States, emphasising on the importance of training, authorisation, and accountability of the transporters. To address the growing trend in globalisation in the absence of worldwide regulation, and to promote full consideration for animal health and welfare during transport globally, additional guidance has been developed by the World Organisation for Animal Health (WOAH, founded as OIE). Both Terrestrial Animal Health Code [8] and Aquatic Animal Health Code [9] have been updated in 2023. They both include a section on trade measures, import/export procedures, and health or veterinary certification (Section 5), with detailed considerations related to animal or public health risk, for instance, on quarantine measures applicable to non-human primates (in "Terrestrial Code", Section 5, Chapter 5.9). As part of the section on animal welfare (Section 7), specific chapters apply to welfare during transport. The Terrestrial Animal Health Code provides more specific considerations depending on whether animals are transport by sea (Chapter 7.2), land (Chapter 7.3), or air (Chapter 7.4).

With regard to air transport, the overarching rules are set by IATA, the International Air Transport Association. IATA ensures that both safety and animal welfare are addressed in all regulatory issues pertaining to the transportation of live animals by air. IATA coordinates the Live Animals and Perishables Board (LAPB) and provides key input to the airline industry on issues such as animal welfare, identification, and animal behaviour based on modern science. Considering proposals made from IATA members, Convention on International Trade in Endangered Species (CITES), WOAH, EU, and national legislative authorities, and other interested parties, LAPB has developed and is constantly updating the IATA Live Animals Regulations (LAR) as the worldwide standard for transporting live animals by commercial airlines [10]. Whereas it is the role of governments to set and enforce the rules concerning the transportation of live animals,

IATA members are expected to adhere to the LAR to "ensure that live animals are handled and transported in such a way that their welfare is top of mind by all parties involved and that they always travel in safe, healthy and humane conditions" [11].

5.1.3 Do Additional References Apply on the Trade of Animals?

As part of the integrated food safety policy of European Union, but impacting well outside the EU, EU law requires consignments of animals, animal products, certain food and feed of non-animal origin, and the majority of plants to be accompanied by official certificates, attesting compliance with the applicable requirements in the food safety and quality, animal health and welfare, and plant health sectors, and ensuring traceability of animals' and goods' movements within the EU and in non-EU countries in relation to their exports to the EU. Various actions and systems are implemented to assure effective control and evaluate compliance. The EU established a single tool to facilitate the exchange of data, information, and documents between all involved trading parties and control authorities and therefore simplifies and speeds up the administrative procedures: TRACES [12].

TRACES is the European Commission's online platform for sanitary and phytosanitary certification required for the importation of animals, animal products, food and feed of non-animal origin, and plants into the European Union, and the intra-EU trade and EU exports of animals and certain animal products.

Nowadays, TRACES is an indispensable tool used in about 90 countries, with more than 55,000 users worldwide for the issuance of sanitary and phytosanitary certificates and official documents required for imports, exports, and intra-EU movements of live animals and goods. The main objective of TRACES is to streamline the certification process and all linked entry procedures and to offer a fully digitised and paperless workflow.

The TRACES platform enhances cooperation and coordination between the competent authorities of EU countries and non-EU countries, but also between the traders themselves and their competent authorities. When a decision is taken on a consignment, the involved parties are notified and have access to the relevant documents. Such coordination also helps rapid reactions in case of health threats.

The trade of animals (and plants) is also regulated under an international wildlife protection programme. CITES, the Convention on International Trade in Endangered Species of Wild Fauna and Flora, is an international agreement between governments under the United Nations Environment Programme [13]. Its aim is to ensure that international trade in specimens of wild animals and plants does not threaten the survival of the species. CITES was first drafted as a result of a resolution adopted in 1963 at a meeting of members of the International Union for Conservation of Nature (IUCN). The text of the Convention, the so-called Washington Convention was finally agreed at a meeting of representatives of 80 countries in Washington, DC, United States of America, on 3 March 1973, and, on 1 July 1975, CITES entered in force. It was amended since then [14].

Because the trade in wild animals and plants crosses borders between countries, the effort to regulate it requires international cooperation to safeguard certain species from over-exploitation. CITES was conceived in the spirit of such cooperation. CITES is an international agreement to which States and regional economic integration organisations adhere voluntarily. States that have agreed to be bound by the Convention (i.e. that "joined" CITES) are known as Parties. Although CITES is legally binding on the Parties—in other words they have to implement the Convention—it does not take the place of national laws. Rather it provides a framework to be respected by each Party, which has to adopt its own domestic legislation to ensure that CITES is implemented at the national level. For many years, CITES has been among the conservation agreements with the largest membership, with now 184 Parties.

Today, CITES accords varying degrees of protection to more than 40,000 species of animals and plants, whether they are traded as live specimens, fur coats, or dried herbs. The species are grouped in the three Appendices to the Convention according to how threatened they are by international trade [15]. They include some whole groups, such as Primates spp. which are included in Appendix II (not necessarily threatened with extinction, but in which trade must be controlled), except individual species included in Appendix I (i.e. species threatened with extinction). But in some cases, only a subspecies or geographically separate population of a species (for example, the population of just one country) is listed. The CITES permit system is the backbone of the regulation of trade in specimens of species, included in the three Appendices to the Convention. Such trade should normally be accompanied by a CITES permit or certificate. The document is the confirmation by the issuing authority that the conditions for authorising the trade are fulfilled; this means that the trade is legal, sustainable, and traceable in accordance with Art. III, IV, and V of the Convention. For instance, for primates (live animals and biological samples), an export permit and an import permit must be obtained prior to shipment.

5.1.4 Which Standards Apply to Research Animals' Health and Welfare?

Based on the above, one shall understand that general applicable regulation and standards are (1) mostly relevant to farm animals, either terrestrial or aquatic, (2) for some, more focused on food safety considerations than actual animal welfare, and (3) species-specific independently from the context of breeding and use. However, guidelines do exist that are directly relevant to animals used in science.

First, WOAH recognises that transportation of animals between institutes is a specialised and important activity supporting scientific research. A specific section on transportation is developed in their chapter on "use of animals in research and education" in Chapter 7.8 of the "Terrestrial Code" [8], emphasising the specific physiological and behavioural needs, and highly defined health status (e.g. pathogen free) such animals have. In particular, if, as a consequence of scientific procedures or because of specific study requirements, welfare of such animals might be compromised, transport might still be needed, and thus undertaken with highest level of consideration for animal welfare. As far as behaviour is concerned, animals transported in compatible pairs or social groups shall be maintained in the same social organisation on arrival. In addition, so as to improve consistency across geographies, WOAH has adopted in 2012 their "Model veterinary certificate for international trade in laboratory animals" in Chapter 5.13 of the "Terrestrial Code" [8] in which specific information can be provided with regard to animals' pathogen free status and to conditions which could impact animals' fitness for transport.

In the 8th edition of The Guide for the Care and Use of Laboratory Animals [16], animal procurement and transportation is addressed as part of the veterinary care programme, emphasising the importance of planning, coordination, responsibility, training, procedures, and documentation. Earlier, in 2006, the US National Research Council (NRC) also published "Guidelines for the Humane Transportation of Research Animals" providing a comprehensive review of the topic [17]. The book includes a set of good practices based on the extensive body of literature on transportation of agricultural animals, universal concepts of physiology, and a scientific understanding of species-specific needs and differences. They address thermal environment, space requirements, food and water requirements, social interaction, monitoring of transportation, emergency procedures, handling, personnel training, and biosecurity. In addition, in a similar set of recommendations, the UK Laboratory Animal Science Association (LASA) Transport Working Group published their guidance where additional specific requirements were included for species and species groups [18]. Although anterior to NRC and other publications, the "LASA guidance" remains one of the most known and relevant pieces of information for laboratory animal transport to date. Both NRC and LASA guidelines have been used as reference documents for the transportation section of the

Canadian Council on Animal Care (CCAC) guidelines on the procurement of animals used in science [19]. General considerations related to transport of animals are embedded in the animal care and management section of the Australian code for the care and use of animals for scientific purposes [20]. In the last edition of the Universities Federation for Animal Welfare (UFAW) Handbook on the Care and Management of Laboratory and Other Research Animals, a full section provides guidance on the transportation of laboratory animals [21].

Based on these many general and specific standards, and other publications, the following sections will seek to dive more into practical details of what needs to be taken into consideration before, during, and after transporting animals, end to end. Relevant to each specific situation, one shall not fail to involve logistics, security, and occupational health and safety teams.

5.2 What Are the End-to-End Transport Aspects to Consider?

Research animals will most often be transported by several routes and means, including numerous steps and involving multiple stakeholders. Addressing different questions, this section seeks to illustrate this complexity and allude to the various nature and severity of potential incidents so as to avoid them.

5.2.1 What Are the Most Common Transport Means and Routes?

Due to the very specific conditions and requirements and the length of journey, animals used for scientific purposes may only rarely be transported by sea, except over short distances (crossing bays or inlets, if there is no other practical option).

The most common means of transporting research animals typically include:

- Road transport is one of the most commonly used methods for transporting animals from breeding to research facilities, between research institutions, and technical service platforms (e.g. imaging platform). Animals are usually transported in specially designed vehicles equipped with appropriate ventilation, temperature control, and secure containment facilities.
- Air transport may be used for transporting animals over long distances or between countries. Air transport has constantly increased due to the specialisation and concentration of breeding activities, far from research facilities, and to the development of collaborations between research institutions across the globe.
- Transporting animals by air across the globe must be subject to the highest animal welfare and logistics considerations, especially due to climate and weather conditions, and need most careful anticipation and planification. For instance, attention to weather forecast is a must when flying primates from the tropical breeding sites to North hemisphere locations in winter, as snowstorms may occur and delay flight arrival or even refrain flights from landing.
- Animals are typically transported in specially designed containers or crates within the cargo hold of commercial or chartered aircraft. Air transport requires careful planning to ensure the animals' welfare and compliance with aviation regulations. IATA guidelines have become the most commonly recognised standards for transporting animals.
- Rail transport is quite infrequent and may be used for transporting animals over medium to long distances, particularly in regions with well-developed railway infrastructure. Animals are usually transported in specially designed containers or compartments within dedicated trains, as for livestock transport.
- Courier services may be used for transporting animals over short distances or for urgent shipments. Animals are usually transported in specially designed containers or crates within vehicles operated by courier companies.
- Specialised Transport Providers: Some research institutions may contract specialised transport providers that offer dedicated services for transporting animals. These providers often have expertise in handling and transporting animals safely and comply with relevant regulations and standards.

Each of these transport methods has its advantages and considerations, and the choice of transport means depends on factors such as the distance of transport—hence transport duration, the urgency of shipment, regulatory requirements, and logistical considerations in relation to the specific needs of the animals being transported. Regardless of the transport method used, ensuring the welfare, safety, and compliance of animals during transport is paramount. Users shall pay attention to various local regulations that apply when planning transport on their own.

5.2.2 What Are the Expectations for Animal Transport Vehicles and Crates?

Vehicles and crates must be designed to provide a safe, secure, and comfortable environment for animals during transport, as well as compliance with relevant regulations and standards. The design of an animal transport crate may vary depending on factors such as the species, size, and specific requirements of the animals being transported. Obviously, with regard to resistance and durability, crates designed for rodents highly differ from those for primates. However, there are some common features and considerations for designing an animal transport vehicle and crate:

- Size and Space: The vehicle and crate should provide sufficient space for the animals to stand, lie down, turn around, stretch, and exhibit natural behaviours comfortably. Adequate space allowance is essential to prevent overcrowding and minimise stress during transit. The crate should be sized appropriately based on the size and breed of the animal being transported.
- Ventilation: Proper ventilation is critical to maintain air quality and prevent heat stress or respiratory problems in the animals. To ensure sufficient airflow without causing drafts or temperature fluctuations, the vehicle should be equipped with ventilation systems and the crate should have adequate ventilation openings or slats on multiple sides.
- Temperature Control: Temperature control systems, such as heating, cooling, or insulation, should be incorporated into the vehicle design to maintain a comfortable temperature range for the animals, regardless of external conditions. With regard to temperature management, one should consider the temperature inside the crate will tend to be higher than in the vehicle.
- Flooring and Surfaces: The vehicle and crate should have a solid, non-slip flooring and smooth surfaces that are easy to clean and disinfect. Flooring materials should be comfortable for the animals to stand or lie on during transit.
- Comfort and Security: The crate should be designed to provide a comfortable and secure environment for the animal during transit. It may include features such as padding, bedding, or partitions to reduce stress and provide support during travel.
- Security, Containment, and Restraint: To prevent the animals from escaping or injuring each other during transit, the vehicle should be equipped with secure containment facilities, such as cages, stalls, or partitions. Restraint systems, such as tie-downs or dividers, may be necessary to ensure the animals' safety. Likewise, the crate should be designed to securely contain the animal and should have a secure locking mechanism, such as latches or bolts, to prevent accidental opening or tampering.
- Durability and Strength: The crate should be constructed from durable, high-quality materials that can withstand the rigours of transport and provide adequate protection for the animal. It should be sturdy and resistant to bending, breaking, or collapsing during transit. Maintaining crate integrity all along the journey is a priority to ensure animal health status is preserved. Crates must be checked upon arrival (Pritchett-Corning KR in [22]).
- Accessibility and Loading: The vehicle and crate should have accessible entry and exit points to facilitate the loading and unloading of animals (e.g. such as ramps or loading docks on vehicles). Consideration should be given to minimising the height and angle of

entry to reduce the risk of injury during loading and unloading. The crate should have a door or gate that can be easily opened and closed without causing stress or injury to the animal.
- Safety Features: Safety features, such as emergency exits, lighting, and alarms, should be incorporated into the vehicle design to ensure the safety of both the animals and handlers in the event of an emergency.
- Hygiene and Waste Management: The vehicle and crate should be designed for easy cleaning and disinfection to maintain hygiene standards and prevent the spread of diseases. Adequate facilities for waste management, such as drainage systems or waste storage areas, should also be provided.
- Compliance with Regulations: The design of the transport vehicle and transport crate should comply with relevant regulations and standards governing animal transport, including those related to vehicle construction, crate dimensions, ventilation requirements, temperature control, and animal welfare.

By carefully considering these factors and incorporating them into the design of the transport vehicle and the transport crate, transporters can ensure the welfare and safety of the animals being transported while maintaining compliance with regulatory requirements.

Industry Best Practices

IATA Guidelines for the Design and Construction of Animal Transport Crates

The International Air Transport Association (IATA) has established guidelines for the design and construction of animal transport crates used in air travel. These guidelines, known as the IATA Live Animals Regulations (LAR), provide standards and recommendations to ensure the safety, welfare, and comfort of animals during air transport [10]. LAR is updated annually.

Some key aspects of the IATA crate guidelines include:

- Size and Dimensions: The crate should be sized appropriately to accommodate the size, breed, and species of the animal being transported. There should be sufficient space for the animal to stand, turn around, and lie down comfortably.
- Construction Materials: The crate should be constructed from durable, non-toxic materials that are capable of withstanding the rigours of air travel. Common materials include rigid plastic, fibreglass, or metal.
- Ventilation: The crate should have adequate ventilation openings on multiple sides to ensure sufficient airflow and prevent overheating or suffocation. Ventilation openings should be covered with mesh or bars to prevent escape or injury.
- Door Design: The crate should have a secure door or gate that can be easily opened and closed by airline personnel. The door should be equipped with a locking mechanism to prevent accidental opening during transit.
- Flooring: The crate should have a solid, leak-proof floor surface that is easy to clean and disinfect. Bedding material, such as absorbent pads or shredded paper, may be added for comfort and hygiene.
- Labelling and Identification: The crate should be clearly labelled with the owner's contact information, as well as information about the animal being transported, including species, breed, age, and any special handling instructions. This helps airline personnel identify and care for the animal appropriately.
- Food and Water Containers: The crate should be equipped with securely attached food and water containers to provide for the animal's nutritional and

hydration needs during transit. These containers should be accessible to airline personnel for replenishment as needed.

- Handling Instructions: The crate should include clear instructions for handling and transporting the animal, including recommendations for loading, unloading, and securing the crate within the aircraft.
- Compliance with Regulations: The design and construction of the crate should comply with relevant regulations and standards established by aviation authorities, as well as any specific requirements or recommendations outlined by the airline.

5.2.3 Short-/Mid-/Long-Term Transport: What Are We Talking About?

Animal transport durations can be categorised based on the length of time the animals spend in transit. These categories may vary depending on factors such as the species of animals being transported, the mode of transport, and the distance travelled. However, common categories of animal transport durations include:

- Short-Distance Transport typically involves journeys of a few hours or less, such as local or regional trips within a city, town, or nearby area.
  Examples of short-distance transport include transporting animals between farms, veterinary clinics, or research facilities between institutions or between departments or facilities in the same institution.
- Medium-Distance Transport involves journeys lasting several hours to a day, covering distances within a region or country.
  Examples of medium-distance transport include transporting animals between different states or provinces, regional distribution centres, or neighbouring countries.
- Long-Distance Transport encompasses journeys lasting more than a day, often involving interstate or international travel over significant distances.
  Examples of long-distance transport include transporting animals between countries or continents, export/import shipments, or transcontinental journeys.
- Extended or Prolonged Transport refers to journeys lasting multiple days or weeks, where animals may be in transit for an extended period.
  Examples of extended transport include livestock shipments, migratory movements, or relocation of animals to distant locations for breeding, exhibition, or research purposes.
- Permanent or Relocation Transport involves moving animals to a new permanent location where they will reside long term.
  Examples include relocating pets or animals to a new home (rehoming!), transferring animals to a sanctuary or rescue facility, or moving breeding stock to a new breeding facility.

More specifically, according to Council Regulation (EC) No 1/2005 (article 2 (m)), **"long journey" means a journey that exceeds 8 h** starting from when the first animal of the consignment is moved [6]. Specific regimen applies for long journeys: transporters' authorisation, prior inspection and approval of means of transport, competent authority checks before, during, and after the journey, and specific journey log.

5.2.4 What Are the Different Steps and Requirements When Planning a Long-Distance Transport? An Example Based on Transporting Animals by Air

Transporting animals by air involves several steps and requirements to ensure the safety, welfare, and compliance of the animals during transit. Everything starts with planning. Here are the different steps and requirements for transporting animals by air:

- Preparation and Planning:
  - Identify the type, species, and number of animals being transported.
  - Determine the destination and route of travel.
  - Verify the specific requirements and regulations for transporting animals by air, including those of the airline, aviation authorities, and destination country.
- Container and Crate Preparation:
  - Select an appropriate transport container or crate that meets the size, ventilation, and security requirements for the species and size of the animal.
  - Ensure the crate is clean, sanitised, and equipped with bedding, food, water containers, and any necessary accessories.
  - Label the crate with the owner's contact information, animal identification details, and handling instructions.
- Health Certification and Documentation:
  - Obtain health certificates and documentation from a licensed veterinarian confirming that the animal is fit for travel and complies with health and vaccination requirements.
  - Ensure all required permits, import/export licenses, and other documentation (e.g. Material Transfer Agreement, MTA) are in compliance with regulatory requirements.
- Booking and Reservation:
  - Make a reservation with the airline for transporting the animal, ensuring that the airline's policies and procedures for transporting animals are understood and followed.
  - Provide the airline with all necessary documentation and information about the animal's transport requirements.
- Check-in and Inspection:
  - Arrive at the airport within the designated time frame for check-in and inspection of the animal.
  - Present the animal and accompanying documentation to airline personnel for verification and inspection.
  - Ensure that the animal is securely contained in the transport crate and properly labelled with identification and handling instructions.
- Loading and Boarding:
  - Accompany the animal to the designated loading area or cargo facility for boarding onto the aircraft.
  - Ensure that the transport crate is safely and securely loaded onto the aircraft according to airline and aviation authority regulations.
- In-Flight Care and Monitoring:
  - During the flight, airline personnel may monitor the animal's welfare and condition, including temperature, ventilation, and comfort.
  - Food and water containers may be replenished as needed, depending on the duration of the flight and the species of the animal.
- Arrival and Disembarkation:
  - Upon arrival at the destination airport, the animal will be unloaded from the aircraft and transferred to the designated cargo or animal handling area.
  - Clear customs procedures, presenting all required documentation for inspection and clearance.
  - Retrieve the animal from the transport crate and ensure its safe transfer to the final destination.
- Post-Arrival Care:
  - Provide post-arrival care and accommodations for the animal, including access to food, water, and shelter as needed.
  - Monitor the animal for any signs of stress, illness, or injury following the journey and seek veterinary care if necessary.

Following these numerous steps and requirements necessarily involves multiple participants whose roles and responsibilities must clearly be defined, in advance, to ensure the safe and humane transport of animals and avoid incidents.

On-site Transport

While the above dispositions will more obviously be considered for long-distance transport, similar attention shall also be paid to very short movement, i.e. moving an animal from one building to another or to a new room within a building. Despite short duration, on-site transport can still cause stress, especially if animals are removed from their home cage or enclosure and placed in another temporary or definitive accommodation. Preparedness is as well important to ensure smooth process, avoid noise, vibrations, and unnecessary transit times [18].

Although more reduced in time, animals shall have an acclimatisation period for recovery and physiological and behavioural stabilisation, after intra-site transfers, even within the same building [23].

5.2.5 What Are the Most Frequent Incidents and Risks During Animal Transport?

Incidents during animal transport can vary in nature and severity, but some of the most frequent incidents reported include:

- Handling Injuries: Incidents involving handling injuries occur when animals are improperly handled during loading, unloading, or transit, resulting in injuries such as bruises, cuts, or fractures.
- Stress-Related Conditions: Animals are susceptible to stress during transport, which can lead to various physiological and behavioural issues, including elevated heart rate, respiratory distress, dehydration, and gastrointestinal disturbances.
- Temperature Fluctuations: Temperature fluctuations inside transport vehicles can pose risks to the welfare of animals, especially if they are exposed to extreme heat or cold during transit. This can lead to heat stress, hypothermia, or other temperature-related health problems.
- Ventilation Issues: Poor ventilation or inadequate airflow inside transport containers can result in respiratory distress or suffocation for animals, particularly during long journeys or when animals are transported in crowded conditions.
- Escape Attempts: Incidents involving escape attempts may occur if transport containers or crates are not properly secured or if animals become agitated or distressed during transit. Escaped animals can pose risks to themselves, handlers, and the public.
- Illness or Injury: Animals may experience illness or injury during transport due to pre-existing health conditions, stress, or environmental factors. This can include conditions such as respiratory infections, injuries from fighting or overcrowding, or exacerbation of existing health issues.
- Regulatory Compliance Issues: Incidents related to non-compliance with regulatory requirements or transport guidelines may occur, such as improper documentation (especially at border inspection post adding avoidable delays), failure to provide adequate care and accommodations, or violations of animal welfare standards.
- Vehicle Accidents or Delays: Vehicle accidents or delays during transit can disrupt transport schedules and pose risks to the safety and welfare of animals. Accidents may result in injuries or fatalities for both animals and personnel involved in the transport; they may also result in animal escape. Delays or even interruptions might be due to extreme weather conditions, preventing animals to be delivered properly to final destination. The impact on animal welfare will vary in degrees depending on each specific situation, and the decision on the fate of animals shall be made on a case-by-case basis, depending on whether the crates can be opened or returned to the sender or not.

Delays may also frequently happen at inspection posts, for administrative (missing or wrong documents) or practical (limited hours of service) reasons. These shall be avoided with appropriate planning, anticipation, and organisation.

- Equipment Malfunctions: Incidents involving equipment malfunctions, such as failures in temperature control systems, ventilation systems, or crate latches, can compromise the safety and welfare of animals during transport.
- Interference or Disruption by Animal Right Activists: Protests and demonstrations are on the rise to raise awareness about animal experimentation or to disrupt the transport of animals. In some cases, activists may attempt to block or interfere with the transportation of animals by physically obstructing vehicles, accessing restricted areas, or chaining themselves to transport containers. In more extreme cases, they may engage in direct action or sabotage.

To mitigate the risks of incidents during animal transport, it is essential to implement appropriate measures, including proper handling techniques, adequate training for personnel, adherence to transport guidelines and regulations, regular vehicle maintenance, contingency planning for emergencies, and appropriate security measures to protect animals, personnel, and facilities from potential threats or disruptions. Additionally, ongoing monitoring and evaluation of transport practices can help identify and address potential risks to improve the safety and welfare of animals during transit.

5.3 What Are the Roles and Responsibilities to Consider?

Before transporting animals for research purposes, in reference to article 7.8.10 of the Terrestrial Animal Health Code [8], the very first responsibility lies with the requestor so that the source of animals and therefore the mode and conditions of transport should be considered in the project proposal review. As a consequence, the consigner and consignee should coordinate the means, route, and duration of transport with emphasis on the potential impact on the health and welfare of the animal(s). WOAH also emphasises on the importance of training: "Personnel handling animals throughout the planned journey should be trained in the basic needs of animals and in good handling practices for the species to facilitate the loading and unloading of animals".

Such considerations are equally embedded in The Guide for the Care and Use of Laboratory Animals [16]: "Movement of animals within or between sites or institutions should be planned and coordinated by responsible and well-trained persons at the sending and receiving sites to minimize animal transit time or delays in receipt. Shipping should be coordinated to ensure that animals arrive during normal business hours or, if delivery occurs outside of this time, that someone is available to receive them. Defining and delegating responsibility to the appropriate persons, who are knowledgeable about the needs of the species being shipped, will help ensure effective communication and planning of animal transport".

This section will focus on key aspects about roles and responsibilities before, during, and after transport.

5.3.1 How Are Ownership and Responsibility for Animals Handled During Transport?

The ownership and responsibility for animals during transport depend on various factors, including the terms of agreements between parties involved, the mode of transportation, and applicable regulations. In general, ownership and responsibility may fall to one or more of the following parties:

- Animal Owners: The owners of the animals are typically responsible for their welfare and well-being, including during transport. They may arrange and oversee transportation themselves or hire third-party transporters to handle the logistics.
- Transporters: If animals are transported by a third-party transportation company or individual transporter, they assume responsibility

for the animals' welfare and safety during transit. Transporters are typically required to comply with relevant regulations, ensure proper handling and care, and maintain appropriate documentation.
- Handlers and Attendants: Individuals responsible for directly handling and caring for animals during transport, such as drivers, attendants, or livestock handlers, have a duty of care to ensure the animals' welfare and safety. They must follow proper handling procedures, provide necessary care, and respond to any emergencies or issues that arise during transit.
- Regulatory Authorities: Government agencies or regulatory bodies may also have oversight and enforcement responsibilities regarding animal transport. They establish and enforce regulations governing animal welfare, transportation standards, and biosecurity measures to safeguard animal health and prevent the spread of diseases.
- Consignees or Receivers: Upon arrival at the destination, the party receiving the animals assumes responsibility for their further care, handling, and compliance with any additional requirements or regulations applicable at the destination.

Ultimately, the specific roles and responsibilities of each party involved in animal transport should be clearly defined and agreed upon in advance to ensure the welfare and safety of the animals throughout the transportation process, especially in terms of ownership between the shipper (e.g. breeder) and the consignee (e.g. end user). Compliance with applicable regulations and industry standards is essential to uphold animal welfare and mitigate risks during transport.

5.3.2 What Are the Responsibilities of Animal Transporters?

Animal transporters have several key responsibilities to ensure the welfare and safety of the animals under their care throughout the transportation process. These responsibilities include:

- Compliance with Regulations: Animal transporters must comply with relevant national and international regulations governing animal welfare during transportation. They must hold a license, vehicles must be authorised, and staff must be trained. This includes also adhering to standards for vehicle design, handling practices, journey duration, and provision of water, feed, and rest.
- Vehicle Maintenance and Safety: Transporters are responsible for ensuring that transport vehicles are properly maintained, clean, and safe for transporting animals. This includes regular inspections, maintenance of temperature control systems, adequate ventilation, and secure containment to prevent injury or escape.
- Animal Handling and Care: Transporters must handle animals with care and respect, using gentle and appropriate handling techniques to minimise stress and injury during loading, unloading, and transit. They should ensure that animals have access to water, feed, and rest as needed during the journey.
- Monitoring and Intervention: Transporters should monitor animals throughout the journey, looking for signs of distress, illness, or injury. Prompt intervention may be necessary to address any health or welfare concerns, including providing veterinary care or making adjustments to transport conditions.
- Documentation and Record-Keeping: Transporters are responsible for maintaining accurate records of transported animals, including their origin, destination, health status, and any treatments administered during transit. Documentation should also include details of journey duration, rest stops, and any incidents or deviations from planned routes.
- Communication and Collaboration: Transporters may need to communicate with animal owners, producers, veterinarians, and regulatory authorities to coordinate transport arrangements, address concerns, or obtain necessary permits or certifications.
- Training and Education: Transporters should receive appropriate training in animal handling, welfare requirements, biosecurity pro-

tocols, and emergency response procedures. Ongoing education and professional development are essential for maintaining high standards of care and compliance with regulations.

Overall, animal transporters play a critical role in ensuring the welfare and safety of animals during transportation, requiring careful attention to regulatory compliance, vehicle maintenance, animal handling, monitoring, and collaboration with stakeholders involved in the transport process.

5.3.3 Which Training Is Required for Drivers Transporting Animals?

Training requirements for drivers transporting animals vary depending on the jurisdiction, type of animals being transported, and specific regulations governing animal welfare during transport. However, common areas of training that may be required or recommended for drivers transporting animals include:

- Animal Handling Techniques: Drivers should receive training in proper animal handling techniques to ensure the safety and welfare of the animals during loading, unloading, and transit. This includes understanding how to move animals calmly and effectively, recognise signs of stress or illness, and respond appropriately to behavioural cues.
- Transport Regulations and Standards: Drivers should be familiar with relevant regulations, standards, and best practices governing animal transport in their jurisdiction. This may include understanding requirements related to vehicle design and maintenance, journey duration, temperature control, ventilation, and provision of water, feed, and rest.
- Health and Biosecurity Protocols: Drivers should be trained to recognise and respond to health issues or emergencies that may arise during transport, including administering basic first aid, contacting veterinary authorities as needed, and implementing biosecurity measures to prevent the spread of diseases.
- Emergency Response Procedures: Drivers should be prepared to handle emergencies or accidents that may occur during transport, such as vehicle breakdowns, adverse weather conditions, or animal escapes. Training in emergency response procedures, including evacuation protocols and communication with emergency services, is essential for ensuring the safety of both the animals and the driver.
- Documentation and Record-Keeping: Drivers should understand the importance of accurate documentation and record-keeping in animal transport, including maintaining records of journey details, health checks, and any incidents or deviations from planned routes.
- Driver Welfare and Well-Being: Training programmes may also address the welfare and well-being of drivers themselves, including strategies for managing stress, fatigue, and mental health issues associated with long hours on the road and the responsibilities of caring for live animals.
- Continuing Education and Professional Development: Ongoing training and professional development opportunities should be provided to drivers to keep them updated on new regulations, technologies, and best practices in animal transport.

Overall, comprehensive training programmes for drivers transporting animals are essential for ensuring the welfare and safety of both the animals and the individuals responsible for their care during transit.

5.3.4 Which Steps Are Taken at a Border Inspection Post?

At a border inspection post (BIP), several steps are typically taken to ensure the safety, health, and compliance of animals, animal products, and other goods entering a country. These steps may vary depending on the specific regulations and requirements of the importing country, but common procedures at a BIP include:

- Documentary Checks: Inspectors review accompanying documentation, such as import permits, health certificates, and other relevant paperwork, to verify that the consignment meets the importing country's requirements.
- Identity Checks: Inspectors verify the identity of the consignment and ensure that it matches the information provided in the accompanying documentation.
- Physical Inspection: Physical inspection of the consignment may be conducted to check for signs of disease, contamination, or other issues. This inspection may include visual examination, sampling, or testing of goods.
- Health Certification: Inspectors may require health certificates issued by a competent authority in the exporting country, confirming that the consignment meets health and sanitary requirements.
- Quarantine Procedures: If there are concerns about the health or safety of the consignment, it may be subject to quarantine measures, such as isolation or further testing, to prevent the spread of diseases or pests.
- Sampling and Testing: Samples of the consignment, such as animal tissues, feed, or other products, may be collected for laboratory testing to detect the presence of pathogens, contaminants, or prohibited substances.
- Documentation and Record-Keeping: Inspectors maintain detailed records of inspections, findings, and any actions taken at the BIP. Documentation is essential for traceability, accountability, and regulatory compliance.
- Clearance or Rejection: Based on the results of inspections and tests, the consignment may be cleared for entry into the country if it meets all requirements. Alternatively, if there are significant concerns or violations, the consignment may be rejected, returned to the country of origin, or subject to corrective actions.

Overall, the primary objective of a border inspection post is to safeguard public health, animal health, and the environment by ensuring that imported goods meet regulatory standards and do not pose risks of introducing diseases, pests, or contaminants into the importing country.

To conclude on roles and responsibilities, coordination is key, and one should care not only for the animals, but also for the accompanying documentation, and for the health and welfare of the drivers and handlers.

5.4 What Are the Transport-Related Health and Welfare Considerations?

The health and welfare integrity of an animal can significantly be impaired by several factors during transport; this is why on a case-by-case basis, one must evaluate if each individual is fit for transport.

In addition, depending on the work practices and the health status of the animals, there are aspects to be taken care of for the health and safety of the staff involved.

5.4.1 Which Factors Most Likely Affect Animal Condition on the Way?

In short: animal condition can most likely be affected at every single step and by every single aspect of a transport journey if not well taken care of, end-to-end. For each individual animal, journey starts as soon as it is removed from its home cage and will only end after stabilisation in a new housing environment at final destination, whether it is a long intercontinental journey or an inter-institutional transfer.

Several factors that significantly impact animal welfare during transport include:

- First and foremost is the duration of the journey, as longer trips increase the potential for stress, exhaustion, and dehydration in animals.
- Secondly, the design and maintenance of vehicles and the design of transport crates play a crucial role, ensuring adequate ventilation, temperature control, and space allowance to minimise discomfort and injury.

- Handling practices during loading, unloading, and transit also greatly influence welfare, with gentle, skilled handling reducing the risk of injury and stress.
- Additionally, the health and fitness of the animals prior to transport are vital, as sick or injured animals may suffer exacerbated distress during transit.
- Regulatory compliance and enforcement of standards further contribute to welfare, ensuring that transport conditions meet minimum requirements for humane treatment.

Overall, a combination of factors such as journey duration, vehicle design, handling practices, animal health, and regulatory oversight collectively determine the welfare outcomes of transported animals.

Upon arrival, quarantine and acclimatisation are essential to allow animal to recover from stress and potential body weight loss due to transport, and get accustomed to the new environment (change in natural and artificial light/dark cycle, change in food and water regimens, change in micro- and micro-environment: temperature, humidity, cage size and density, environmental enrichment, and last but not least, change in group or pair-housing). The less changes from one end to another, the better.

5.4.2 What Are the Animal Fitness Conditions to Be Considered for Transport?

Animal fitness for transport refers to the physical and behavioural condition of an animal, ensuring it is suitable for safe and humane transportation. Several factors contribute to determining whether an animal is fit for transport. Exceptions to the following conditions shall be examined carefully on a case-by-case basis:

- Health Status: Animals should be free from illness, injury, or any condition that may compromise their welfare during transport. They should be assessed by a competent person familiar with the species to ensure they are in good health. This is important for welfare reasons and also because latent infections may become clinically apparent due to the stress during transport (Pritchett-Corning KR in [22]).
- Fitness for the Journey: Consideration should be given to the specific requirements of the journey, including duration, mode of transport, and environmental conditions. Animals should be physically capable of enduring the journey without experiencing undue stress, discomfort, or harm.
- Age and Condition: Young, old, or otherwise vulnerable animals may have different transport needs. Special considerations should be made for animals that may be more susceptible to the stresses of transport.
- Handling and Behaviour: Animals should be calm, well-behaved, and accustomed to handling and transportation procedures. Aggressive or excessively fearful animals may pose risks to themselves, other animals, and handlers during transport.
- Regulatory Requirements: National and international regulations often define criteria for animal fitness for transport. These regulations may specify health certifications, veterinary inspections, or other requirements to ensure animals are fit for transport.
- Transport Conditions: The design and condition of the transport vehicle, including ventilation, temperature control, and space allowance, should be suitable for the species being transported. Animals should have access to water, feed, and rest as needed during the journey.

Overall, determining animal fitness for transport requires careful consideration of the individual animal's health and behavioural characteristics, as well as compliance with relevant regulations and standards aimed at safeguarding animal welfare during transport.

5.4.3 What Are the Considerations to Feed and Water Animals During Transport?

Rules and regulations regarding the provision of feed and water to animals during transport vary depending on the jurisdiction and the specific species being transported. However, several common principles and guidelines that apply in many regions include:

- Access to Water: Animals must have access to clean and fresh water throughout the journey. Water must be provided at regular intervals, and containers should be designed to prevent spillage and contamination.
- Access to Feed: For longer journeys, animals may require access to feed to meet their nutritional needs. The type and frequency of feeding depend on the species, age, and duration of the journey. Feeding practices should minimise spillage and waste and ensure that animals can comfortably access the feed.
- Duration of Transport: Regulations often specify maximum journey times without access to water and feed. If the journey exceeds these limits, mandatory rest stops with provisions for water and feed may be required.
- Transportation Conditions: Transport vehicles must be equipped to safely provide water and feed to animals. This includes secure containers, proper ventilation to maintain feed freshness, and measures to prevent contamination.

Overall, the aim of these rules is to ensure that animals are provided with adequate nutrition and hydration to maintain their health and welfare throughout the transport process.

5.4.4 What Are the Health Risks to Be Considered for Animals During Transport?

Transporting animals poses various health risks, and these risks can vary depending on factors such as species, age, individual health status, transport conditions, and duration of the journey. Some common health risks for animals during transport include:

- Stress: Transportation can be inherently stressful for animals due to unfamiliar environments, sounds, and movements. Prolonged stress may weaken the immune system, making animals more susceptible to diseases.
- Injuries: Rough handling, inadequate space, or poorly designed transport vehicles can lead to injuries such as bruises, fractures, or abrasions. Animals may also injure themselves or others during loading and unloading.
- Dehydration: Insufficient access to water during transport can lead to dehydration, especially in hot or humid conditions. Dehydration can have serious health consequences and affect the overall well-being of the animals.
- Heat Stress or Hypothermia: Extreme temperatures inside transport vehicles can cause heat stress or hypothermia, depending on weather conditions. Lack of proper ventilation and temperature control can exacerbate these risks. Depending on 1) the design of the crates, their density in the container and the space around for air circulation and 2) the variation in air temperature and animal density in the crate, body temperature may be subject to a very high degree of variation.
- Respiratory Issues: Poor ventilation in transport vehicles can result in respiratory problems, particularly if the air quality is compromised by dust, ammonia, or other pollutants. This is especially relevant for animals with respiratory sensitivities.
- Disease Transmission: Close proximity to other animals during transport increases the risk of disease transmission. Contagious diseases can spread easily, particularly if animals are not adequately separated or if biosecurity measures are lacking.
- Motion Sickness: Animals may experience motion sickness during transport, leading to symptoms such as nausea, vomiting, and discomfort.
- Exhaustion: Long journeys without sufficient rest breaks or inadequate space for animals to lie down and rest can lead to exhaustion and physical fatigue.
- Compromised Immune Function: The stress of transportation can suppress the immune system, making animals more susceptible to infections and diseases.

- Parturition Issues: Pregnant animals may face complications during transport, particularly if close to the time of giving birth. Stress and discomfort can increase the risk of parturition-related issues.

Minimising these health risks requires careful planning, adherence to animal welfare standards, appropriate handling practices, and compliance with relevant regulations governing the transport of animals. Regular monitoring and prompt intervention in case of issues are crucial to ensuring the health and well-being of transported animals.

5.4.5 What Are the Health Risks to Be Considered for the Staff Transporting and Handling Animals?

Staff involved in transporting and handling animals face several health risks, which can vary depending on the species being handled, the nature of the work, and the environment in which it takes place. Some common health risks for staff involved in animal transport and handling include:

- Physical Injuries: Handling large or unpredictable animals can pose risks of physical injuries such as bites, kicks, or crush injuries. Improper lifting techniques or accidents during loading and unloading may result in strains, sprains, or musculoskeletal injuries.
- Allergic Reactions: Exposure to animal dander, fur, feathers, or other allergens can trigger allergic reactions in susceptible individuals, leading to symptoms such as respiratory distress, skin irritation, or asthma attacks.
- Zoonotic Diseases: Staff may be at risk of contracting zoonotic diseases. Examples include brucellosis, salmonellosis, Q fever, or avian influenza, which can be transmitted through direct contact with infected animals, their excreta, or contaminated surfaces.

  This same health risk could be of concern for the general public in case (an) animal(s) would escape from the transport crate or container.
- Occupational Stress: Working with animals, particularly in high-pressure or challenging situations, can contribute to occupational stress, burnout, or mental health issues such as anxiety or depression.
- Chemical Exposures: The use of disinfectants, pesticides, or other chemicals in animal transport and handling facilities may pose risks of chemical exposure to staff, leading to respiratory irritation, skin sensitisation, or other adverse health effects.
- Biological Hazards: Handling animal waste, bedding, or carcasses may expose staff to biological hazards such as bacteria, fungi, parasites, or viruses, increasing the risk of infections or other health problems.
- Noise and Vibrations: Working in noisy or vibrating environments, such as during transportation or within facilities with heavy machinery, can lead to hearing loss, stress, or other health issues over time.
- Injury from Equipment: Operating machinery or handling equipment such as gates, chutes, or restraining devices poses risks of crush injuries, entanglement, or other accidents if proper safety protocols are not followed.

To mitigate these health risks, staff should receive appropriate training in animal handling techniques, use personal protective equipment (PPE) as necessary, follow hygiene protocols, and receive vaccinations or prophylactic treatments against relevant zoonotic diseases. Regular health monitoring, ergonomic assessments, and access to support services for mental well-being can also help safeguard the health and safety of staff involved in animal transport and handling.

5.5 What Are the Specific Considerations for the Safe and Humane Transport of Research Animals?

Animals used for scientific purposes differ from animals in general because (1) they belong to a more limited number of species, (2) they have a more defined health status, and (3) of additional considerations related to the research they are used for as models (fragile or genetically modified animals, contaminated animals). While most rules and guidelines described above apply to all animals, this section will seek to address dispositions that are specifically relevant to animals used for scientific purposes, depending on their (defined/undefined) health status, (modified) genetic status and phenotype, (intact/impaired) physiological condition, the presence or absence of (biological, radioactive…) hazard.

Until new relevant rules or guidelines are published, for all general and species-specific considerations for transporting research animals, including feeding and watering, careful handling and loading, one shall refer to the Guidance on the transport of laboratory animals [18].

5.5.1 What Are the Particularities to Be Considered for Transporting Research Animals?

Transporting research animals requires careful planning and adherence to specific considerations to ensure their welfare, safety, and compliance with regulatory requirements. Some of the key considerations for transporting research animals include:

- Animal Welfare Regulations: Laboratory animals are typically subject to stringent welfare regulations, including those outlined in laws such as the Animal Welfare Act [3] in the United States or corresponding legislation in other countries. Transporters must ensure compliance with these regulations regarding housing, handling, and transport conditions.
- Transport Container Requirements: Transport containers for research animals must be suitable for the species being transported and meet regulatory standards for size, ventilation, temperature control, and security. Containers should provide adequate space and protection to minimise stress and injury during transit. So as to minimise stress, animals should be habituated to the transport boxes in advance by placing the containers in their holding pen (e.g. for dogs and primates), and even to be moved in the transport boxes, to be accustomed to motion and unfamiliar stimuli (sounds, smells…). One shall also consider giving animals enough time to leave the transport box after arrival and discover their new environment at their own pace.
- Health Status, Health Monitoring and Certification: Research animals often require health monitoring and certification before transport to ensure they are free from infectious diseases and meet health requirements. To facilitate international transfer of rodents between facilities, a joint US-Europe working group agreed on minimum health monitoring recommendations and proposed harmonised health monitoring formats accompanied by instructions for users [24].

  In addition, health certificates issued by a veterinarian or regulatory authority may be required for interstate or international transport. Verification of animals' health status, before departure and safeguard animal facilities' microbiological status integrity of animal facilities, microbiological status, and the quality of animals as research models. IATA has defined health status categories for laboratory animals in order to dictate selection of appropriate transport means and containers that maintain health status during transport [10, 21].
- Biosecurity Measures: To prevent the spread of diseases between animal facilities, transporters must implement appropriate biosecurity measures, including cleaning and disinfection of transport containers, and protocols for preventing cross-contamination between animals. So as to preserve animals' health status, transport duration should be as short as possible, and the inner part of containers or crates should not be exposed to potential contaminants. Such practical considerations may be in contradictions with specific legal requirements, as illustrated in next section.

- Transportation Routes and Timing: Transport routes and timing should be carefully planned to minimise stress and discomfort for the animals. Consideration should be given to factors such as journey duration, temperature and weather fluctuations, and potential delays to ensure the animals' welfare during transit. Total transport time, including all steps, should be minimised, especially as the journey often requires changes in transport modes (land–air–land) and clearance by various authorities.
- Separation of Animals by Species, Sexes, and Origins: In order to avoid unnecessary stress, preserve animals' health status, and minimise the risk of cross-contamination, animals of different species, sexes, and different origins should be transported separately.
- Handling and Training of Staff: Staff responsible for handling research animals during transport should receive training in proper handling techniques, animal welfare regulations, and biosecurity protocols. They should be equipped to respond to emergencies and ensure the animals' welfare throughout the journey.
- Emergency Response Preparedness: Transporters should have contingency plans and protocols in place to address emergencies such as accidents, vehicle breakdowns, or adverse weather conditions. Plans should include procedures for evacuating animals safely and seeking veterinary care if needed.
- Documentation and Record-Keeping: Accurate documentation of transport details, health certificates, and any incidents or deviations from planned routes is essential for regulatory compliance and traceability.
- Acclimatisation and Quarantine at Destination: In order to present all the characteristics expected for their use in scientific research, the animals shall recover from the stress of transport and acclimatise to their new environment before being used. The acclimatisation time must allow the animals to recover from the physiological effects of transport and the change of environment or diet (e.g. diarrhoea, cardio-respiratory rhythm, hormonal secretions) so that the physiological constants stabilise. This should also be a time for observing behavioural traits to check that they return to normal, as far as possible, and for gradual habituation between the animals and the staff.

  The duration of acclimatisation time shall vary according to the species and the duration of transport before animals reached the final destination.

  Exemptions shall only be granted on a case-by-case basis, in relation to project evaluation and authorisation.

  In addition, depending on the situation, where there is a proven or potential health risk, it will be imperative, for regulatory reasons and/or to protect the health of people and animals and/or the integrity of research models, to observe a quarantine period and carry out appropriate analyses before releasing the animals for use in research.

5.5.2 What Are the Species- and Status-Specific Considerations to Be Considered for Transporting Research Animals?

In this section are being illustrated or emphasised key features related to the transport of relevant animal species or species groups, either because of aspects that are not covered by regulation but embedded in specific guidelines, or because a regulatory requirement exists but is not relevant to them (Table 5.1).

Table 5.1 Species- and health status-specific considerations applying to animals transported for research purposes

Species/Species group	Specific considerations
Rodents	Specific pathogen free conditions shall be sought for the transport of laboratory rodents, regardless of their microbiological status, to protect them from pathogens carried by any other (companion or wild) animals, either transported on the same vehicle, or crossing the transport crates pathway in a waiting area [18] Transport crates should be made of lightweight though robust material, particularly resistant to the sharp teeth of rodents, and fitted with filters to allow good air circulation so as to avoid too great a rise in temperature in the crate while preserving the microbiological status of the animals, and therefore avoiding exposure to external microbiological agents. However, the animals must be able to be observed at all times and have sufficient feed and hydration without having to open the crate. Finally, the animals must be provided with clean and dry bedding materials, free from contaminants. Rodent transport crates should be handled gently and carefully during loading, unloading, and transit to minimise stress and prevent injuries. Transport personnel should be trained in proper handling techniques to ensure the welfare of the animals. Depending on the physiological and behavioural parameters considered, and the type and duration of transport, acclimatisation of rodents at destination should be a minimum of 3 days [25] to up to 2 weeks [26–28].
Genetically modified animals The transport of live GM animals should be replaced, wherever possible, by the transfer of fresh embryos, or cryopreserved embryos and gametes [29].	Compliance must be assured with relevant national and international regulations governing the transport of genetically modified organisms (GMOs), including GM animals. Any necessary permits or approvals required for the transport of GM animals across borders or between facilities must be obtained prior to transport. In conjunction with the recommendations for preserving the health status of rodents, the provisions relating to genetically modified animals must enable them to be kept confined to the outside environment and prevent them from escaping. Appropriate biosecurity measures must be implemented to prevent the escape or unintentional release of genetically modified animals during transport. Secure transport containers or vehicles shall be used that prevent unauthorised access and minimise the risk of unintended contact with other animals or the environment. Transporters must have contingency plans in place to address emergencies and be trained accordingly. Any special requirements or considerations related to the transport of GM animals shall be communicated to all parties involved.
Effect of phenotype and state of health (e.g. disease models)	Rodents' ability to cope with the impact of transport (stress, disease onset…) is typically impacted by the phenotypic effects of inbreeding, genetic mutations or modifications, age, and state of health. Inbred animals or those with a genetic mutation, or a condition that has been induced (to replicate a disease model) are less able to tolerate transport constraints. It is vital that effective contingency plans are in place for these animals to cope with likely delays. For instance, stocking densities during transport shall be adjusted depending on the animals' ability to cope with potential temperature fluctuations: higher density for juveniles to ease grouping, lower density for obese animals because their ability to dissipate body heat can be limited. Water, food, and bedding supply shall be adjusted to the condition of diabetic animals.

(continued)

Table 5.1 (continued)

Species/Species group	Specific considerations
Animals after surgery	Transporting animals after surgery requires special care and attention to ensure their comfort, safety, and recovery. Good recovery from surgery shall be assured before animals are considered fit for transport (Lynn Anderson in [22]). Should animals be transported in short delays after surgery, they should be closely monitored after surgery to ensure they are recovering well and to identify any signs of complications or distress. Transporters should be trained to recognise signs of pain, discomfort, or surgical complications, respond promptly with appropriate care, and report any abnormalities or concerns to the veterinarian promptly. Animals may experience pain or discomfort after surgery, so transporters should follow any prescribed pain management protocols and ensure that the animal receives any necessary medications or treatments during transport. They should also offer the recovering animal access to water and, if appropriate, small amounts of food during transport to support hydration and recovery, following any dietary restrictions or recommendations provided by the veterinarian. Transport accommodations should minimise stress and discomfort for the recovering animal. Transport containers or vehicles should be spacious enough to allow the animal to move and lie down comfortably, with appropriate bedding and ventilation. Vehicle or container temperature must be controlled and monitored to prevent overheating or chilling of the recovering animal. Handling and stressors shall be minimised during loading, unloading, and transit to reduce the risk of post-surgical complications or discomfort. Transporters should have contingency plans in place to address emergencies such as surgical complications, adverse reactions to anaesthesia or medications, or accidents during transport.
Pregnant animals	In general, pregnant females for whom 90% or more of the expected gestation period has already passed, or females who have given birth in the previous week shall not be considered fit for transport [6, 7]. For research animals as well, transporting pregnant animals shall be avoided to prevent additional complications related to transport. It is however sometimes preferable compared to transporting newborn or juvenile animals. Guidelines recommend that pregnant laboratory animals should not normally be transported during the last fifth of gestation, or even the last third in the case of rabbits, which are more prone to abortion [18, 21]. Before transport, pregnant animals should be assessed by a veterinarian to ensure they are fit for travel. Animals in advanced stages of pregnancy or experiencing complications may not be suitable for transport and may require alternative arrangements. Transport containers or vehicles should be spacious enough to allow the animal to move and lie down comfortably, with appropriate bedding and ventilation. Low stocking densities may be necessary for pregnant animals because of their limited ability to dissipate body heat. Pregnant animals require access to water and feed at regular intervals throughout the journey. Gentle handling techniques and minimal disturbances can help keep pregnant animals calm and comfortable during transport and reduce the risk of complications or premature labour. Transporters should have contingency plans in place to address emergencies such as premature labour, complications, or accidents during transport. Plans should include procedures for providing emergency veterinary care and ensuring the safety of both the pregnant animal and her unborn offspring.

(continued)

Table 5.1 (continued)

Species/Species group	Specific considerations
Newborn animals	In general, newborn mammals in which the navel has not completely healed shall not be considered fit for transport [6]. However, specific situations may occur where pre-weaned animals would have to be transported, along with their mother. Newborn animals are often sensitive to temperature fluctuations. Transport environment must be neither too hot nor too cold, maintaining a comfortable temperature range suitable for the species. Proper ventilation is essential to prevent heat stress and maintain good air quality within the transport vehicle. Suitable bedding or substrate should be provided to ensure the newborn animals have a comfortable surface to lie on during transport. This helps prevent injuries and provides cushioning during movements. Newborn animals shall be handled with care to minimise stress and prevent injuries during loading, unloading, and transport. Appropriate restraint methods should ensure their safety and security during transit. Access to food and water shall be provided as appropriate for the species and age of the newborn animals, so as to meet their nutritional and hydration needs during transport. The health and well-being of newborn animals shall be monitored throughout the transport process, being vigilant for signs of distress, illness, or injury, and taking prompt action to address any issues that arise.
(Mini)Pigs & piglets	For pigs that are to be loaded and unloaded directly in the transport mean (and not handled with crates), refer to "farm animals" (Mini)Pigs should have adequate space to stand, lie down, and turn around comfortably during transport. Overcrowding can lead to stress, fatigue, and injury. Bedding helps maintain hygiene and prevents injuries during transport. Bedding materials should be absorbent and comfortable for pigs. (Mini)Pigs shall be transported in transport boxes with a minimum of two other animals from the same pen of origin. (Mini)Pigs are sensitive to temperature extremes and shall not be exposed to extreme temperatures or temperature fluctuations. During transport, their environment shall be kept to a temperature between 18–22 °C, and 20–24 °C for piglets. (Mini)Pigs being very sensitive by nature, acclimatisation and gentle handling are particularly important for them. Habituation applies both to the initial familiarisation with the crate and other transport modalities before departure, and to the adaptation to the new accommodation at destination. It is important to approach them calmly, give them fresh water, food and bedding, and leave them time to get out of the transport crate themselves, at their own pace. Although necessary, the clinical examination can wait until the day after arrival, when interaction and socialisation with the (mini)pigs may begin. Piglets are more sensitive than adult pigs. Gentle handling is essential to minimise stress and prevent injuries to piglets. Rough handling can lead to bruising, fractures, or other injuries. Piglets should not be transported until at least 2 weeks after weaning, so they can eat dry pellets and drink water from a bowl during transportation. Current regulatory provisions allow pigs to be transported for long journeys only over a minimum body weight, whereas a minimum age limit would be a better fit for minipigs, as opposed to farm pigs to which the general case apply. Minipigs for laboratory use are frequently transported as young, weaned animals by road in rigid containers within climate-controlled vehicles.
Farm animals	For pigs, ruminants, and other farm species, acclimatisation, quarantine, and transport are key components of an integrated health management programme that starts with the selection of the breeder/supplier and ends at the user establishment to ensure regulatory compliance, preserve animal health and welfare, and relevance for the purpose of use [30]. Ensure that vehicles are clean, well-ventilated, and equipped with appropriate flooring, partitions, and temperature control systems. Loading and unloading facilities should be designed to minimise stress and injury. Ramps and vehicle floor should be non-slippery, with appropriate slope angles. Suitable ramps, chutes, or loading docks should facilitate the movement of animals onto and off of transport vehicles. Loading densities should be carefully managed to avoid overcrowding, and thus prevent injuries, heat stress, and aggression among animals.

(contttinued)

Table 5.1 (continued)

Species/Species group	Specific considerations
Dogs	Each dog should be properly identified Ensure appropriately sized container for the dog's breed and size, which allow the dog to stand, turn around, and lie down comfortably. Dogs should be transported in pairs (by air) or established, compatible groups (by truck), to reduce stress and improve welfare. Familiar items such as blankets or toys can provide minimum comfort to the dog during transit. Gentle handling, positive reinforcement, and fostering human–animal interaction can help reduce stress and ensure a better experience for the dog. Dogs should be given an acclimatisation period of at least 7 days following transport involving a journey in a vehicle and between sites, and at least 3 days when moved in individual containers between buildings on-site. At least 24 h should be permitted for acclimatisation following a permanent change of pen location, assuming a similar husbandry and care regime exist [31].
Primates	Primates requires special considerations due to their complex social structures, cognitive abilities, and susceptibility to stress. Studies have demonstrated that, as a whole, the process of international air transport and re-housing in laboratory conditions may result in the compromising of the welfare of the study animals and suggest measures to reduce stress and mitigate behavioural impact [32]. Early collaboration with the breeders and other stakeholders on the supply chain is of key importance to give full consideration to animal behavioural traits and social structures of the groups, as early as possible before transport and to allow animals to adjust as much as possible after arrival at destination. Primates are subject to national and international regulations governing animal welfare, conservation, and trade. Different species of non-human primates have specific physiological and behavioural needs that must be considered during transport. Containers should fit to animal size depending on the species and age. Crates should be designed and locked with primates' manual dexterity and agility in mind to avoid animal escape. Primates should undergo health screening and quarantine procedures before transport to prevent the spread of diseases between individuals and facilities. Handling and restraint should be minimum and gentle, so as to minimise stress and avoid injury for both animals and staff. Emergency situations should be anticipated and staff should be aware of health and safety instructions related to the specific sanitary aspects of handling primates during transport [33]. Upon arrival, quarantine shall be implemented with procedures that allow to preserve the social groups as they were established before and during transport (single/pair/group housing), and interactions between animals shall be carefully monitored to avoid problems of incompatibility and disrupted social relationships. Intervention, with minimal observation, shall be limited during a recovery time of minimum of 3 days at destination. Due to the variety of situations and the complex nature of these animals, ideal acclimatation time is not well defined for primates, but should at least ensure food and water consumption are normal, animals have normal behavioural patterns and interactions with each other, their environment and care staff [34].

(continued)

Table 5.1 (continued)

Species/Species group	Specific considerations
Cephalopods Shipping eggs shall be the preferred option, if possible.	Due to the lack of legal requirement or existing standards, professional organisations have developed their own guidelines based on the increasing level of evidence that fostering the care and welfare of cephalopods was needed, not only for their use in research [35], but also for their capture and transport [36]. Essentially: Transporting eggs should be preferred to transporting juvenile and adult cephalopods. Transport shall always be performed in well-oxygenated seawater, in appropriate volume and quality throughout the journey. Above 2 h, transport will be considered as long duration experience for the animals. Food deprivation (before shipment) and water cooling may be desirable practices to be considered. After transport, Care should be provided to avoid any difference in salinity and water temperature between the transport container and the environment where the animals will be placed. It is important to allow time for cephalopods to recover from transport-related effects, to acclimatise to the new conditions including possible differences in water quality, temperature, illumination, diet, and the shape and arrangement of the water tank. More work may be needed to assess and validate recommended methods, develop guidance, and implement training programmes accordingly.
Zebrafish Shipping embryos shall be the preferred option, if possible.	As for cephalopods, professional organisations have published guidelines for the housing and husbandry of zebrafish, including recommendations for transportation [37]. Specific guidelines for shipping zebrafish can be found online [38]. As for other species, but with specific relevance for fish, to transfer fish between institutions: safe shipment should be organised, compliance with fish welfare national and international regulations should be assured, and fish pathogens shall not be spread across borders and between laboratories. For genetically modified zebrafish lines, GM organisms rules shall apply. During shipment, the challenge is to keep temperature and water quality parameters within a suitable range in particular with respect to oxygen, CO2, and nitrogen. Shipment of adult fish shall preferably be organised with relatively low fish density. Reception and acclimatisation of adult fish must be well organised. Upon arrival, to preserve water quality of the new environment, and avoid ammonia poisoning, fish shall be transferred into the new tank using a net without transferring the water from the transport container.

5.6 What Are the Conclusions and Perspectives for the Future?

5.6.1 What Few Tips and Tricks About Animal Transport Can Be Used?

- **Key aspects to consider when planning lab animal transport—a check list proposal:**
  - Logistics, transport means and steps, live monitoring, and back-up plans
  - Security, preparedness, crisis management
  - Many applicable regulations (animal protection, hazards, CITES…)
  - Paperwork/inspections
  - Weather forecast, in all geographies, at all steps
  - Animal welfare, animal health
  - Transporters and handlers' health and safety
  - Public health…
- and bear in mind: Incidents do happen!
- **Documents**
  - At inspection posts, documents can be considered more important than animals. Animals may not be released if a document is missing or unreadable.
  - All original documents should be included with the shipment.
  - Save spare copies. Send copies to the recipient. Pack multiple copies of all licenses

with the shipment to prepare for loss at the borders…

- **Coordination and responsibility**
  - Journeys generally involve several transporters and brokers.
  - Overall responsibility of the organiser and individual responsibilities of parties involved must be clearly defined and agreed upon.
  - Develop local or institutional policies, guidelines, procedures, checklists, and working instructions to anticipate and address animal welfare concerns, security and safety issues (e.g. attitudes in case of vehicle accident, animal escape, bite or scratch…) and ensure they are read and understood, on a "need to know" basis.
  - Communication! Awareness! Training! Communication!…
- **Anticipation will be key to success**
  Anticipation is a must:
  - Because of the unavoidable preparation and coordination that are needed for each shipment.
  - Because animals will not be ready for use in research upon arrival, and a minimum acclimatisation time, if not a long quarantine period, will be needed for them to recover from transport.

What if …?

Although one fully recognises that animal needs may be particular, just considering an anthropomorphic view can help identifying a list of aspects that one should fully consider when planning an animal transport.

Just ask yourself "where do the animals I order come from"? and put yourself in traveller mode. How do you get prepared for an international flight? How long in advance would you book your flight and make sure everything's ready? How would you make sure not to forget your boarding pass, passport, luggage, and… drinks and snacks? How many hours would you have to leave home before reaching the airport and then wait and queue before boarding and taking off?? Was the taxi comfortable? Any traffic jam?

Were you allowed access to the "lounge" or did you have to wait in a crowded, uncomfortable, over- or under-air-conditioned hall, with a club sandwich and a hot drink from the vending machine?

I'm sure you have already experienced flight delay or cancellation…Did you had back-up plans or at least at your mind ready to think about Plan B should it be needed because you had to reach destination??

How much would you like to be cared for before boarding, during boarding and the whole flight, before and at arrival? And what if you had to take a connecting flight and wait few more hours ….? Wouldn't you treat yourself with a drink and a snack, hopefully in a comfortable and quite place, again …?

Just imagine … and make sure you still have your boarding pass and passport ready for next connecting flight … or you will get stuck … maybe for quite a while!

5.6.2 What Are the Perspectives About Animal Transport in a Changing Environment?

With the high specialisation level of breeding activities, the increasing demand in highly specific models such as genetically modified mice or fish, and the globalisation of research collaboration, the demand for animal transport has dramatically increased. Although performed by highly specialised transporters, this remains a very complex activity because of the sensitive nature of animal beings, of the variety of species with defined health and genetic status used in research, and the diversity of applicable standards and regulations. The complexity and challenges of transporting laboratory animals have been highlighted with recent and ongoing supply chain disruptions, contrasting with providers', transporters', and users' commitment to maintain high welfare standards [39].

To deal with the diversity of regulatory texts, and sometimes their inadequacies when it comes to animals used for scientific purposes, professional organisations have drawn up guidelines that apply specifically to this area. Although the legal requirements are bound to change regularly, as illustrated by the revision of the European Regulation initiated by the EU Commission in 2023 [5], it is unlikely that they will make much of an impact on laboratory animals specifically. It is therefore appropriate, not to say essential, for the community to get to grips with the subject, as with the specific recommendations for zebrafish and cephalopods. After all, who can do more can do less: applying the highest standards of animal welfare during transport, based on guidelines developed and endorsed by professionals and animal welfare experts, is a guarantee of quality and compliance that goes beyond the regulations, so that animals can continue to be transported to laboratories for as long as they are and remain necessary.

References

1. European Parliament and Council of the European Union. 2010. Directive 2010/63/EU of the European Parliament and of the Council of 22 September 2010 on the protection of animals used for scientific purposes. Off J Eur Union: L276/33-79. Directive - 2010/63 - EN - EUR-Lex (europa.eu), last accessed 11/03/2024.
2. Council of Europe. 2006. Appendix A of the European Convention for the Protection of vertebrate Animals Used for Experimental and other Scientific Purposes (European Treaty Series No. 123), Guidelines for Accommodation and Care of Animals (article 5 of the Convention). https://www.coe.int/en/web/conventions/full-list/-/conventions/treaty/123, last accessed 11/03/2024.
3. US Department of Agriculture, Animal and Plant Health Inspection Service. 2023. Animal Welfare Act and Animal Welfare Regulations. Animal Welfare Regulations, Part 3 - Standards. https://www.aphis.usda.gov/animal_welfare/downloads/AC_BlueBook_AWA_508_comp_version.pdf, last accessed 11/03/2024.
4. Eurogroup for Animals. 2024. Live animal transport: due time to change the rules. https://www.eurogroupforanimals.org/files/eurogroupforanimals/2024-02/2024_february_efa_live%20animal%20transport%20due%20time%20to%20change%20the%20rules_white%20paper_eng.pdf, last accessed 11/03/2024.
5. European Commission. 2024. Revision of the animal welfare legislation. https://food.ec.europa.eu/animals/animal-welfare/evaluations-and-impact-assessment/revision-animal-welfare-legislation_en, last accessed 11/03/2024.
6. Council of Europe. 2019. Council Regulation (EC) No 1/2005 of 22 December 2004 on the protection of animals during transport and related operations and amending Directives 64/432/EEC and 93/119/EC and Regulation (EC) No 1255/97. https://eur-lex.europa.eu/legal-content/en/ALL/?uri=CELEX%3A32005R0001, last accessed 11/03/2024.
7. Council of Europe. 2003. European Convention for the Protection of Animals During International Transport (Revised). European Treaty Series No. 193. https://www.coe.int/en/web/conventions/full-list/-/conventions/treaty/193, last accessed 11/03/2024.
8. World Organisation for Animal Health. 2023a. Terrestrial Animal Health Code. https://www.woah.org/en/what-we-do/standards/codes-and-manuals/terrestrial-code-online-access/, last accessed 11/03/2024.
9. World Organisation for Animal Health. 2023b. Aquatic Animal Health Code. https://www.woah.org/en/what-we-do/standards/codes-and-manuals/aquatic-code-online-access/, last accessed 11/03/2024.
10. International Air Transportation Association. Live animals regulations. 50th ed. Montreal: IATA; 2024.
11. International Air Transportation Association. 2024. IATA programs and policies – cargo – live animals. https://www.iata.org/en/programs/cargo/live-animals/, last accessed 11/03/2024.
12. European Commission. 2024. TRACES. https://food.ec.europa.eu/horizontal-topics/traces_en, last accessed 11/03/2024.
13. United Nations Environment Programme. 2024. Convention on international trade in endangered species of Wild Fauna and Flora. https://cites.org/eng, last accessed 11/03/2024.
14. Convention on International Trade in Endangered Species of Wild Fauna and Flora. 1983. Text of the Convention. https://cites.org/sites/default/files/eng/disc/CITES-Convention-EN.pdf, last accessed 11/03/2024.
15. Convention on International Trade in Endangered Species of Wild Fauna and Flora. 2023. Appendices I, II and III to the Convention. https://cites.org/sites/default/files/eng/app/2023/E-Appendices-2023-11-25.pdf, last accessed 11/03/2024.

16. National Research Council (US) Committee for the Update of the Guide for the Care and Use of Laboratory Animals. 2011. Guide for the Care and Use of Laboratory Animals, 8th edition. Washington, DC: National Academies Press (US). Available from: https://www.ncbi.nlm.nih.gov/books/NBK54050/, doi: 10.17226/12910.
17. National Research Council (US) Committee on Guidelines for the Humane Transportation of Laboratory Animals. 2006. Guidelines for the Humane Transportation of Research Animals. Washington, DC: National Academies Press (US). Available from: https://www.ncbi.nlm.nih.gov/books/NBK19637/, doi: 10.17226/11557.
18. Swallow J, Anderson D, Buckwell AC, et al. Guidance on the transport of laboratory animals. Report of the Transport Working Group established by the Laboratory Animal Science Association (LASA). Lab Anim. 2005;39(1):1–39. https://doi.org/10.1258/0023677052886493.
19. Canadian Council on Animal Care. 2007. CCAC guidelines on: procurement of animals used in science. https://ccac.ca/en/guidelines-and-policies/the-guidelines/general-guidelines.html, last accessed 11/03/2024.
20. National Health and Medical Research Council. 2013. Australian code for the care and use of animals for scientific purposes, 8th Edition. https://www.nhmrc.gov.au/about-us/publications/australian-code-care-and-use-animals-scientific-purposes, last accessed 11/03/2024.
21. Universities Federation for Animal Welfare. 2024. UFAW Handbook on the Care and Management of Laboratory and Other Research Animals, 9th edition. Editors Golledge H & Richardson C. Wiley-Blackwell. ISBN: 978-1-119-55525-4, 978-1-119-55524-7.
22. National Academies of Sciences, Engineering, and Medicine; Division on Earth and Life Studies; Institute for Laboratory Animal Research; Roundtable on Science and Welfare in Laboratory Animal Use. 2017. Transportation of Laboratory Animals: Proceedings of a Workshop. Washington, DC: National Academies Press (US). Available from: https://www.ncbi.nlm.nih.gov/books/NBK464310/, doi: 10.17226/21734.
23. Castelhano-Carlos MJ, Baumans V. The impact of light, noise, cage cleaning and in-house transport on welfare and stress of laboratory rats. Lab Anim. 2009;43(4):311–27. https://doi.org/10.1258/la.2009.0080098.
24. Pritchett-Corning KR, Prins JB, Feinstein R, Goodwin J, Nicklas W, Riley L. AALAS/FELASA Working Group on Health Monitoring of rodents for animal transfer. J Am Assoc Lab Anim Sci. 2014;53(6):633–40.
25. Capdevila S, Giral M, Ruiz de la Torre JL, Russell RJ, Kramer K. Acclimatization of rats after ground transportation to a new animal facility. Lab Anim. 2007;41(2):255–61. https://doi.org/10.1258/002367707780378096.
26. Arts JW, Kramer K, Arndt SS, Ohl F. The impact of transportation on physiological and behavioral parameters in Wistar rats: implications for acclimatization periods. ILAR J. 2012;53(1):E82–98. https://doi.org/10.1093/ilar.53.1.82.
27. Arts JW, Oosterhuis NR, Kramer K, Ohl F. Effects of transfer from breeding to research facility on the welfare of rats. Animals (Basel). 2014;4(4):712–28. https://doi.org/10.3390/ani4040712.
28. Stemkens-Sevens S, van Berkel K, de Greeuw I, Snoeijer B, Kramer K. The use of radiotelemetry to assess the time needed to acclimatize guineapigs following several hours of ground transport. Lab Anim. 2009;43(1):78–84. https://doi.org/10.1258/la.2007.007039.
29. BVAAWF/FRAME/RSPCA/UFAW Joint Working Group on Refinement. Sixth Report of the BVAAWF/FRAME/RSPCA/UFAW Joint Working Group on Refinement. 24 Transport of GM mice. Lab Anim. 2003;37(1_suppl):43–4. https://doi.org/10.1258/002367703766452967.
30. Berset C (Convenor Felasa Working Group on Farm Animals), Caristo ME, Ferrara F, Hardy P, Oropeza-Moe M, Waters R. Federation of European Laboratory Animal Science Associations recommendations of best practices for the health management of ruminants and pigs used for scientific and educational purposes. Lab Anim. 2021;55(2):117–28. https://doi.org/10.1177/0023677220944461.
31. Prescott MJ, Morton DB, Anderson D, et al. Refining dog husbandry and care. 15 Transport. Lab Anim. 2004;38(1_suppl):63–7. https://doi.org/10.1258/002367704323146219.
32. Honess PE, Johnson PJ, Wolfensohn SE. A study of behavioural responses of non-human primates to air transport and re-housing. Lab Anim. 2004;38(2):119–32. https://doi.org/10.1258/002367704322968795.
33. Weber H, Berge E, Finch J, et al. Sanitary aspects of handling non-human primates during transport: Report of the Federation of European Laboratory Animal Science Associations (FELASA) Working Group on Non-human Primate Health accepted by the FELASA Board of Management, April 1997. Lab Anim. 1997;31(4):298–302. https://doi.org/10.1258/002367797780596185.
34. Jennings M, Prescott MJ, et al. Refinements in husbandry, care and common procedures for non-human primates: Ninth report of the BVAAWF/FRAME/RSPCA/UFAW Joint Working Group on Refinement. Lab Anim. 2009;43(1_suppl):1–47. https://doi.org/10.1258/la.2008.00714.
35. Fiorito G, Affuso A, Basil J, et al. Guidelines for the care and welfare of cephalopods in research – a consen-

sus based on an initiative by CephRes, FELASA and the Boyd Group. Lab Anim. 2015;49(2_suppl):1–90. https://doi.org/10.1177/0023677215580006.

36. Sykes AV, Galligioni V, Estefanell J, et al. 2023. FELASA Working Group report: capture and transport of live cephalopods – recommendations for scientific purposes. Lab Anim 0(0). doi:https://doi.org/10.1177/00236772231176347.

37. Aleström P, D'Angelo L, Midtlyng PJ, et al. Zebrafish: housing and husbandry recommendations. Lab Anim. 2020;54(3):213–24. https://doi.org/10.1177/0023677219869037.

38. Zebrafish International Resource Center (ZIRC). 2023. Shipping Zebrafish Protocols [ZIRC Public Wiki]. https://zebrafish.org/wiki/protocols/start, last accessed 12/03/2024.

39. Kundu M. Addressing the current challenges of transporting laboratory rodents. Lab Anim (NY). 2022;51:210–2. https://doi.org/10.1038/s41684-022-01018-8.

Husbandry

6

Delphine Denais-Lalieve, Jean-Philippe Mocho, and Elodie Bouchoux

Abstract

Husbandry is a general term that gathers several aspects in relation to the housing and basic care of laboratory animals. In this chapter, we will explore essential aspects of husbandry for laboratory animals, emphasizing the pivotal role of optimal conditions to ensure animal well-being and care and to meet experimental requirements. It highlights the significance of providing animals with an environment that not only meets regulatory standards but also contributes to their welfare, while taking into account their respective features and specificities.

Some topics will also be discussed in other chapters of this book; reference to these other chapters is indicated.

Keywords

Husbandry · Housing practices · Food · Water · Sanitation · Care · Waste management

D. Denais-Lalieve (✉)
IRSN, Fontenay-aux-Roses, France
e-mail: delphine.denaislalieve@irsn.fr

J.-P. Mocho
Joint Production System Ltd, Potters Bar, UK
e-mail: jpmocho@daniovet.com

E. Bouchoux
Sanofi, Vitry-sur-Seine, France
e-mail: elodie.bouchoux@sanofi.com

6.1 What Are Husbandry Practices and How Can They Be Refined?

6.1.1 What Are the Links Between Husbandry Practices and Care of Animals?

Husbandry practices are defined as all actions performed in regard to the housing and basic care of laboratory animals. These actions are mostly performed daily to ensure the welfare of animals. Frequency of actions will depend on species and/or specific requirements linked to research models. They are also performed during the day in accordance with the working schedule of animal care staff.

Providing water, food, bedding, and enrichment (see Chap. 7 on Environmental Enrichment) are the main husbandry practices. These practices can also be viewed as an opportunity to interact with animals, creating bonds with them. Therefore, this could allow for habituation and training of animals. In addition, human–animal interaction is also a major component of the social enrichment.

Care practices, as other techniques and procedures performed on animals, are subject to continuous refinement. Practices could be discussed within the animal care staff, the Animal Welfare Body (AWB), or equivalent Oversight Body (OB), and even between establishments when sharing good practices.

J. Guillén, V. Galligioni (eds.), *Practical Management of Research Animal Care and Use Programs*, Laboratory Animal Science and Medicine 3, https://doi.org/10.1007/978-3-031-65414-5_6

Husbandry practices through the link established between animals and caretakers enhance compassion and impact the reproducibility of research data [1, 2].

6.1.2 Where to Find New Ideas for Husbandry and Care Improvements?

New ideas for husbandry and care improvements are often discussed at professional network levels. Discussions with suppliers and experience sharing with other establishments, either during informal meetings or as congress presentations and posters remain essential sources of information. Attendance to scientific and training events is encouraged since it constitutes Continued Professional Development (CPD), of which a minimum regular participation is sometimes compulsory. Reviewing literature, another source of CPD, provides the most valuable source of information when sharing new ideas within AWB/OB, in the view of husbandry refinement implementation within facilities. National and international networks and 3R centres (https://norecopa.no/global3r) propose websites and databases regularly updated with examples of 3R initiatives (https://www.ri.se/en; https://norecopa.no/; https://wiki.norecopa.no/) and selection of publications to dedicated topics. Laboratory animal science and technology associations also propose guidance (https://felasa.eu/; https://www.aaalac.org/; https://science.rspca.org.uk/sciencegroup/researchanimals) and organize congresses, webinars, and forum for experience sharing. For example, the Royal Society for the Prevention of Cruelty to Animals (RSPCA) (https://science.rspca.org.uk/sciencegroup/researchanimals/implementing3rs/refininghousing) and the Federation for European Laboratory Animal Science Associations (FELASA) are well-recognized sources for expert working group recommendations on housing, husbandry, and care management for a wide range of laboratory animal species (https://felasa.eu/working-groups) and education of personnel for that purpose.

6.1.3 How to Implement Husbandry Refinements?

Although implementing refinements is a must in the laboratory animal settings, we should consider the potential impacts of these on different aspects.

Refining husbandry practices can impact users by significantly increasing their workload. It can also impact the budget: cost of the refinement itself, additional cost needed to handle or set up the proposed refinement, etc. … New refinements would also require staff training and to ensure they accept the new technique and implement it.

For instance, the use of bedding materials (wood shaving, shredded paper, etc. …) in dog pens is well-known as an environmental enrichment, an enhancer in playing behaviour and provides a dry and comfortable area [3]. However, the removal of the dirty bedding increases workload or requires the purchase of specific equipment. Using non-aversive handling methods (i.e. tunnel and cup) for mice might increase workload [4], but with adequate training these methods do not add time to husbandry or procedures [5, 6].

Impact on research should be thoroughly assessed to avoid any interference.

Therefore, refinements must be evaluated on all aspects, considering a cost/benefit analysis.

Implementing a new refinement in husbandry must be an informed decision. This means that this would need justification of the costs, explanation of the expected benefits for animal welfare, training of staff, and daily observations. Once the refinement implemented, a retrospective assessment would help to decide whether this new refinement has a positive impact on the animals. Moreover, if the proposal comes from the ground, it might help all staff to adhere to the change. Ideally opportunities (e.g. regular meetings and discussions, suggestion box …) should be offered to staff to propose new ideas to refine husbandry practices.

This is also an important part of the continuous improvement of animal care and use programme. This topic could be regularly discussed at AWB/OB meetings.

6.1.4 What Are the Husbandry Procedures Required During Weekends and Times of Restricted Staff Availability?

In the European Union, the Directive 2010/63/EU [7] has set up a new requirement in 2010 for all animal facilities: "*Animals shall be checked at least daily by a competent person. These checks shall ensure that all sick or injured animals are identified, and appropriate action is taken*". However, daily tasks must be defined at the level of the animal facilities depending on the species housed, and precise instructions must be set up to ensure complete check of animals. It can be possible to add specific checks or actions on animals with special needs or requiring a clinical check.

Minimal tasks include actions to ensure that animals have access to food and water, that they are not in presence of dead or moribund animals, that there is no animal with obvious health impairment or sign of distress, and that their environment is suitably clean. In addition, environmental parameters must be checked to ensure they are in line with requirements. Usually, these daily inspections do not require handling of animals, and they have limited impact on animals [8].

A procedure for systematic check of defined points at the housing unit level can be implemented. This will allow to ensure full check-up of all housing units. Depending on the quality system in place, records of these verifications can be required. Checks should also include observations when entering room (sound, smell, etc.).

All these checks result in better animal welfare by avoiding any stress or suffering for animals.

Training of personnel in charge of these checks is crucial: if personnel are not correctly trained to recognize clinical signs, animal welfare can be impaired. Information on clinical signs and how to report them are available in a FELASA report [9] and could serve as a basis for internal training.

6.1.5 How to Refine Identification?

As group-housing is considered as the standard housing of animals, we need to be able to individually identify animals when required.

Animal identification is essential for traceability and research quality. The Directive 2010/63/EU shall not apply to practices undertaken for the primary purpose of identification of an animal. However, identification methods have various degrees of invasiveness [10]. As there is no gold standard method, choosing the most appropriate method would need to consider several aspects:

- What is the impact of the methods on animal welfare (e.g. microchip vs. marking pen)?
- How many animals to identify: at the cage/tank/pen level? at the batch level?
- What is the duration of the study (e.g. permanent vs. temporary)?
- Is the identification method compatible with the procedures (e.g. metal-containing tags cannot be used in animals undergoing some imaging techniques)?
- How frequently the identification will be checked?
- Is the identification method combined with a genotyping technique (only for rodents)? [11, 12]

Refinement of identification methods could be made at the level of the procedure itself: anaesthesia or restraint? use of local anaesthesia/analgesic?

New identification techniques are continuously developed by suppliers; therefore, staff is encouraged to seek information.

Note that for some species, individual identification is a legal requirement to follow their movements and ensure a sanitary traceability. A refinement could be to use this primary identification to track animals for experimental procedure and thus to avoid double identification.

6.1.6 How to Quality Control Husbandry Practices?

Ensuring quality control in laboratory animal facilities relies on several aspects: training, audit, action plan, indicators, etc. … A strong quality programme should cover all aspects, including husbandry practices.

- Training and competency are part of everyday life in the modern laboratory, and husbandry is no exception. Staff handling animals or responsible for cleaning duties must demonstrate competency, and continuing education will contribute to further enhance competences and knowledge.
- Records of all accomplished tasks must be completed and kept; this is essential for further investigation of contamination or any animal welfare concern, or data reproducibility.
- Standard Operating Procedures (SOP) are designed to standardize husbandry practices, and checklists are created to prevent mistakes and facilitate fast recording. Checklists are very useful to define tasks to be done on a daily or weekly basis. It could serve as a reminder to the team. To facilitate comprehension and implementation, it is recommended to design them collectively. This will ensure that the checklist is tailor-made to the tasks. Regular review of such documents is also recommended.
- Veterinary and clinical records, as well as morbidity and mortality or breeding performance are very relevant tools to monitor changes of pattern or to compare animal rooms or facilities. For example, a relevant indicator can be the proportion of animals euthanized on welfare grounds (i.e. having reached a humane endpoint) amongst the whole mortality, i.e. including animals found dead.
- Audits can be a useful tool to assess husbandry output in the animal facility. For example, the smell in the animal room, the cleanliness of surfaces, and the provision of sufficient environmental enrichment to all animals are useful indicators. Audits can be performed by several bodies such as AWB/OB or the Quality Assurance Unit. Rules for such audits should be set up. To ensure positive impact of such audits, reports should be done and made available, as well as a clear detailed action plan. Establishments interested in accreditation/certification schemes (e.g. AAALAC International, Good Laboratory Practices, ISO) must comply with further requirements ([13], see also Chap. 18). In addition, inspections regularly done by national competent authorities could also participate in this process. Action plan based on reports could be implemented accordingly (see Chap. 18 on Quality Systems).

6.1.7 How to Reduce the Environmental Impact of Husbandry?

The environmental impact of the care of animals in research is an ethical concern, in addition to other societal concerns on the use of animals for research. Laboratory strategic discussions on the topic should involve all stakeholders with sustainability in mind, for example when designing a new facility and deciding on husbandry, disinfection, sterilization, and biosecurity barriers. Accreditation schemes are available to assess eco-responsible laboratories, and the schemes are usually very popular amongst personnel. Resources are available to help identify new green initiatives (https://felasa.eu/about-us/library/3rs-reduce-reuse-recycle) or designate a green champion in the animal facility to lead assessment and initiatives (https://www.ucl.ac.uk/sustainable/staff/labs/take-part-leaf).

Specific husbandry concerns are consumables (e.g. single-use vs. re-usable cages and environmental enrichment items) and waste of energy and resources (e.g. routine disposal of diet and water). For example, reverse osmosis for automatic watering or aquatic housing systems may consume five times more water than a simple carbon filtered supply. The choice of a caging system, e.g., individually ventilated cages (IVC) versus open cages, solicits green global thinking since IVC reduce the frequency of cage changing but consume more energy for their ventilation. Autoclaving also consumes much more water and electricity than alternatives (e.g. washer equipped with thermal disinfection). Another concern has been raised by anaesthetists: the greenhouse effect of gas anaesthetics [14]. All these green initiatives can be re-grouped under a different 3Rs orientation: Reduce, Re-use, Recycle [15].

6.1.8 How to Adapt Sanitation Process, Including Disinfection and Sterilization, to Animal Models, Experimental Requirements While Avoiding Waste of Resources?

The animal facility can be split into different zones requiring dedicated husbandry practices. This defines the flows for equipment, animals, and staff in the biosecurity programme. Animal models are then attributed to the zone providing the husbandry conditions required to optimize the reproducibility of the animal model. For example, immune-compromised mice should be kept behind a bio-exclusive barrier, in IVC with positive pressure. Cages from this barrier are autoclaved before re-use and animals are never exposed to unfiltered air. On the other hand, for some models and colonies, immune-competent mice can be kept in open cages or in IVC and exposed to ambient unfiltered air during procedures. Cages used for this zone do not need to be autoclaved. But flows must be defined to minimize cross-contamination, for example to ensure cages from quarantine do not enter this zone, unless they have been autoclaved, etc. Such an organization, restricting biosecurity equipment to the necessary cases allows a significant reduction of resource waste. Cages still need to be washed, and if a further reduction of microbial load is required, the washer can be equipped with thermal disinfection, or a hydrogen peroxide chamber can be used, and resource waste remains well reduced compared to using an autoclave for every purpose blindly [16]. Regular assessment of autoclave, disinfection chamber, and washer performance is also useful to ensure the processes perform as expected and resources are not wasted [17, 18].

When designing the biosecurity zones, further questions must be asked for each zone: the need to autoclave or irradiate bedding, nesting, water, and food; which personal protective equipment should be used (e.g. disposable or not); how staff will protect themselves against laboratory animal allergens. Some barrier options may be costly and only required when very high containment is required. Spending extensive resources to afford such options may provide a false sense of security. Indeed, the microbiological status of the animal facility depends only on the weakest point of the biosecurity barrier, not on the stronger ones.

6.2 How to Adapt Husbandry Practices to Animals' Needs?

6.2.1 How to Enter an Animal Room?

In animal facilities, entering an animal room is done frequently: e.g., husbandry activities, daily checks, for study purposes, technical interventions. To avoid disturbing animals, human activities in animal rooms might need to be limited depending on the species housed. Rodents need a quiet environment during the day (as nocturnal animals), whereas dogs appreciate human presence.

The way to enter animal rooms could depend on the housed species. It could be recommended to announce the entry in the room by knocking on the door, so that animals are conditioned to the entrance. However, even before entering the room, animals may detect human presence (especially noise) and be on alert state. Knocking on the door could be done with all terrestrial species.

Before entering, some checks can be done to minimize the impact on the animals in the room:

- Check information displayed on the door (ongoing experiments, specific requirements, health status …).
- Check pressure if device is available.
- Listen to the noise coming from the room.
- Check the behaviour of the animals without entering the room through video surveillance or oculus.

Once in the room, additional checks can be done:

- Use all your senses: sight, hearing, and smelling.
- Smell the environment to detect any abnormality or change.
- Listening to animals can help detect aggressive behaviour or any other abnormality.
- Look at cages/pens/tanks and animals.
- Check any stain or leak on the floor or in the cage.
- Check the light intensity.
- Check if music is on and its volume (in case music is part of the enrichment programme) [19, 20].
- Check the sound of any apparatus including Heating, Ventilation, and Air Conditioning (HVAC) and water flows.
- Check any change in animal behaviour after you enter the room.

Finally, staff need to be informed and trained to these practices to ensure full implementation.

6.2.2 How Long Should I Let Animals Acclimatize to New Husbandry Practices and/or Facility Settings?

Following transport and reception in the facility, animals need to get an appropriate and adequate period of acclimatization to their new environment. Transport (see Chap. 5 on Animal Procurement & Transport) is a source of stress for animals, even if special care is in place to limit impact on animals. As collaborations between establishments tend to develop, the impact of the transport and the acclimatization to the new conditions should be considered.

This period allows for restoring homeostasis and having physiological measures return to normal and thus to avoid any impact on research results. Depending on the parameters measured and on the general state of animals, measures can return to normal after 1 to 7 days, but in some circumstances and/or for some parameters several weeks might be needed [21–23]. Therefore, a thorough review of the literature is needed before starting a project to define the best duration for acclimatization.

During this period, animals will get acclimatized to their new environment and surroundings: housing conditions, food/bedding, environmental parameters, animal care staff, etc. Special attention needs to be given to water, as some animals might not be accustomed to automatic sipper or water bottles [23].

The duration will also depend on the species [24, 25], e.g. minimal 3 days for rodents and rabbits, 7–14 days for dogs.

Finally, microbiome might be impacted by transportation. Studies showed that at least 1 week is needed to stabilize gut microbiota of mice after transportation [26].

By allowing animals to be accustomed to the new environment, better animal welfare and thus more reliable experimental results will be promoted.

6.2.3 How Husbandry Practices Impact on Microbiome?

The microbial populations in the gut or on the animal body constitute the microbiome and are influenced by the animal's genotype, immunity, and environment. The microbiome is mainly defined during the first weeks of life, when the immune system is gaining competency. Husbandry conditions in the facility of birth are therefore key for the establishment of the adult's microbiome. In practice, it means that animals purchased from different suppliers and different facilities have different microbiome. Differences in bedding, water, and diet can explain these differences. Once animals are set in the facility, factors like age, length of acclimation after arrival, housing conditions (IVC versus open cages) may also explain microbiome variation between animals and cages [27–30].

The biosecurity programme and husbandry practices will further influence the microbiome by allowing or avoiding cross-contamination between cages, e.g. IVC hood disinfection practice, breeding schemes, and equipment, staff and animal flows.

6.2.4 Which Rodent Handling Techniques Should We Use for Routine Husbandry?

For the past years, emphasize has been put on improving handling techniques to enhance animal welfare. Multiple studies have demonstrated that routine handling is a source of stress for animals [31]. Among improved handling techniques, we can cite tickling [32], tunnel handling [5], 3-digits scuffing [33], and animal training [34, 35]. By having positive impact on animal welfare, these techniques have also impact on experiments' reproducibility.

However, to limit variability, these techniques must be performed consistently among persons in contact with animals. This could be achieved through initial and regular training, as well as discussion within the animal care staff and/or the animal welfare body. This topic is subject to continuous refinement.

Regarding the change of animals or the cleaning of their cages/pens, depending on the species, this action could be performed differently and offers a way to interact with animals, such as playtime with dogs and human socialization with Non-Human Primates (NHP).

In the case of rodents, handling techniques are regularly refined, for example the use of cup handling or tunnel for cage change [4]. Improvements of the handling techniques aim to minimize animal stress. In some circumstances (animal in pain or impaired), specific attention to the way animals are handled is utmost.

These handling techniques might also impact positively on the human/animal bound by increasing interractions [36].

6.2.5 How to Train Users and Animals on Restraining Techniques?

Stress due to restraining techniques can bias research data [37]. Proper training and development of non-aversive restraining techniques present benefits for animals, for handlers, and for the reliability of experimental results (www.ri.se/en/what-we-do/expertises/3r-focus-on-animal-welfare).

There are several ways to limit impact of restraining techniques on animal welfare through refinements: gradual habitation to the procedure, training of animals to cope with the procedure without restraint, improvements made to the restraining devices to limit harm on animals, positive reinforcement, literature research, and staff meetings [38, 39]. The possibility to perform the restraint under slight anaesthesia could also be considered.

If an animal failed to cope with the restraining technique, it would be possible to not use this animal for the procedure requiring restraint. This animal could then be used for another procedure, not implying restraint. It could be interesting to record how animals react during and after the habituation or the restraint itself. Each animal reacts differently, and the habituation needs to be adapted individually depending on the progress of each animal. As for any topic in relation to animal behaviour, knowing the natural behaviour of the animals helps to better assess their welfare.

Implementing such changes has a positive impact on animals and on technicians as well.

6.2.6 How to Manage Exposure to Hazardous Materials When Performing Husbandry Procedures?

Waste products, including autoclaved waste, must be removed from the facility and disposed of to ensure a safe workplace for personnel and to prevent the contamination of work areas with waste materials.

This must be done in an efficient and safe manner. Staff must protect themselves and avoid contaminating other areas of the facility while disposing of waste materials.

Waste management will depend on the intrinsic risk of the waste: chemical, biologic, radioactive. As risk can be combined, the hierarchy of risks should be considered.

Risks need to be clearly identified and known to be correctly handled by staff: clear and accurate identification, staff training, and procedures established in accordance with the risk. Staff meetings before the start of such experiments could be useful to inform and remind good practices.

Husbandry practices could also be modified to ease the handling of the risk. For example, while animals are administered a chemical compound (e.g. tamoxifen), it could be decided to lower the cage change frequency to limit hazardous waste. Disposable cages could also be used when working, for instance, with isotopes, but the use of such cages has an ecological impact and might impact animals as well [40].

In case of accident, incidental exposure should be considered, and emergency care is tailored to the risk. The aspects are to be discussed and implemented in accordance with the risk assessment and the occupational health and safety (OHS) department.

6.2.7 How to Adapt Lighting to Animals' Needs?

Light in terms of cycle and of intensity impacts on the regulation of circadian, physiologic, and behavioural systems of animals, especially in animal facilities where usually there is no natural light [41]. Therefore, designing and building the lighting system of an animal facility should be adequately addressed, considering all parameters (light cycle, light intensity, distribution in the space and spectrum).

For animals housed in racks, such as rodents or rabbits, light intensity level can be different depending on location. Attention should be brought to animals at the top of the rack, and shaded tops could be added to limit light intensity, especially for albino animals susceptible to retinal degeneration [42].

Regular light measurements could be implemented to ensure avoiding exposition of animals to too high light intensity and to ensure that the light cycle is still adequate. This could also be done if some changes in breeding or in behaviour have been recorded.

When the transition between day and night is done, system mimicking dawn and dusk could avoid disturbance of animals, especially in large species.

The use of LED lighting is more and more common in animal facilities for various reasons. They are more environment-friendly and last longer, their intensity can be easily handled, and they do not emit ultrasound. All these features make them more adequate than fluorescent lighting [43, 44]. A particular attention should be paid also to the spectrum of light [45, 46].

Some facilities could also allow for work in reverse cycle, using red light to assess animal behaviour in various settings [47]. However, rodents are not red-light blind, and a period of complete darkness should be preserved [48].

Finally, careful attention should also be paid to any light pollution such as external window, flying insect control units, illuminated screen. However, external windows can provide enrichment to large species and be beneficial for personnel.

6.2.8 How to Adapt Husbandry Practices to Specific Pathological Conditions of Animals?

Some animal models aim to mimic human pathology or disease, and this might lead to physiologic and metabolic changes. In case of such adverse effects, tailoring of husbandry practices could be needed.

The better the model and its adverse effects are known, the better practices could be adapted.

For example, diabetic animals will urinate more frequently with larger volumes. Thus, they will require more frequent cage changing, higher quantity of bedding, and/or more absorbent bedding, bigger water bottles, etc.

Other husbandry adjustments could be like longer bottle sippers, food in the bedding, soft food, softer bedding, higher cage temperature, limited entrances in the room, quiet and dim environment, etc. … ([49–52]; https://focusonseveresuffering.co.uk/reports/).

These improvements could be discussed and decided during AWB/OB meetings. They can also be identified when performing retrospective assessment of projects.

Monitoring the effects of proposed improvements is of utmost importance whether they have a positive or a negative impact on animal welfare.

6.2.9 How to Adapt Husbandry Practices to Reduce Noise and Vibration?

The relation between noise and vibration is species dependent [53, 54]. Both can trigger stress and have acute or chronic consequences. Inaudible (for human) sounds (e.g. ultrasound), such as fluorescent lights, computers and screens, should be considered and can be mitigated by housing systems (e.g. IVC, light casing, anti-vibration pads). Acute noises can be reduced when performing routine husbandry tasks like feeding and cleaning.

For large animals, metallic bowls could be avoided and replaced by plastic or equipment less likely to bang loudly and warn far away lab mates that it is feeding time and to induce impatience. When cleaning pens, instead of exposing animals to the disturbance, they can be set in a separate playroom with toys and human interaction.

6.2.10 How to Implement the Use of External Monitoring, Digital Technologies, and Automated Systems?

Last decades have seen the development of digital technologies and their use in the animal facilities.

Video monitoring could be used to observe laboratory animals without unnecessarily disturbing them. It is particularly useful to monitor hierarchical and aggressive dynamics at group level. At cage and pen level, video is used in a species-specific context to monitor mating (e.g. opossum) and farrowing (large animals). It is also a useful tool to score behaviours due to environmental changes or procedures (e.g. rabbits hide pain from humans [55]).

Similarly, infrared thermography allows group and individual body temperature monitoring [56]. Radiofrequency identification (RFID) based systems allow an individual follow-up compatible with group-housing. Sensor plate systems allow the detection of the animals' location in the cage, the distance travelled, or other behaviours related to the animal's activity [57]. Such technologies are sometimes integrated into the rodent (mice) rack and cage structure to assess, for example, the circadian rhythm, the animals' behaviour, locomotor activity, or physicochemical parameters live in the home-cage [57, 58]. These systems enable a remote detection, without human interference, of these parameters and a 24/7 monitoring of the cages. Some of them can also be configured to send automated alerts concerning the housing conditions (e.g. bottle leak, bedding condition) and the animals' welfare (e.g. anomaly in the activity pattern). This "home cage monitoring" helps refine husbandry, care, and model exploration [59]. The next step could be the use of artificial intelligence in facility management.

As any recording system, it might capture people's activity. Therefore, personnel must be informed and reassured that the system is in place to check on animals, not on them. Legal aspects must be studied before implementing such surveillance.

6.3 How to Provide the Right Diet?

6.3.1 What Do I Need to Know About for Laboratory Animals?

Diet has many impacts on the scope of laboratory animal science: it impacts animal health, but also experimental results [60]. The nutritive quality is to be known, as well as type, form, and distribution mode. The food is to be adapted to the physiological status of animals (e.g. breeding, growth, maintenance), the age, the clinical condition, the body condition score. Animals should be fed with palatable, uncontaminated diets that meet their nutritional and behavioural needs, or according to their particular requirements (e.g. any pathological state).

Common diets can be classified into three main categories according to their ingredients and their level of refinement [17]:

Natural-ingredient diets are manufactured with agricultural products and by-products, therefore nutrient composition may vary, and contaminants may also be present. Most of diets in animal facilities are in this category.

Certified or purified diets have been tested for contaminants and can be used in Good Laboratory Practice (GLP) studies.

Chemically defined diets are made from chemically pure nutrients, and they can be used for studies on specific nutrient alteration.

Regarding species-specific nutrient needs, complete recommendations are available for some species [61]. These recommendations set up best practices on nutrients for food formula. According to species, some nutrients are essential or non-essential, as some species may not be able to synthetize some particular nutrients (e.g. guinea pig food has to be supplemented with vitamin C).

The whole process from the manufacturer to the animal facility including transport and storage has also an impact and therefore needs to be known.

Once you have identified and selected adequate composition of the feed, formulas and types are to be selected: pelleted, extruded, flaked, powdered, dry, soft/moist, supplemental fibre, live. Additional treatments could occur for storage and sterilization purposes: e.g., autoclaving, gamma-irradiation; however, care should be taken to preserve the nutritional value of the treated food.

For experimental purposes, specific food could be provided to animals: e.g., tamoxifen enriched food to promote a specific phenotypic modification [62], high fat diet to study the impact of such regimen on physiology or to induce obesity [63] and other diet-induced pathologies [64].

Finally, once you have chosen food for the animals, consideration should be paid in case the food is changed with trials to ensure a transition period, valid controls, and that the change will not impact further results.

Species-specific needs will be addressed in the further questions.

6.3.2 How to Preserve Nutritive Quality and Hygiene of Animal Food?

Storage can impact food and bedding leading to potential impact on animals or experimental results. The Directive and the National Research Council (NRC) Guide set recommendations on the storage of food and bedding [7, 17]. Particular attention should be made to avoid contamination or deterioration (e.g. pest control). A specific storage area with controlled temperature and humidity level is recommendable, especially with natural-ingredient diets and fresh vegetables.

Usual rules of storage apply: follow-up of stocks according to use, respect of expiry dates, first-in/first-out, check of integrity of bags/buckets upon delivery, etc.

Food can be processed to ensure longer shelf life and to limit microbial contamination [65]. Nonetheless, some nutrients are fragile, for example vitamins can be degraded by heat. Therefore, feeds destined to specific treatments (e.g. autoclaving) should be enriched in these nutrients and ordered specifically.

Double bags are often used to respect barrier rules. Feed can be transferred in various containers to ease distribution. This container should be regularly cleaned, and information about the food is to be kept, such as batch number, manufacturing date, and expiry date.

6.3.3 Why Is It Important to Take Dominance into Account When Dealing with Food Distribution?

Dominant animals prevent others to access food and water. On the opposite, dominant animals may spend excessive time and energy defending their territory and lose body condition compared to others. The dynamic is sometimes complex and must be analysed in the context of the whole building, pen, or cage.

For example, it is essential that farm animals have wide access to several water and feed troughs. If a narrow corridor leads to a single access point, a dominant animal can easily obstruct the way. The Directive 2010/63/EU sets access space required within the troughs, but the number and disposition of troughs within the building are sometimes a more relevant factor [7].

To take a canine example, dogs eat at different speeds. To prevent ration stealing, it is very useful to feed each dog in a separate area. The same applies for pigs and minipigs.

6.3.4 How to Make the Best of Feeding Time as an Opportunity to Check Animal's Welfare?

Feeding time can be an excellent opportunity to assess laboratory animal welfare and monitor their health and well-being. First, this allows for animal–human interaction, without necessarily entering the enclosure. Animals' behaviours can be closely observed, focusing on normal eating habits such as eagerness to eat, normal chewing and swallowing. Any abnormal behaviour, like reduced appetite, disinterest in food, or difficulty eating, may indicate potential issues. General appearance, individual and group behaviour (e.g. dominant hierarchy) can also be observed, and this will help to detect the need for routine care (claw trimming, dental care …) or further intervention. This interaction time could also be used as positive reinforcement.

Attention should also be paid to not disturb animals too much at this moment, as it might impact on its food intake.

When an automated system is used for food distribution, a specific time for the close observation of the animals should be decided.

Food distribution could also vary with time to ensure animals eat the adequate food ratio. A schedule could be food pellets in the morning and vegetables in the afternoon.

Finally, veterinary reason or experimental procedure could require fasting of the animals. This requirement setting needs to be clearly indicated and recorded. If only one animal is required as to fast in a group of animals, it may be advisable to fast the whole group. As a result, the animal in question can remain in the group and, if unsuitable, another animal from the group can be used.

6.3.5 What Is Specific About Rodent and Lagomorph Diets?

While choosing the right diet, nutrient requirements for rodents and lagomorphs first need to be known, and recommendations are available for each species [61]. The choice of a specific composition should be made upon the physiological status of the animals. Animals in breeding or just after weaning will require a higher percentage of proteins, in comparison with animals in stock or in studies. The sanitary status of the animal facility and hygienic rules are also to be considered: a specific treatment of the diet might be required before entering the facility. For example, diets could be autoclaved or gamma-irradiated. These treatments will impact the heat-labile nutrients such as thiamine or vitamin A, B12, and E [65], and some enriched diets are designed to compensate this deterioration. The choice of the food is of utmost importance as it might impact experimental data [66]; therefore, a literature search is highly recommended before changing a diet formula.

In most of the cases, pelleted food is provided to rodents: this allows for the densest and highest energy content per weight. This process has multiple advantages: less waste, less storage space, easy handling when distributed, better stability in time, less dust, and the diet's hardness induces the gnawing and tooth abrasion required to keep healthy rodents [65]. Extruded food can also be provided: the initial process is the same, but the pellets are expanded leading to a less dense food requiring more storage space. Extrusion allows higher levels of fat in the diet and more digestibility. Extruded diets are less hard to eat and more suitable for autoclaving. In some cases, such as post-operative time or for specific animal models, soft food can be provided. Powered food will be useful in case additives need to be added, or when using metabolic cages.

If animals are fed with a less hard diet for a long period (e.g. extruded pellets, high fat diets, soft food), additional enrichment items such as wood blocks should be provided to animals, and regular tooth checks performed.

Usually, food will be provided *ad libitum*, with regular check of the quantity in the food hoppers. However, in some specific situations, animals might be restricted to avoid excessive bodyweight.

When imaging techniques using bioluminescence are performed on animals, specific diets chlorophyll- or alfalfa-free are recommended [67, 68].

6.3.6 How to Ensure Access to Food and Water for Ruminants and Poultry?

For poultry, access to feed and water must first be adapted to the animals' age and height; it is thus adapted as the animals grow. Feed and water must be high enough to avoid soiling from feet, urine, and faeces, but not too high to ensure animals can reach them as necessary.

In ruminants, the challenges are mainly for adults where hay (or similar) and water must be made easily accessible, despite social dominance relationship. Dominant animals will prevent others from accessing key points like water troughs and hay racks. Therefore, corridors must be wide enough to allow free movement of more than one animal, and several water troughs are set in various parts of the stable. Access to hay should be wide enough to accommodate animals with horns, and numbers of hay access points must be higher than the number of animals to feed, to count for animals obstructing access for others.

6.3.7 How to Provide the Diet Right for Aquatic Animals?

Besides farmed species, there is little knowledge regarding nutritive requirements for other laboratory aquatic species. However, feed distribution must be controlled to avoid disease and water pollution and address animal needs.

Techniques to feed larvae are specific as animals can be more resistant to water chemical pollution and are over-fed at this developmental stage: tanks hold a condensed soup of nutrients for the first days of feeding. The rationale is to reduce energy waste by reducing movement and food seeking behaviour. Thus, water stream is reduced as long as larvae do not need more oxygen. As fish grows, water stream increases to restore oxygen and more suitable chemical conditions, and biofilm is removed to avoid build-up of pathogens [69].

Larvae are fed very fine diets and live feed (e.g. *Paramecium* spp.) that fit in their small mouth [70]. As animals grow, diet size increases. For predator species (e.g. zebrafish), live feed (e.g. *Artemia* spp.) is necessary to develop the corresponding behaviour (Aleströmet al., 2020, [71, 72]). When a change of diet is required, a smooth transition must be implemented; otherwise, enteritis may set and induce an acute gas production interfering with buoyancy regulation from the swim bladder. Buoyancy would then be disturbed for a few hours post-prandial; the clinical signs would not show the next morning before feeding.

When an increased feed consumption is sought, since stomachs are not expendable but may empty in a few hours, it is often a better option to feed more often rather than to feed a larger meal. Otherwise, feeding larger meals is likely to induce more waste and biofilm development, which would require more cleaning duties (i.e. no time saving).

6.3.8 How to Provide NHP with Appropriate Diet?

In their natural environment, monkeys spend most of their time searching food, mainly fruits, leaves, seeds, bugs. It is therefore very important to provide them with the opportunity to forage and make feeding complex [73, 74]. For instance, staff can put fruits or vegetables in places difficult to reach for the animals (feeder puzzles, or on the top of the grid in the aviaries …). Seeds can be spread in the bedding or in a foraging box if there is no bedding on the ground.

Laboratory macaques are usually fed with specific commercial pelleted food, distributed once a day in different points of the enclosure or cages, to avoid competitive behaviour. In addition, animals should be provided daily with various fruits and vegetables.

Pelleted food should be distributed separately from the fruits/vegetables, as it is less palatable. For instance, pellets are distributed in the morning, whereas fruits and vegetables are distributed in the afternoon. Fruits and vegetables should be washed prior to distribution. However, it is recommended to leave monkeys with the opportunity to remove inedible parts, and to "prepare" their feed before eating.

Food enrichment is essential for monkeys and can be provided by a diversity of fruits, vegetables, and treats, used in rotation according to a pre-established schedule. It is important to record what fruits or vegetables are eaten or not by the animals.

Sugar levels must be checked to prevent teeth cavities or abscesses. As NHP could also be subject to obesity, quantity of food might need to be tailored to the body score condition and other aspects [75]. Some species, like marmosets, are very sensitive to the variety of food provided and food distribution systems are to be considered as enrichment [76, 77].

Feeding time is a unique occasion to observe animals and make sure that all individuals are eating. Distribution of food might be adapted to ensure all animals are eating, while not disturbing the group cohesion.

Treats and juice can be used as a positive reinforcement and animals can be trained to specific tasks. Training the animals to drink to the syringe, for instance, can also be leveraged for the administration of medication with animal cooperation.

Staff can feed some monkeys by hand, which creates a positive human–animal interaction.

6.3.9 How to Provide the Right Diet to Carnivores (Dogs, Ferrets, Cats)?

Cats and ferrets are fed ad libitum, and group-housing means that it is often difficult to monitor individual consumption. Dogs receive one or two meals a day depending on their age and breed. They are fed individually, separated from others, and consumption should be fast, ensuring that others do not steal their meal.

In routine, dry diets are preferred for dental hygiene since they are designed to apply a mechanical action on the teeth and help remove dirt as the animal chews. However, soft diets can be useful to stimulate appetite and rehydrate or medicate animals when necessary.

Treats (e.g. ice cubes for dogs) can be used for positive reinforcements. Foraging and puzzles are particularly interesting for ferrets. When healthy, ferrets usually enjoy a wide variety of food and treats (e.g. egg, custard). When suffering adverse effects of an experiment, their behaviour significantly changes, they do not welcome as much human interaction, and they easily lose appetite or interest for novelty. It is therefore particularly useful to habituate the animals to eat the media used for potential oral treatment during or after procedure (e.g. oseltamivir crushed in custard when suffering from flu) [78].

6.3.10 How to Provide the Right Diet for Pigs Right?

When providing diet to pigs, frequency of distribution over the day is to be thought, as pigs will probably eat quickly. Feeding twice daily could allow for more interaction between staff and animals, enhancing bonding between them. Attention should also be paid to the dominance and therefore it could be advisable to distribute feed at several places in the pen, allowing food access to all animals. In some instances, it could be decided to singly housed animals during feeding time.

Pigs are also known to gain weight easily, thus providing food ad libitum is not recommended.

Feed quantity needs to be strictly adapted to gender, age, and weight, as recommended by the feed manufacturer.

Another way to provide pigs with food could be based on their natural habit for foraging. Food puzzle could be used, also providing enrichment, and enhancing welfare [79]. Hay can also be provided as a complementary high-fibre diet, and enrichment opportunity.

6.4 How to Adapt Water Provision to the Animals' Needs?

6.4.1 What Water Treatments May Be Considered?

Pollutants such as chloramines and other by-products of the chlorination process, pesticides, toluene and other volatile organic compounds, and some heavy metals are common in municipal drinking water and may have an impact on research and animal welfare. Also, despite being treated with chlorine, municipal water remains microbiologically contaminated. Therefore, the treatment of water supplied to laboratory animals can be relevant.

The first objective would be to remove contaminants (i.e. pollutants and/or microbes) from the water. Carbon filtration is the minimum to remove chlorine, organic pollutants, and some pesticides from water. Reverse osmosis, or more refined processes, can complete pollutant removal with action on ions and metals, other pesticides, and particles. When reverse osmosis is used for aquatic housing system, the water is either conditioned before entering the system or the recirculating water is dosed with salts to compensate pH and other parameter variations [69, 80].

Regarding microbiological control, de-ionization, reverse osmosis, ultra-violet treatment, fine filtration, irradiation, and autoclaving can be used to disinfect and eventually sterilize water. The issue remains of post-treatment contamination, starting with bacteria in the air. Disinfected water can be kept in reservoirs equipped with ultra-violet, before or after conditioning for supply to aquatic housing systems. For drinking water, chlorination and acidification are the two main options to reduce bacterial growth when the water is finally made available to animals. Acidification has the longest efficacy, whereas chlorine will either evaporate or react with residual organic matter, and active chlorine concentration will be reduced to nil in a few days in bottles or pouches [27, 81].

6.4.2 How to Monitor Water Quality?

Considering the load of chlorine, pollutants and microbes commonly contaminating municipal water, it is useful to analyse the water supplied to the establishment and to the animals. For example, pollutants are worth testing regularly to monitor the efficacy or life expectancy of the carbon filtration and reverse osmosis membrane, and to document potential impact on animal models [82]. These tests require specific assays, and samples are usually sent to a specialized water analysis laboratory. Alternatively, the water supplier might be able to provide detailed analysis to document the chemical and microbial quality of the water supplied to the establishment.

Chlorine content can be measured with dipstick or more precise electronic devices (preferred). Due to its capacity to evaporate, sending samples to laboratory for fine titration is challenging.

6.4.3 What Are the Different Systems to Provide Drinking Water to Animals?

Drinking water is always provided ad libitum. It can be provided in a trough, e.g., carnivores, ruminants, and birds, although waste and soil may contaminate the water and the trough become a medium of transmission for pathogens, e.g. coccidian parasites. Hence, poultry water troughs are elevated at increasing heights as birds grow. For other species, drinking waterspouts and nipples must be adapted to animals' species and size, i.e. mouth shape, strength, and flow.

Access to water is a key issue. This can be compromised by dominant behaviours, and the housing area must either be designed to prevent obstruction or propose several drinking points. Environmental enrichment, nesting material, bedding, and other housing equipment and items must not hide or be in the way to the water supply. A particular attention should also be given to enrichment in rodent cages with automatic watering, in which context the risk of flooding must allow be mitigated. If cage items are not chosen adequately, they might trigger the nipple continuously and induce a cage flood. Thus, when considering a change from bottles to automatic water, the whole cage environment must be re-assessed. The animals must also adapt to the new water distribution system; this is sometimes helped by triggering the nipple with a finger to ensure it works and to leave it wet. Animals must then be checked more frequently for signs of dehydration or drinking behaviour.

6.4.4 Can Water Be Used as Enrichment?

Water can be used as an enrichment in some species: e.g., swimming pool for NHP [83], shower for pigs, ice cubes containing fruits or vegetables for NHP, dogs, and pigs. Animals, especially NHP, but also guinea pigs, are known to love playing with water nipples. Attention should be paid to ensure nipples are not blocked or leak.

Moreover, for some species, such as ducks, geese, farm animals, or amphibians, the Directive 2010/63/EU requires to provide animals with a pool of specific size [7]. The size and the height will depend on species and on animal density, to avoid any incident.

As for any enrichment, the animal care staffs and/or the animal welfare body can propose new items and test it on animals.

6.4.5 How to Adapt Husbandry to the Housing Systems of Aquatic Animals: Static Tanks, Flow-Through, or Recirculating Aquaculture Systems (RAS)?

In all cases, it is essential to prevent contamination of aquatic housing systems by chlorine and chloramine, as aquatic animals are very sensitive to these chemicals. The supplied water must therefore be left to evaporate for 24-48 h to let chlorine evaporate, tested and/or filtered by carbon filtration and/or reverse osmosis before reaching aquatic animals [69, 80].

In static conditions, a frequent change of water is necessary to control pH and concentrations of nitrogen pollutants. Oxygen is provided with an air pump. In flow-through, parameters are dictated by supplied water and do not need action at the tank level but a good control of the supplied water. In RAS, the systems re-use the water after filtration. The daily system care is therefore mainly focused on controlling the filters, and dosing pumps provide the right water quality [69]. To prevent issues, aquatic husbandry must also consider the link between feeding and cleaning: for example, build-ups of algae can damage bio-filter and induce water chemical pollution, and biofilm accumulation increases infection pressure [69, 82, 84–86].

6.4.6 What Are the Filters in a Recirculating System?

Mechanical filtration removes solid particles. Bio-filter uses bacteria called bio-media to recycle nitrogen pollutants (ammonia and nitrite). Water exchange is mainly used to remove nitrate, in absence of denitrification systems. Ultra-violet filtration reduces microbial load. Carbon filtration adsorbs mainly large organic molecules, this is particularly useful to capture molecules that are released to the water by fish (e.g. residual anaesthetics), feed (e.g. phyto-oestrogens), or equipment (e.g. bisphenol A) [69, 80, 82, 87–89].

6.4.7 How to Control the Water Parameters in Aquatic Housing Systems?

It is tempting to supply reverse osmosis to aquatic housing systems to ensure the systems rely on a clean water—chemically and microbiologically. However, it can be very challenging to reconstitute specific water requirements, and a simple carbon filtration is sometimes sufficient to ensure a safe water supply [69, 80].

In RAS, pH is controlled by the addition of sodium bicarbonate as pH usually decreases with feeding. Water parameters are monitored by devices integrated to the RAS (e.g. pH, conductivity), and often the RAS self-dose until the chosen settings are reached. For species with more demanding needs, specific dosing pumps need to be added to decrease pH or reach the right levels of hardness or alkalinity. Conductivity is of lesser importance, unless the species is marine, and in that case the term salinity is used to indicate the quantity of salt in water [88].

Oxygen must always be provided in enough quantity, and carbon dioxide concentration must be limited. Most importantly, gas must not reach saturation point in water. This can be monitored with probes for oxygen saturation or total dissolved gas. In case of super-saturation, animals may suffer gas bubble disease, a lethal condition with often non-pathognomonic clinical signs [82, 87, 89].

In all aquatic housing systems, water parameters such as temperature and pH should be monitored at least daily. Salinity can also be very important for marine species, whereas other animals can usually undergo reasonable conductivity variations without suffering. Electronic probes allowing continuous monitoring are available for temperature, pH, conductivity/salinity, ammonia, and total dissolved gas; all relevant parameters to control, considering that increase in ammonia or total dissolved gas may kill animals [69, 80, 82, 87–89]. Water chemistry is monitored regularly, either daily when monitoring bio-filtration performance and resulting ammonia and nitrite levels, or weekly for stable systems (e.g. ammonia, nitrite, nitrate, hardness, alkalinity, dissolved gas). Water parameters can be tested by drop tests or electronic measurements. Dipsticks are not recommended [69, 89].

Pollutant screening and bacterial counts by serial dilution are useful to monitor the supplied or recirculating water. Dedicated media culture, microscopy, or PCR can be used to identify specific pathogens [81, 82, 86, 90, 91].

6.5 How to Improve the Animal's Micro-Environment with Bedding and Nesting?

6.5.1 What Is the Role of Bedding?

The role of bedding for laboratory animals is to provide a comfortable, clean, and suitable environment for their well-being. It should be adapted to their species-specific needs; giving them the possibility to express their behavioural repertoire. It has various functions: it absorbs excreta, is used for nest building, allows thermoregulation, and is part of the environmental enrichment programme. Like feed, bedding can also impact experimental results [65].

As for the food distribution, bedding change is the opportunity to check animals for their general appearance and individual and group behaviour, and to detect the need for routine care (claw trimming, dental care …) or further intervention.

Bedding change frequencies would depend on housing systems. Open cages will require more frequent changes, whereas in IVC, the frequency could be reduced. Several parameters are to be considered when deciding on frequencies: species, housing density, type of bedding, but also microenvironmental conditions (ammonia and CO2, microbiologic load) and animal behaviour.

Some rodent strains, such as diabetic animals, often require higher change frequencies due to increased urine production.

To minimize animal stress at bedding change, it is essential to transfer some dirty bedding and/or enrichment with its marking scent to the clean cage. Soiled bedding can also be collected for health monitoring (dirty bedding sentinels or environmental monitoring on in-cage filters). Bedding should be provided in adequate quantity, depending on species. Gerbils and ferrets will prefer large amounts of bedding where they can create tunnels. Thus, the adequate quantity of bedding depends on its role: absorbent material and/or enrichment. Moreover, the bedding type must be adapted to models and procedures like soft bedding for neuropathic pain, or cellulose bedding for post-operative care (to avoid slowing down the healing process and to detect any bleeding).

Bedding generates dust, and it is a hazard contributing to laboratory animal allergies [92, 93]. To mitigate this risk, the use of automated systems for dispensing clean bedding and/or collecting soiled bedding can be implemented. The bedding type must be chosen with care to avoid any blockage and clogging.

6.5.2 Why Providing Bedding Is Important for Mammals?

Bedding contributes to animal welfare in all species [65].

In the general recommendations of Directive 2010/63/EU, it is indicated that "*bedding materials or sleeping structures adapted to the species shall always be provided*" [7]. Therefore, if no bedding is provided, a sleeping structure shall be provided. Sleeping structure can be a solid and comfortable resting area.

Even if it is highly recommended to provide bedding, it depends on species housed, e.g. it is hardly imaginable to house rodents in cages without bedding. In the rare cases when bedding could not be provided (for veterinary or scientific reasons: e.g., fasting, use of metabolic cages, post-operative period), an increase in cleaning frequency might be necessary to ensure adequate hygienic conditions for the animals. When no bedding is provided, there is a higher risk of injuries, of pododermatitis.

It can be decided to limit the bedding to a limited space in the cage/pen, to limit the quantity provided, the workload, or any obstruction of the drains.

Providing bedding might be considered by animal care staff as additional workload, e.g. change, waste management. For dogs, if no bedding is provided, the pen should be cleaned every day, and if bedding is provided, soiled bedding should be removed daily. Thus, any change could have an impact. As for any change in husbandry practices, it is recommended to explain, to collegially discuss, and decide, and finally to accompany and ensure adequate implementation.

6.5.3 What Are the Different Beddings Available?

Bedding is an important component of the environment of the animals. Providing animals with suitable bedding and nesting material is an essential husbandry practice. This practice can lower stress in animals and improve their microenvironment [65].

The principal characteristics of an adequate bedding are dry, absorbent, dust-free, nontoxic, and free from infectious agents or vermin and other forms of contamination. Particular attention should be paid to the wood-based beddings.

Bedding can be classified as contact bedding (such as wood chips), in direct contact with animals or as noncontact bedding like the paper sheets placed under the cages. Both will collect and absorb urine and faeces.

Bedding is derived from plants like wood, cotton, and corncob, and it involves several processes such as chopping, shredding, or shaving, leading to a variety of beddings. There is also a possibility to mix different beddings, like shavings and granulate, or a mix of bedding with various granulometry.

Wood bedding can come from aspen, beech, maple, birch, or any mix of them [65, 94]. Materials derived from wood that has been chemically treated or containing toxic natural substances as well as products which cannot be clearly defined and standardized should be avoided to limit potential impact on research [17].

When choosing a bedding, several criteria are to be considered: preference of the animals [95], capacity to absorb excreta, ease of handling, dispensing and collecting, level of dustiness and exposure to particles as potential source of airborne contaminants [96], availability, storage and, of course, cost. The best way to select the most appropriate bedding is to perform tests to assess its adequacy. Like feed, bedding can also impact directly or indirectly experimental results [65, 97].

If a centralized vacuum system is in place, compatibility of the bedding with the system needs to be tested to avoid clotting and deterioration of the equipment.

6.5.4 What Is the Role of Nesting?

Several options are available as nesting materials: paper-based materiel such as paper towel, tissues, folded paper strips, or wood-based like wood-wool, wood-shaving (see Chap. 7 on Environmental Enrichment). The choice should be made according to known species preferences [98, 99], and via in-house trials too.

Nesting material and/or nest boxes are provided to animals to give them the opportunity to control their own microclimate. It could also give them the opportunity to withdraw from the whole group, especially around parturition, or in case of fighting or aggressive behaviour [100]. This could allow for the protection of the litter.

As other enrichment, nesting aims to reply to behavioural needs of the different species; however, the choice of the nesting should be based on the species preference. For example, rodents appreciate to manipulate the provided material and to construct their own nest, whereas other species (such as new world monkeys) prefer a nest box.

Nest construction and the complexity of the nest can be used as a welfare indicator in rodents [101].

Like for other enrichment, a strategy of assessment and validation should be implemented when using a new enrichment, as well as a periodic review.

Attendances to congresses and other meetings, but also publication review and discussion of practices is helpful to collect ideas, e.g. new materials or devices.

6.5.5 How to Ensure the Best Air Quality?

The purpose of ventilation at the level of the cage is to ensure that animals are kept in an atmosphere with adequate air quality, i.e. meaning dust levels and gas concentrations (e.g. ammonia) are kept below harmful levels for the housed animals. Same applies in pen and aviaries. The environment should be ventilated adequately to limit heat, particles levels, and odours for the animals.

The European legislation does not fix a rate for the number of air changes per hour (ACH); thus, common sense should apply. The most important is to ensure that the atmosphere does not negatively impact the animal welfare. Usually, a rate of 10 ACH is the minimal needed to ensure this [17]. The use of IVC is getting more and more common for rodents housing. These systems allow for high ACH level, up to 120. To achieve such a high rate, air is blown in the cage at a high-speed rate, and this must be considered to avoid any impact on animal physiology [102]. By blowing air, ultrasound can be generated, and they could disturb animals. Regular ultrasound checking in the facility could be performed, although no recommendations are provided [103].

The air provided at enclosure level can be 100% fresh air, fully recycled or any percentage in between. Recycled air can be an energy-saving solution, but it increases the risk of contamination, especially cross-contamination between rooms.

Ventilation is of utmost importance, but there are other ways to ensure the best air quality, e.g. regular bedding change, adequate bedding (that generates lower level of particles), air filtration in supply and exhaust, respecting housing density limits. Very limited recommendations are available to define limits in terms of air pollution or standards [104]. Therefore, performance-based approach should be implemented considering animal welfare and evaluating potential impact on animals.

6.6 Conclusion

In conclusion, while considering experimental requirements, it is necessary to adapt husbandry practices to meet the specific needs of the housed species.

Husbandry involves multiple factors (diet and water, housing, environmental enrichment) that must first be understood and then tailored with care to create a (micro)environment adapted to the species and the individual. Striking a balance between providing a naturalistic environment for the animals and meeting the demands of scientific investigation is essential for ethical and effective research. Through thoughtful consideration and constant refinement, the animal welfare and advance in scientific knowledge can be equally enhanced in a responsible manner.

Effective communication and coordination among animal technicians, veterinarians, and research team members are fundamental to ensure both animal welfare and the quality of scientific research. By maintaining open lines of communication, these professionals can share information and updates about the specific needs and well-being of the animals, which in turn allows for appropriate adjustments to husbandry practices and experimental procedures.

Moreover, proper communication helps in aligning research objectives with animal welfare guidelines and regulations, ultimately contributing to the credibility and reliability of the scientific findings. It also fosters a culture of care within the animal facility [105, 106].

References

1. Fontoura-Andrade JL, Amorim RF, Sousa JB. Improving reproducibility and external validity. The role of standardization and data reporting of laboratory rat husbandry and housing. Acta Cir Bras. 2017;32(3):251–62. https://doi.org/10.1590/S0102-865020170030000010.
2. Hasenau JJ. Reproducibility and comparative aspects of terrestrial housing systems and husbandry procedures in animal research facilities on study data. ILAR J. 2020;60(2):228–38. https://doi.org/10.1093/ilar/ilz021. Erratum in: ILAR J 2020;60(2):298
3. BVAAWF/FRAME/RSPCA/UFAW Joint Working Group on Refinement. Refining dog husbandry and care. Eighth report of BVAAWF/FRAME/RSPCA/UFAW Joint Working Group on Refinement. Lab Anim. 2004;38(Suppl 1):1–94. https://doi.org/10.1258/002367704323145742.
4. Doerning CM, Thurston SE, Villano JS, Kaska CL, Vozheiko TD, Soleimanpour SA, Lofgren JL. Assessment of mouse handling techniques during cage changing. J Am Assoc Lab Anim Sci. 2019;58(6):767–73. https://doi.org/10.30802/AALAS-JAALAS-19-000015.
5. Henderson LJ, Dani B, Serrano EMN, Smulders TV, Roughan JV. Benefits of tunnel handling persist after repeated restraint, injection and anaesthesia. Sci Rep. 2020;10(1):14562. https://doi.org/10.1038/s41598-020-71476-y.
6. Hurst JL, West RS. Taming anxiety in laboratory mice. Nat Methods. 2010;7(10):825–6. https://doi.org/10.1038/nmeth.1500.
7. The European Parliament and the Council of the European Union. Directive 2010/63/EU of the European Parliament and of the Council of 22 September 2010 on the protection of animals used for scientific purposes. Off J Eur Union. 2010;L276:33–79.
8. Clancy BM, Theriault BR, Turcios R, Langan GP, Luchins KR. The effect of noise, vibration, and light disturbances from daily health checks on breeding performance, nest building, and corticosterone in mice. J Am Assoc Lab Anim Sci. 2023;62(4):291–302. https://doi.org/10.30802/AALAS-JAALAS-23-000002.
9. Fentener van Vlissingen JM, Borrens M, Girod A, Lelovas P, Morrison F, Torres YS. The reporting of clinical signs in laboratory animals: FELASA Working Group Report. Lab Anim. 2015;49(4):267–83. https://doi.org/10.1177/0023677215584249.
10. Dahlborn K, Bugnon P, Nevalainen T, Raspa M, Verbost P, Spangenberg E. Report of the Federation of European Laboratory Animal Science Associations Working Group on animal identification. Lab Anim. 2013;47(1):2–11. https://doi.org/10.1177/002367712473290.
11. Bonaparte D, Cinelli P, Douni E, Hérault Y, Maas M, Pakarinen P, Poutanen M, Lafuente MS, Scavizzi F. Federation of European Laboratory Animal Science Associations Working Group. FELASA guidelines for the refinement of methods for genotyping genetically-modified rodents: a report of the Federation of European Laboratory Animal Science Associations Working Group. Lab Anim. 2013;47(3):134–45. https://doi.org/10.1177/0023677212473918.
12. European Commission. Directorate-General for Environment, Framework for the genetically altered animals under Directive 2010/63/EU on the protection of animals used for scientific purposes. Publications Office of the European Union; 2022. https://data.europa.eu/doi/10.2779/499108
13. Guillen J, Medina CL, Denais-Lalière DG. Assessment of animal care and use programs. In: Hau J, Schapiro SJ, editors. Handbook of laboratory animal science: essential principles and practices. 4th ed. CRC Press; 2021. https://doi.org/10.1201/9780429439964.
14. Jones RS, West E. Environmental sustainability in veterinary anaesthesia. Vet Anaesth Analg.

2019;46(4):409–20. https://doi.org/10.1016/j.vaa.2018.12.008.
15. Lopez JB, Jackson D, Gammie A, Badrick T. Reducing the environmental impact of clinical laboratories. Clin Biochem Rev. 2017;38(1):3–11.
16. Compton SR, Macy JD. Effect of cage-wash temperature on the removal of infectious agents from caging and the detection of infectious agents on the filters of animal bedding-disposal cabinets by PCR analysis. J Am Assoc Lab Anim Sci. 2015;54(6):745–55.
17. Guide NRC … Institute for Laboratory Animal Research. Guide for the care and use of laboratory animals. 8th ed. Washington, DC: National Academies Press; 2011.
18. McCormick PJ, Schoene MJ, Dehmler MA, McDonnell G. Moist heat disinfection and revisiting the A0 concept. Biomed Instrum Technol. 2016;50(S3):19–26.
19. Alworth LC, Buerkle SC. The effects of music on animal physiology, behavior and welfare. Lab Anim (NY). 2013;42(2):54–61. https://doi.org/10.1038/laban.162.
20. Barcellos HHA, Koakoski G, Chaulet F, Kirsten KS, Kreutz LC, Kalueff AV, Barcellos LJG. The effects of auditory enrichment on zebrafish behavior and physiology. PeerJ. 2018;6:e5162. https://doi.org/10.7717/peerj.5162.
21. Bundgaard CJ, Kalliokoski O, Abelson KS, Hau J. Acclimatization of mice to different cage types and social groupings with respect to fecal secretion of IgA and corticosterone metabolites. In Vivo. 2012;26(6):883–8.
22. Obernier JA, Baldwin RL. Establishing an appropriate period of acclimatization following transportation of laboratory animals. ILAR J. 2006;47(4):364–9. https://doi.org/10.1093/ilar.47.4.364.
23. Tardif S, Bales K, Williams L, Moeller EL, Abbott D, Schultz-Darken N, Mendoza S, Mason W, Bourgeois S, Ruiz J. Preparing New World monkeys for laboratory research. ILAR J. 2006;47(4):307–15. https://doi.org/10.1093/ilar.47.4.307.
24. Conour LA, Murray KA, Brown MJ. Preparation of animals for research--issues to consider for rodents and rabbits. ILAR J. 2006;47(4):283–93. https://doi.org/10.1093/ilar.47.4.283.
25. Meunier LD. Selection, acclimation, training, and preparation of dogs for the research setting. ILAR J. 2006;47(4):326–47. https://doi.org/10.1093/ilar.47.4.326.
26. Montonye DR, Ericsson AC, Busi SB, Lutz C, Wardwell K, Franklin CL. Acclimation and institutionalization of the mouse microbiota following transportation. Front Microbiol. 2018;9:1085. https://doi.org/10.3389/fmicb.2018.01085.
27. Bidot WA, Ericsson AC, Franklin CL. Effects of water decontamination methods and bedding material on the gut microbiota. PLoS One. 2018;13(10):e0198305. https://doi.org/10.1371/journal.pone.0198305.
28. Ericsson AC, Davis JW, Spollen W, Bivens N, Givan S, Hagan CE, et al. Effects of vendor and genetic background on the composition of the fecal microbiota of inbred mice. PLoS One. 2015;10(2):e0116704. https://doi.org/10.1371/journal.pone.0116704.
29. Ericsson AC, Gagliardi J, Bouhan D, Spollen WG, Givan SA, Franklin CL. The influence of caging, bedding, and diet on the composition of the microbiota in different regions of the mouse gut. Sci Rep. 2018;8(1):4065. https://doi.org/10.1038/s41598-018-21986-7.
30. Long LL, Svenson KL, Mourino AJ, Michaud M, Fahey JR, Waterman L, Vandegrift KL, Adams MD. Shared and distinctive features of the gut microbiome of C57BL/6 mice from different vendors and production sites, and in response to a new vivarium. Lab Anim (NY). 2021;50(7):185–95. https://doi.org/10.1038/s41684-021-00777-0.
31. Balcombe JP, Barnard ND, Sandusky C. Laboratory routines cause animal stress. Contemp Top Lab Anim Sci. 2004;43(6):42–51.
32. LaFollette MR, O'Haire ME, Cloutier S, Blankenberger WB, Gaskill BN. Rat tickling: a systematic review of applications, outcomes, and moderators. PLoS One. 2017;12(4):e0175320. https://doi.org/10.1371/journal.pone.0175320.
33. Norecopa. Video “Three fingers better than two“. 2021. Available: https://vimeo.com/290857433 (27/07/2021)
34. Hanson LR, Fine JM, Svitak AL, Faltesek KA. Intranasal administration of CNS therapeutics to awake mice. J Vis Exp. 2013;74:4440. https://doi.org/10.3791/4440.
35. O’Malley CI, Hubley R, Moody C, Turner PV. Use of nonaversive handling and training procedures for laboratory mice and rats: attitudes of American and Canadian laboratory animal professionals. Front Vet Sci. 2022;9:1040572. https://doi.org/10.3389/fvets.2022.1040572.
36. Neely C, Lane C, Torres J, Flinn J. The effect of gentle handling on depressive-like behavior in adult male mice: considerations for human and rodent interactions in the laboratory. Behav Neurol. 2018;2018:2976014. https://doi.org/10.1155/2018/2976014.
37. Labitt RN, Oxford EM, Davis AK, Butler SD, Daugherity EK. A validated smartphone-based electrocardiogram reveals severe bradyarrhythmias during immobilizing restraint in mice of both sexes and four strains. J Am Assoc Lab Anim Sci. 2021;60(2):201–12. https://doi.org/10.30802/AALAS-JAALAS-20-000069.
38. Hall LE, Robinson S, Buchanan-Smith HM. Refining dosing by oral gavage in the dog: a protocol to harmonise welfare. J Pharmacol Toxicol Methods. 2015;72:35–46. https://doi.org/10.1016/j.vascn.2014.12.007.
39. McMillan J, Bloomsmith MA, Prescott MJ. An international survey of approaches to chair

restraint of nonhuman primates. Comp Med. 2017;67(5):442–51.
40. Ferguson DR, Bailey MM. Reproductive performance of mice in disposable and standard individually ventilated cages. J Am Assoc Lab Anim Sci. 2013;52(3):228–32.
41. Dauchy RT, Blask DE. Vivarium lighting as an important extrinsic factor influencing animal-based research. J Am Assoc Lab Anim Sci. 2023;62(1):3–25. https://doi.org/10.30802/AALAS-JAALAS-23-000003.
42. Li F, Cao W, Anderson RE. Protection of photoreceptor cells in adult rats from light-induced degeneration by adaptation to bright cyclic light. Exp Eye Res. 2001;73(4):569–77. https://doi.org/10.1006/exer.2001.1068.
43. Allen AA, Pierce AT, Dauchy RT, Voros GB, Dobek GL. Influence of light phase exposure to LED lighting on circadian levels of neuroendocrine hormones in Sprague-Dawley rats. J Am Assoc Lab Anim Sci. 2022;61(4):333–43. https://doi.org/10.30802/AALAS-JAALAS-21-000123.
44. Voros GB, Dauchy RT, Myers L, Hill SM, Blask DE, Dobek GL. Effects of daytime blue-enriched LED light on physiologic parameters of three common mouse strains maintained on an IVC system. J Am Assoc Lab Anim Sci. 2021;60(3):259–71. https://doi.org/10.30802/AALAS-JAALAS-20-000109.
45. de Alba G, Carrillo S, Sánchez-Vázquez FJ, López-Olmeda JF. Combined blue light and daily thermocycles enhance zebrafish growth and development. J Exp Zool A Ecol Integr Physiol. 2022;337(5):501–15. https://doi.org/10.1002/jez.2584.
46. Jaadane I, Boulenguez P, Chahory S, Carré S, Savoldelli M, Jonet L, Behar-Cohen F, Martinsons C, Torriglia A. Retinal damage induced by commercial light emitting diodes (LEDs). Free Radic Biol Med. 2015;84:373–84. https://doi.org/10.1016/j.freeradbiomed.2015.03.034.
47. Yang M, Weber MD, Crawley JN. Light phase testing of social behaviors: not a problem. Front Neurosci. 2008;2(2):186–91. https://doi.org/10.3389/neuro.01.029.2008.
48. Niklaus S, Albertini S, Schnitzer TK, Denk N. Challenging a myth and misconception: red-light vision in rats. Animals (Basel). 2020;10(3):422. https://doi.org/10.3390/ani10030422.
49. Daniels Gatward LF, Kennard MR, Smith LIF, King AJF. The use of mice in diabetes research: the impact of physiological characteristics, choice of model and husbandry practices. Diabet Med. 2021;38(12):e14711. https://doi.org/10.1111/dme.14711.
50. Hawkins P, Armstrong R, Boden T, Garside P, Knight K, Lilley E, Seed M, Wilkinson M, Williams RO. Applying refinement to the use of mice and rats in rheumatoid arthritis research. Inflammopharmacology. 2015;23(4):131–50. https://doi.org/10.1007/s10787-015-0241-4.
51. Lilley E, Andrews MR, Bradbury EJ, Elliott H, Hawkins P, Ichiyama RM, Keeley J, Michael-Titus AT, Moon LDF, Pluchino S, Riddell J, Ryder K, Yip PK. Refining rodent models of spinal cord injury. Exp Neurol. 2020;328:113273. https://doi.org/10.1016/j.expneurol.2020.113273.
52. Wolfensohn S, Hawkins P, Lilley E, Anthony D, Chambers C, Lane S, Lawton M, Robinson S, Voipio HM, Woodhall G. Reducing suffering in animal models and procedures involving seizures, convulsions and epilepsy. J Pharmacol Toxicol Methods. 2013;67(1):9–15. https://doi.org/10.1016/j.vascn.2012.09.001.
53. Lara RA, Vasconcelos RO. Characterization of the natural soundscape of Zebrafish and comparison with the captive noise conditions. Zebrafish. 2019;16(2):152–64. https://doi.org/10.1089/zeb.2018.1654.
54. Turner JG. Noise and vibration in the vivarium: recommendations for developing a measurement plan. J Am Assoc Lab Anim Sci. 2020;59(6):665–72. https://doi.org/10.30802/AALAS-JAALAS-19-000131.
55. Pinho RH, Justo AA, Cima DS, Fonseca MW, Minto BW, Rocha FDL, Leach MC, Luna SPL. Effects of human observer presence on pain assessment using facial expressions in rabbits. J Am Assoc Lab Anim Sci. 2023;62(1):81–6. https://doi.org/10.30802/AALAS-JAALAS-22-000056.
56. Franco NH, Gerós A, Oliveira L, Olsson IAS, Aguiar P. ThermoLabAnimal - a high-throughput analysis software for non-invasive thermal assessment of laboratory mice. Physiol Behav. 2019;207:113–21. https://doi.org/10.1016/j.physbeh.2019.05.004.
57. Voikar V, Gaburro S. Three pillars of automated home-cage phenotyping of mice: novel findings, refinement, and reproducibility based on literature and experience. Front Behav Neurosci. 2020;14:575434. https://doi.org/10.3389/fnbeh.2020.575434.
58. Baran SW, Bratcher N, Dennis J, Gaburro S, Karlsson EM, Maguire S, Makidon P, Noldus LPJJ, Potier Y, Rosati G, Ruiter M, Schaevitz L, Sweeney P, LaFollette MR. Emerging role of translational digital biomarkers within home cage monitoring technologies in preclinical drug discovery and development. Front Behav Neurosci. 2022;15:758274. https://doi.org/10.3389/fnbeh.2021.758274.
59. Golini E, Rigamonti M, Raspa M, Scavizzi F, Falcone G, Gourdon G, Mandillo S. Excessive rest time during active phase is reliably detected in a mouse model of myotonic dystrophy type 1 using home cage monitoring. Front Behav Neurosci. 2023;17:1130055. https://doi.org/10.3389/fnbeh.2023.1130055.
60. Baker DA, Lipman NS. Factors that can influence animal research. In: Fox JG, Anderson LC, Otto G, Pritchett-Corning KR, Whary MT, editors. Laboratory animal medicine. 3rd ed. Oxford: Academic Press; 2015. p. 1441–96.

61. National Research Council (US) Subcommittee on Laboratory Animal Nutrition. *Nutrient Requirements of Laboratory Animals*: Fourth Revised Edition. Washington, DC: National Academies Press; 1995.
62. Yoshinobu K, Araki M, Morita A, Araki M, Kokuba S, Nakagata N, Araki K. Tamoxifen feeding method is suitable for efficient conditional knockout. Exp Anim. 2021;70(1):91–100. https://doi.org/10.1538/expanim.19-0138.
63. Speakman J, Hambly C, Mitchell S, Król E. Animal models of obesity. Obes Rev. 2007;8(Suppl 1):55–61. https://doi.org/10.1111/j.1467-789X.2007.00319.x.
64. Dube P, Aradhyula V, Lad A, Khalaf FK, Breidenbach JD, Kashaboina E, Gorthi S, Varatharajan S, Stevens TW, Connolly JA, Soehnlen SM, Sood A, Marellapudi A, Ranabothu M, Kleinhenz AL, Domenig O, Dworkin LD, Malhotra D, Haller ST, Kennedy DJ. Novel model of oxalate diet-induced chronic kidney disease in Dahl-salt-sensitive rats. Int J Mol Sci. 2023;24(12):10062. https://doi.org/10.3390/ijms241210062.
65. Carter RL, Lipman NS. Feed and bedding, Chapter 27. In: Weichbrod RH, Thompson GA, Norton JN, editors. Management of animal care and use programs in research, education, and testing. 2nd ed. Boca Raton, FL: CRC Press/Taylor & Francis; 2018.
66. Pellizzon MA, Ricci MR. Choice of laboratory rodent diet may confound data interpretation and reproducibility. Curr Dev Nutr. 2020;4(4):nzaa031. https://doi.org/10.1093/cdn/nzaa031.
67. Bhaumik S, DePuy J, Klimash J. Strategies to minimize background autofluorescence in live mice during noninvasive fluorescence optical imaging. Lab Anim (NY). 2007;36(8):40–3. https://doi.org/10.1038/laban0907-40.
68. Inoue Y, Izawa K, Kiryu S, Tojo A, Ohtomo K. Diet and abdominal autofluorescence detected by in vivo fluorescence imaging of living mice. Mol Imaging. 2008;7(1):21–7.
69. Aleström P, D'Angelo L, Midtlyng PJ, Schorderet DF, Schulte-Merker S, Sohm F, Warner S. Zebrafish: housing and husbandry recommendations. Lab Anim. 2020;54(3):213–24. https://doi.org/10.1177/0023677219869037.
70. Harper C, Lawrence C, editors. The laboratory zebrafish. Boca Raton, FL: CRC Press; 2011.
71. Filosa A, Barker AJ, Dal Maschio M, Baier H. Feeding state modulates behavioral choice and processing of prey stimuli in the zebrafish tectum. Neuron. 2016;90(3):596–608. https://doi.org/10.1016/j.neuron.2016.03.014.
72. Gerlai R. Reproducibility and replicability in zebrafish behavioral neuroscience research. Pharmacol Biochem Behav. 2019;178:30–8. https://doi.org/10.1016/j.pbb.2018.02.005.
73. Gore MA. Effects of food distribution on foraging competition in rhesus monkeys, *Macaca mulatta*, and hamadryas baboons, *Papio hamadryas*. Animal Behaviour. 1993;45(4):773–86. https://doi.org/10.1006/anbe.1993.1091.
74. Jennings M, Prescott MJ; Members of the Joint Working Group on Refinement (Primates); Buchanan-Smith HM, Gamble MR, Gore M, Hawkins P, Hubrecht R, Hudson S, Jennings M, Keeley JR, Morris K, Morton DB, Owen S, Pearce PC, Prescott MJ, Robb D, Rumble RJ, Wolfensohn S, Buist D. Refinements in husbandry, care and common procedures for non-human primates: Ninth report of the BVAAWF/FRAME/RSPCA/UFAW Joint Working Group on Refinement. Lab Anim. 2009;43(Suppl 1):1–47. https://doi.org/10.1258/la.2008.007143.
75. Bauer SA, Pearl DL, Leslie KE, Fournier J, Turner PV. Causes of obesity in captive cynomolgus macaques: influence of body condition, social and management factors on behaviour around feeding. Lab Anim. 2012;46(3):193–9. https://doi.org/10.1258/la.2012.011120.
76. Layne DG, Power RA. Husbandry, handling, and nutrition for marmosets. Comp Med. 2003;53(4):351–9.
77. Roberts RL, Roytburd LA, Newman JD. Puzzle feeders and gum feeders as environmental enrichment for common marmosets. Contemp Top Lab Anim Sci. 1999;38(5):27–31.
78. Reddy MB, Yang KH, Rao G, Rayner CR, Nie J, Pamulapati C, Marathe BM, Forrest A, Govorkova EA. Oseltamivir population pharmacokinetics in the ferret: model application for pharmacokinetic/pharmacodynamic study design. PLoS One. 2015;10(10):e0138069. https://doi.org/10.1371/journal.pone.0138069.
79. Huntsberry ME, Charles D, Adams KM, Weed JL. The foraging ball as a quick and easy enrichment device for pigs (*Sus scrofa*). Lab Anim (NY). 2008;37(9):411–4. https://doi.org/10.1038/laban0908-411.
80. Green SL, editor. The laboratory Xenopus sp. Boca Raton, FL: CRC Press; 2010. Supplementary
81. Molk DM, Karr-May CL, Trang ED, Sanders GE. Sanitization of an automatic reverse-osmosis watering system: removal of a clinically significant biofilm. J Am Assoc Lab Anim Sci. 2013;52(2):197–205.
82. Mocho JP, Collymore C, Farmer SC, Leguay E, Murray KN, Pereira N. FELASA-AALAS recommendations for monitoring and reporting of laboratory fish diseases and health status, with an emphasis on zebrafish (*Danio Rerio*). Comp Med. 2022;72(3):127–48. https://doi.org/10.30802/AALAS-CM-22-000034.
83. Robins JG, Waitt CD. Improving the welfare of captive macaques (Macaca sp.) through the use of water as enrichment. J Appl Anim Welf Sci. 2011;14(1):75–84. https://doi.org/10.1080/10888705.2011.527605.
84. Chang CT, Lewis J, Whipps CM. Source or sink: examining the role of biofilms in transmission of mycobacterium spp. in laboratory zebrafish. Zebrafish. 2019;16(2):197–206. https://doi.org/10.1089/zeb.2018.1689.

85. Mason T, Snell K, Mittge E, Melancon E, Montgomery R, McFadden M, Camoriano J, Kent ML, Whipps CM, Peirce J. Strategies to mitigate a *Mycobacterium marinum* outbreak in a zebrafish research facility. Zebrafish. 2016;13(Suppl 1):S77–87. https://doi.org/10.1089/zeb.2015.1218.
86. Mocho JP. Three-dimensional screen: a comprehensive approach to the health monitoring of zebrafish. Zebrafish. 2016;13(Suppl 1):S132–7. https://doi.org/10.1089/zeb.2015.1200.
87. Cartner SC, Eisen JS, Farmer SC, Guillemin KJ, Kent ML, Sanders GE, editors. The zebrafish in biomedical research. San Diego, CA: Elsevier; 2020.
88. Ostrander GK, editor. The laboratory fish. San Diego, CA: Academic Press; 2000.
89. Wildgoose WH, editor. BSAVA manual of ornamental fish. 2nd ed. Gloucester: British Small Animal Veterinary Association; 2001.
90. Collymore C, Giuliano F, Banks EK. Head tilt in immunodeficient mice due to contamination of drinking water by *Burkholderia gladioli*. J Am Assoc Lab Anim Sci. 2019;58(2):246–50. https://doi.org/10.30802/AALAS-JAALAS-18-000106.
91. Mocho JP, Martin DJ, Millington ME, Saavedra TY. Environmental screening of *Aeromonas hydrophila*, *Mycobacterium* spp., and *Pseudocapillaria tomentosa* in zebrafish systems. J Vis Exp. 2017;130 https://doi.org/10.3791/55306.
92. Bush RK, Stave GM. Laboratory animal allergy: an update. ILAR J. 2003;44(1):28–51. https://doi.org/10.1093/ilar.44.1.28.
93. Stave GM. Occupational animal allergy. Curr Allergy Asthma Rep. 2018;18(2):11. https://doi.org/10.1007/s11882-018-0755-0.
94. Potgieter FJ, Wilke PI. Laboratory animal bedding: a review of specifications and requirements. J S Afr Vet Assoc. 1991;62(3):143–6.
95. Blom HJ, Van Tintelen G, Van Vorstenbosch CJ, Baumans V, Beynen AC. Preferences of mice and rats for types of bedding material. Lab Anim. 1996;30(3):234–44. https://doi.org/10.1258/002367796780684890.
96. Kaliste E, Linnainmaa M, Meklin T, Torvinen E, Nevalainen A. The bedding of laboratory animals as a source of airborne contaminants. Lab Anim. 2004;38(1):25–37. https://doi.org/10.1258/00236770460734362.
97. Jackson E, Demarest K, Eckert WJ, Cates-Gatto C, Nadav T, Cates LN, Howard H, Roberts AJ. Aspen shaving versus chip bedding: effects on breeding and behavior. Lab Anim. 2015;49(1):46–56. https://doi.org/10.1177/0023677214553320.
98. Van de Weerd HA, Van Loo PL, Van Zutphen LF, Koolhaas JM, Baumans V. Preferences for nesting material as environmental enrichment for laboratory mice. Lab Anim. 1997;31(2):133–43. https://doi.org/10.1258/002367797780600152.
99. Windsor Z, Bate ST. Assessing the safety and suitability of nesting material for singly housed mice with surgically fitted head plates. Heliyon. 2019;5(7):e02097. https://doi.org/10.1016/j.heliyon.2019.e02097.
100. Amendola L, Xu N, Weary DM. Rats move nesting materials to create different functional areas: short report. Lab Anim. 2023;57(1):75–8. https://doi.org/10.1177/00236772221122132.
101. Jirkof P, Fleischmann T, Cesarovic N, Rettich A, Vogel J, Arras M. Assessment of postsurgical distress and pain in laboratory mice by nest complexity scoring. Lab Anim. 2013;47(3):153–61. https://doi.org/10.1177/0023677213475603.
102. Krohn TC, Hansen AK, Dragsted N. The impact of cage ventilation on rats housed in IVC systems. Lab Anim. 2003;37(2):85–93. https://doi.org/10.1258/00236770360563714.
103. Parker A, Hobson L, Bains R, Wells S, Bowl M. Investigating audible and ultrasonic noise in modern animal facilities. F1000Res. 2022;11:651. https://doi.org/10.12688/f1000research.111170.1.
104. Kacergis JB, Jones RB, Reeb CK, Turner WA, Ohman JL, Ardman MR, Paigen B. Air quality in an animal facility: particulates, ammonia, and volatile organic compounds. Am Ind Hyg Assoc J. 1996;57(7):634–40. https://doi.org/10.1080/15428119691014693.
105. Brown MJ, Symonowicz C, Medina LV, Bratcher NA, Buckmaster CA, Klein H, Anderson LC. Culture of care: organizational responsibilities, Chapter 2. In: Weichbrod RH, Thompson GA, Norton JN, editors. Management of animal care and use programs in research, education, and testing. 2nd ed. Boca Raton, FL: CRC Press/Taylor & Francis; 2018.
106. Ferrara F, Hiebl B, Kunzmann P, Hutter F, Afkham F, LaFollette M, Gruber C. Culture of care in animal research - expanding the 3Rs to include people. Lab Anim. 2022;56(6):511–8. https://doi.org/10.1177/00236772221102238.

7 How to Enrich/Refine Lab Animal's Housing and Environment by Environmental Enrichment Programs and Training?

Sabine Chourbaji, Alberto Elmi,
Jan A. M. Langermans, Annet L. Louwerse,
Martina Stocker, Yannick Raeves,
and Jean-Philippe Mocho

Abstract

Provision of environmental enrichment has become a basic consideration for the animals used in research. Societal concerns, ethical aspects, legal requirement, and quality of research have made animal housing conditions evolve significantly in recent years. Barren cages have been replaced by a variable spectrum of enriched environments. This poses several challenges for both animal care staff and researchers, and therefore, for institutions. In this chapter, responses to some practical questions on provision of environmental enrichment to several of the most commonly used species (rodents, rabbits, dogs, pigs, and macaques) are offered. The general concepts in the rodent section are applicable to all species.

Keywords

Environment · Enrichment · Animal welfare · Housing refinement

S. Chourbaji (✉)
University of Heidelberg, Heidelberg, Germany
e-mail: chourbaji@uni-heidelberg.de

A. Elmi
University of Pisa, Pisa, Italy

Jan A. M. Langermans
Biomedical Primate Research Centre, Rijswijk, The Netherlands
Department of Population Health Sciences, Animals in Science and Society, Faculty of Veterinary Sciences, Utrecht University, Utrecht, The Netherlands

A. L. Louwerse · M. Stocker
Biomedical Primate Research Centre, Rijswijk, The Netherlands

Y. Raeves
Janssen Pharmaceutical NV, Johnson & Johnson, Beerse, Belgium

J.-P. Mocho
Joint Production System Ltd, Potters Bar, UK

7.1 General Thoughts on Enrichment, and More Specific for Laboratory Rodents: How to Refine Environment for Mice and Rats

7.1.1 Introduction

Laboratory rodents, but also other lab species represent highly valuable opportunities to model human diseases. However, along with great opportunities for science come great ethical responsibilities, which researchers have to shoulder. As a consequence of such principal concerns, but also poor reproducibility, in vivo research is under controversial debate.

Systematic standardization of animal housing (at least in theory) aims at resolving difficulties

J. Guillén, V. Galligioni (eds.), *Practical Management of Research Animal Care and Use Programs*, Laboratory Animal Science and Medicine 3, https://doi.org/10.1007/978-3-031-65414-5_7

of irreproducible data. However, animals cannot be fully standardized.

Mouse housing and breeding facilities do have rather universal processes fixed by standard operating procedures (SOPs). Most terms and conditions, such as cage density, humidity, and temperature are legally specified and regularly monitored by the respective authorities. Some terms are rather facility-specific, such as breeding and weaning procedures. Overall, it is common to comply with recommendations of expert organizations and accreditation associations.

This chapter will describe general housing aspects, which need to be addressed for enrichment programs, that animal facilities, nowadays, must have installed with regard to the "3R" philosophy.

7.1.2 Environmental Enrichment: A "Must Have" *or* "Nice to Have?"

The use of environmental enrichment in housing programs of experimental animals is a controversially debated topic [1–3]. While it is embedded in current legal regulations and an essential refinement aspect in the context of the 3R philosophy, there is an ongoing discussion about the danger of enrichment to have an influence on scientific data [4, 5]. The resulting problem is not easy to address since the use of enrichment primarily addresses the welfare of the animals in captive conditions, seemingly two opposite itineraries. On the other hand, the validity of science cannot be missed out and the use of animals requires appropriate ethical consideration balanced to the gain of knowledge [6]. Appropriate enrichment programs considering the scientific focus is therefore essential to avoid discussion about potential "danger of enrichment."

Environmental enrichment is not equally enrichment, though, its use is the prerequisite for compliance with European Union (EU) legislation (Directive 2010/63/EU) [7]. With a huge market of commercially available enrichments items, each animal facility has its individual setup with different constellations of bedding, enrichment items, and nesting material. All of them may be used in different contexts though, e.g. tunnels as housing or handling items. However mostly there is an overall use regarding animals of different sexes, animals in different social constellations in different live phases.

7.1.3 What Do We Mean When We Talk About Environmental Enrichment?

"Enriched" environmental conditions should oppose "impoverished" conditions and *per definitionem* "realize environmental modification of captive animals that seeks to enhance their physical and psychological well-being by providing stimuli meeting the animals' species-specific needs" [8, 9]. It is essential to differentiate here between "standard" and "enriched" environmental settings, since there is no overall strategy to imply enrichment in large-dimensioned animal facilities. While it is common sense to improve housing conditions for laboratory animals and ethical considerations, legal requirements and the wide-acknowledged 3R principle led to certain approaches, e.g., nesting material as a minimum standard for rodents, there is no general conformity.

Enrichment, therefore, may be considered as addition of any type of items beyond the provision of minimum requirements such as bedding, food, water and meanwhile also nesting material, which, nowadays, should be considered standard, as it is mandatory in certain areas such as the European Union.

If enrichment claims to be meaningful for the animal to enhance its welfare, enrichment has to be biologically relevant to the subject. This may be reached by the provision of stimuli, e.g., structures, objects ("structural enrichment"), but also by the social constellation, dependent on the social organization of the species ("social enrichment") [10–13]. Enrichment may also be any kind of food enrichment, interaction with caretaker staff, or training programs.

It is critical to be aware that changes in the enrichment provided may result in different types of stimulation for the animal. In summary, enrichment has to be considered as biologically relevant element that is associated with refinement of the living conditions of the animals enhancing its welfare.

7.1.4 Concept of Five Freedoms: Sufficient to Fulfill the Criteria of an Enriched Environment?

The biological needs of domesticated animals, including laboratory animals, often apply the concept of the so-called five freedoms, an idea originally derived from the use of farm animals in 1979. The five freedoms include *Freedom from (1) hunger and thirst, (2) discomfort, (3) pain, injury, and disease, (4) fear and distress, and (5) freedom to express normal behavior* [14, 15]. What, however, has to be kept in mind is, that the five freedoms somewhat state, what should be prevented, rather than what enriches the lives of laboratory animals.

Moreover, there are some limitations with regard to the application of the five freedoms in the sense of refinement, which are worthy of consideration. Enriching the lives of captive animals with the provision of well-balanced food "ad libitum" may even have challenging effects, i.e. animals tend to overeat, foraging behavior becomes unnecessary, and the restricted possibilities to exercise may lead to overweight problems. While the exclusion of discomfort mainly addresses physical discomfort, psychological distress is rather barely considered by the concept of the five freedoms. Discomfort is prevented by strictly standardized housing programs with regulated climatic conditions, standardized dark-light cycles, temperature and humidity controls. Homogeneous bedding substrates permit low-dust conditions and absorb urine and feces. Respective handling routine and daily health controls ensure hygienic and healthy conditions for the animals. By standard cage designs and SOP-regulated procedures pain, injuries, and diseases can be handled soundly. What, however, commonly occurs when housing male mice together is aggression, which can lead to compromised health and distress. The freedom of fear and distress represents another challenge when housing, especially male mice in groups of certain size or constellation [16, 17]. Particularly the period after maturation represents a critical phase in male mice if conditions do not allow respective coping strategies, e.g. escape, hiding, or avoiding dominant conspecifics.

7.1.5 What Are the Legal Requirements for the Use of Enrichment?

Animal welfare in the context of animal experimentation is under precise scrutiny and becomes a more and more politically relevant issue [18]. While there is no common way on how to implement environmental enrichment in large-dimensioned animal facilities, in Europe it is legally binding to provide conditions, which allow the animals to hide and find shelter (Directive 2010/63/EU, ETS123, Council of Europe 2006). Usually, legal requirements are fulfilled by the use of commercial bedding and nesting material. Alternatively, mouse igloos may be applied to fulfill such criteria; however, again, especially the use for male animals may create problems due to increased territorial behavior and increased aggression. While there are no patents on enrichment articles, there is also no systematic evaluation of newly introduced enrichment items. Scientific evaluation, on the other hand, requires a formal application and approval at the local authorities.

7.1.6 How Can Enrichment Be Considered in the Context of Toxicology Studies?

While in academia one may be rather creative defining a fit for purpose enrichment program, involving animal caretaker staff, scientists, but also consider infrastructural circumstances, e.g., storing, cage cleaning, and sterilization processes, CROs (Clinical Research Organization) need to address different challenges [19]. Here, clients do have opinions about contract research that limits creativity, even choosing enrichment items among those that are certified for, e.g. toxicology studies. This, of course, eventually leads to discussions with other clients about the standards in such institutions, which are really much affected by culture and mentality of different countries, even inside the EU. Enrichment choices are sometimes made based on availability of certified enrichment items or belief that experimental outcomes could be affected with the placement of enrichment.

7.1.7 How Does Enrichment Affect Animal Welfare?

Assessing animal welfare represents a puzzling task since animals may not communicate verbally and animal's needs and behavior are often misinterpreted due to a quite high degree of anthropocentrism. Whether the well-meant stimuli are meaningful to the animals, fulfill the criteria of biological relevance, or are even harmful/stressful for them is not easy to rank.

Nowadays, there is a huge market of "new" enrichment offered by several commercial providers, which is often not systematically evaluated according to scientific parameters, but more assessed by caretakers and facility managers, who may sometimes also be biased because of additional work. Examples include different sizes of gnawing material, usually biting sticks, which are easy to include in the operation of cage management, but also suspended material, like tunnels, which require more time to put in place and manage respective cleaning. It has to be noted that sustainability of such decisions should not be forgotten. Also, it has to be considered that different strains of rodents may have strain-specific needs and requirements.

When defining categories for poor, moderate, or good welfare, one can get some orientation considering the five freedoms. While four freedoms may be easily applied for judgement of welfare, i.e., exclusion of starvation, weight loss, sickness signs, wounds or changes in stress physiological parameters, e.g., release of stress hormones, changes in heart rate, the assessment of "normal behavior" is rather difficult [18]. Since artificial conditions in the laboratory housing setup do not require certain facets of the entire behavioral repertoire, normal behavior can never be comparable to the natural conditions, which are not standardized. Particular ways to enrich the lives of laboratory rodents may be functional (Fig. 7.1).

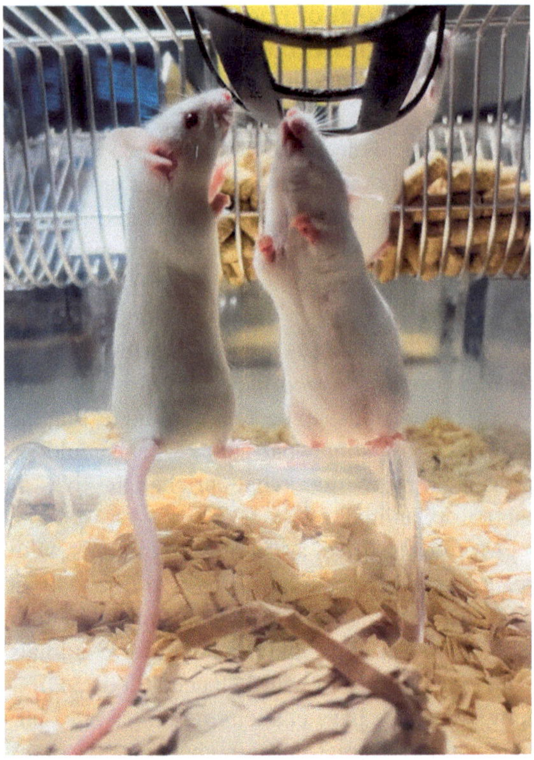

Fig. 7.1 Suspended enrichment: Mouse enrichment provided by suspended additional plastic climbing structures, sometimes with tunnels to adapt animals to potential handling equipment. Animals make use of these structural enrichment elements and use it when climbing up to lid grids, using it individually or together with other counterparts, with which they share such refining cage additions. Animals approach without neophobic attitudes, which underlines the biological relevance of such measures inside given cage environment, but intake of plastic particles when using it has to be taken under consideration

7.1.8 What Is the Impact of Nesting Material?

Despite general discussions about the definition of enrichment and minimum standards, nesting material fulfills several needs of the animals, which should evoke enhanced welfare. Nest building represents a behavior that is shown by male and female mice, respectively, and allows the normal nesting behavior of the animals. It reduces increased intermale aggression behavior without affecting physiological parameters [16]. The animals may manipulate their environment in a mouse-comfortable manner, they can split the nesting material and therefore avoid each other's direct physical presence. Nest building contrasts the under-stimulation by boredom, which is considered a major concern of animal welfare. It furthermore offers the animals the chance to separate the cage in different thermozones with higher temperatures than the usu-

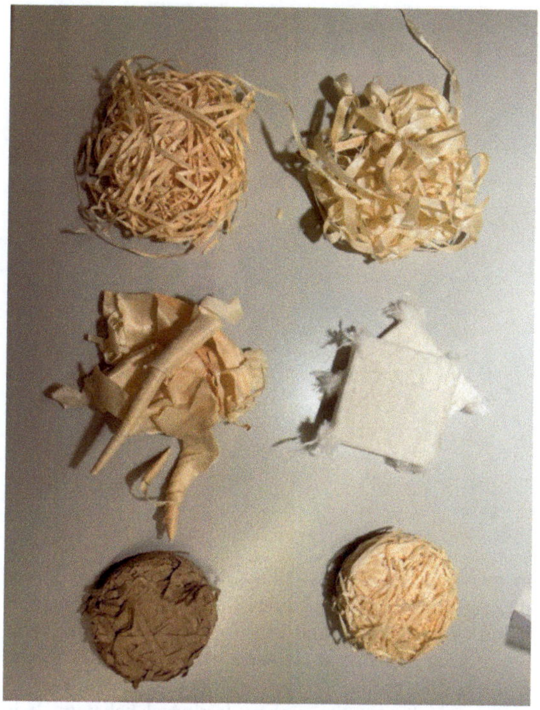

Fig. 7.2 Nesting material: Nesting material may be provided in different shapes consisting of different material. It has to be kept in mind that caretakers need to control the health status of animals in their day-to-day business; therefore, the amount of nest material has to be considered. Dust as potential allergen for humans as well as danger of pups becoming struggled has to be evaluated. Furthermore, it has to be considered that material flow may be constraint by nesting material blocking filters during cage washing processes

ally predicted 21 °C inside the nest itself [20, 21]. Since higher temperatures around 30 °C are preferred by mice, nests can be considered as beneficial for the well-being. Quality of mouse nests has, furthermore, evolved as valid and reproducible indicator for well-being and adequate behavioral performance [22, 23]. Temperature modulation seems to be important for mice [20].

Nesting material is available in various volumes, shapes, and doses, it can be easily autoclaved and stored; however, visibility of the animals may be compromised due to the amount of material in the cage, which needs to be addressed.

It has to be noted that nesting material is not synonym with "Enrichment" per se, since it is assumed to be part of the standard housing cage (Fig. 7.2).

7.1.9 What Is the Impact of Mouse Igloos, Tunnels, and Huts?

Mouse shelters provide protected areas inside the cages, represent a standardized and hygienic enrichment item, and allow proper daily inspections due to the fact that most of them are made of red transparent plastic. Especially during breeding the use of such enrichment is advantageous because the litter is surrounded by the shelter, which has positive effects on lactating dams and number of pups weaned [24]. While such positive effects speak for the use of this type of enrichment, there are side effects such as increased aggression that are not trivial [25, 26]. One more problem could be the fact that mice are rodents (with the habit to gnaw). Here it is essential to estimate the effects of longtime intake of plastic against the value of this type of environmental enrichment [27].

Plastic enrichment is easy to handle, liked by the caretaker staff, and can be reused many times. Combinations of igloos with running dishes allow simultaneous options to find shelter and exert physical activity. More appropriate alternatives, if there are worries about plastic enrichment, are cardboard huts, igloos, and tunnels that are available at different vendors in different sizes (Fig. 7.3).

7.1.10 What Is the Impact of Running Wheels?

Lack of activity and exploration may result in manifested behavioral abnormalities including self-injurious behavior, stereotypies, or apathetic behavior. Running wheels are a widely used tool to measure activity in the homecage. In this case, running wheels may be regarded as experimental tool, where activity is monitored and used as correlate for the respective research question [28]. The usage as enrichment tool is rather arguable, because it is said that running wheels may not induce but promote stereotypic behavior for certain strains in certain conditions [29]. Furthermore, many experimental setups using running wheels require isolated housing, a debatable fact since mice and rats are considered to be social species. Natural habitats require certain activity of the ani-

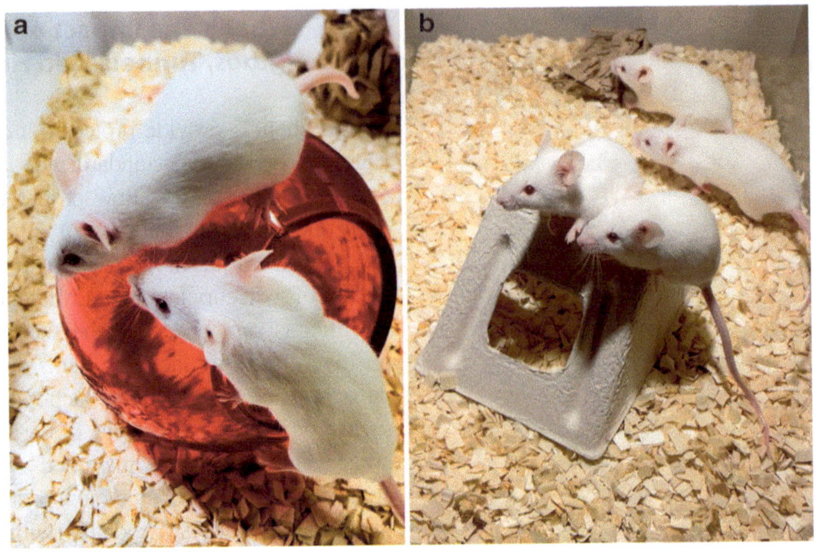

Fig. 7.3 (**a**, **b**) Mouse igloos and shelters: Rodent shelters and areas to hide are essential elements to fulfill the needs of mice and rats behavioral repertoire and are therefore recommended to include in the facility's enrichment programs. Different variations of shape and material require consideration/evaluation which one is the one of choice for different purposes. Plastic material allows observation of animals, without the need to lift or destroy the hiding zone, which may evoke stress. But rodents like to gnaw. Other materials may be more appropriate for these species to allow an animal-fitting/-adapted manipulation of enrichment and cage space without long-term use of such enrichment elements. All is welcomed by the animals, but needs careful consideration when used in males, which sometimes show territorial behavior. It is therefore a prerequisite that such structures possess more than one entrance/exit

mals to run and climb, be it to guard the territory, to search for nutrition, or in the context of interaction with counterparts. In the wilderness activity is very individual due to social status, fitness, life phase, which may lead to very variable use of items like running wheels. Under laboratory conditions individual use of running wheels may increase the variance of data, which goes along with increased numbers of experimental animals contradicting the aspect of "reduction."

While the use of running wheels in the context of experimental housing is therefore debated, wild mice show interest in this kind of activity when installed in natural settings and frequently use it without a reason to develop stereotypies [30] (Fig. 7.4).

7.1.11 What Is the Impact of Climbing Structures?

Climbing represents an important element in the behavioral repertoire of rodents. Adequate structures in the homecage allow to keep track about the surrounding environment, promote physical activity, and serve as structure to escape on or hide under. Depending on the structure of the enrichment object, familiarity may be an additional plus, which is the case if, e.g., cage lids are used, to which the animals are used to [31]. The so-called cage-climbers" are a positive stimulus when exposed in a novel context, they are utilized by group-housed animals in a way that no changes in variation occur and are accepted by males and females in a comparable manner. What however needs to be taken in mind is that different designs of climbing structures may affect variation of different experimental parameters and exert different effects according to sex [5] (Fig. 7.5).

7.1.12 What Is the Impact of Cage Dividers?

Group-housing, especially of adult male mice states a major problem in nearly all animal facili-

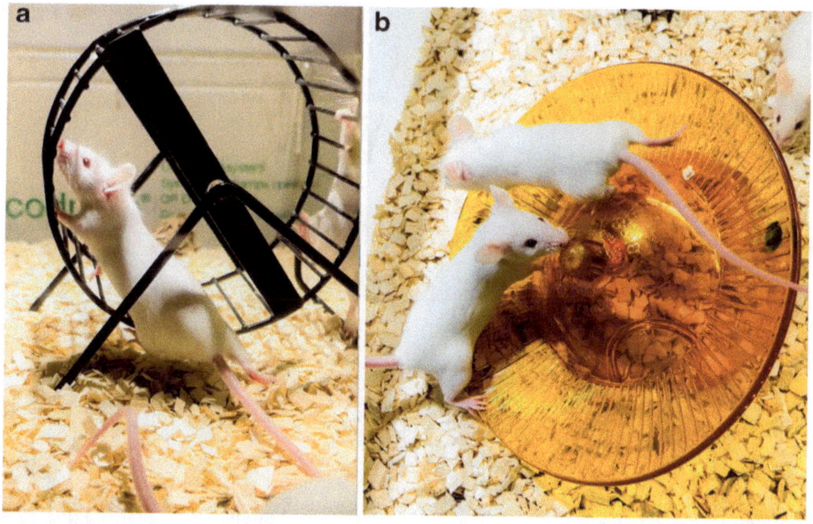

Fig. 7.4 (a, b) Running wheels: Running and physical activity within regulated and limited cage space represent essential parts in enrichment programs and may be restricted by using IVC cages, where the cage lid grid is reduced by the cage type. It has to be taken under consideration that the use of running wheels may be different between counterparts, which in some studies needs clear monitoring to be able to correlate activity with certain scientific outcome. Therefore, it definitely needs to be included in the experimental design. Problems may occur due to squeaking of wheels, which may be perceived as stress for the animals. Consumption of plastic has to be evaluated in the context of respective studies. Furthermore, risk of injury by getting stuck in such structures needs to be excluded

ties [32, 33]. The problem not only correlates with cage- or group size, but often with the social constellation of the group [16, 34]. While igloos and huts always comprise limited access to the most attractive parts, be it inside to hide or on top to be able to secure the territory, cage dividers follow a different concept. The idea behind this structural enrichment is the possibility to avoid contact and aggressive interaction with same conditions for all mice of a group [35, 36]. What has to be kept in mind using such enrichment is that not only shape plays a role, but also the color. Opaque material may even increase agonistic interaction, possibly because coping is restricted by the lack of visibility of the opponent. Transparent dividers may therefore be the better option. The use of two stuctural enrichment items may be recommendable to give more options for coping behavior (Fig. 7.6).

7.1.13 What Is the Impact of Semi-naturalistic Environment?

Semi-naturalistic environments can be considered as a kind of "super-enrichment" [37], in which a large range of items is offered, i.e. enrichment of different materials (wood, stone, different bedding), multiple levels, tunnels, connections between different areas or in between cages and haptic elements like rope and different feeding areas. Nest boxes and the multiple availability of several potentially attractive enrichment items allow social avoidance, but also sociability plus a great offer of resources for physical activity. This type of enrichment is thought to model the natural habitat of non-captive animals wide, more closely than standard conditions [38]. The practicability is rather problematic despite this very interesting approach. Besides challenges in the day-to-day business of caretakers and technicians one needs to keep in mind the hygienic restraints of some material, which would be optimal in the sense of enriching the rodent's life, but contrast the rules of animal facilities with high hygienic standard operation procedures. With the raise of "wildlings," in which the hygienic status is defined in a different way addressing, e.g., approaches in immunology, such type of enrichment may represent a promising way to improve animal welfare in such animals (Fig. 7.7).

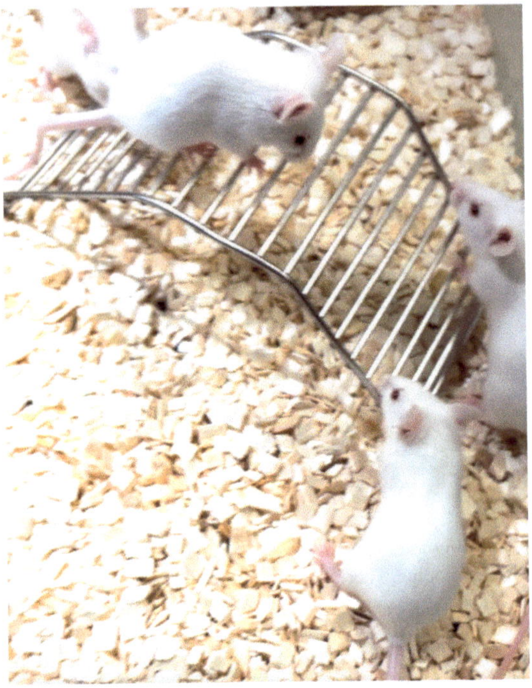

Fig. 7.5 Climbing structures: Rodents of all age and strain spend more or less time climbing the lid of cage covers, which is limited by the use of IVC cages with less opportunities to do so. Many mice used in experiments are bred at sites of commercial breeders and are familiar with such environment and opportunities to exert activity. Therefore "cage climbers" may be contemplated as refinement, because they do not induce neophobia; mice use it to include such structures in nest building and there is no indication that the use of such enrichment leads to higher variation of data by individual use

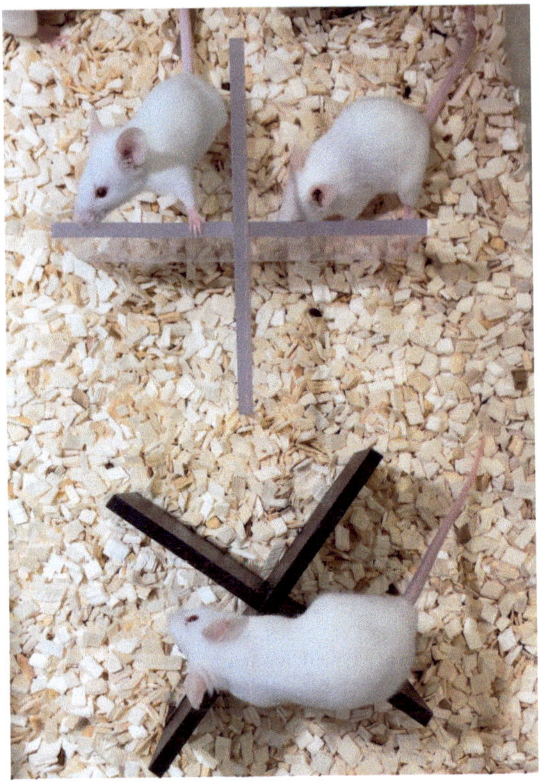

Fig. 7.6 Cage dividers: Cage dividers may be provided in different ways, being part of the cage itself or as structures made of wood or plastic. Wooden cage dividers often contain holes through which animals can transit or interact with other cage mates. The visibility of counterparts plays an essential role. Stress, e.g. by cohousing adult male mice together, may be reduced if appropriate ability to cope exists

One option is the use of Nestpaks, a commercial product available at stores of many professional sellers in the animal welfare branch. Systematic analyses published in the literature are lacking, but the concept of this category of enrichment is, the standardized supply with defined amounts of bedding material of choice, which is enclosed by an outer paper bag. The instinct of the animals to shredder the paper ensures both, the accessibility to nesting material and physical activity during manipulation. Nestpaks therefore provide an easy-to-handle enrichment option, a hygienic and standardizable enrichment item; however, visibility of animals with a strategy to hide inside of the bags is critical (Fig. 7.8).

7.1.14 What Are the Challenges and Limitations of Elaborate Enrichment Programs?

Establishing an enrichment program in a large facility that addresses all agendas is quite tricky. Enrichment must fulfill several criteria from different points of view:

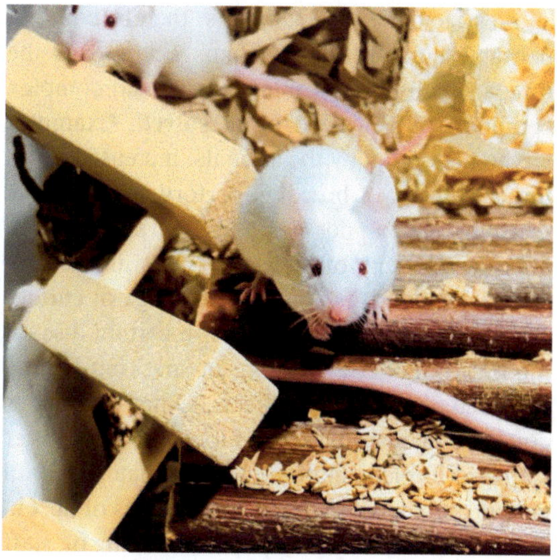

Fig. 7.7 Semi-naturalistic environment: Semi-naturalistic environment is very well accepted by rodents, which may make use of different areas with different opportunities to hide and gnaw. Environments displaying a natural habitat surely serve to counteract boredom of standard caging, but go along with problems of the hygienic standards and workload of caretakers. Material needs to be consciously defined to avoid hygienic challenges. Standardization and biometric planning of potentially higher variance have to be taken under consideration. Equally the need that animals have to have daily health checks, which may compromise well-being by lifting up enrichment-elements to find them has to be kept in mind

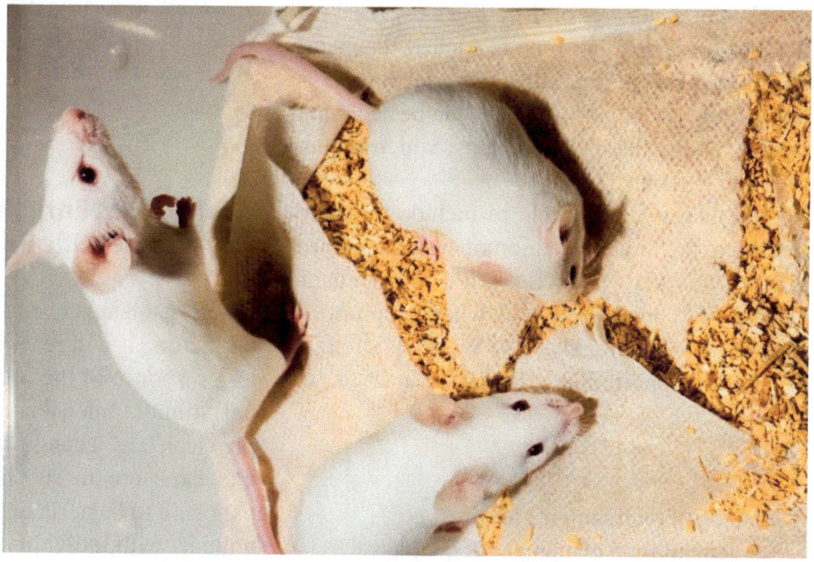

Fig. 7.8 Nestpacks: Nestpacks combine the natural need of mice to perform nest-building behavior with the idea of standardization, i.e. provide a defined amount of bedding material and nesting material. With differing sizes of nestpacks it may be managed to handle various cage types. Different types of bedding may be provided on demand

Animals	Caretaker	Scientist	Facility manager
• Biologically relevant • Stimulating • No risk of injuries	• Easy to handle • Easy to apply to the animal • Good adoption by the animals • Easy to store • Easy to dispose • Good visibility of the animals • Non-allergic	• No influence of variance • Good background knowledge about the effects on a certain research question • Information about housing conditions to apply to the ARRIVE and PREPARE guidelines [39]	• Good compliance of staff and researchers • Constant availability • Easy storing • Stable costs • Hygienic flawless • Sustainable • Compatible with occupational safety in animal- and washing area • Compatible with technical conditions in the facility

A systematic evaluation is therefore indispensable since many problems occur over the time and can turn out in expensive and complex conditions which need to be solved. Examples are non-adoption by the animals, increased fighting or cutback of breeding performance or litter weaning due to poor nest building performance or entanglement of newborn pups in nesting material which is not suitable. Change of enrichment can affect the phenotype in certain disease models by either provoking or masking behavioral and physiological effects. Other challenges comprise increased dust development when, after stepwise implementation, nesting materials in a certain amount leads to increased levels of dust in the air, which may compromise health of staff and problems with technical equipment. Handling enrichment at all sites of the chain can create difficulties because more time is needed than actually thought, e.g. if nesting material has to be dosed or is hard to portion. This can be accompanied by additional cleaning steps, which require time and personnel.

It is therefore advisable to include all stakeholders in the implementation of enrichment programs and start stepwise with a systematic catalog of requirements and where appropriate include a SWOT analysis (SWOT = Strength, Weakness, Opportunities, Threats).

Catalog of requirements for the implementation of animal-adequate enrichment

1. The introduction of enrichment must be **biologically relevant** for the animal and being steadily adopted for utilization. The animal should not show aversion or anxiety/neophobia
2. It should be possible for the animal to regulate their **microclimate**
3. The enrichment should **not induce competition for resources**, e.g. evoke aggressive behavior
4. It should be possible to **portion** enrichment, e.g., nesting material, to be able to standardize the housing conditions
5. **Disposal** has to be easy-to-handle and environmentally sound
6. The **storage** has to be easy and space-saving
7. Use of enrichment by the animals should still allow adequate **daily inspection** and warrant disturbances of the animals, i.e., by lifting the element
8. The enrichment needs to fulfill all criteria for **hygienic measures** in the facility organization
9. Enrichment should **not evoke health compromises** due to injuries, e.g. by constraint or oral absorption, e.g. by gnawing
10. It has to be ensured that there is no danger for the caretaker staff, e.g. increased **risk of allergies due to high development of dust**

7.1.15 Does Enrichment Affect Scientific Results?

If an organism is exposed to certain environmental factors, it will react by changing its condition as a response of the organism to the given external stimuli. Such exposure may include either physical, e.g. change in temperature; chemical, e.g. exposure to substances; or biological, e.g. exposure to bacteria or viruses [40]. Humans and animals with individual and particular genotypes show different susceptibility to cope with environmental conditions [41], which can be reached by active or passive responses. Based on this concept, one can assume that the interaction between genes and environment can cause different impact of the environment on disease risk and vice versa. The genotype can be decisive in how far the environment, e.g., enrichment may it be structural or social, can exert an effect on the organism and its susceptibility.

With many genetically modified animals involved in answering research questions, this presents quite a challenge, since the environment in animal facilities is rather underestimated. While the PREPARE and ARRIVE guidelines

[42, 43] represent important tools to consider potential factors impacting study validity by addressing whole checklists, including the environment, many researchers still do not comply with such guidelines. This is somewhat dangerous, because published work about, e.g., the effects of all kinds of mutations screened, e.g., in mice may be masked by environmental conditions [44]. In this context, enrichment may hide a phenotype on one hand side, whereas, on the other hand, impoverished conditions may evoke a phenotype in animals with respective predisposition [11]. If this is kept in mind and included in the scientific hypotheses, environmental conditions, e.g., enrichment, can be perfectly used to address certain hypotheses by a more holistic analysis including the effects of "gene X environment" interactions. The effects of enrichment on neural functioning have been topic of many reviews during the last decades [41, 45, 46]. These reviews illustrate the impaired brain development when animals are deprived from enrichment; furthermore, stereotypies and effects on the behavioral profile are described, such as changes in anxiety and depressive-like behavior. With insufficient awareness for respective facts misinterpretation of data is a risk because the results may be the consequence of the environment (rich or poor) and not the result of the research hypothesis or treatment.

Other examples for environmental influencing are given by certain temperature ranges, under which phenotypes may occur, which is not the case when the same experiment is conducted under different conditions, e.g. standard housing temperatures [47]. Many recommendations about temperature are not evaluated, but it is known that rodents need to adapt anatomically, physiologically, and behaviorally to maintain stable body temperature in thermoneutrality and keep their preferred range [48]. This affects cardiovascular parameters [49]. Essential for breeding is also humidity, which can be regulated not only technically and by group size, but also by type of enrichment in shape of bedding and nesting material [21, 50, 51]. Being able to build nest therefore represents a valuable strategy to provide a thermal compensation mechanism to reach a thermoneutral microclimate [20], which controls also the experimental outcome in many disciplines.

With regard to cancer growth it was described that an enriched environment, even in a simplified form affected tumor development and affected body temperature [52]. This prevention may explain the mechanistic background of eustress induced by an enriched cage environment. However, it has to be kept in mind that (in not considered appropriately in the experimental design) this form of housing may exert a "masking" effect.

There are other examples from the field of immunology, where enrichment has been shown to buffer the reactivity of the immune system in response to stress when enrichment was provided in form of cage toys (nesting material, crawl tubes, and running wheels) [53, 54]. When considering social components of enrichment it is, likewise, known that there are differences in many scientific parameters, depending on how the animals' social constellations are, e.g. food consumption and associated body weight being reduced in group-housed rats of both genders [55], but there are contractionary findings, which suggest increased food intake in group-housed animals. In these animals, increased blood-glucose and triglyceride levels were noted [56]. Also, findings in the field of experimental psychiatry may be changed depending on how the animals are housed. Here there are findings of group-housed mice being more prone to develop symptoms [11, 57].

It is therefore essential and worthy considering potential effects of enrichment to manipulate parameters of interest as additional scientific variable, even if it is generally expected to exert positive effects on the well-being of animal.

7.1.16 One Size Fits All? Is There a Necessity for Individual Enrichment?

Facing the problems of aggression only in males poses the question whether male and female mice should not be handled in a more "gender-appropriate" manner. Usually, vivariums use one type of enrichment, evaluated by their individual enrichment programs and only those animals, which are part of an experimental design using environment as a factor may be housed differently. While different conditions like breeding or experimental treatment include individual management including warming, nutrition, and increased numbers of inspections it is rather normal that enrichment is handled in a standardized manner. Looking at recent discussions about the scientific validity of standardization in *in vivo* studies open the chance to be more creative in the installation of enrichment programs, e.g. by enrichment rotation, which is considered to be more stimulation to the animals. However, also in this context, a comprehensive evaluation is needed to exclude, e.g. neophobia, agonistic behavior, or destabilization of experiments, which address defined environmental conditions such as gene x environment interaction. The use of different types of enrichment (rotation) could therefore be more appropriate in terms of animal welfare; it would however challenge a direct comparison of both sexes. One therefore needs to balance and include different perspectives—the one addressing the nature of the animals, the other one focusing on scientific gain of knowledge.

7.1.17 How Important Is Social Enrichment?

The question, how to handle group-housing of rodents in the best possible way, seems to be not easy to handle. Rodents are said to be social animals, but while rats have a social system that allows group-housing of both genders, group-housing of male mice states a problem due to severe aggression among the group members [58, 59]. It seems therefore difficult to define a social group composition as "social enrichment" in mice in this sex; however, in females, it is indispensable and social isolation may be treated as impoverished environment [60, 61]. What obviously plays a role for successful group housing is the age when the group is composed and in male mice early socialization with littermates is the mostly suggested way to handle the situation [54]. Own unpublished observations and those of others revealed also the importance or the time of separating a certain social constellation, i.e. early weaning may exert significant effects on the animals' behavior [62], which can go along with compromised welfare and increased stress hormone release depending on the sex of the animals. Earlier weaning, therefore, has a different impact for male and female mice, for which the social environment obviously plays an important role. For the day-to day buisness in animal facilities that would mean to group-house females compulsory either with littermates or by pooling with counterparts from different litters (except the experimental setup does not allow this setting).

7.1.18 How Important Is the Human Factor?

Former and recent literature proves that the human factor needs to be considered in the context of sex of who handles animals or perform experiments with them. There is strong evidence that being male or female when interacting with rodents plays an essential role when it comes to behavioral or pain-related readouts in the animals [63]. What, however, may not be assessed is the compassion of, e.g., caretakers or scientists, who conduct caregiving of experiments. While some (according to personal experience in training) demonstrate a high level of bonding and responsibility, especially at the beginning of their career, there is sometimes less identification with the animal after a certain time when working with them. This is when we talk about compassion fatigue [64], a demanding aspect in the field of animal research. Interacting with a person in a positive anticipation manner may represent an enriched environment per se, also known as medical training, where, e.g., zoo animals learn to associate cooperative behavior with a certain reward [65]. A potential way to overcome the "personal" individuality when handling animals is the use of tunnel handling [66], since animals which had learned to interact in a positive way with the person who handles them may have a broader self-determined choice when interaction takes place. Furthermore, tunnels are more standardized than other handling effects like the force of fingers, when animals are picked up by hand. An individual style of how to use tunnel handling can, however, also not be excluded. Proper training on

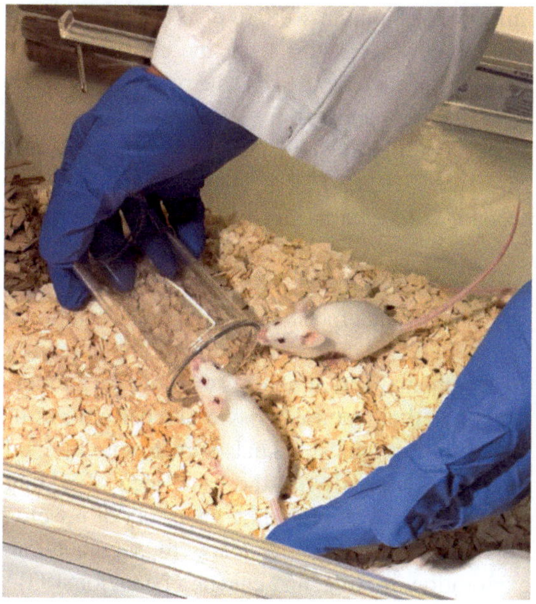

Fig. 7.9 "Human Factor": Interaction with caretakers and scientists represents an often underestimated base for animal well-being. Cage changes may vary between facilities depending on cage systems and SOPs and may be performed by hand, forceps or by tunnel handling. Mice being trained to enter tunnels tolerate handling and interaction with less hyperactivity, and transparent tunnels allow holistic vision of the condition of the animals

not only how to use physical enrichment but also to consider personal involvement in the well-being of animals is therefore an essential prerequisite for enrichment programs [67] (Fig. 7.9).

7.1.19 What About Tunnel Enrichment in the Context of Handling?

The above mentioned tunnel handling also needs to evaluate the use of such tunnels in the housing of animals [68]. An appropriate way to implement such handling techniques requires the consideration of tunnels, available in opaque and red or clear, in the enrichment program of the respective institution. This may not be underestimated since (according to personal observation) tunnels represent a structural element inside of rodent cages. Animals tend to structure their environment according to elements provided in the cages and change "mouse-relevant use" of the cage. A fact that may be dependent on sex, age, and the social environment. Again, there needs to be a fair balance between the gain regarding animal welfare and compliance, e.g. regarding toxicology studies (rodents gnaw, material may not be certified for such purposes). However, considerations of such new innovations need to be implemented in enrichment programs—even, if at a first sight they seem trivial.

7.1.20 What Other General Aspects of Housing Conditions of Laboratory Animals Should Be Considered?

Scientists may have limited knowledge of the biology and housing history of their model organisms. Coming from disciplines such as medicine or molecular biology, their background from curricular lessons may not have enough focus in regard to animal behavior and welfare. Laboratory animal professionals should work with scientists to ensure there is a complete understanding related to the biology, behavior, repro cycle, etc., of the models they are using. This underlines how much important it is to secure proper interfaces between theoretical disciplines and the importance to promote the potential influences of the day-to-day business of animal facilities. Approaches could consider implementation of other questionnaires apart from the PREPARE and ARRIVE guidelines [43, 69]. Essential information about housing has to be provided in the context of clear compliance and communication strategies, being part of the institutional public relation departments. There are certainly approaches by scientific societies to provide recommendations, but as long as this is not an obligation, it is probably an insufficient approach. There is a trend that such requirements come from the industrial section. Still many institutions in academia remain very rigid about it. Communication and a sense for transparency regarding all kind of processes are widely missing. There is neither a way to find out how animals are euthanized, nor any information about the qualification of staff or the implementation of the 3Rs as a legal requirement. More engagement of researchers with any of the 3Rs could be better illuminated when marketing a human, ethical, and scientific image of animal housing within large research institutions, in which the use of animals is still a prerequisite for excellent science—also taking into account the economic aspects and public image.

7.1.21 Lessons Learned?

There seems to be no general agreement on how to appropriately enrich animals' environments in a proper and standardized way. There are, even within one community, different perspectives and opinions, which makes it challenging to fulfill all needs of different stakeholders—keeping an eye on animal welfare. It is therefore essential to be aware of these different aspects and go for adequate considerations and reporting systems, which may help to overcome the obstacles of the widely discussed reproducibility crisis [70]. There is not cooking recipe or "one-fits-all" solution, when addressing the challenge of the use of enrichment. Efforts have to be taken to promote the dialogue between stakeholders, profile and improve the sense for such seemingly trivial issues, and the need to implement housing conditions in the experimental design has to be communicated in a convincing way. In the context of a "Culture of Care" one needs to be aware of different cultures, a diverse understanding of the role of such aspects, and the will to promote, grant, and publish research and findings in this sector. It is worth it!

7.2 Thoughts on Enrichment for Laboratory Pigs: Why Enrichment Means Refinement for Pigs Used in Research

7.2.1 From Farms to Experimental Setup: What Do We Know About Environmental Enrichments in Pig?

Basic knowledge regarding environmental enrichments for swine species originated and developed mainly from the pork industry and conventional farms where animal welfare does not only represent an ethical request from the consumers, but also an improvement of production quality standards. When addressing environmental enrichments for pigs, alongside with the European Directive 2010/63/EU, it is pivotal to take into account the Commission Recommendation (EU) 2016/336 on the application of the Council Directive 2008/120/EC regarding the categories and types of materials that may be used to improve pig welfare [71, 72]. The goal of implementing environmental enrichments is to allow the animals to express their natural behavioral repertoire, stimulating the animals' visual, somatosensory, and olfactory systems, with the basic idea of adding objects capable of providing an aspect of novelty. Pigs have an innate tendency to socialization, exploration, rooting, and chewing behaviors [73].

The enrichment materials, in the case of pigs, should always be edible, chewable, investigable, and manipulable [74]. According to the Directive, the Environmental Enrichment (EE) should be safe and clean, and animals should have free access to a sufficient amount of enrichments. The most common materials, when it comes to pigs, are chopped straw bedding, suspended ropes, wood and chains, plastic and wooden toy (e.g., Dog toys), colored plastic object, rubber tubing, table tennis balls, balls, and strings [75]. Considering these elements, the environmental enrichments are divided into: (a) optimal materials, possessing all the required characteristics, as straw; (b) suboptimal materials as wood bark or biodegradable flavored chewing toys; and (c) materials of marginal interest (e.g., plastic toys) that only fulfill their essential needs, thus addition of optimal or suboptimal materials should also be granted. In light of the different categories of enrichment, straw as well other edible bedding materials as hay, green fodder, miscanthus pressed or chipped, and root vegetables, can be considered as optimal for enrichment of pig facilities. Indeed, several studies showed how the use of straw or other edible bedding, in comparison to the use of other materials alone, can improve pigs welfare reducing the display of negative behavior and the effects of the stress syndrome. As for suboptimal EEs for porcine facilities, these include peanuts shells, fresh wood, corn cobs, natural ropes, com-

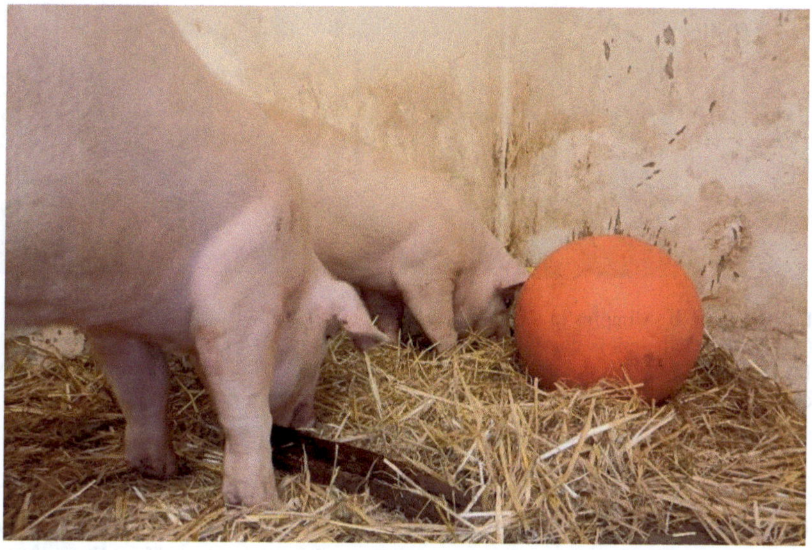

Fig. 7.10 Optimal enrichment for pigs: Straw as bedding and additional materials as woods and plastic toys (marginal enrichments)

pressed straw cylinders, shredded paper, and pellets. When provided in a rack or in a dispenser, also straw is classified as a suboptimal enrichment. The marginal materials include chains, rubber, soft plastic, pipes, hard woods, and balls [76].

7.2.2 Providing Materials as Environmental Enrichment Is Not Always Enough .... What Else?

As reported for the other animal species, the types of environmental enrichments not only include occupational and physical enrichments but also nutritional and social ones. In the case of the pig, it has to be considered that the diet is very standard, often boring, without any type of flavor stimuli nor variation. Additional nutritional enrichment such as fruits, vegetables, yogurt, or juices can be used to improve and to enrich the diet and, at the same time, may represent an important rewarding tool to train the animals. Edible toys (with different flavors) and bedding (as straw) can be supplied as adequate nutritional stimuli [77]. In addition, it is important to remember that the porcine one is a social species, so it is mandatory to guarantee social interspecific behavior. The group of animals must be stable and, in case of redistribution of pigs, it is pivotal to improve the availability of occupational enrichments and grant the animals enough time to establish hierarchy, trying to reduce the potential related stress. When isolation of an animal is required by the given experimental protocol of other compelling reasons, it is always recommended to try and maintain some degree of social connection, mostly by housing other animals in adjoining pens divided by bars or at least in the same room, so that visual, olfactory, and auditory interactions can be granted.

Overall, especially for pigs, intraspecific social interactions are fundamental for animals enrolled in research [78, 79]. As for the personnel working in the facility, constant interaction and dedicated training sessions with pigs not only are important to get the latter accustomed to manipulations but can be also considered as excellent enrichments capable of positively stimulating the animals. The role of animal caretakers in the management, handling, and training of pigs can be seen as a daily social enrichment for the animal, especially important for isolated animal and during specific experimental procedures [80–82] (Fig. 7.10).

7.2.3 How Can We Balance When Choosing the Best Enrichment? A Matter of Compromising

The porcine model is used for several purposes including regulatory ones, infectious diseases

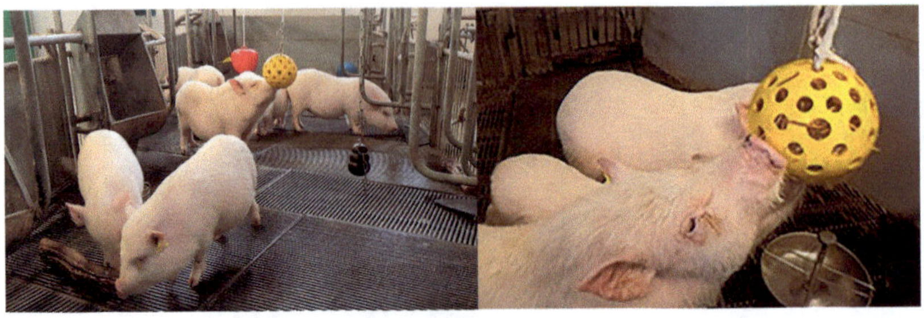

Fig. 7.11 (**a**, **b**) Minipigs in a Biological Safety Level 2 (BLS2) cage, where it is not possible to use the bedding. In figure xA, there are different types of suspended and chewable enrichments. Some of the enrichments present different flavors or, as reported in figure Xb, is possible to add straw in the suspended ball (suboptimal enrichment). In addition, wooden are provided as edible enrichment

aims, basic sciences and also surgical modelling. In such scenario, it is possible to find pigs/minipigs with different health profiles generally ranging from conventional to SPF (specific pathogen free), but also up to Gnotobiotic/SOPF (specific opportunistic pathogen free) animals in isolators/biobubbles [83, 84]. As for all the other laboratory animals' species, the choice of materials and types of enrichment have to take into account the health status of the animals, their physiological stage as well as the type of procedures they will be enrolled in, while always maintaining the highest standards in terms of standardization of the study design. Because the most commonly used natural materials, as straw or wooden toys, can house different pathogens, it is mandatory, also in conventional facilities, to consider the potential biohazard and to select sterilized materials (e.g., irradiated) [85]. Overall, the best materials to expose experimental animals to, should be cleanable, sanitizable, and/or autoclavable [76]. For this reason, there are many commercially available solutions on the market of certified sterile bedding and materials. The type of the enrichment of choice also needs to be adapted to the status of the animals, be it physiological (e.g., sows during the peripartum, where it is necessary to provide nest-building materials to guarantee their maternal behavior), or naturally occurring/induced pathological (e.g., choice of specific bedding materials when managing animals with abdominal surgical wound or isolated for specific procedures) [86, 87].

7.2.4 One Enrichment Is Not Enough! How Can You Develop an Environmental Enhancement Plan?

Taking into consideration the fact that pig/minipig may lose attention and interest toward the newly offered objects within few days, frequent replacement or renewal of environmental enrichment is recommended to decrease the risk of boredom, thus negative behaviors. This is one of the reasons why the sole use of toys or chain is considered marginal or suboptimal. As reported for nonhuman primates, it is important to maximize and standardize the enrichments in the swine facility, by developing, documenting, and following an appropriate plan for environment enhancement capable of promoting the psychological well-being. The plan must include information on social housing, environmental enrichment and, if relevant, sections on animals with special considerations, use of restraint devices, and exemptions. For best results, when bedding cannot be provided, the combination of different kinds of enrichment materials should be used. Importantly, environmental enrichment plans should be delivered in a consistent and systematic manner so as not to become a source of uncontrolled variation [88, 89] (Fig. 7.11).

7.3 Thoughts on Enrichment for Macaques: Examples of Housing and Enrichment for Macaques in Scientific Laboratory Settings

7.3.1 Introduction

Macaques are still indispensable as important animal models in biomedical research. Although the exact number is not known, it is estimated that globally more than 100,000 NHP are used each year, with an excess of this number kept in the breeding colonies [90, 91]. To minimize harm to these animals, it is essential that the animal management in such facilities is aimed at promoting positive welfare states and mental well-being. Providing social and environmental enrichment is an essential component for promoting a healthy mental and physical state.

7.3.2 Welfare

7.3.2.1 How to Define Welfare?

With the use of macaques for biomedical research comes also our responsibility to ensure their welfare in breeding and experimental facilities to the highest standards possible. To effectively assess and enhance animal welfare, it is essential to establish conceptual frameworks that can be applied across different contexts in which these animals are kept. Animal welfare can be described as the ability of animals to react to both negative and positive circumstances in their environment and to adapt to these environmental settings in such a way that a positive mental state is achieved. Earlier concepts such as the Five Freedoms served as a fundamental framework for animal welfare assessment, but mainly focused on the absence of negative aspects. The Five Domains concept has expanded on this and takes besides the physical experiences also the mental experiences into account, focusing more on the ability of the animals to adapt to the circumstances. The domains in this model are nutrition, physical environment, health, behavioral interactions (including human–animal interactions), and mental state [14, 92]. The recently introduced Dynamic Animal Welfare Concept (DAWCon) considers the principle that an animal's welfare is positive when it possesses the mental and physical capacity to effectively respond to both favorable and unfavorable internal and external stimuli, events, and conditions in dynamic ways [93]. These various concepts show that animal welfare depends on various aspects and is of a dynamic rather than static nature (Fig. 7.12).

7.3.2.2 How Can Welfare Be Assessed?

One of the main challenges lies in effectively assessing the welfare of animals [94]. A recent survey among facilities housing macaques for research purposes revealed some practical and valid welfare indicators [95] as was a novel practical primate welfare assessment tool [96]. Behavior is in general one of the important indicators for the well-being of an animal. Hence, it is crucial for staff working with these animals to be acquainted with the typical behavior of macaques and proficient in utilizing ethograms (see, e.g., [97, 98]. Most facilities use a combination of indicators. These indicators include physical observations (e.g., coat and body condition), physiological measurements (e.g., body temperature), and behavior (e.g., activity budget and behavioral repertoire) (Table 7.1). Offering high-quality, species-specific enrichment is one of the key opportunities for promoting positive welfare.

7.3.3 Housing

7.3.3.1 What Are the Housing Conditions for Macaques?

A good guideline for housing requirements for macaques as laboratory animals is provided by Appendix A of EU Directive 2010/63 EU, (http://data.europa.eu/eli/dir/2010/63/oj). These guidelines describe general issues regarding the housing of these animals, such as ventilation,

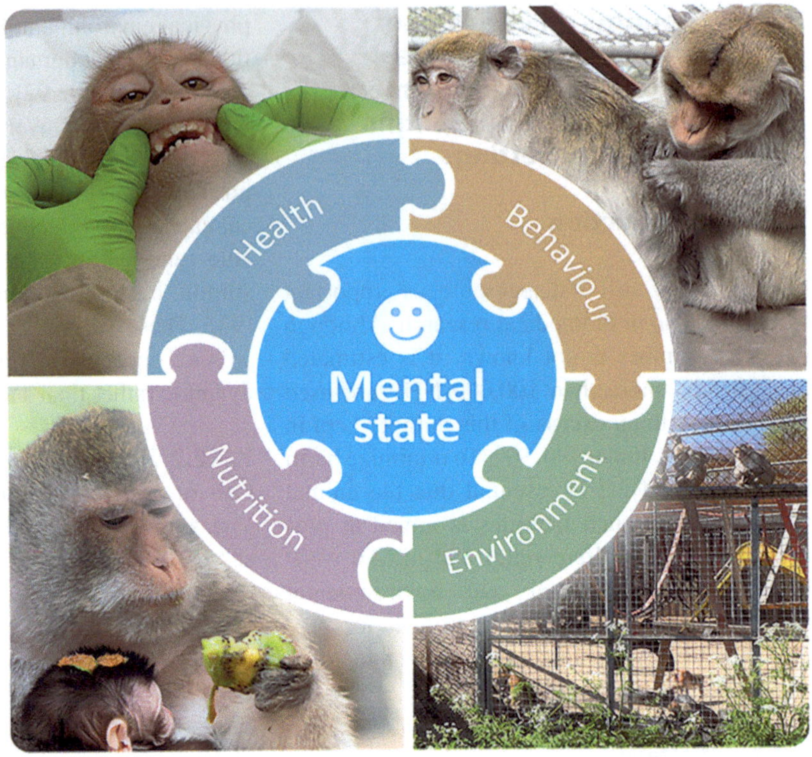

Fig. 7.12 The five domains

Table 7.1 Some examples of welfare indicators

Indicators of poor welfare	Indicators of good welfare
Self-inflicted body damage	Social play
Frequent conflicts	Allogrooming
Reduced growth and breeding success	Normal growth and breeding success
Stereotypic behavior	Large variety of normal behavior
Low activity	Exploration

temperature, humidity, light, and noise, but also specific issues such as minimum cage dimensions, and provide the mandatory minimal standards for all EU member countries.

Cages in experimental facilities are typically constructed from metal with wire mesh walls or parallel metal bars for easy cleaning. However, materials that are warmer to the touch, chew-resistant, and provide a quieter environment than clanking metal cages are preferred and should be used when possible. Ideally, cages should include a separate area, like a balcony, where animals can be individually trained.

Breeding facilities typically encompass larger spaces and house larger groups of animals compared to experimental facilities. Ideally, animals in breeding groups should have access to both indoor and outdoor enclosures, if feasible. In a breeding configuration, animals can be housed in peer groups where all animals are of the same age, or in multigenerational groups. While it may be legally permissible to remove infants from their mothers and peer-house them already from the age of 8 months, this practice diverges from their species-specific behavior and negatively impacts their welfare [99]. Preferably, animals in breeding groups should be housed in multigenerational groups that closely mimic the species' natural group composition as much as possible, and young males should only be removed from their natal group at a juvenile age [100].

The structural layout of macaque enclosures is crucial. Both the size and complexity must be sufficient to prevent intimidation by cage mates. It is vital that animals can utilize as much of the volume as possible and have access to high perches. Incorporating large structures to create a 3D environment ensures optimal use of the enclosure. Environmental enrichment, such as swings, perches, climbing opportunities, and bedding for foraging, should be provided (see below). Foraging is a natural and beneficial behavior that can occupy a significant portion of time, reducing boredom and the occurrence of stereotypic behaviors. Therefore, substrates like sawdust, woodchips, hemp, or shavings should be used to scatter food for foraging. Additionally, hay, straw, or shredded paper can be offered for further enrichment.

Careful design and positioning of drains and air vents are essential to ensure optimal functionality, facilitate easy maintenance, and maintain a healthy climate for the animals, e.g. [101]. Visual barriers and escape routes should be integrated into cage systems to enable animals to be out of sight of each other and to provide means for escaping from dominant individuals. Flexibility is essential to separate animals when required, such as for treatments or when animals are injured.

7.3.3.2 Is Single Housing of Macaques Acceptable?

Macaques are social animals and housing them individually can lead to abnormal behavior. This has not only impact on their well-being but also on research outcomes [102]. Therefore, providing social housing for macaques in both breeding and experimental settings is among the most crucial forms of enrichment and represents an essential aspect of their well-being. Single housing should only be considered for a short time and under compelling circumstances, such as illness or specific short-term experimental requirements. All efforts should focus on actively managing the environment and group composition to maintain social stability. A critical element of this approach is to start with suitable compatible individuals. Whenever feasible, engaging in effective communication with the breeding colony from which the animals originate can aid in selecting compatible animals. Because social housing is crucial, there are occasions when it becomes necessary to introduce unfamiliar animals to each other. This situation may arise when an animal in a pair-housing arrangement must be euthanized due to health or welfare concerns, when animals engage in fights and need to be separated, or when new animals are introduced to the facility. Introducing unfamiliar animals should be undertaken by staff members with extensive behavioral knowledge and the expertise to assess the introduction process accurately.

7.3.3.3 What Are the Possibilities for Social Enrichment?

It is essential that macaques are housed in social groups. When considering social enrichment, bear in mind that introduction processes are sometimes easy, other times very challenging. Knowing your animals, proper planning, selection of partners, and good observation skills are key to achieve a compatible pair or group. Bear in mind that no introduction is the same. Sometimes everything seems to be going smoothly until you leave the animal room and the animals start fighting. Even the presence of a familiar observer can inhibit their behavior. Introduction success and formation of stable compatible pairs or groups are also dependent on the group size and composition. Important aspects, are, e.g., how are existing groups related to each other? Have they been stable for a while? Have animals been tried to pair up before or have they never met each other? (Figs. 7.13 and 7.14)

7.3.4 Physical Enrichment: Structure and Changing Items

7.3.4.1 How Essential Is Environmental Enrichment?

Given the natural behavior of macaques and their highly social and cognitive capabilities, environmental enrichment is not a choice but a must. Environmental enrichment is a dynamic process that requires ongoing review, assessment, and adjustment. It is pivotal in shaping and modifying an animal's environment to offer behavioral

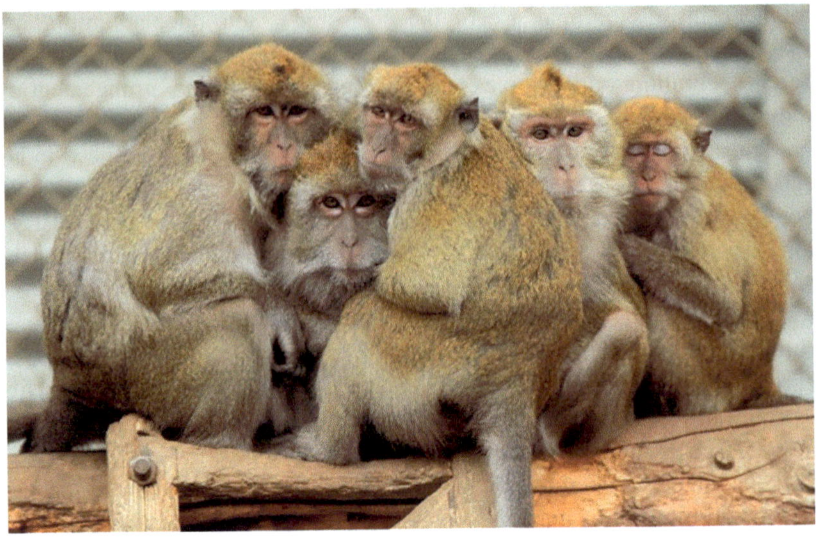

Fig. 7.13 Social housing of macaques

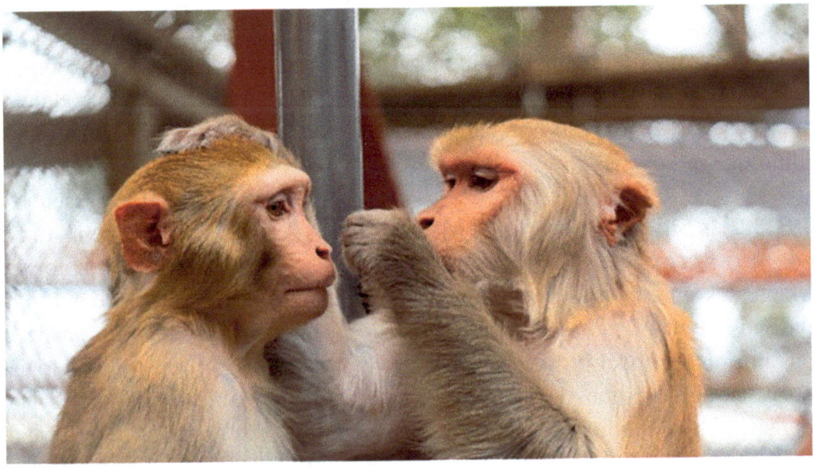

Fig. 7.14 Macaques: importance of social interaction

options and elicit species-specific behaviors and abilities, thereby enhancing their welfare. Whereas it is good to have everything controllable to provide the animal a sense of control through predictability, changes and variation of the environmental enrichment are required to keep it interesting and unpredictable to the animal. It is essential to acknowledge that the optimal enrichment varies for each individual macaque.

There are several approaches that can be used to implement environmental enrichment. Especially in breeding facilities approaching the natural wild environment of the animals is a feasible possibility. This is an approach that resembles the situation in zoos to some extent. This is more difficult in experimental facilities in which cages are usually smaller and social groups are less naturalistic. Here, specific enrichment items and approaches can be used, including the regular changing of food and non-food enrichment. In the following paragraphs, we provide some examples of environmental enrichment that can be used in breeding and experimental facilities housing macaques.

7.3.4.2 How to Use Perches and Climbing Structures to Enrich the Physical Environment?

The physical habitat includes all elements related to the housing of the animals. In breeding facilities, these include a variety of large, more complex constructions, such as climbing and perching structures. Importantly, durability and usability of such constructions must be taken into consideration. Safety is also an important element for all constructions/items, consult the veterinarian when there is any doubt. When applying wood in an enclosure, it should be realized that macaques will eat and destroy the wood. It is important to be aware that wood from certain trees can be toxic when consumed in larger quantities. However, this also grants animals a higher level of control over the environment, as they have the option to choose whether to engage in destructive behaviors or not. It also increases the level of control over the environment for the animals since they can choose to destroy something or not. Hard plastic can be a viable alternative that is less easily destroyed and better cleanable. Especially in experimental facilities, such as those studying infectious diseases, it is crucial to consider cleanability as well. In both, experimental and breeding facilities, fire hoses or ropes can be an option for more flexible climbing structures. A variation in length of the ropes might make it even more attractive for the animals in that they can choose what they prefer. Other examples of items that can be used, especially in larger cages, are car tires, larger food or storage containers, or rubber grilles, where they can sit with conspecifics. When dealing with older or very young animals, careful consideration of the implications for cage design is essential. Universal access to all perches must be ensured. Strategies such as incorporating ladders or minimizing jumping distances required to reach perches should be explored.

Large outdoor facilities have more possibilities for enrichment. Even climate can have positive impact, provided that the animals have a possibility to choose where they want to be and can seek shelter for rain, sun, and warm or cold weather. On nice winter days, especially rhesus macaques are often observed to play in the snow and with ice (Figs. 7.15 and 7.16).

7.3.4.3 How to Use Water as Enrichment?

Macaques, especially long-tailed macaques (*Macaca fascicularis*), like to play with water and, if possible, to swim. In outdoor facilities small ponds can be used as enrichment [103]. Especially in breeding or larger groups younger animals will use water to play and interact with each other, resulting in a positive group dynamic. Also in experimental facilities, this can be used, e.g., by providing, just before or after cleaning, deep containers filled with water in areas where bedding is not present at that moment. Adding baby bubblesoap makes it possible to play with foam (Fig. 7.17).

7.3.5 Food and Foraging

7.3.5.1 How to Stimulate Foraging Behavior?

Macaques are omnivores and in wilderness such primates spend more time in foraging than they invest in any other activity. In captivity, the main

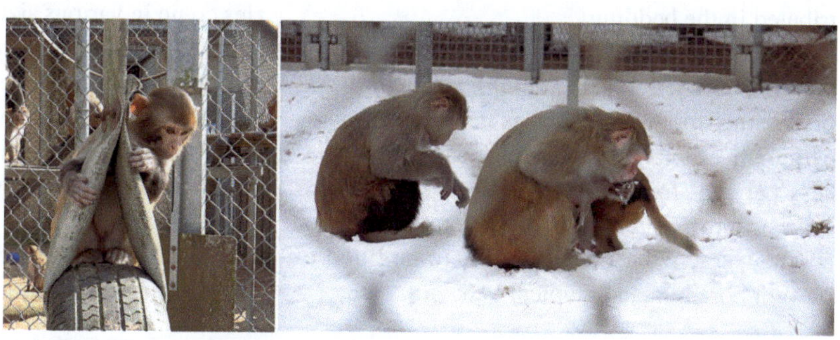

Fig. 7.15 Physical environment: (**a**) use of tires and (**b**) climate, macaques in the snow

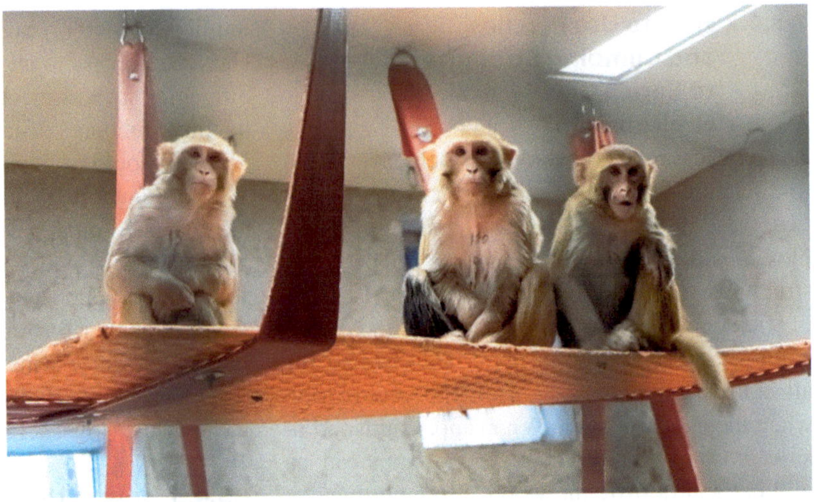

Fig. 7.16 Physical environment: Use of rubber grilles (tenderfoot)

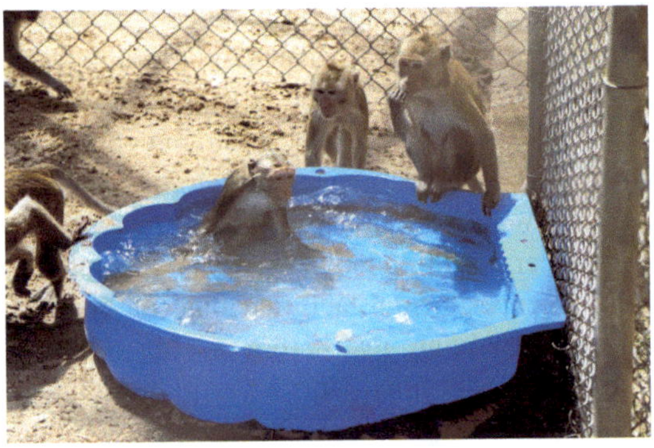

Fig. 7.17 Water as enrichment for macaques (courtesy of Sacha Dumay, BPRC)

source of food is commercially available pellets that contain all necessary nutrients. Since food gathering in captivity is much less needed, it is advisable to have several feeding times throughout the day during which vegetables, grains, and fruit can be offered. With regard to the latter, care must be taken to limit the amount of sugar-rich food. To further stimulate foraging behavior, it is advisable to provide herbs and grains that are distributed in the bedding.

The availability of and ease to get food reduces the time needed for searching, retrieving, and processing food. This makes captive primates extremely efficient foragers, as measured by success per unit foraging time. However, this also leaves captive primates with much more time for alternative activities, which needs to be filled to prevent boredom and atypical behavior.

By providing primates with food enrichment, food searching, food retrieving, and food processing behaviors are promoted. Food enrichment can include the provision of new food items and providing food in such a way that it takes time and efforts for the animals to obtain the food. Novelty as well as complexity will trigger exploratory behaviors, next to the other behaviors that are paired with providing food enrichment (being food searching, food retrieving, and food processing). When providing animals with novelty, it must be ensured that there is also a possibility for them to avoid and ignore the novel item, to minimize fearful reactions. Furthermore, it is important to keep in mind that not all individuals have had the same rearing conditions and experiences and that what is new for some individuals is not new for others.

For familiar food items, enrichment solutions can be found in alternative food presentation.

Some daily pellet food can be presented in a puzzle feeder or in a rolled-up paper bag, which makes food retrieval more complex. Food puzzles come in various sizes and forms. They can be easily crafted from materials like bottles, empty food containers, etc., as long as they afford the animals the opportunity to engage in food-related activities and are safe for their use. Another option is to scatter feed. Especially small food items, such as grains, herbs, or corn scattered over a bedded floor (woodchips, sawdust, or biofloor) promote foraging behaviors.

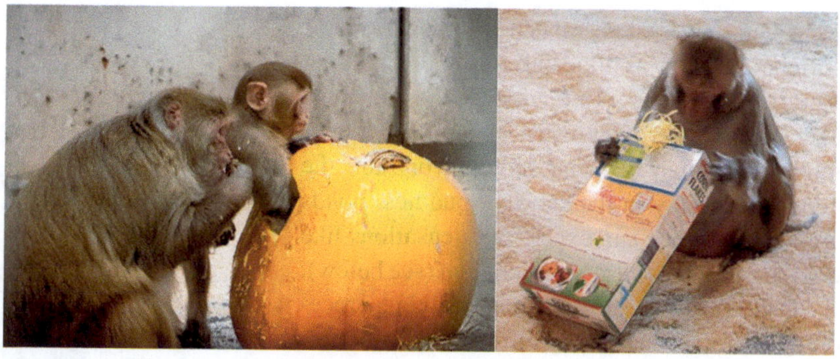

Fig. 7.18 Food enrichment: novel food (**a**) and hiding of food (**b**)

Finally, alternative presentation can be found in hiding, freezing, or burying food. This makes not only food retrieval more difficult but also its processing, resulting in increased time that is spent on feeding. Providing small or larger cups with frozen water containing small particles of fruit, grains, or sunflower seeds is easy and will occupy the animals for some time. In all cases, care must be taken that the food enrichment items are not monopolized by high-ranking individuals. To prevent this, many smaller food (but also non-food) enrichment items can be distributed at different sites in the enclosures to spread out competition. Additionally, hiding various items in hard-to-reach areas helps to reduce the effects of monopolization (Fig. 7.18).

7.3.5.2 Can Substrate Be Used to Stimulate Foraging Behavior?

Foraging is an essential pastime for the macaques. In outdoor-indoor facilities, this is relatively easy to reach. Although many facilities have concrete floors in their outdoor facility this can also be replaced by sand or bedding. Indoor facilities are usually using bedding, such as sawdust, woodchip, or biofloors. In experimental cages, having a good overview of the animals' dietary intake and fecal characteristics is crucial, with cleanliness being a particularly important aspect to address. Therefore, biofloors are usually not a good choice, and in general wood chips or sawdust dedicated for animal facilities is used. To promote foraging, some straw or hay can be added to increase the height of the substrate and increase the difficulty to find small grains or food items (see below). All this bedding material can be autoclaved/destroyed when used in high-containment facilities. Important aspects to consider for bedding are: cleanability, absorption of feces and urine, and quality for foraging (Fig. 7.19).

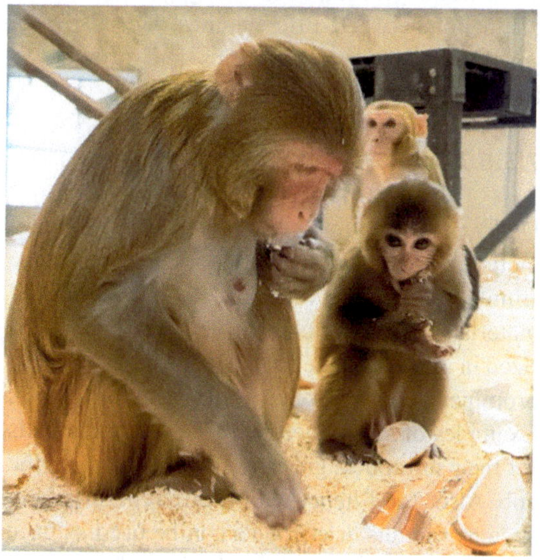

Fig. 7.19 Foraging possibilities

7.3.6 Engaging Mind and Sensory Systems

7.3.6.1 What About Cognitive Enrichment?

Like all animals, macaques require novel experiences and mental stimulation. Cognitive enrichment is one of the categories of enrichment. Cognitive enrichment is not an isolated enrichment item but is often related to other forms of enrichment such as food puzzles. For breeding facilities with access to outdoor enclosures also changing weather circumstances are part of cognitive enrichment. During snowfall or rain, the animals can play in the snow or puddles, ponds are frozen or they can experience sensations like cold weather and sensory enrichment (see below). By using positive reinforcement training procedures, there are many ways to interact with animals, by having them step on items (e.g., a scale), drink from syringes, follow targets, and make a distinction between different cues. This also triggers their cognitive capacities and provides a form of enrichment.

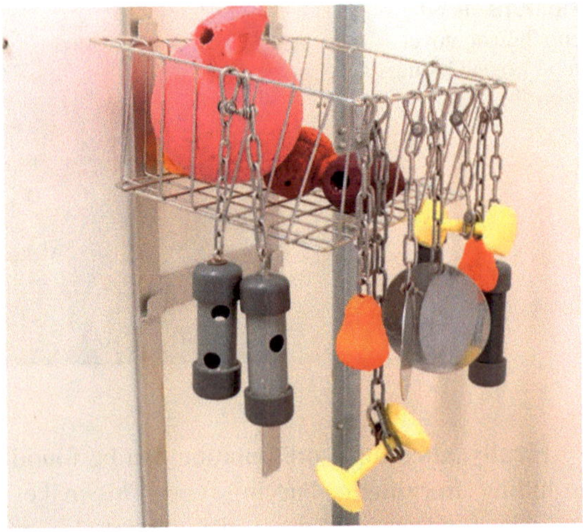

Fig. 7.20 Sensory enrichment: examples of enrichment items

7.3.6.2 What About Sensory Enrichment?

Different forms of sensory enrichment may include visual, auditory, olfactory, and gustatory stimuli, as well as variations in the texture of materials. Every enrichment item can be categorized in more than one way, but some have a more prominent feature, like a certain smell or texture. Examples of sensory enrichment are tennis balls for their soft touch, grooming mats or corn on the cob. Also, food items with a different structure, such as walnuts or coconuts can be used as taste and sensory enrichment. Addition of olfactory stimuli can be achieved by providing/adding scenting herbs like garlic or anise. Further sensory enrichment includes provision of bright colored objects or visual enrichment such as movable mirrors (Fig. 7.20).

7.3.7 Concluding Remarks

There are many ways to provide environmental enrichment to macaques. Given the high cognitive capacities of these animals, it is necessary to have an enrichment program in place where the enrichment items are regularly rotated to prevent habituation and boredom. Because macaques are outbred animals, raised in various breeding settings, and due to a strict dominance hierarchy which influences their upbringing (low-ranking or high-ranking individuals have easy/difficult access to enrichment), it is impossible to make enrichment comparable for all animals. Therefore, unlike in the case of mice, it is much less relevant which specific type of enrichment a macaque has access to. What is far more important is that there is always sufficient social and environmental enrichment available.

Please be aware that this chapter does not provide an in-depth review regarding housing and environmental enrichment for macaques or other nonhuman primate species. For more information on various enrichment possibilities, you can refer to resources like, e.g., the BPRC enrichment manual (https://www.bprc.nl/sites/default/files/downloads/Enrichment%20Manual.pdf) [104] and the NC3R macaque website (https://macaques.nc3rs.org.uk).

7.4 Thoughts on Enrichment for Laboratory Dogs and Rabbits: How to Address the Needs of These Species in Enrichment Programs?

7.4.1 How Does Housing Larger Species Differ from the More Commonly Used Rodents?

Housing larger species such as rabbits and dogs brings with it different challenges compared to housing rodents. Their larger size not only requires larger housing needs but also larger equipment, enrichment items, more expansive cleaning workload, and a larger time investment from personnel per animal. Since these species are larger, they often require more physically intensive handling, and as such, investing in a training schedule [105] can benefit both animal welfare and ease of handling in the long run. Staff require training in how to handle these larger animals, as inappropriate handling increases the risk of distress and injury to the animals and can possibly cause harm and ergonomic concerns for the people working with them [106]. Difficult handling of larger animals can also contribute to work dissatisfaction [107].

Housing larger species may also require the need for additional barriers and practices to prevent escape, as the animals can damage their surroundings or even learn how to open doors and pens. Providing sufficient enrichment prevents boredom and can reduce instances of animals damaging the housing environment.

Veterinary treatment options for larger species are more expansive compared to what is possible for rodents. Basic medical and surgical treatment for illnesses must be possible, and staff must be trained and equipped to provide the necessary care for each species.

7.4.2 What Are Specific Considerations When Housing Dogs?

Legislation such as the EU directive 2010/63/EU and the USDA include requirements on the housing of dogs. However, housing practices for dogs should include more than what is legally required. Similar to rodents, dogs are social animals that should be housed in groups as much as possible. These groups can vary in size but using small, stable groups is preferred. Staff should be familiar with dog behavior and should know how and when to adjust groups when incompatibility between individuals is observed. Usually, dog groups are easily adjusted if needed [108]. Primary enclosures for dogs should be of sufficient size to allow the dogs in the group to be able to be together, to hide from others if desired, and should allow for sufficient physical exercise. Being able to observe the room, including other animals and points of entry, helps to reduce loud vocalizations and instances of aggression toward other dogs in the same room. Reduced vocalizations also presents less risk for hearing damage to staff and reduces distress to the dogs [109]. Other species, especially prey species, can be disturbed by the noises generated by dogs and should be housed separately and distant as a mitigation method.

Female dogs have on average two estrus cycles per year, though there are variations. During these cycles, intact males may display more instances of aggression or other unwanted behavior. The fertile periods are also not always clearly observable; care must be taken to avoid males coming into contact with females to avoid unwanted pregnancies. Separating males and females into different rooms is best practice.

Depending on the type of research, dogs can be housed in facilities long term, and routine health maintenance is necessary. As dogs age, frequent prophylactic treatments, regular veterinary health checks [110], and routine dental care are more frequently necessary. Proper veterinary care for dogs also requires the necessary infrastructure, such as surgical facilities, in-house medication supplies, and equipment such as X-ray, ultrasound, and dental facilities. More extensive veterinary care such as specialist surgeries may require cooperation with veterinary clinics or specialty centers. When maintaining older dogs, additional care is needed, such as more frequent health checks, long-term treatments, or modified housing, and as such this should only be considered when scientifically necessary. Treatments may be needed for common canine maladies and might conflict with research goals. In these cases, veterinarians, care staff, and researchers must determine the best way forward on a case-by-case basis, with the animal's welfare always taking precedence [105].

7.4.3 What Special Considerations Are There When Designing an Enrichment Program for Dogs?

Dogs are intelligent, social, and curious and can be prone to boredom if not properly provided with enrichment. Insufficient enrichment and minimal social interactions may cause welfare and behavioral problems in the animals [111]. Enrichment for dogs includes toys, treats [112], socialization [113] (both with other dogs and with humans), and diverse resting spaces. Toys [114] should be of high quality, easily cleaned, and sturdy enough to remain intact with active use but also soft enough not to cause damage to their teeth. Toys should be rotated to avoid disinterest. If dogs are not provided with materials for chewing, they might seek other ways of expressing this need, which could result in damage to the environment [115] and injury to the animal. A wide variety of treats are available but should be used sparingly and when not in conflict with the study goals. It is good practice to have treats distinct from regular food. Resting places, such as baskets or dog beds, are highly desired by the animals, but must also be of high quality and easily cleanable.

Enrichment items should be frequently rotated, routinely cleaned, regularly inspected and replaced as needed. The number of items per dog must be sufficient to not cause conflict within the group. This also can conflict with the need to standardize all environmental parameters; however, not doing so will negatively impact animal welfare and as mentioned above, might result in boredom and unwanted behaviors.

Providing dogs with play areas, both inside and outside, is a good form of enrichment. These can be outfitted with exercise equipment and novel toys, allow for more freedom of movement and exploration, and the animals can socialize with a larger group. Of course, these play areas bring an additional need for maintenance and time spent transporting and supervising the animals. Having outdoor play areas may invite public curiosity and an appropriate communication plan should be developed. While in the play areas, dogs should have unlimited access and handling should be limited to necessity to foster the positive impact of the play areas.

A walking program for dogs can also be considered. This can be contained to the facility grounds or even go outside of the perimeter. This can provide an opportunity for staff that do not work with these animals to get acquainted with the animals and the research program and is often well perceived. For the dogs, this provides an opportunity to explore novel environments and get accustomed to typical outside factors like cars, bikes, and pedestrians, which helps them acclimate should they be adopted. Again, this requires time, effort, planning, and additional prophylaxis (deworming, vaccination, treatment for ectoparasites), and not all dogs will eagerly join such walks. Dogs will require training for these walks to get accustomed to walking on a leash. While actively participating in study, dogs may not be able to participate in outdoor walks as this brings them outside of the controlled environment. There are also risks that need to be considered, such as potential contact with pathogens.

7.4.4 What Is Needed to Train and Socialize Dogs?

Both pet dogs and research dogs require socialization and training to be well acclimated and adjusted [113, 116]. Behavioral issues often stem from poor or improper training and socialization. Although dogs purposefully bred for research tend to be docile, social, and not aggressive, there are benefits to having a well-thought-out training plan in place for dogs. Training animals to willingly participate in procedures reduces stress and anxiety, stereotypic behavior, and aggression in the animals, which will benefit welfare and provide more accurate results. An additional benefit of training and socialization is that staff working with these animals have more positive interactions, increasing work satisfaction [117]. One of the pitfalls of training is that staff can misread [118] or even (often unintentionally) encourage behaviors in the animals that are actually signs of stress [119]. A dog that lays down instantly when approached is easily picked up, but this behavior is actually a sign of distress in the animal. Similarly, a training plan that is not well thought out can potentially increase discomfort in the animals and can make animals less compliant. Having a robust training plan with measurable goals is encouraged. Staff should also be encouraged to seek routine opportunity for interaction with the animals [120], while not encouraging poor behaviors. Having staff formally trained in dog behavior or hiring external specialist consultants is preferred and will help in avoiding the use of incorrect training techniques.

7.4.5 How Do You Start an Adoption Program?

An adoption program should be considered [121], especially for dogs and other amenable non-rodent species. While adoption is possible for all species, dogs, as commonly housed pets, are generally easy to find a suitable home for. Animals can be adopted both within and outside of the institution. Working with an intermediary such as a rehoming organization or humane society can make it easier to find homes for the animals. Since these animals will be placed in private homes, proper, open communication with the adoption agency or foster homes is a must. Animals considered for adoption must be healthy, well-adjusted and should have received appropriate prophylaxis. However, animals with health or behavioral abnormalities may also be adopted with the proper evaluations and under appropriate conditions [122]. Careful consideration of the long-term well-being of these animals is key, and while one must consider the public perception of animal research, this alone is not reason to not rehome these animals. These instances should be discussed on a case-by-case basis with veterinarians, management and care staff and should first and foremost have the animal's best interest in mind.

Working with an adoption agency, local shelter or other intermediaries help to shape the adoption program, as they can provide feedback on the typical challenges these animals face when rehomed and have experience in rehoming animals. Often times these animals go from a very regulated, stable, and predictable environment to the chaos of an ordinary home. These can often present as the new owner comparing the animals to pets already acclimated to living in an ordinary home and may believe any behavioral challenges are the result of research, rather than the animal simply being unfamiliar with the new environment [122]. Walking the dogs outside on a leash while they are in the facility, for instance, and having them get accustomed to cars, bikes, pedestrians, and outside noises, will improve their adaption to retirement. Having the animals well accustomed to handling and petting will also help reduce fear and anxiety in the new environment.

7.4.6 How Can the Public Perception of Research Dogs Best Be Handled?

While the public [123] generally understands the need for animals in research (within ethical and legal limitations), the public acceptance of the study of dogs compared to rodents is more challenged, likely due to their status as loyal and well-liked pets. Having a very strong Culture of Care within the research program will help alleviate some public concerns surrounding the study of dogs. Going beyond the minimum requirements for housing dogs and providing strong enrichment are a must within a program that has a strong Culture of Care and may help alleviate some public concerns. Adoption programs are a good method of interacting with the public [121], as the dogs that were previously involved in research then become part of the public sphere. Having well-adjusted, social, and healthy dogs in the public view will support an institute's commitment to strong animal welfare in research. Having outside activities such as play areas or walking programs might invite questions and curiosity from the general public. Instead of avoiding these types of outside activities, they can be opportunities to engage and educate the public on the high standard of care that is provided within research institutions.

7.4.7 Do Dogs Require Specific PPE?

There are diseases that can transmit between dogs and humans, such as leptospirosis [124], dermatophytosis [125], and Methicillin-Resistant *Staphylococcus aureus* (MRSA) [126]. The risk of transmission is fairly low when the dogs are acquired from reputable sources, are treated with appropriate prophylaxis, and with appropriate hygiene. The nature of dogs as pets might encourage staff to be a bit careless though, and they might, for instance, let dogs lick one's face, which can potentially transmit disease. Unless the research requires otherwise, appropriate work clothing and gloves should be sufficient. Dogs that go outside should receive additional prophylaxis as mentioned above, which reduces the dog's risk of acquiring disease and transmitting diseases to staff.

Aggression can be a concern when working with dogs. Distress, pain, research compound, or study setup (such as when using stimulants) can increase the risk of dog-to-dog and dog-to-human aggression. The staff in charge of the day-to-day care of the dogs often know these animals, but even then there can be a risk of a biting incident. Appropriate training and socialization, warnings on the cage, staff training, and use of aids such as muzzles can reduce the risk of a biting incident. Dog bites should always be taken seriously and be reported. They should be followed by action to prevent the animal from biting others and determine potential causes and methods on how this could have been prevented. Dog bites also require medical intervention [127], as they can be a cause for bacterial infection, such as *Pasteurella* spp.

7.4.8 How Do You Approach Housing of Rabbits?

Rabbits are preferably housed in groups, though it is well known that both males and females can be aggressive [128], so there should be room to separate individuals if needed. When grouping rabbits, it is normal for the animals to establish hierarchy and this does not always require separating the animals [129]. Group-housing should still be considered the standard, and where possible, castration and sterilization can help reduce aggression. This is a consideration when housing rabbits for a longer period. Separating males and females in different rooms will also help reduce aggression. Unless housed together from a young age, grouping older animals, especially males, can trigger aggression. Careful observation when regrouping is needed [130], as fighting rabbits can cause serious, even life-threatening injuries to one another. The risk of injury is reduced if the animals have sufficient space to avoid one another when needed. When rabbits are single-housed one needs to ensure that they can visualize other animals which helps to reduce distress and boredom [131]. The cages can also be provided with separators that still allow the animals a small amount of physical contact such as nose-to-nose without risk of harm, though in certain situations this can increase distress between incompatible individuals. However, this gradual contact can improve the chances of successful group-housing later.

Housing can be done in cages, both conventional and IVC, or on floor pens. Cages are limited in space and capacity for enrichment but are more efficiently managed, and make it easier to house animals in small groups and isolate aggressive individuals or animals with health issues. IVC systems reduce exposure to allergens as well. Floor pens allow for more space for enrichment, larger groups, and freedom of movement, but are more labor-intensive, and must have provisions for staff to easily handle the animals when needed. Still, from a Culture of Care perspective, floor pens are the preferred housing method. As mentioned, sufficient freedom to avoid others and retreat can reduce aggression and the risk of injury [130]. Providing sufficient opportunities for food and water can also help avoid conflict over resources. When housing in cages, animals should be provided time in more open play areas or have increased human interaction. Cages should also be tall enough to allow the animals to rear and scan their environments.

Pest control is as important here as it is in other species, but for rabbits specifically, diseases such as myxomatosis [132] and myiasis that are transmitted by arthropods are important to consider.

7.4.9 What Enrichment Can Rabbits Be Given?

Typical enrichment [133] for rabbits consists of gnawing [134] materials, manipulanda, shelters, and elevations. When housing animals individually or in cages, having a designated play area with enough space to exercise and climb should be considered as enrichment. Cardboard shelters and items can be considered but require frequent replacement to avoid becoming soiled and too damaged. Researchers might also have concerns regarding the animals eating too much cardboard which can interfere with intestinal uptake. Having solid shelters is a must since rabbits seek a place to hide in times of stress [130]. Providing rabbits with hay [135] can stimulate foraging behavior, add needed roughage to the diet, and give the animals material to play and build nests with. Rabbit teeth [136] continuously grow, so providing suitable gnawing materials such as gnawing blocks helps prevent dental overgrowth and provides an additional play item.

Rabbits can be given fresh produce as treats, though this must be done in moderation and without interfering with research. Foods and treats too high in fats and carbohydrates, and low in fiber, can cause life-threatening gastrointestinal signs [137].

Mirrors have been suggested as enrichment for rabbits [138], though response can vary and as such, their use requires validation in most cases.

As described above, rabbits also benefit from training and habituation, though the approach in these animals can be a bit different. As prey species, they can be harder to motivate. Sufficient habituation to handling and human contact will help with this.

7.4.10 What Special Considerations Do Rabbits Need?

Similar to rodents, rabbits are prey species and as such will try to escape, especially when handled inappropriately. Their larger size and delicate bone structure means these animals are more prone to injury [139–141], for instance, due to kicking. Inappropriate handling can result in skin lesions or degloving injuries of tails. Staff need to be well trained in handling rabbits to reduce the animals' distress and avoid injury. Habituating the rabbits to handling and procedures from a young age will help reduce stress and fear responses [142].

7.4.11 Do Rabbits Require Special Personal Protective Enrichment (PPE)?

Laboratory animal allergy is a well-known occupational hazard in animal research [143]. As rabbits can be housed in floor pens or open cages and are often provided hay and/or straw, there can be a large concentration of allergens [144, 145] associated with rabbit housing. A risk assessment [146] must be made when housing rabbits to protect staff from unacceptable exposure to allergens. Measurements of rabbit allergens are possible and should be done to assess the risks and required PPE. There exist IVC systems for rabbits but by their nature often are restricted in space and room for enrichment, as mentioned earlier. Ventilation, PPE, workflows, and Laminar Air Flow (LAF) roofs will reduce the risks of exposure to allergens.

7.5 Thoughts on Enrichment for Aquatics: What About Environmental Enrichment for Our Aquatic Animals?

7.5.1 Introduction

The housing conditions for aquatic animals are obviously very different to terrestrial species, but similar questions must be addressed regarding their welfare and the enrichment of their environment. The topic is barely studied in most species, and the impact on science remains unknown. However, practical observations in the animal facility and experimental data from zebrafish (*Danio rerio*) and *Xenopus* spp. studies correlate on what appears to be beneficial to the animals in their physical and social environment, sometimes making it into a compulsory provision under national regulations. In general, social animals must be kept group housed, and isolation of a singly-housed animal in a tank is only tolerated for short periods. As natural behaviors are to be promoted, providing live feed to predators seems a relevant feeding option, as long as nutritional values and biosecurity constraints are observed [147]. Regarding the physical environment, regulations insist mainly on the water quality (See chapter "Husbandry (food, water, sanitation, waste, identification)"). Little is known regarding the light spectrum that best adapted to each species. However, ensuring a gradual light intensity variation to simulate dawn and dusk is a popular approach in aquatic facilities. Limiting vibration is also a concern often raised in the laboratories, whereas the provision of music is a topic of investigation. No general rule can be set regarding the addition of devices and the occupation of the space in the tanks, these are species-dependent matters.

7.5.2 How to Enrich the Environment of Zebrafish?

The first rule to observe regarding zebrafish is to avoid singly-housing. If singly-housing is not avoidable, then it is recommended to add enrichment devices to the housing tanks [148]. When group-housing zebrafish, the animal can be set with other fish of visibly identifiable markings (e.g., spots vs stripes, long or short fins, males with females, nacre or transparent fish with wild types). However, keeping zebrafish in pairs long term is not the preferred solution as it can lead to aggression. Therefore, zebrafish are kept of groups of three fishes as a bare minimum, for social enrichment to provide a robust environmental enrichment. Note that it can be a regulatory requirement to keep a maximum of 5 to 10 adult zebrafish per liter of tank water.

Even when zebrafish are group housed, only a few facilities add enrichment devices in their housing tanks. Many facilities fear to follow this step which requires supplementary technician time to clean the devices to prevent biofilm build-up. There is also report that aggression due to territorial behavior may be triggered by the addition of enrichment devices to the tank, although these behaviors are sometimes seen in absence of such devices [148]. Items can also be added at the bottom of or underneath the zebrafish tanks [149]. Again, the addition of marbles might constitute a valuable environmental enrichment at the cost of significant additional cleaning duties. A common alternative is to focus on procedural and husbandry events for which fish tanks are removed from their housing shelves and set on a bench of a vivid color contrast, for example from black shelf to white bench. To tame the contrast, a picture of gravels or of a suitable color can be set on the bench and prevent fish from displaying signs of stress such as swimming at the tank bottom.

The last points to bear in mind regarding environmental enrichment for zebrafish are linked to the swimming activity of the fish. To support the animals' predatorial behavior, and to provide adequate nutrition at early developmental stages, live feeds are provided from 5 days post fertilization, when zebrafish becomes able to swim, chase, and bite freely moving targets. Brine shrimp or similar are usually provided to later stages, although avoiding routine daily provision to adults may be an arguable option to avoid habituation. With the rapid standardization of the housing systems in the laboratory facilities, variations of flow strengths and of spaces available to zebrafish have not been studied extensively, despite both being adjustable at tank level. For example, experience shows that a stressed group of fish in a small tank sometimes shows relief when set in a larger tank, potentially signalling that increasing tank sizes could be a valuable environmental enrichment for zebrafish.

7.5.3 How to Enrich the Environment of *Xenopus* spp.?

Xenopus tropicalis are smaller animals than *Xenopus laevis*. When provided with the right environmental enrichment, such as nenuphar-type devices creating supports at the surface of the tank water, *X. tropicalis* are commonly seen out of the water resting on the supports, or potentially hiding floating within the enrichment device. *X. laevis* are too heavy to be carried by soft plastic, but they show a strong preference for environmental enrichment devices providing them with many hiding places. For example, this can be large enough PVC pipes or complex plants. The most important is to provide many hiding places and avoid empty tanks [150].

The number of *X. laevis* in a tank should be adapted to the animals' behaviors. For example, when too many males are housed together, they stay plugged to each other for too long and skin injury appear. An easy solution is to add some males to the female tanks; this does not seem to reduce the egg quality or quantity. Another example is when the access to the feed distribution point is too narrow (i.e., the side of the tank accessed by the technician at feeding time), *X. laevis* fight and bite each other forelimbs. The behavior is easily recognizable for such an otherwise calm animal. Moreover, it leaves typical wounds on the forelimbs (Fig. 7.21). When the access to feed cannot be widened, the only solution is to reduce the number of *Xenopus* spp. in the tank.

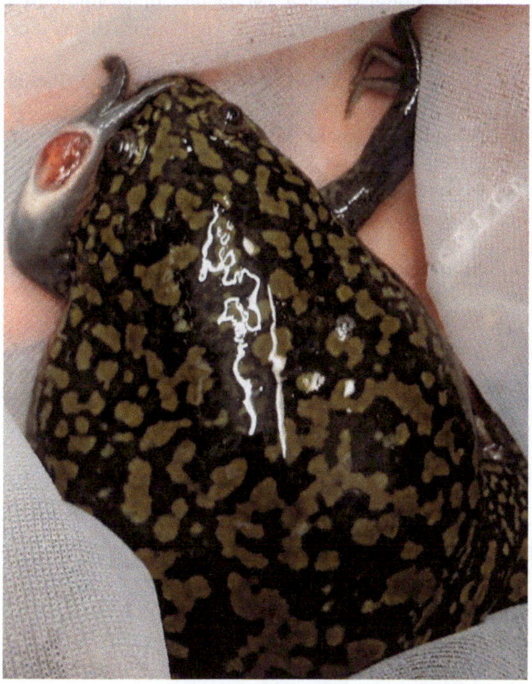

Fig. 7.21 Wound on the forelimb of a *Xenopus laevis* following a fight at feeding time

References

1. Bailoo JD, Murphy E, Boada-Sana M, Varholick JA, Hintze S, Baussiere C, et al. Effects of cage enrichment on behavior, welfare and outcome variability in female mice. Front Behav Neurosci. 2018;12:232.
2. Augustsson H, van de Weerd HA, Kruitwagen CL, Baumans V. Effect of enrichment on variation and results in the light/dark test. Lab Anim. 2003;37(4):328–40.
3. Wolfer DP, Litvin O, Morf S, Nitsch RM, Lipp HP, Wurbel H. Laboratory animal welfare: cage enrichment and mouse behaviour. Nature. 2004;432(7019):821–2.
4. Reardon S. A mouse's house may ruin experiments. Nature. 2016;530(7590):264.
5. Tsai PP, Stelzer HD, Hedrich HJ, Hackbarth H. Are the effects of different enrichment designs on the physiology and behaviour of DBA/2 mice consistent? Lab Anim. 2003;37(4):314–27.
6. Andre V, Gau C, Scheideler A, Aguilar-Pimentel JA, Amarie OV, Becker L, et al. Laboratory mouse housing conditions can be improved using common environmental enrichment without compromising data. PLoS Biol. 2018;16(4):e2005019.
7. Chlebus M, Guillen J, Prins JB. Directive 2010/63/EU: facilitating full and correct implementation. Lab Anim. 2016;50(2):151.
8. Baumans V. Environmental enrichment for laboratory rodents and rabbits: requirements of rodents, rabbits, and research. ILAR J. 2005;46(2):162–70.
9. Baumans V. Science-based assessment of animal welfare: laboratory animals. Rev Sci Tech. 2005;24(2):503–13.
10. Branchi I, D'Andrea I, Fiore M, Di Fausto V, Aloe L, Alleva E. Early social enrichment shapes social behavior and nerve growth factor and brain-derived neurotrophic factor levels in the adult mouse brain. Biol Psychiatry. 2006;60(7):690–6.
11. Chourbaji S, Zacher C, Sanchis-Segura C, Spanagel R, Gass P. Social and structural housing conditions influence the development of a depressive-like phe-

notype in the learned helplessness paradigm in male mice. Behav Brain Res. 2005;164(1):100–6.
12. Curley JP, Jensen CL, Mashoodh R, Champagne FA. Social influences on neurobiology and behavior: epigenetic effects during development. Psychoneuroendocrinology. 2011;36(3):352–71.
13. So N, Franks B, Lim S, Curley JP. A social network approach reveals associations between mouse social dominance and brain gene expression. PLoS One. 2015;10(7):e0134509.
14. Mellor DJ. Moving beyond the "five freedoms" by updating the "five provisions" and introducing aligned "animal welfare aims". Animals (Basel). 2016;6(10)
15. Mellor DJ. Updating animal welfare thinking: moving beyond the "five freedoms" towards "a life worth living". Animals (Basel). 2016;6(3)
16. Van Loo PL, Mol JA, Koolhaas JM, Van Zutphen BF, Baumans V. Modulation of aggression in male mice: influence of group size and cage size. Physiol Behav. 2001;72(5):675–83.
17. Van Loo PL, Van Zutphen LF, Baumans V. Male management: coping with aggression problems in male laboratory mice. Lab Anim. 2003;37(4):300–13.
18. Lewejohann L, Schwabe K, Hager C, Jirkof P. Impulse for animal welfare outside the experiment. Lab Anim. 2020;54(2):150–8.
19. Bratcher NA, Allen CM, McLahan CL, O'Connell DM, Burr HN, Keen JN, et al. Identification of rodent husbandry refinement opportunities through benchmarking and collaboration. J Am Assoc Lab Anim Sci. 2022;61(6):624–33.
20. Gaskill BN, Garner JP. Letter-to-the-editor on "Not so hot: Optimal housing temperatures for mice to mimic the thermal environment of humans". Mol Metab. 2014;3(4):335–6.
21. Gaskill BN, Gordon CJ, Pajor EA, Lucas JR, Davis JK, Garner JP. Impact of nesting material on mouse body temperature and physiology. Physiol Behav. 2013;110–111:87–95.
22. Gaskill BN, Karas AZ, Garner JP, Pritchett-Corning KR. Nest building as an indicator of health and welfare in laboratory mice. J Vis Exp. 2013;82:51012.
23. Deacon RM. Assessing nest building in mice. Nat Protoc. 2006;1(3):1117–9.
24. Whitaker JW, Moy SS, Pritchett-Corning KR, Fletcher CA. Effects of enrichment and litter parity on reproductive performance and behavior in BALB/c and 129/Sv Mice. J Am Assoc Lab Anim Sci. 2016;55(4):387–99.
25. Marashi V, Barnekow A, Sachser N. Effects of environmental enrichment on males of a docile inbred strain of mice. Physiol Behav. 2004;82(5):765–76.
26. Haemisch A, Gartner K. Effects of cage enrichment on territorial aggression and stress physiology in male laboratory mice. Acta Physiol Scand Suppl. 1997;640:73–6.
27. Moghaddam HS, Samarghandian S, Farkhondeh T. Effect of bisphenol A on blood glucose, lipid profile and oxidative stress indices in adult male mice. Toxicol Mech Methods. 2015;25(7):507–13.
28. Weegh N, Funer J, Janke O, Winter Y, Jung C, Struve B, et al. Wheel running behaviour in group-housed female mice indicates disturbed wellbeing due to DSS colitis. Lab Anim. 2020;54(1):63–72.
29. Richter H, Ambree O, Lewejohann L, Herring A, Keyvani K, Paulus W, et al. Wheel-running in a transgenic mouse model of Alzheimer's disease: protection or symptom? Behav Brain Res. 2008;190(1):74–84.
30. Meijer JH, Robbers Y. Wheel running in the wild. Proc Biol Sci R Soc. 2014;281(1786)
31. Vogt MA, Mertens S, Serba S, Palme R, Chourbaji S. The 'Cage Climber' - a new enrichment for use in large-dimensioned mouse facilities. Appl Anim Behav Sci. 2020:230.
32. Theil JH, Ahloy-Dallaire J, Weber EM, Gaskill BN, Pritchett-Corning KR, Felt SA, et al. The epidemiology of fighting in group-housed laboratory mice. Sci Rep. 2020;10(1):16649.
33. Zidar J, Weber EM, Ewaldsson B, Tjader S, Lilja J, Mount J, et al. Group and single housing of male mice: collected experiences from research facilities in Sweden. Animals (Basel). 2019;9(12)
34. Paigen B, Svenson KL, Von Smith R, Marion MA, Stearns T, Peters LL, et al. Physiological effects of housing density on C57BL/6J mice over a 9-month period. J Anim Sci. 2012;90(13):5182–92.
35. Mertens S, Gass P, Palme R, Hiebl B, Chourbaji S. Effect of a partial cage dividing enrichment on aggression-associated parameters in group-housed male C57BL/6NCrl mice. Appl Anim Behav Sci. 2020;224:104939.
36. Tallent BR, Law LM, Rowe RK, Lifshitz J. Partial cage division significantly reduces aggressive behavior in male laboratory mice. Lab Anim. 2018;52(4):384–93.
37. Mazarakis NK, Mo C, Renoir T, van Dellen A, Deacon R, Blakemore C, et al. Super-enrichment' reveals dose-dependent therapeutic effects of environmental stimulation in a transgenic mouse model of huntington's disease. J Huntingtons Dis. 2014;3(3):299–309.
38. Lewejohann L, Reefmann N, Widmann P, Ambree O, Herring A, Keyvani K, et al. Transgenic Alzheimer mice in a semi-naturalistic environment: more plaques, yet not compromised in daily life. Behav Brain Res. 2009;201(1):99–102.
39. Animal research: reporting in vivo experiments: the ARRIVE guidelines. J Physiol. 2010;588(Pt 14):2519–21.
40. Ottman R. Gene-environment interaction: definitions and study designs. Prev Med. 1996;25(6): 764–70.
41. Chourbaji S, Brandwein C, Gass P. Altering BDNF expression by genetics and/or environment: impact for emotional and depression-like behaviour in laboratory mice. Neurosci Biobehav Rev. 2011;35(3):599–611.

42. Drummond GB, Paterson DJ, McGrath JC. ARRIVE: new guidelines for reporting animal research. J Physiol. 2010;588(Pt 14):2517.
43. Smith AJ, Clutton RE, Lilley E, Hansen KEA, Brattelid T. PREPARE: guidelines for planning animal research and testing. Lab Anim. 2018;52(2):135–41.
44. Chourbaji S, Brandwein C, Vogt MA, Dormann C, Hellweg R, Gass P. Nature vs. nurture: Can enrichment rescue the behavioural phenotype of BDNF heterozygous mice? Behav Brain Res. 2008;192(2):254–8.
45. Dahlqvist P, Ronnback A, Bergstrom SA, Soderstrom I, Olsson T. Environmental enrichment reverses learning impairment in the Morris water maze after focal cerebral ischemia in rats. Eur J Neurosci. 2004;19(8):2288–98.
46. Wurbel H. Ideal homes? Housing effects on rodent brain and behaviour. Trends Neurosci. 2001;24(4):207–11.
47. Ganeshan K, Chawla A. Warming the mouse to model human diseases. Nat Rev Endocrinol. 2017;13(8):458–65.
48. Gonder JC, Laber K. A renewed look at laboratory rodent housing and management. ILAR J. 2007;48(1):29–36.
49. Swoap SJ, Overton JM, Garber G. Effect of ambient temperature on cardiovascular parameters in rats and mice: a comparative approach. Am J Physiol Regul Integr Comp Physiol. 2004;287(2):R391–6.
50. Gordon CJ, Aydin C, Repasky EA, Kokolus KM, Dheyongera G, Johnstone AF. Behaviorally mediated, warm adaptation: a physiological strategy when mice behaviorally thermoregulate. J Therm Biol. 2014;44:41–6.
51. Butler-Struben HM, Kentner AC, Trainor BC. What's wrong with my experiment?: The impact of hidden variables on neuropsychopharmacology research. Neuropsychopharmacology. 2022;47(7):1285–91.
52. Watanabe J, Kagami N, Kawazoe M, Arata S. A simplified enriched environment increases body temperature and suppresses cancer progression in mice. Exp Anim. 2020;69(2):207–18.
53. Kingston SG, Hoffman-Goetz L. Effect of environmental enrichment and housing density on immune system reactivity to acute exercise stress. Physiol Behav. 1996;60(1):145–50.
54. Grifols R, Zamora C, Ortega-Saez I, Azkona G. Postweaning grouping as a strategy to reduce singly housed male mice. Animals (Basel). 2020;10(11)
55. Potrebic MS, Pavkovic ZZ, Srbovan MM, Dmura GM, Pesic VT. Changes in the behavior and body weight of mature, adult male wistar han rats after reduced social grouping and social isolation. J Am Assoc Lab Anim Sci. 2022;61(6):615–23.
56. Perez C, Canal JR, Dominguez E, Campillo JE, Guillen M, Torres MD. Individual housing influences certain biochemical parameters in the rat. Lab Anim. 1997;31(4):357–61.
57. Karolewicz B, Paul IA. Group housing of mice increases immobility and antidepressant sensitivity in the forced swim and tail suspension tests. Eur J Pharmacol. 2001;415(2–3):197–201.
58. Weber EM, Zidar J, Ewaldsson B, Askevik K, Uden E, Svensk E, et al. Aggression in group-housed male mice: a systematic review. Animals (Basel). 2022;13(1)
59. Kappel S, Hawkins P, Mendl MT. To group or not to group? good practice for housing male laboratory mice. Animals (Basel). 2017;7(12)
60. Hohlbaum K, Merle R, Frahm S, Rex A, Palme R, Thone-Reineke C, et al. Effects of separated pair housing of female C57BL/6JRj mice on well-being. Sci Rep. 2022;12(1):8819.
61. Moreno-Jimenez EP, Jurado-Arjona J, Avila J, Llorens-Martin M. The social component of environmental enrichment is a pro-neurogenic stimulus in adult c57BL6 female mice. Front Cell Dev Biol. 2019;7:62.
62. Richter SH, Kastner N, Loddenkemper DH, Kaiser S, Sachser N. A time to wean? Impact of weaning age on anxiety-like behaviour and stability of behavioural traits in full adulthood. PLoS One. 2016;11(12):e0167652.
63. Grimm D. Animal research. Male scent may compromise biomedical studies. Science. 2014;344(6183):461.
64. Ferrara F, Hiebl B, Kunzmann P, Hutter F, Afkham F, LaFollette M, et al. Culture of care in animal research - expanding the 3Rs to include people. Lab Anim. 2022;56(6):511–8.
65. Mattison S. Training birds and small mammals for medical behaviors. Vet Clin North Am Exot Anim Pract. 2012;15(3):487–99.
66. Hurst JL, West RS. Taming anxiety in laboratory mice. Nat Methods. 2010;7(10):825–6.
67. Gouveia K, Hurst JL. Improving the practicality of using non-aversive handling methods to reduce background stress and anxiety in laboratory mice. Sci Rep. 2019;9(1):20305.
68. Oatess TL, Harrison FE, Himmel LE, Jones CP. Effects of acrylic tunnel enrichment on anxiety-like behavior, neurogenesis, and physiology of C57BL/6J mice. J Am Assoc Lab Anim Sci. 2021;60(1):44–53.
69. Kilkenny C, Browne W, Cuthill IC, Emerson M, Altman DG. Animal research: reporting in vivo experiments: the ARRIVE guidelines. Br J Pharmacol. 2010;160(7):1577–9.
70. Fitzpatrick BG, Koustova E, Wang Y. Getting personal with the "reproducibility crisis": interviews in the animal research community. Lab Anim (NY). 2018;47(7):175–7.
71. EUR-Lex - L:2009:047:TOC - EN - EUR-Lex [WWW Document], n.d. URL https://eur-lex.europa.eu/legal-content/EN/TXT/?uri=OJ%3AL%3A2009%3A047%3ATOC (accessed 2.25.24a).

72. EUR-Lex - L:2016:062:TOC - EN - EUR-Lex [WWW Document], n.d. URL https://eur-lex.europa.eu/legal-content/EN/TXT/?uri=OJ%3AL%3A2016%3A062%3ATOC (accessed 2.25.24b).
73. Giuliotti L, Benvenuti MN, Giannarelli A, Mariti C, Gazzano A. Effect of different environment enrichments on behaviour and social interactions in growing pigs. Animals. 2019;9:101. https://doi.org/10.3390/ani9030101.
74. Kittawornrat A, Zimmerman JJ. Toward a better understanding of pig behavior and pig welfare. Anim Health Res Rev. 2011;12:25–32. https://doi.org/10.1017/S1466252310000174.
75. Mkwanazi MV, Ncobela CN, Kanengoni AT, Chimonyo M. Effects of environmental enrichment on behaviour, physiology and performance of pigs — A review. Asian Australas J Anim Sci. 2018;32:1–13. https://doi.org/10.5713/ajas.17.0138.
76. Godyń D, Nowicki J, Herbut P. Effects of environmental enrichment on pig welfare—a review. Animals. 2019;9:383. https://doi.org/10.3390/ani9060383.
77. Rørvang MV, Schild S-LA, Stenfelt J, Grut R, Gadri MA, Valros A, Nielsen BL, Wallenbeck A. Odor exploration behavior of the domestic pig (Sus scrofa) as indicator of enriching properties of odors. Front Behav Neurosci. 2023;17
78. Guevara RD, Pastor JJ, Manteca X, Tedo G, Llonch P. Systematic review of animal-based indicators to measure thermal, social, and immune-related stress in pigs. PLoS One. 2022;17:e0266524. https://doi.org/10.1371/journal.pone.0266524.
79. Herskin MS, Jensen KH. Effects of different degrees of social isolation on the behaviour of weaned piglets kept for experimental purposes. Anim Welf. 2000;9:237–49. https://doi.org/10.1017/S0962728600022727.
80. Paredes-Ramos P, Diaz-Morales JV, Espinosa-Palencia M, Coria-Avila GA, Carrasco-Garcia AA. Clicker training accelerates learning of complex behaviors but reduces discriminative abilities of yucatan miniature pigs. Animals. 2020;10:959. https://doi.org/10.3390/ani10060959.
81. Rydén A, Manell E, Biglarnia A, Hedenqvist P, Strandberg G, Ley C, Hansson K, Nyman G, Jensen-Waern M. Nursing and training of pigs used in renal transplantation studies. Lab Anim. 2020;54:469–78. https://doi.org/10.1177/0023677219879169.
82. Thomsen AF, Kousholt BS. Transition of farm pigs to research pigs using a designated checklist followed by initiation of clicker training - a refinement initiative. J Vis Exp. 2021:e62099. https://doi.org/10.3791/62099.
83. Smith ME, Gopee NV, Ferguson SA. Preferences of minipigs for environmental enrichment objects. J Am Assoc Lab Anim Sci. 2009;48:391–4.
84. Swindle MM, Smith AC, editors. Swine in the laboratory: surgery, anesthesia, imaging, and experimental techniques. 3rd ed. Boca Raton, FL: CRC Press; 2015.
85. Wagner KM, Schulz J, Kemper N. Examination of the hygienic status of selected organic enrichment materials used in pig farming with special emphasis on pathogenic bacteria. Porc Health Manag. 2018;4:24. https://doi.org/10.1186/s40813-018-0100-y.
86. Chaloupková H, Illmann G, Neuhauserová K, Šimečková M, Kratinová P. The effect of nesting material on the nest-building and maternal behavior of domestic sows and piglet production1. J Anim Sci. 2011;89:531–7. https://doi.org/10.2527/jas.2010-2854.
87. Markland L, Johnson JS, Richert BT, Erasmus MA, Lay DC Jr. Investigating the effects of jute nesting material and enriched piglet mats on sow welfare and piglet survival. Transl Anim Sci. 2023;7:txad076. https://doi.org/10.1093/tas/txad076.
88. Casey B, Abney D, Skoumbordis E. A playroom as novel swine enrichment. Lab Anim. 2007;36:32–4. https://doi.org/10.1038/laban0307-32.
89. Coleman K, Novak MA. Environmental enrichment in the 21st century. ILAR J. 2017;58:295–307. https://doi.org/10.1093/ilar/ilx008.
90. Vermeire T, Hoet P, Krätke R, Testai E, Badin RA, Epstein M, Flecknell PA, Hudson-Shore M, Jones D, Langermans JAM, Prescott MJ, Simonnard A (2017) Final Opinion on The need for non-human primates in biomedical research, production and testing of products and devices (update 2017). SCHEER.
91. Yost OC, Downey A, Ramos KS. Nonhuman primate models in biomedical research: state of the science and future needs. In: Yost OC, Downey A, Ramos KS, editors. *Nonhuman primate models in biomedical research: state of the science and future needs*. Washington, DC: The National Academies Press; 2023.
92. Mellor DJ, Beausoleil NJ, Littlewood KE, Mclean AN, Mcgreevy PD, Jones B, Wilkins C. The 2020 five domains model: including human-animal interactions in assessments of animal welfare. Animals (Basel). 2020;10
93. Arndt SS, Goerlich VC, Van Der Staay FJ. A dynamic concept of animal welfare: the role of appetitive and adverse internal and external factors and the animal's ability to adapt to them. Front Anim Sci. 2022;3
94. Truelove MA, Martin JE, Langford FM, Leach MC. The identification of effective welfare indicators for laboratory-housed macaques using a Delphi consultation process. Sci Rep. 2020;10:20402.
95. Prescott MJ, Leach MC, Truelove MA. Harmonisation of welfare indicators for macaques and marmosets used or bred for research. F1000Res. 2022;11:272.
96. Paterson EA, O'Malley CI, Abney DM, Archibald WJ, Turner PV. Development of a novel primate welfare assessment tool for research macaques. Anim Welf. 2024;33:1–15.
97. Hage SR, Ott T, Eiselt AK, Jacob SN, Nieder A. Ethograms indicate stable well-being dur-

ing prolonged training phases in rhesus monkeys used in neurophysiological research. Lab Anim. 2014;48:82–7.
98. Polanco A, Mccowan B, Niel L, Pearl DL, Mason G. Recommendations for abnormal behaviour ethograms in monkey research. Animals (Basel). 2021;11
99. Prescott MJ, Nixon ME, Farningham DAH, Naiken S, Griffiths MA. Laboratory macaques: when to wean? Appl Anim Behav Sci. 2012;137:194–207.
100. Rox A, Waasdorp S, Sterck EHM, Langermans, J.a.M., and Louwerse, A.L. Multigenerational social housing and group-rearing enhance female reproductive success in captive rhesus macaques (Macaca mulatta). Biology (Basel). 2022;11
101. Maaskant A, Janssen I, Wouters IM, Eerdenburg F, Remarque EJ, Langermans JAM, Bakker J. Assessment of indoor air quality for group-housed macaques (Macaca spp.). Animals (Basel). 2022;12
102. Poole T. Happy animals make good science. Lab Anim. 1997;31:116–24.
103. Robins JG, Waitt CD. Improving the welfare of captive macaques (Macaca sp.) through the use of water as enrichment. J Appl Anim Welf Sci. 2011;14:75–84.
104. Vernes M, Louwerse AL (2010) BPRC's enrichment manual for macaques and marmosets
105. Voipio H-M, et al. Guidelines for the veterinary care of laboratory animals: Report of the FELASA/ECLAM/ESLAV Joint Working Group on Veterinary Care. Lab Anim. 2008;42(1):1–11.
106. Steelman ED, Alexander JL. Laboratory animal workers' attitudes and perceptions concerning occupational risk and injury. J Am Assoc Lab Anim Sci. 2016;55(4):419–25.
107. Adams KM, et al. A canine socialization and training program at the national institutes of health. Lab Anim. 2004;33(1):32–6.
108. Grigg EK, et al. Evaluating pair versus solitary housing in kennelled domestic dogs (Canis familiaris) using behaviour and hair cortisol: a pilot study. Veterinary Record Open. 2017;4(1):e000193.
109. Hewison LF, et al. Short term consequences of preventing visitor access to kennels on noise and the behaviour and physiology of dogs housed in a rescue shelter. Physiol Behav. 2014;133:1–7.
110. Willems A, et al. Results of screening of apparently healthy senior and geriatric dogs. J Vet Intern Med. 2017;31(1):81–92.
111. Kiddie JL, Collins LM. Development and validation of a quality of life assessment tool for use in kennelled dogs (Canis familiaris). Appl Anim Behav Sci. 2014;158:57–68.
112. Schipper LL, et al. The effect of feeding enrichment toys on the behaviour of kennelled dogs (Canis familiaris). Appl Anim Behav Sci. 2008;114(1):182–95.
113. McEvoy V, et al. Canine socialisation: a narrative systematic review. Animals. 2022;12(21):2895.
114. Wells DL. The influence of toys on the behaviour and welfare of kennelled dogs. Anim Welf. 2004;13:367–73.
115. Arhant C, Winkelmann R, Troxler J. Chewing behaviour in dogs – a survey-based exploratory study. Appl Anim Behav Sci. 2021;241:105372.
116. Meunier LD. Selection, acclimation, training, and preparation of dogs for the research setting. ILAR J. 2006;47(4):326–47.
117. Van Hooser JP, et al. Caring for the animal caregiver—occupational health, human-animal bond and compassion fatigue. Front Vet Sci. 2021:8.
118. Grigg EK, et al. Stress-related behaviors in companion dogs exposed to common household noises, and owners' interpretations of their dogs' behaviors. Front Vet Sci. 2021:8.
119. Pedretti G, et al. Appeasement function of displacement behaviours? Dogs' behavioural displays exhibited towards threatening and neutral humans. Anim Cogn. 2023;26(3):943–52.
120. Pullen AJ, Merrill RJN, Bradshaw JWS. The effect of familiarity on behaviour of kennel housed dogs during interactions with humans. Appl Anim Behav Sci. 2012;137(1):66–73.
121. Skidmore T, et al. Researching animal research. Researching animal research: What the humanities and social sciences can contribute to laboratory animal science and welfare, in 'The place for a dog is in the home': Why does species matter when rehoming laboratory animals? Manchester University Press; 2024.
122. Döring D, et al. Behavior of laboratory dogs before and after rehoming in private homes. ALTEX - Alternatives to animal experimentation. 2017;34(1):133–47.
123. Petetta F, Ciccocioppo R. Public perception of laboratory animal testing: historical, philosophical, and ethical view. Addict Biol. 2021;26(6):e12991.
124. Sykes JE, et al. 2010 ACVIM small animal consensus statement on leptospirosis: diagnosis, epidemiology, treatment, and prevention. J Vet Intern Med. 2011;25(1):1–13.
125. Paryuni AD, Indarjulianto S, Widyarini S. Dermatophytosis in companion animals: a review. Vet World. 2020;13(6):1174–81.
126. Khairullah AR, et al. Pet animals as reservoirs for spreading methicillin-resistant Staphylococcus aureus to human health. J Adv Vet Anim Res. 2023;10(1):1–13.
127. Morgan M, Palmer J. Dog bites. BMJ. 2007;334(7590):413–7.
128. Gerencsér Z, et al. Aggressiveness, mating behaviour and lifespan of group housed rabbit does. Animals. 2019;9(10):708.
129. Thurston S, et al. Methods of pairing and pair maintenance of New Zealand white rabbits (Oryctolagus Cuniculus) via behavioral ethogram, monitoring, and interventions. J Vis Exp. 2018;133
130. DiVincenti L Jr, Rehrig AN. The social nature of European rabbits (Oryctolagus cuniculus). J Am Assoc Lab Anim Sci. 2016;55(6):729–36.
131. Podberscek AL, Blackshaw JK, Beattie AW. The behaviour of group penned and individually

caged laboratory rabbits. Appl Anim Behav Sci. 1991;28(4):353–63.
132. Varga M. Infectious diseases of domestic rabbits. In: Textbook of rabbit medicine; 2014. p. 435–71. https://doi.org/10.1016/B978-0-7020-4979-8.00014-5.
133. Coda KA, Fortman JD, García KD. Behavioral effects of cage size and environmental enrichment in New Zealand white rabbits. J Am Assoc Lab Anim Sci. 2020;59(4):356–64.
134. Crowell-Davis SL. Behavior problems in pet rabbits. J Exot Pet Med. 2007;16(1):38–44.
135. Clauss M, Hatt JM. Evidence-Based rabbit housing and nutrition. Vet Clin North Am Exot Anim Pract. 2017;20(3):871–84.
136. Harcourt-Brown F. Dental disease in pet rabbits. In Pract. 2009;31(8):370–9.
137. Oglesbee BL, Lord B. Gastrointestinal diseases of rabbits. Ferrets Rabbits Rodents. 2020:174–87. https://doi.org/10.1016/B978-0-323-48435-0.00014-9.
138. Mastellone V, et al. Mirrors improve rabbit natural behavior in a free-range breeding system. Animals. 2019;9(8):533.
139. Hetterich J, et al. Treatment options, complications and long-term outcomes for limb fractures in pet rabbits. Vet Rec. 2023;192(3):e2344.
140. Keeble E. Common neurological and musculoskeletal problems in rabbits. In Pract. 2006;28(4):212–8.
141. Malley D. Safe handling and restraint of pet rabbits. In Pract. 2007;29(7):378–86.
142. Bradbury AG, Dickens GJE. Appropriate handling of pet rabbits: a literature review. J Small Anim Pract. 2016;57(10):503–9.
143. Jones M. Laboratory animal allergy in the modern era. Curr Allergy Asthma Rep. 2015;15(12):73.
144. Choi JH, Kim HM, Park HS. Allergic asthma and rhinitis caused by household rabbit exposure: identification of serum-specific IgE and its allergens. J Korean Med Sci. 2007;22(5):820–4.
145. Laura W, Howard JM. The development of methods to measure exposure to a major rabbit allergen (Ory c 1). AIMS Public Health. 2018;5(2):99–110.
146. Gordon S, Preece R. Prevention of laboratory animal allergy. Occup Med. 2003;53(6):371–7.
147. Mocho JP, Collymore C, Farmer SC, Leguay E, Murray KN, Pereira N. FELASA-AALAS recommendations for biosecurity in an aquatic facility, including prevention of zoonosis, introduction of new fish colonies, and quarantine. Comp Med. 2022;72(3):149–68. https://doi.org/10.30802/AALAS-CM-22-000042.
148. Stevens CH, Reed BT, Hawkins P. Enrichment for laboratory zebrafish-a review of the evidence and the challenges. Animals (Basel). 2021;11(3):698. https://doi.org/10.3390/ani11030698.
149. Schroeder P, Jones S, Young IS, Sneddon LU. What do zebrafish want? Impact of social grouping, dominance and gender on preference for enrichment. Lab Anim. 2014 Oct;48(4):328–37. https://doi.org/10.1177/0023677214538239.
150. Ramos J, Ortiz-Díez G. Evaluation of environmental enrichment for Xenopus laevis using a preference test. Lab Anim. 2021 Oct;55(5):428–34. https://doi.org/10.1177/00236772211011290.

Health Management and Monitoring

8

Stefanie Hansborg Kolstrup,
Axel Kornerup Hansen,
and Tina Brønnum Pedersen

Abstract

The concept of "health" in laboratory animal science is a crucial link that brings together ethical, scientific, and practical considerations. It plays a central role in ensuring the successful and responsible conduct of experiments involving laboratory animals. Comprehensive care of laboratory animals depends on effective health management and requires close co-operation between those working with the animals. Persons working with laboratory animals must be qualified, and the supervision of animals by trained personnel is essential to ensure animal health. This chapter provides examples of how to establish effective communication and identifies key personnel responsible for animal health.

Microbiological health monitoring is a fundamental aspect of the operation of an animal research facility. It provides the ability to identify and control the presence of microorganisms, which is important for both research integrity and animal welfare. This chapter serves as a practical guide to assist veterinarians at every stage, from planning and implementation to interpretation of results. It also provides guidelines for outbreak management and biosecurity programs, which are essential to prevent the spread of disease and protect the overall health of laboratory animals. Monitoring the health of laboratory animals in a proactive and facility-specific manner is an essential part of the veterinarian's responsibilities.

Keywords

Health management · Qualification of personnel · Health monitoring · Outbreak management · Biosecurity · Practical guidelines

8.1 Health Management

8.1.1 What Is Animal Health?

The World Health Organization defines "Health as a state of complete physical, mental, and social well-being and not merely the absence of disease

S. H. Kolstrup
Faculty of Health Sciences, Biomedical Laboratory, University of Southern Denmark, Odense C, Denmark
e-mail: skolstrup@health.sdu.dk

A. K. Hansen (✉)
Faculty of Health and Medical Sciences, Department of Veterinary and Animal Sciences, University of Copenhagen, Frederiksberg C, Denmark
e-mail: Akh@sund.ku.dk

T. B. Pedersen
H. Lundbeck A/S, Valby, Denmark
e-mail: tibp@lundbeck.com

J. Guillén, V. Galligioni (eds.), *Practical Management of Research Animal Care and Use Programs*, Laboratory Animal Science and Medicine 3, https://doi.org/10.1007/978-3-031-65414-5_8

and infirmity" [1]. Ensuring that healthy animals are used in research is an important responsibility. This includes ensuring that animals are free from infection, housed in enriched and socially appropriate environments, and provided with a safe physical environment to prevent injury. It also requires adherence to best practices in laboratory animal science, ensuring that animals are cared for by trained staff on a daily basis. Laboratory animal facilities play a key role in providing optimal housing, care, and management of research animals, complementing the responsibilities of the laboratory animal veterinarian in monitoring health, ensuring good animal welfare, providing scientific support, managing pain, and making euthanasia decisions when necessary. In addition, seamless communication between the competent authority, researchers, veterinarians, and animal technicians is essential to ensure animal health.

This chapter focuses on the practical aspects of rodent health management.

8.1.2 How Can We Ensure Health Issues Are Promptly Detected and Who Is Key Staff?

Laboratory animals are not only captive animals but also animals that may have a harmful phenotype and are subject to experimental procedures. They are therefore highly dependent on competent and compassionate staff (animal technicians, veterinarians, and researchers) with the attitude and skills to ensure a high level of animal care and welfare. Under the EU Directive 2010/63, the training and education of staff is mandatory, and staff must be supervised until they have achieved and demonstrated the necessary competence. From an animal welfare perspective, the staff needs to be familiar with the normal behavior of the animal species they are working with to be able to recognize signs of abnormal behavior that may indicate disease, pain, or distress. As prey species, mice and rats may hide signs of pain and distress, making welfare monitoring even more difficult.

All laboratory animals should be subject to inspection by a competent person at least once a day. The daily inspection must include the general condition of the animal and the housing conditions, such as free access to food and water. In most animal facilities, it is the animal technician who carries out the daily routine checks on the animals. They work with the animals on a day-to-day basis and are therefore very well-trained to spot any abnormal behavior. If sick animals are identified, the designated veterinarian must be contacted. For the veterinarian, it is always important to listen to why the technicians experience this animal as sick, as the veterinarian normally does not see the animals on a daily basis. If considered that the disease may turn out be infectious, sick animals should be isolated to prevent the spread. If the animal shows signs of pain or distress as a result of an experimental procedure, the responsible researcher should be contacted and the condition relieved either by treatment or euthanasia. Any animal found dead should be necropsied according to the instructions found in Chap. 12 of the book "Rodent Quality Control: Genes and Microorganisms" [2].

8.1.3 How Can an Efficient Communication Be Established?

Communication between animal technicians, researchers, and the veterinarian(s) is an absolute necessity, and the larger the facility, the more important it is to have a structure in place to facilitate efficient communication (Fig. 8.1). The veterinarian should join meetings with the researcher to understand their research needs and challenge studies for setup, in regard to refinement, replacement, and alignment of humane endpoints. Often the veterinarian becomes the point of contact to help "fix things" as many issues will directly or indirectly affect the health of the animal. Involving the veterinarian in the research project from the planning phase through its conclusion offers significant advantages. In practice, this is accomplished by involving the veterinarian in

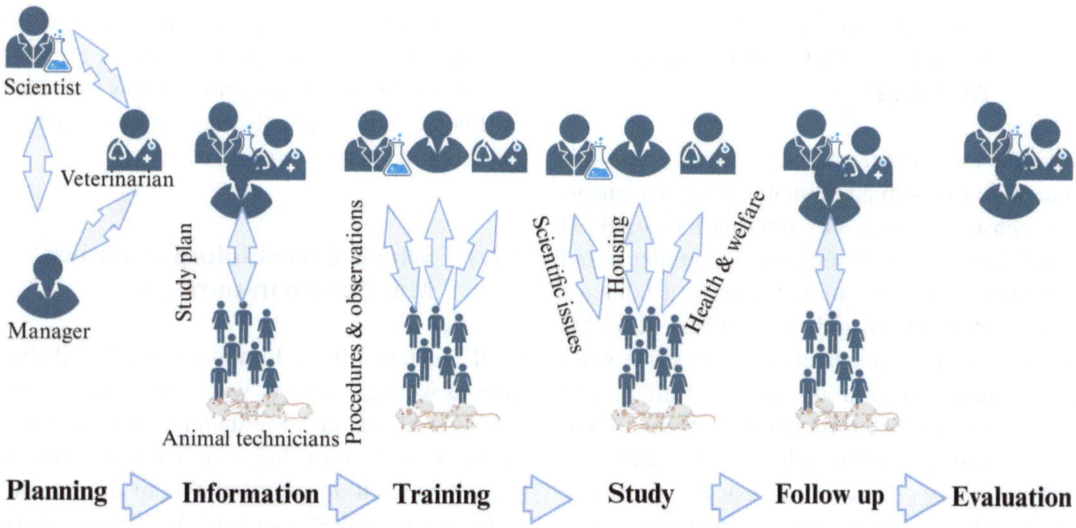

Fig. 8.1 Establishing communication lines
The scientist, the manager, and the veterinarian should have a running and mutual communication during study planning. When a study plan is ready, a meeting between the scientist, the manager, and the animal technicians to be involved should be established, and at this, there should be a mutual communication about procedures, endpoints, observations to be made, welfare, etc., and considerations from the animal technicians should afterwards be discussed and if necessary incorporated in the study plan. During the training phase, the scientist, the manager, and the veterinarian must each of them take responsibility of the training of the technicians for issues relevant for performance of the specific tasks. During the study there should be a current and mutual communication, and, e.g., the technicians should communicate unexpected symptoms to the veterinarian, who communicates back on actions to be taken. After the study, a follow-up meeting should be used for the collection of relevant experiences from the study, and hereafter the scientist, the manager, and the veterinarian make a final evaluation.

reviewing the animal research application before submission to the competent authority, assessing the study protocol, conducting inspections of animals throughout the study, and considering potential improvements after the study has been conducted.

Review of the animal research application prior to submission to the competent authority will ensure that the description is consistent with the standard practice in the animal facility. Furthermore, having the veterinarian propose humane endpoints that correspond to the study's impact on the animal's health is advantageous, ensuring research goals are met without unnecessary harming of the animals. When the project application is approved, a specific study protocol should be aligned with the responsible veterinarian and animal technician. Expected clinical symptoms caused by study interventions or phenotypic alterations due to transgenesis should be reviewed, and study periods when animals are expected to be at highest risk of distress should be clarified. Simultaneously, establishing protocols for unforeseen complications, including who to contact and when, is essential.

Beyond study-specific discussions, regular group meetings within laboratory animal facilities are vital. These gatherings involve animal technicians, accompanied by veterinarians, facilitating the exchange of information and discussions. Department meetings unite all facility staff, fostering collaboration to identify and address common issues. These forums serve to disseminate important updates such as handling unexpected infections, implementing new health monitoring strategies, or outlining renovation plans. In larger facilities, multiple veterinarians may be present, necessitating alignment meetings to ensure cohesive efforts and updated knowledge among them. Balancing these meetings amidst busy schedules remains a challenge. Practical guidelines should be made available for all users as part of training and to help staff to follow compliance.

8.1.4 How Can We Ensure Veterinary Care Is Provided at All Times?

Veterinary assistance is crucial and ideally available at all times in an animal facility. By ensuring constant access to veterinarians, animal technicians can feel supported, confident, and empowered in their roles, fostering a compassionate approach towards the animals they care for. This support contributes to a positive work environment centered on animal welfare and ethical practices. Unfortunately, certain circumstances like quarantine rules or logistical constraints may hinder physical presence. Fortunately, advancements in technology now enable remote veterinary support through video calls or similar applications. This allows veterinarians to guide animal technicians through visual observation and provide instructions over a call if well-trained technicians are present. Practical guidance, including detailed observations and clinical findings, is available in handbooks, helping to define clinical situations. Looking ahead, the future might entail the development of applications specifically designed to offer virtual veterinary assistance. These apps could include features like images, videos, severity assessments, and instructions, facilitating quick decisions and guidance for animal technicians or researchers in need.

8.2 Microbiological Health Monitoring in Practice

An essential aspect of maintaining the health of laboratory animals involves ensuring that the animals are free from infections. This is achieved through routine "health monitoring" (HM) or "microbiological monitoring," which entails regular screening for the absence of pathogenic and in some cases even opportunistic microorganisms within the facility. The EU Directive enforces that "regular health monitoring" should be done, that there should be "plans for dealing with health breakdowns" and that "health parameters and procedures for the introduction of new animals" shall be defined. Typically, these responsibilities fall under the tasks of veterinarians.

8.2.1 Why Is Microbiological Health Monitoring Important?

Until the late fifties, fulminant and lethal diseases as well as zoonoses were commonly occurring in rodents in experimental and breeding facilities eradicating huge numbers of animals [3], which led to the development of the specific pathogen free (SPF) concept [4]. Although there might be differences in the perception of how SPF actually is defined, there is an international understanding that laboratory animals, and especially rodents, must come from an SPF facility and that they should be maintained in this state during the experiments. However, there is an increasing number of examples of how the absence of pathogens results in animals being poor models for humans [5–7], which will lead to a waste of animals as far as results turn out not to be reproducible or translational. Probably, in a not so distant future, larger institutions and companies will have dedicated and isolated facilities, where they would house "dirty" animals as a supplement to their SPF animals [5]. There is, however, no strict solution on how to avoid the increased disease incidence and mortality that re-introduction of the pathogens would lead to. As a secondary purpose, many vets will consider it professionally the most correct to adhere to international standards, such as the guidelines for health monitoring from the Federation of European Laboratory Animal Science Associations (FELASA) [8]. Without adhering to such standards, it would be difficult to exchange animals between facilities. Such exchange without new rederivations is generally not a good idea due to the differences in perception on which infectious agents to monitor, how often to do it, and by which methods. In addition, the level of barrier protection differs between facilities. However, even without exchange with external facilities, running "dirty" non-SPF facilities imposes a risk that samples from the animals may be exchanged by scientists, and, thereby, spread the infections between laboratories or facilities [9]. Finally, according to annex III, point 3.1. of the EU Directive [10], laboratory animal facilities must run a program for microbiological surveillance, so even if some facilities or their vets should be unable to see the benefits of avoiding disease, research interference, and zoonoses, it is simply a legal demand to have a program in place.

8.2.2 Why Is It Important to Test Both Healthy and Sick Animals?

One of the arguments for the SPF concept is that disease and mortality among the animals obviously disturbs research and imposes an animal welfare issue. Therefore, there are good reasons for a thorough examination of sick animals and eventually a necropsy with microbiological sampling if animals are found dead or euthanized. However, there are also bunches of examples on how latent infections, which are not necessarily a disease problem, can disturb or ruin animal studies [11]. Therefore, a facility cannot solely rely on being able to diagnose any relevant pathogen intruder from sick animal examination. Any facility would need to prioritize resources to run a screening program for pathogens based upon the routine sampling of healthy animals. Even if some infections at some time point would lead to some clinical indications, these may be that discrete that it may take a substantial time for the facility staff to realize the problem, e.g. as it is often the case for the increase pup mortality in mouse breeding colonies infected with mouse hepatitis virus. Often, the better the management the more discrete the symptoms of infections will be.

8.2.3 What to Test for in a Microbiological Monitoring?

The FELASA recommendations are a good starting point for the evaluation of which agents to test for. It is worth bearing in mind that the recommendations are named so, as they are in fact recommendations. Quite often, the HM program is referred to as "performed according to FELASA," however, unless specified, such a FELASA certificate may vary between institutional health monitoring programs. It is important to consider the type of research and studies performed at the facility to be health monitored. It is also important to consider how the facility is structured in terms of "microbiological units," defined as a self-contained microbiological entity with separate space and traffic for animals, personnel, and materials. If strict measures apply, the entire animal facility as one unit can be broken down into smaller microbiological subunits, which must be decided for each animal facility.

The person responsible for the health monitoring program should ask themselves the following questions:

- What would be the consequence if an unwanted agent is present?
- Can the presence of an unwanted agent be avoided, and can its re-occurrence be avoided by implemented mitigation strategies, such as having barriers, cleaning and disinfection procedures, changed routines in the facility, etc.?
- Is there support from the management for the execution of mitigation strategies?

By asking these questions, the agents to be tested for, can be grouped into five categories:

1. *Not accepted unwanted agents* which cause zoonoses, animal disease, and/or interference of the research leading to immediate culling strategies.
2. *Temporarily accepted unwanted agents*, for which it is not necessary to terminate the studies or the breeding immediately.

3. *Acceptable unwanted agents* that per se is unwanted but will be accepted in case they are detected.
4. *Accepted agents* with no impact or interference.
5. *Wanted agents* for which presence is required.

Unwanted agents in the first two categories should be tested for, and the execution of the risk mitigation strategies will come with a high cost. It is, therefore, imperative to have management support, a clear communication path, and defined roles and responsibilities to be able to execute quickly and diligently in the unfortunate event of positive findings within these categories.

Temporarily accepted unwanted agents could be finding of a virus potentially affecting the research, where studies can be finalized while setting up barriers and movement restrictions to prevent further contamination and spreading in the facility. In this case, it is necessary to consider how to investigate whether the finding had an effect by correlating positive findings with study outcomes. For example, if the presence of a virus resulted in 30% of all animals being infected, the result of serological samples from each animal can be correlated with one or more study parameters to determine the cause of the effect.

Agents unwanted but not critical and thus acceptable could be agents typically found at the breeder. The benefits of testing should be considered, and testing should only be initiated if the animals show clinical signs consistent with that particular agent. It should be considered whether it is necessary to spend any costs on testing for agents for which there is not risk of any impact or interference, and for which a positive finding will have no consequences in the facility.

The "wanted agents" category is opposite, as the experimental facility may have a need for certain bacteria to be present in a particular animal model, making monitoring for such bacteria important.

The categorization of infectious agents must be reviewed regularly, as the type of research may change, or if investigations show that the presence of an infection did not affect the type of study, or if it did, the agent may become re-categorized. Examples are given in Table 8.1.

The book "Rodent Quality Control: Genes and Bugs—Monitoring Health and Genetics of Laboratory Animals" [3] has a chapter with further information on Health monitoring programs and international standards [4].

8.2.4 How Many Animals Should Be Tested?

On the one hand, the FELASA guidelines give some clear numbers on how many animals should be tested, while it, on the other hand, states that this should be assessed individually for the different agents. The book "Rodent Quality Control: Genes and Bugs—Monitoring Health and Genetics of Laboratory Animals" [3] has a chapter on estimating statistically valid sample sizes for health monitoring [12], which states that the sample size for each agent depends on the expected prevalence that the infection would reach in a colony of that particular species, the risk of a false negative result, the sensitivity of the assay applied, and for smaller colonies, such as experimental colonies, the colony size [12]. The prevalence that a certain infectious agent may reach also depends on some environmental and eventually some genetic factors (Table 8.2). Normally very infectious agents also spread easily in IVC cages, but if housing is run with very strict hygienic measurements between the cages, the prevalence might be lower. Some strains of mice are more sensitive to some infections than other strains, and some infections mostly spread vertically and are therefore less likely to spread in experimental facilities (Table 8.2). Such factors should therefore also be considered when estimating prevalence.

8.2.5 How Should the Samples Be Taken, and Which Samples Can Be Obtained for Different Detection Methods?

When planning a health monitoring program, you need to consider the routes of transmission between animals in a colony, and in particular, the type of animal housing. When housing ani-

Table 8.1 Examples on how an experimental facility can set up of a scheme to categorize agents, the expected risk impact if accepted, and mitigation strategies. This should be evaluated for each microbiological unit and will not be general for all facilities

Agent	Risk			Acceptance	Mitigation strategies
	Zoonosis	Clinical disease of animals	Interference with research		
Mouse Hepatitis Virus	No	None in immune-competent animals	Yes	1. Not accepted unwanted agents	Set up barriers to prevent spreading of infection, no deliveries of animals with a positive HM result, culling of animals with infection or the risk of being infected, do risk assessment on stored animal samples
Helicobacter spp.	No	In some sensitive transgenic strains	In case of clinical disease in some models	2. Temporarily accepted unwanted agents	Isolation of critical strains as *Helicobacter*-free in dedicated units
Staphylococcus aureus	Opportunistic pathogen	Mostly after trauma	In case of clinical disease	3. Accepted unwanted agents	Treat/euthanize animals with abscesses
Klebsiella oxytoca	Opportunistic pathogen	Not in immune-competent animals	No	4. Accepted agents	None
Bifidobacterium spp.	No	No	Lacking effect of prebiotics if not present	5. Wanted agents	Ensure animals are positive by careful vendor selection or own pretesting

Table 8.2 Examples of estimated prevalences and sensitivities of two viruses, two bacteria, and two parasites with different expected prevalences, and, thereby, need for different sample sizes for health monitoring

Infectious agent	Approximately estimated prevalence	Conditions eventually affecting prevalence	Sensitivity of typical testing method	References
Mouse hepatitis virus	100%	Strain, housing	Serology: High PCR: High	[13–18]
Lymphocytic choriomeningitis virus	20%	Breeding	Serology: High PCR: Low	[19]
Clostridium piliforme	50–60%	Strain, housing	Serology: High PCR: High Histopathology: Low	[14, 20, 21]
Klebsiella oxytoca	15- 20%	Housing, hygiene	Cultivation: Moderate	[14]
Syphacia obvelata	50 – 100%	Age	Microscopy: High PCR: High	[13, 14, 22]
Giardia muris	15–75%	Sex, strain	Direct fluorescence antibody assay: High PCR: High	[23–25]

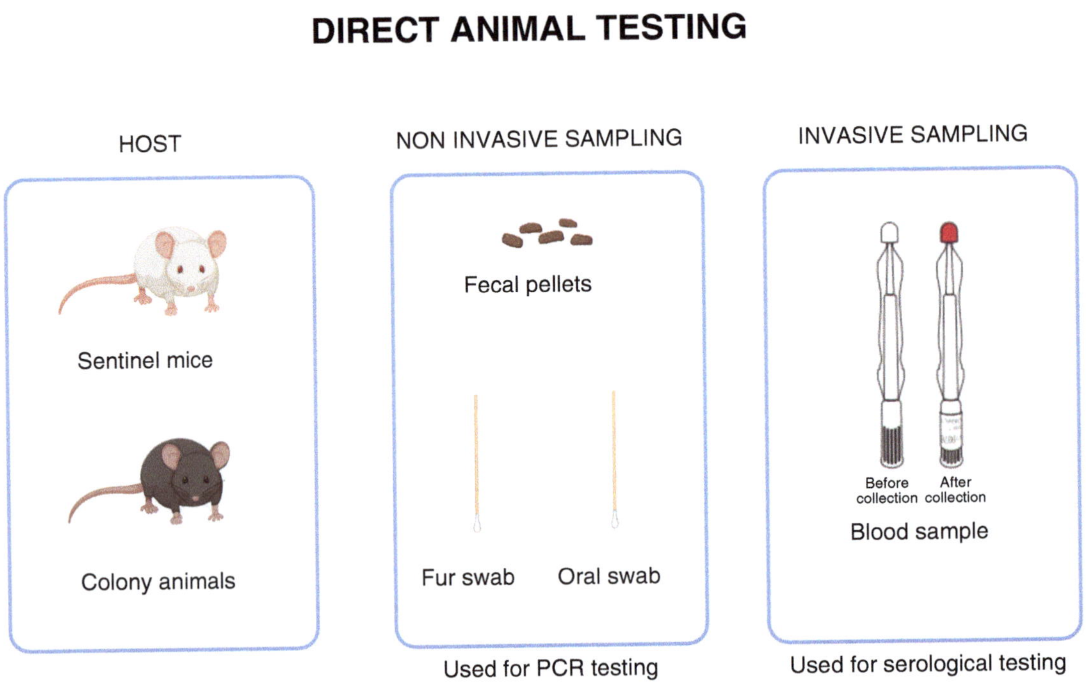

Fig. 8.2 Illustration of direct animal testing options, including host, non-invasive sampling for PCR testing and micro-sampling of blood as a minimally invasive sampling method for serological testing. Created with BioRender.com

mals in open top cages, microorganisms are very likely to be transmitted by fomites or aerosols, and infections transmitted in this way can easily and quickly spread throughout a colony. If not possible to sample directly from the animals (Fig. 8.2), soiled bedding sentinels (SBS) are often used for health monitoring when animals are housed in open top cages. SBS receive soiled bedding from the cages they represent and should be placed near and preferably below these cages to increase the risk of microorganism transmission. However, recent research has shown that several pathogens, such as *Helicobacter* spp. and *Rodentibacter* spp. [26], are poorly transmitted through soiled bedding, especially when rodents are kept in individually ventilated cages (IVC),

Table 8.3 The typical testing methodology, age of animals when testing, and sampling errors when monitoring for viruses, bacteria, and parasites

Agent	Methodology	Animal sample	Sampling error
Viruses	Serology	Immunocompetent animals often old animals/breeders	Immunodeficient animals (false negative) Maternal antibodies (false positive) if samples are obtained from young animals
	PCR	Newly infected animals, most often young animals	Animals that have recovered from the infection (false negative)
Bacteria	PCR	All ages	Animals that have recovered from the infection (false negative) Contamination of sample (false positive)
Parasites	PCR	Around weaning	Adult animals that have recovered from the infection (false negative)

resulting in unreliable results from the health monitoring program. Because of this, SBS are used less frequently in IVC facilities, in which colony animal testing and environmental testing are more often used, as discussed below.

When using SBS for health monitoring, sentinels are euthanized after repeated exposure to soiled bedding, and a full necropsy of tissues and organs must be performed. Previously, selected tissue specimens, gastrointestinal content, and blood were collected for microbiological investigation by direct microscopic examination or cultural isolation. Today, due to PCR, collection of non-invasive samples such as feces pellets, fur-, and oral swabs are widely used to screen for changes in microbiological status in rodent colonies. With non-invasive testing methods it is possible to include samples from colony animals and thus significantly increase the sample size. The PCR technique exponentially amplifies targeted microbial genomic DNA sequences, resulting in high sensitivity and analytic specificity compared to other testing methods for most agents. It also enables the detection of small amounts of targeted microbial genomic sequences, allowing feces, fur-, or oral swabs from various animals to be pooled in one sample. PCR testing of animals reveals the microbial status of the animal at the time of testing. It is important to know that many infections are non-persisting, and it is, therefore, impossible with this method to know if the animal has previously been exposed to microorganisms.

Today's serological methods require only a few blood drops (25 μl) from un-anesthetized animals, which can be done either on filter paper or by a HemaTIP™, depending on the method used by the testing laboratory. Animals used for serologic monitoring must be immunocompetent and able to produce antibodies, which may not necessarily be the case for all the facility's transgenic animals.

For each type of microorganisms, carefully consider which animals to use for testing, and which test to apply (Table 8.3) [3]. As an alternative to samples obtained from SBS, colony animals or research animals may be sampled by agreement with the scientist (Fig. 8.2). The most typical scenario is to perform health monitoring every 3 months to ensure that the SBS have been exposed to a potential infection and have seroconverted, although the FELASA guidelines only recommends that SBS are housed for minimum 6 weeks prior to testing using the same husbandry conditions in the same unit as resident animals and exposed. When selecting SBS it is recommended to use an immunocompetent strain such as BALB/c and CD1 mice as they are more susceptible to infection than B6 mice; however, lack of seroconversion has been demonstrated in the BALB/c strain for Mouse parvovirus type 1 infection [27]. Following pathogen exposure of viral infection in naive animals, persistence of infection and shedding can be quite variable depending on the agent. Some viral infections are cleared or persist latently in host tissues, resulting in reduced and later cessation of viral shedding in, e.g., feces. In these cases, the animals will be seropositive for the virus, but detection by PCR will be impossible. Other viruses, such as

Murine Norovirus (MNV), are continuously shed in the feces of seropositive mice for at least 35 days after inoculation [28].

Bacterial cultivation may be done at most ages. However, since some bacterial infections are cleared over time, detection of bacteria requires sample collection during the shedding period. When detecting parasites in laboratory animals, it is important to consider the age of the animal, as adult mice show a lower burden compared to younger mice, possibly due to differences in immune responses between young and old animals. For certain pinworms, the burden may even change from positive in young mice to negative in adult mice, without any anthelmintic treatment [29].

8.2.6 How to Perform Environmental Sampling?

The use of environmental sampling techniques has increased over time. This method is advantageous because from a 3R perspective, as it can replace or reduce the use of animals for testing, or it can in combination with animal testing increase the probability of detecting infectious agents. Depending on the type of housing system used in the facility, there are different application methods. The first to be developed, and currently the most widely used, involves the collection of exhaust air dust (EAD) from IVC cage systems. This is done by placing a filter in the air-handling unit just before the pre-filter (Fig. 8.3a), exposing one filter to dust from one to multiple racks, or by placing a plenum attachment (Fig. 8.3b, c) with a filter at each rack. It is recommended to test and replace the filter quarterly. Environmental testing by this method reveals whether there have been infections in the colony during the exposure period, and previous studies have shown that this method is more sensitive for the detection of pathogens such as Mouse norovirus [30], *Helicobacter* spp., and *Rodentibacter* spp. [26] than SBS. In addition, environmental health monitoring through an EAD program has been shown to be 26% less expensive and significantly less time-consuming than traditional SBS programs [26]. The limitation of this method is that it cannot be used when animals are housed in open cages or racks with cage-level filtration, e.g. Innovive housing system. When these cage systems are used, another method of environmental sampling is required to replace the use of animal testing. A relatively new method has been developed for this purpose, which is similar in principle to the use of SBS. Here, soiled bedding is collected weekly in a cage, but instead of sentinels, a filter material is placed at the bottom of the cage. The filter material is then exposed to microorganisms in the soiled bedding for a period of 3 months. This method has been shown to be similar or more effective in detecting Mouse norovirus, Mouse hepatitis virus, Mouse Parvovirus, *Helicobacter* spp., endoparasites, and fur mites than traditional SBS programs for colony health monitoring and is a viable option when rack-level sampling is ineffective [31–33]. All the evidence suggest that it is possible to replace the use of sentinels with environmental testing and still get valid, and perhaps better, results.

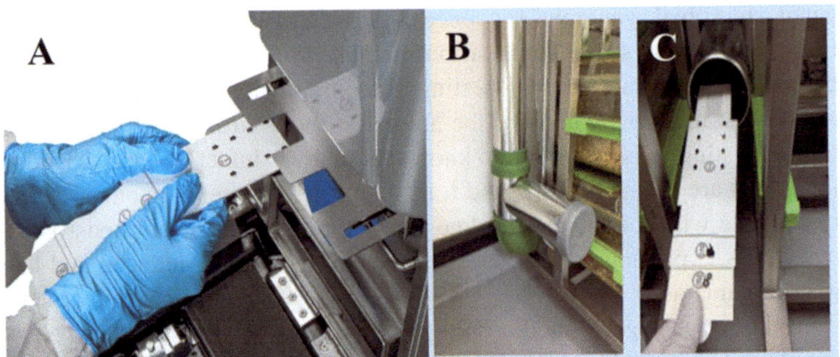

Fig. 8.3 (**a**) Interceptor filter being placed into the air-handling unit. (**b**) Plenum attachment connected to the exhaust plenum on the IVC rack. (**c**) Interceptor filter being placed into the plenum attachment (Courtesy of Tecniplast)

8.2.7 What to Do with the Samples?

Sample condition can affect the accuracy of test results and relies on the sample collection, storage, and shipping procedure. Common pitfalls in sample collection are cross contamination of samples or improper labelling. Most often cross contamination occurs when collection instruments are reused, which highlights the need to decontaminate instruments between samples. Most samples for PCR and whole blood for serological testing can be shipped at ambient temperature. Storage and shipping instructions from the testing laboratory should always be read and followed.

Many commercial laboratories specialized in health monitoring of laboratory animals are available. Selecting a laboratory should depend on your needs for counseling, screening profiles, scientific contribution by the laboratory, testing methods, and price. If positive findings occur in your colony, reconfirming the result by another laboratory is advisable, as results may vary between different diagnostic laboratories.

For some it might be an option to set up various health monitoring assays themselves depending on the qualifications of the responsible person and his/her staff. However, such a set-up should be justified from both a scientific and business point of view. The equipment needs to be available along with expertise on how to use it. Universities and some larger companies do have ELISA and PCR labs, but this does not necessarily mean that there is staff available, who has time and/or competences to run health monitoring assays. For some of the assays, commercial kits are available, but to avoid false positives and negatives cut-off values and cycle threshold (CT) values should be calculated from surely negative samples. Also, there should be a current validation, e.g., in the form of testing positive and negative samples in a ring test involving several laboratories. For a university, and especially veterinary schools, an argument for in-house testing might be that it enables the involvement of students for educational purposes, and some veterinary schools also host and are accredited for the national screening of infectious diseases in farm animals, and including own samples for rodent health monitoring will just be a minor add-on. The same argument can be used for institutions accredited for running assays for the human public health surveillance. From a business point of view, the costs should be calculated also considering the quality and speed of replies. As commercial laboratories often set up their own assays and propagate the antigens for serology themselves, and have access to fully automated laboratory machines, the costs of an in-house testing based upon commercial kits and a certain amount of manual labor power are often not competitive to a commercial price.

8.3 Microbiomic Management

8.3.1 How Should Microbiomics Be Handled?

Today there is increasing attention that not only should pathogens be absent, but there are also some agents which are needed for the induction of certain animal models or are targets for specific interventions [34]. An example of model important bacteria are those popularly called Segment Filamentous Bacteria, whose real name is *Candidatus Savagella*. As stimulators of the T helper cell type 17, they are highly needed for the induction of some models of inflammatory bowel disease [35]. An example of bacteria, which are intervention targets, are *Bifidobacterium* spp., which are propagated by oligosaccharides intensively developed by the food industry over the last decade as anti-inflammatory food components [36].

A simple solution to that challenge is to make a list of bacteria needed for the research in the facility and have the animals screened for those at the vendor. As the presence of such microbes are not likely to change over time, certain colonies can be selected for delivery and further screening can be downscaled to a one or 2-year interval. Likely, also those research groups working with these interventions or models will initiate some screening themselves. Screening can be done for each agent by PCR. However, technologies such as the Oxford Nanopore has made sequencing much more cost efficient, and, therefore, with several wanted bacteria on a list it is a better choice to have fecal samples from the delivering colonies sequenced, which will create a full picture of the gut microbiota. As sequencing will deliver a full list of microbiota members this information can also be used for current evaluation of the applicability of animals from a specific colony, as there is a current stream of new information on bacteria relevant for specific animal studies. In the very ambitious facility, sensitive animal studies, e.g., within the fields of diabetes [37, 38], skin diseases [39], and psychiatry [40], can be appointed, and sequencing can be made routinely for all animals in each study and incorporated in the data evaluation, which is very likely to increase power and reduce group sizes [37].

8.4 Outbreak Management and Biosecurity

8.4.1 How Should We Handle the Microbial Results?

Normally, the anticipation is that everything is negative, so the finding of something positive can come with a bit of thrill. If any positives, the first thing is to look at how the positive finding of an infectious agent is categorized according to Table 8.1. If accepted, do nothing, or at least consider why to spend money on further testing. If not accepted and eliminable, then find out best practice and initiate a strategy, for which there are (at least) two approaches:

1. The infection has most likely been here for a long time, so no hurry, things can run normally until results are verified. How do you interpret if this has been here for a long time? Evaluate the expected disease prevalence and find some more positive samples in different locations. This approach can be taken if animals are not being moved around in the animal facility, but consider to, i.e., put up barriers or movement restrictions of staff or introduce showers after working in "infected" areas before entering a new room to avoid further cross contamination.
2. Immediately set up barriers to prevent further spread of infection, i.e., rooms with animals are now defined as "dirty" and one time use shoe covers, PPE/Coverall, gloves, etc., are put on when entering the room, and discarded when leaving the room. Also consider if showering is needed before any re-entry.

Regardless of the approach, the results deemed not acceptable must be confirmed to ensure the finding is not a false positive.

Call the laboratory and ask how the test has been conducted, e.g. evaluate the used test-profile, whether the appropriate methodology has been used, if the sample has been tested one time or multiple times, ask for the exact reading and the cut-off value to evaluate if the infection is very early or false positive. The best is to do a re-test of the specific sample material. If the analysis is DNA based, then optimally, a new DNA extraction should be made in addition to ensure no cross contamination occurred during the lab work. If still positive, then have the sample validated by another type of test, e.g., if positive by ELISA, verify by immunofluorescence assay, or have another lab to test the sample. If both positive, then you must react based on the risk mitigation strategies laid out.

If the first test result is positive and then tested negative, if re-sampling is not possible, or if it is necessary to know the status on the actual research animals and not the sentinels, consider sampling further to find out if the relevant animals do have an unwanted infection. For calculation of how many animals that need to be sampled for verification of the results the chapter on estimating statistically valid sample sizes for health monitoring [12] in the book "Rodent Quality Control: Genes and Bugs—Monitoring Health and Genetics of Laboratory Animals" [3] should be consulted.

8.4.2 When Should We Inform the Management, Animal Facility, and the Animal Users?

The communication strategy depends on organizational structure and size and is, therefore, unique for each facility. Here it makes sense to have this aligned, and at some point, provide information that there is a positive finding, especially if barriers or restrictions of movements are set up, and at least when the result is verified. It is recommended to set up a task force group to help and ensure everything is considered before executing on the strategy, and this is especially important if the facility is large and have a lot of different types of users (animal caring staff, research staff, laboratory technicians, veterinarians, etc.) that potentially will be affected. It is also advisable to have a "lessons learned" meeting, when the situation has been handled to evaluate all steps in the process, what was done, and if any improvements can be made.

8.4.3 How Can Spreading of the Infection Be Limited?

Get the overview of all the animals, location of these and the animal responsible. If the animals have been moved around inside the facility, then location and time for these are important to find out if other animals have been in the room in the period at risk, as these animals now also might be at risk and therefore need to be included in the evaluation. In case, it is decided that ongoing studies can be completed with restricted access to a housing/laboratory room, take decisions on how to care for the animals, while the result is being confirmed and/or until the animals no longer are being used. Then look at movement of staff and decide, who can enter the facility/room, and to which extent staff may be allowed to enter several rooms, and whether work should be done in a certain order, so the non-infected rooms are entered first and the infected rooms last. Another issue to be discussed is, whether any restrictions should apply for the staff working with the infected tissue in laboratories outside of the animal facility, especially if they also work in vivo. Dependent on the infection, re-entry may be allowed after showering or a specified quarantine period. It should also be considered how equipment is managed when cleaned and disinfected, or whether it may leave the barrier for cleaning and disinfection, to avoid further spreading. For example, if a housing room is infected and has been sealed off, how should the animals be removed, the cages emptied, the waste sealed, the materials and the scantainer/rack be cleaned and disinfected sufficiently to change the status to non-infected room/"clean," and how should staff enter and leave the room while this work is being carried out. As some infectious agents such as parvoviruses may survive in dust and debris in ventilation systems, the cleaning of these in the animal housing and experimental areas should be included as well. All management parameters must be considered to prevent further spread of the unwanted agent. It is perhaps a little depressing to know that even if all measures have been taken and enormous efforts and costs have been expended to eliminate the infection, there is always a risk that the infection has not been eradicated.

8.4.4 Which Information Should Be Given?

Depending on its importance and potential impact, the information may be communicated through a dedicated meeting, or in writing, or preferably both. A meeting is smart because you get an immediate chance to deal with any reaction from the users, while written information is smart because nobody remembers everything said in meetings. Be concise about what has been found and use layman's language. Include which importance the finding has for the animal(s), the staff working with the animals, and the research. Be clear about an eventual zoonotic potential of the infective agent and communicate also clearly, if there is no risk of transmission to humans. If a zoonotic agent has been found, it is important to advice on how to handle the animals to ensure the safety of staff.

8.4.5 How Can We Prevent Positive Results from Coming Back?

Once a positive finding has been verified, various actions are initiated to contain, eradicate, and investigate the contamination with the aim of pre-

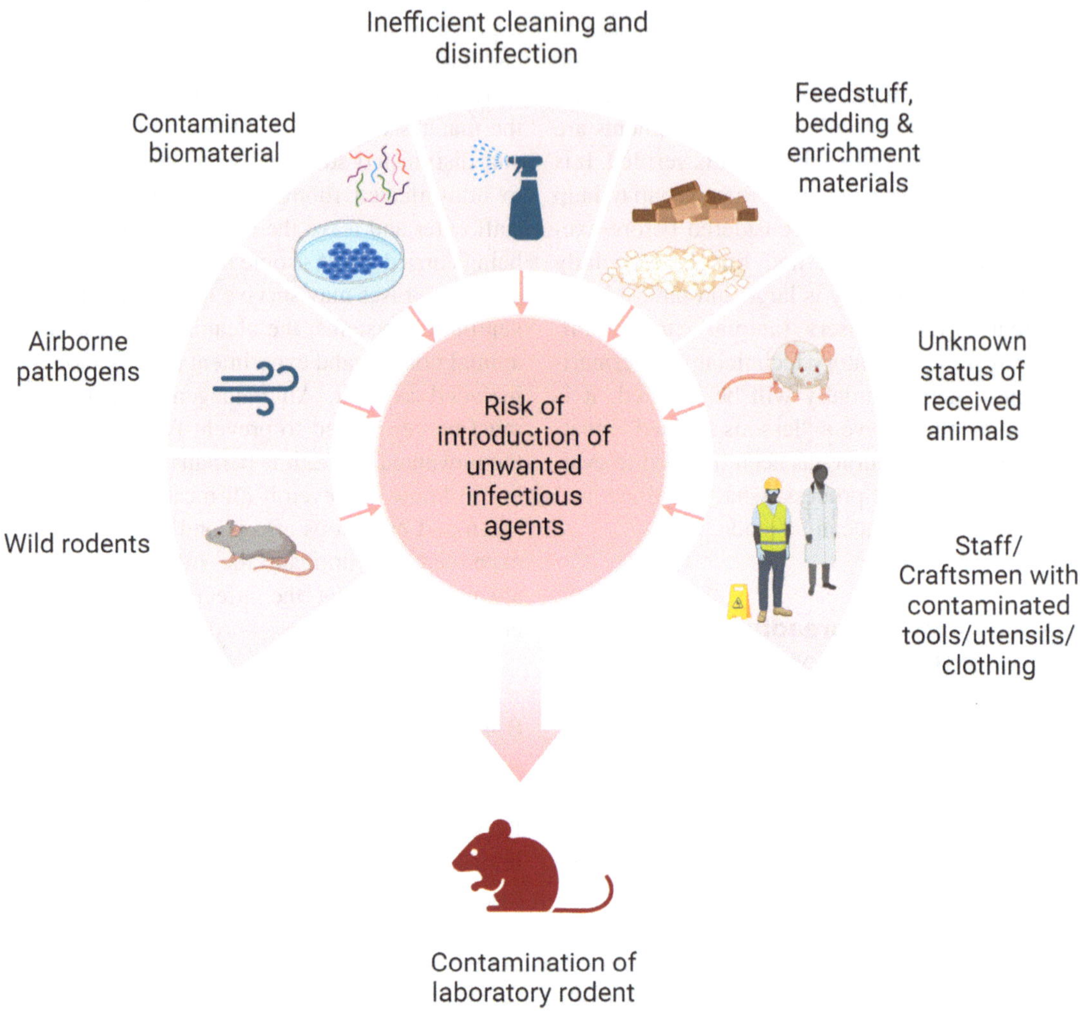

Fig. 8.4 A diagram showing the most common routes of infection for contamination of laboratory animals with unwanted infectious agents. Created with Biorender.com

venting a recurrence. Infectious agents can be introduced to a rodent colony through other rodents, either wild or imported, unrestricted traffic of staff or equipment, or by biological materials such as contaminated cell lines (Fig. 8.4). The source of the infection should be investigated, but still, it may reveal forever undiscovered. However, a proper investigation of procedural breaches and addressing all possible sources of contamination could limit the risk of future outbreaks.

Successful exclusion of pathogens from rodent colonies requires an in-depth understanding of the chain of infection, such as reservoir, source, and modes of transmission. The first step of the eradication program is to identify all animals positive for the infection and plan how to eliminate the infection from the animals. Rederivation is considered the most reliable method to eliminate pathogens, e.g., by the transfer of extensively washed embryos with intact zona pellucida into SPF recipient females, which is a standardized method that minimizes the risks of transferring an infection. As an alternative to rederivation, some infections may be eradicated with antibiotics (which comes with a high a risk of failure) or chemotherapeutic treatments, or a test-and-cull procedure can be used to eliminate charles river

The Jackson Laboratory

EUROPE Mouse SPF/VAF Barrier Room

EUROPEAN

Charles River Laboratories Kent

Location UK A52 Mice

Health Status SPF / VAF

Summary Item	*Method*	*Primary Lab*	*Most Recent*		*Past 18 Months*
			Test Date	*Positive / Tested*	*Positive / Tested*
Viruses					
Minute Virus of Mice (MVM) **ad**	MFIA	RADS US	15-Mar-2023	0 / 16	0 / 320
Mouse Parvovirus (MPV) **ad**	MFIA	RADS US	15-Mar-2023	0 / 16	0 / 320
Mouse Hepatitis Virus (MHV) **ad**	MFIA	RADS US	15-Mar-2023	0 / 16	0 / 320
Mouse Norovirus (MNV) **ad**	MFIA	RADS US	15-Mar-2023	0 / 16	0 / 320
Theiler Virus (TMEV -GDVII) **ad**	MFIA	RADS US	15-Mar-2023	0 / 16	0 / 320
Mouse Rotavirus (EDIM) **ad**	MFIA	RADS US	15-Mar-2023	0 / 16	0 / 320

Fig. 8.5 Example on how a health report can be organized (Charles River Laboratories)

infections in transgenic mouse lines difficult to replace. The next step of the eradication program is to eliminate the pathogen from the environment by a disinfection program designed to kill the pathogen depending on the type of pathogen. Non-enveloped viruses such as parvoviruses, spore-forming bacteria such as Clostridia and parasitic eggs all survive well in the environment and are resistant to some disinfectants, making it necessary to have a tailored disinfection program that targets the specific pathogen. A thorough cleaning of the affected area and contaminated equipment should be performed to remove any soiling before disinfection procedures can begin. The overall goal of the disinfection program is to eradicate infection, and thereby prevent its recurrence.

8.4.6 Reception of Animals and Animal Products

8.4.6.1 What Should Be the Criteria for Receiving Animals?

Rodents of the same or related species may serve as a reservoir of microorganisms and pose a major risk of infecting an SPF colony either by direct contact between animals or indirectly by fomites, such as contaminated food or bedding material. The risk of introducing pathogens when live animals are imported depends on different factors. Most commercial vendors have a good microbiological quality control program, high barrier protection, well defined standard operating procedures, and a controlled SPF transport program, decreasing the risk of infection when importing animals. Other research institutions may have varying qualities of the above-mentioned procedures, which, therefore, needs to be analyzed prior to the approval of import of live animals. For this analysis, the institutional veterinarian should always receive a health monitoring report from the source colony (Fig. 8.5). The health report should include the following five points: (1) a panel of relevant pathogens and opportunistic microorganisms, (2) testing method and frequency of each microorganism, (3) test material for each microorganism (e.g., feces, serology), (4) recent and historical data of the last 18 months, and (5) name of the laboratory performing the testing. The health report should be accompanied by a thorough facility description including the biosecurity level of the facility and information on the methodology for the health monitoring program used to obtain the report.

Animals with a health status approved by the institutional veterinarian are then accepted for import. Some institutions accept animals directly into the facility, while other institutions quarantine the animals to carry out an additional health screening of the animals before they are released into the facility. If this is done, individual deliveries must be isolated separately. In the latter case, samples are taken from the animals 2–3 weeks after arrival at the facility to detect any infections transmitted during the transport of the animals or not reported from the source colony. Health screening of quarantined animals can be done by collecting non-invasive specimens such as feces, fur, and oral swabbing for PCR testing.

8.4.6.2 How Should Animals Be Transported and Received? (For More Information, See Chapter on Transport)

The transport of live animals, and in particular genetically modified mice, places high demands on the breeder and courier to ensure that the animals are transported in an appropriate environment in terms of temperature, humidity, and microbiological protection. The commercial breeders use transport cages specifically designed for keeping the microbiological status of the rodents during shipping, and in the case of transport between in-house but distant facilities such cages should also be used. For distances within Europe, the commercial vendors will mostly use dedicated trucks, which can keep temperature and ventilation on a stable and acceptable level, even if the engine is not running. Public transport, e.g. by airplane, may be necessary for long and eventually inter-continental distance, but if possible it should be avoided.

At reception all animals must be inspected for injuries applied during transport, which for example can be caused by improper ventilation or handling or fighting due to stressful conditions. This will also reveal eventual damages not caused by the transport, but already were present, when the animals left the facility of origin. If such inspection is not done by the veterinarian, clear instructions must be made for the staff on what to look for.

Instead of sending live animals, distribution of frozen sperm or embryos is a way to overcome the logistical challenges and welfare concerns associated with shipping live mice. Shipment of sperm or embryos instead of live animals is also a method to accommodate import of specific strains that do not have an approved health report, e.g., if there are positive findings at the sending facility that cannot be approved by the recipient facility. Once the frozen material is delivered at the receiving facility, transported embryos can be thawed and transplanted to a recipient female or sperm can be used for in vitro fertilization (IVF) followed by embryo transfer.

8.4.6.3 How Should We Address the Risks of Biologicals?

Biological samples, especially those from animals of the same species, brought into the facility with unknown microbiological status increase the risk of contamination of the animals. This is typically the case with serum antibodies and cell transplants, but virtually any biological material injected or applied to animals during experiments has the potential to inadvertently introduce unwanted infectious agents. It is, therefore, important to test biological samples before they are brought into the animal facility. The selection of agents to be tested should correlate with the health monitoring program of the facility. Apart from serology, testing of biological samples can be carried out in the same way as samples for health monitoring, and they can be sent to commercial laboratories for testing.

8.4.6.4 How Should We Address the Risks of Feedstuff, Bedding Material, and Environmental Enrichment?

Feedstuff, bedding material, and environmental enrichment must also be considered as a risk for introduction of unwanted agents. To date, there is no evidence that feedstuff can be the direct cause of virus outbreaks, as virus has never been found in tested feed. Rodent chow is based upon crops from fields with plenty of wild rodents and birds flying over. Pelleted feed for rodents will only be exposed momentarily to temperatures in the range of 60–90 °C during the pelleting process, which will result in a reduction but not a full elimination of bacteria [41]. Extruded products are typically produced at higher temperatures reaching up to 200 °C momentarily. Viruses such as Mouse norovirus and Mouse parvovirus may resist the heat treatment and remain infectious after conditions modelling the rodent chow pelleting process, and, therefore, non-sterilized rodent chow is a potential source of viral outbreaks [42, 43]. Therefore, risk mitigation must be in place and typically, the feedstuff should be autoclaved or irradiated before brought into the animal facility.

Bedding material and environmental enrichment are most often not produced in a heated process as is the rodent chow. Therefore, it is important to evaluate the hygienic measures taken during the production of these materials, such as where does the raw material come from, how is it treated and with what, what is the risk of contamination during process, packaging, and storage, is a wild rodent control program in place, and will the materials come with a certificate stating it free of pathogens. If impossible to evaluate, then sterilization should be considered. A primary choice for this would be autoclaving, while gamma irradiation is a quite expensive alternative.

Diet and bedding may also contain toxic agents, for which the producer regularly make a batch control. The facility must have access to these batch controls, and deliveries should be checked for their batch number, and it should be ensured that there is a clean batch certificate for each delivery.

8.4.6.5 Where Can Background Information on Health Management Be Found?

The first place to look for exact guidance on microbiological health monitoring would be the recommendations from FELASA. There are guidelines for rodents and rabbits [8], ruminants and pigs [44], and non-human primates [45]. FELASA also has guidelines for the accreditation of health monitoring programs and testing laboratories involved in health monitoring [46]. In a collaboration between FELASA and the American Association for Laboratory Animal Science (AALAS), recommendations have also been issued for fish with an emphasis on zebra fish [47], and for health monitoring of rodents for animal transfer [48]. The good thing about such recommendations is that they can be used as a common standard, e.g., when purchasing animals from commercial vendors, and when collaborating between institutions. However, with a critical mindset, it should be noted that mostly such recommendations are the outcome of a consensus from a working group with different interests and expertise, and practices recommended can be both based upon scientific documentation as on traditions, and in some cases commercial interests. When planning a health monitoring program, it is wise always to consider, what makes sense to adapt for the particular institution; a principle, which is in accordance with the recommendations from FELASA [8]. Reading some textbook material is helpful. In this book series, the book "Rodent Quality Control: Genes and Bugs—Monitoring Health and Genetics of Laboratory Animals" covers the aspects of microbiological health monitoring [3]. In most laboratory animal science textbooks, there will also be chapters on health monitoring. However, the information to be obtained from here is too sparse, if being in charge of an institutional health management program.

To obtain a broader understanding of health and well-being of laboratory rodents, it will also be useful to read some textbook material on the basic biology of the animals, such as the UFAW Handbook [49], The Laboratory Mouse [50], or Animal-centric Care and Management [51].

It is also possible to find lots of information on the Internet. The homepage "Diseases of Research Animals" http://dora.missouri.edu/ gives small inputs to a range of the most important agents in laboratory rodents and rabbits. Commercial breeders and diagnostic laboratories have created informative materials and put them on their homepages. These materials are often excellent, but it should always be remembered that materials from commercial sources may also be subject to conflicts of interests, i.e. companies may have an interest in selling a certain service or downscaling the importance of an infection they are struggling with themselves. The annex III of the EU Directive is based upon a comprehensive work from the Council of Europe, and all the background information for proposing certain requirements for the housing of all laboratory animals can be found on their homepage [52]. Also, the chapter on Management of Laboratory Animals from the MSD Veterinary Manual is freely available [53]. Again, it is important to be critical, as materials freely available are often produced as some sort of commercial product or the result of a consensus in a working group.

8.5 Final Remarks

Beyond ethical and regulatory compliance, the health of laboratory animals profoundly affects the reliability and credibility of scientific research outcomes. This obligation encompasses preserving the animal's physical, mental, and social well-being through suitable environments, proper research conditions, and skilled staff who can collaborate across disciplines. Moreover, a robust health management program within the facility's biosecurity framework is essential. This program entails preventive measures to limit infections from entering the facility, a rigorous health monitoring system to rapidly detect unexpected infections, and a practical policy for effectively addressing positive findings. Regular reviews of the biosecurity measures and health monitoring program are vital to pinpoint potential procedural gaps that could compromise animal health.

References

1. World-Health-Organization. Constitution, https://www.who.int/about/governance/constitution (1946).
2. Jensen HE, Leifsson P, Jensen LK. Laboratory animal pathology in relation to spontaneous infections. In: Benavides F, Hansen AK, editors. Rodent quality control: genes and microorganisms. Springer-Nature; 2024.
3. Benavides FJ, Hansen AK. Rodent quality control: genes and bugs - monitoring health and genetics of laboratory animals. Cham: Springer; 2024.
4. Nicklas W, Buchheister S, Bleich A. Health monitoring programs and international standards. In: Benavides F, Hansen AK, editors. Rodent quality control: genes and microorganisms. Springer-Nature; 2024.
5. Masopust D, Sivula CP, Jameson SC. Of mice, dirty mice, and men: using mice to understand human immunology. J Immunol. 2017;199:383–8. https://doi.org/10.4049/jimmunol.1700453.
6. Fiege JK, Block KE, Pierson MJ, et al. Mice with diverse microbial exposure histories as a model for preclinical vaccine testing. Cell Host Microbe. 2021; https://doi.org/10.1016/j.chom.2021.10.001.
7. Rosshart SP, Herz J, Vassallo BG, et al. Laboratory mice born to wild mice have natural microbiota and model human immune responses. Science. 2019;365:461. https://doi.org/10.1126/science.aaw4361.
8. Mahler M, Berard M, Feinstein R, et al. FELASA recommendations for the health monitoring of mouse, rat, hamster, guinea pig and rabbit colonies in breeding and experimental units. Lab Anim. 2014;48:178–92. https://doi.org/10.1177/0023677213516312.
9. Nicklas W, Kraft V, Meyer B. Contamination of transplantable tumors, cell lines, and monoclonal antibodies with rodent viruses. Lab Anim Sci. 1993;43:296–300.
10. European_Union. Directive 2010/63/EU of The European Parliament and The Council of 22 September 2010 on the Protection of Animals used for Scientific Purposes. 2010.
11. Hansen AK. Microbiology and microbiome. Experimental design and reproducibility in preclinical animal studies. Cham: Springer; 2021. p. 77–104.
12. Hansen AK. Statistical aspects of health monitoring in rodents. In: Benavides F, Hansen AK, editors. Rodent quality control: genes and bugs - monitoring health and genetics of laboratory animals. Springer; 2024.
13. Hayashimoto N, Morita H, Ishida T, et al. Microbiological survey of mice (Mus musculus) purchased from commercial pet shops in Kanagawa and Tokyo, Japan. Exp Anim. 2015;64:155–60. https://doi.org/10.1538/expanim.14-0087.
14. Dammann P, Hilken G, Hueber B, et al. Infectious microorganisms in mice (Mus musculus) purchased from commercial pet shops in Germany. Lab Anim. 2011;45:271–5. https://doi.org/10.1258/la.2011.010183.
15. Homberger FR. Enterotropic mouse hepatitis virus. Lab Anim. 1997;31:97–115.
16. Homberger FR, Thomann PE. Transmission of murine viruses and mycoplasma in laboratory mouse colonies with respect to housing conditions. Lab Anim. 1994;28:113–20.
17. Bauer BA, Besch-Williford C, Livingston RS, et al. Influence of rack design and disease prevalence on detection of rodent pathogens in exhaust debris samples from individually ventilated caging systems. J Am Assoc Lab Anim Sci. 2016;55:782–8.
18. Compton SR, Homberger FR, Paturzo FX, et al. Efficacy of three microbiological monitoring methods in a ventilated cage rack. Comp Med. 2004;54:382–92.
19. Knust B, Stroher U, Edison L, et al. Lymphocytic choriomeningitis virus in employees and mice at multipremises feeder-rodent operation, United States,

2012. Emerging infectious diseases. 2014;20:240–7. https://doi.org/10.3201/eid2002.130860.
20. Hansen AK, Andersen HV, Svendsen O. Studies on the diagnosis of Tyzzer's disease in laboratory rat colonies with antibodies against Bacillus piliformis (Clostridium piliforme). Lab Anim Sci. 1994;44:424–9.
21. Furukawa T, Furumoto K, Fujieda M, et al. Detection by PCR of the Tyzzer's disease organism (Clostridium piliforme) in feces. Exp Anim. 2002;51:513–6. https://doi.org/10.1538/expanim.51.513.
22. Goto K, Horiuchi H, Shinohara H, et al. Specific and quantitative detection of PCR products from Clostridium piliforme, Helicobacter bilis, H-hepaticus, and mouse hepatitis virus infected mouse samples using a newly developed electrochemical DNA chip. J Microbiol Methods. 2007;69:93–9.
23. Whary MT, Baumgarth N, Fox JG, et al. Chapter 3 - Biology and diseases of mice. In: Fox JG, Anderson LC, Otto GM, et al., editors. Laboratory animal medicine. 3rd ed. Boston: Academic; 2015. p. 43–149.
24. Kunstýř I, Schoeneberg U, Friedhoff K. Host specificity of Giardia muris isolates from mouse and golden hamster. Parasitol Res. 1992;78:621–2.
25. CDC. Laboratory identification of parasitic diseases of public health concern. In: Malaria GH-DoPDa (Ed.) Atlanta, Georgia: Center for Disease Control, 2013.
26. Mailhiot D, Ostdiek AM, Luchins KR, et al. Comparing mouse health monitoring between soiled-bedding sentinel and exhaust air dust surveillance programs. J Am Assoc Lab Anim Sci. 2020;59:58–66. https://doi.org/10.30802/aalas-jaalas-19-000061.
27. Filipovska-Naumovska E, Thompson MJ, Hopwood D, et al. Strain- and age-associated variation in viral persistence and antibody response to mouse parvovirus 1 in experimentally infected mice. J Am Assoc Lab Anim Sci. 2010:443–9, 447.
28. Thackray LB, Wobus CE, Chachu KA, et al. Murine noroviruses comprising a single genogroup exhibit biological diversity despite limited sequence divergence. J Virol. 2007;81:10460–73. https://doi.org/10.1128/jvi.00783-07.
29. Clerc M, Babayan SA, Fenton A, et al. Age affects antibody levels and anthelmintic treatment efficacy in a wild rodent. Int J Parasitol Parasites Wildl. 2019;8:240–7. https://doi.org/10.1016/j.ijppaw.2019.03.004.
30. Zorn J, Ritter B, Miller M, et al. Murine norovirus detection in the exhaust air of IVCs is more sensitive than serological analysis of soiled bedding sentinels. Lab Anim. 2017;51:301–10. https://doi.org/10.1177/0023677216661586.
31. Hanson WH, Taylor K, Taylor DK. PCR testing of media placed in soiled bedding as a method for mouse colony health surveillance. J Am Assoc Lab Anim Sci. 2021;60:306–10. https://doi.org/10.30802/aalas-jaalas-20-000096.
32. O'Connell KA, Tigyi GJ, Livingston RS, et al. Evaluation of in-cage filter paper as a replacement for sentinel mice in the detection of murine pathogens. J Am Assoc Lab Anim Sci. 2021;60:160–7. https://doi.org/10.30802/aalas-jaalas-20-000086.
33. Henderson KS, Perkins CL, Havens RB, et al. Efficacy of direct detection of pathogens in naturally infected mice by using a high-density PCR array. J Am Assoc Lab Anim Sci. 2013;52:763–72.
34. Hansen AK, Nielsen DS, Krych L, et al. Bacterial species to be considered in quality assurance of mice and rats. Lab Anim. 2019;53:281–91.
35. Ivanov II, Frutos RD, Manel N, et al. Specific microbiota direct the differentiation of IL-17-producing T-helper cells in the mucosa of the small intestine. Cell Host Microbe. 2008;4:337–49. https://doi.org/10.1016/j.chom.2008.09.009.
36. Christensen EG, Licht TR, Leser TD, et al. Dietary xylo-oligosaccharide stimulates intestinal bifidobacteria and lactobacilli but has limited effect on intestinal integrity in rats. BMC Res Notes. 2014;7:660. https://doi.org/10.1186/1756-0500-7-660.
37. Bondarenko V, Løkke CR, Dobrowolski P, et al. Controlling the uncontrolled variation in the diet induced obese mouse by microbiomic characterization. Sci Rep. 2022;12:13767. https://doi.org/10.1038/s41598-022-17242-8.
38. Hansen CHF, Krych L, Nielsen DS, et al. Early life treatment with vancomycin propagates Akkermansia muciniphila and reduces diabetes incidence in the NOD mouse. Diabetologia. 2012;55:2285–94.
39. Zachariassen LF, Krych L, Engkilde K, et al. Sensitivity to oxazolone induced dermatitis is transferable with gut microbiota in mice. Sci Rep. 2017;7:44385. https://doi.org/10.1038/srep44385.
40. Pyndt Jorgensen B, Hansen JT, Krych L, et al. A possible link between food and mood: dietary impact on gut microbiota and behavior in BALB/c mice. PLoS One. 2014;9:e103398. https://doi.org/10.1371/journal.pone.0103398.
41. Steghöfer S, Limburn R, Margas E. Microbiological assessment of heat treatment of broiler mash at laboratory scale to evaluate Salmonella reduction during feed conditioning. J Appl Poult Res. 2021;30:100122. https://doi.org/10.1016/j.japr.2020.100122.
42. Adams SC, Myles MH, Tracey LN, et al. Effects of pelleting, irradiation, and autoclaving of rodent feed on MPV and MNV infectivity. J Am Assoc Lab Anim Sci. 2019;58:542–50. https://doi.org/10.30802/aalas-jaalas-18-000142.
43. Watson J. Unsterilized feed as the apparent cause of a mouse parvovirus outbreak. J Am Assoc Lab Anim Sci. 2013;52:83–8.
44. Berset Convenor F, Caristo ME, Ferrara F, et al. Federation of European Laboratory Animal Science Associations recommendations of best practices for the health management of ruminants and pigs used for scientific and educational purposes. Lab Anim. 2021;55:117–28. https://doi.org/10.1177/0023677220944461.
45. Balansard I, Cleverley L, Cutler KL, et al. Revised recommendations for health monitoring of non-

human primate colonies (2018): FELASA Working Group Report. Lab Anim. 2019;53:429–46. https://doi.org/10.1177/0023677219844541.
46. Nicklas W, Deeny A, Diercks P, et al. FELASA guidelines for the accreditation of health monitoring programs and testing laboratories involved in health monitoring. Lab Anim. 2010;39:43–8. https://doi.org/10.1038/laban0210-43.
47. Mocho JP, Collymore C, Farmer SC, et al. FELASA-AALAS recommendations for biosecurity in an aquatic facility, including prevention of zoonosis, introduction of new fish colonies, and quarantine. Comp Med. 2022;72:149–68. https://doi.org/10.30802/aalas-cm-22-000042.
48. Pritchett-Corning KR, Prins JB, Feinstein R, et al. AALAS/FELASA Working Group on Health Monitoring of rodents for animal transfer. J Am Assoc Lab Anim Sci. 2014;53:633–40.
49. Kirkwood J, Hubrecht R. The UFAW handbook on the care and management of laboratory and other research animals. London: Wiley-Blackwell; 2010.
50. Hedrich H. The laboratory mouse. Elsevier; 2012.
51. Sørensen DB, Cloutier S, Gaskill BN. Animal-centric care and management. CRC Press; 2020.
52. Council-of-Europe. Revision of Appendix A, https://www.coe.int/t/e/legal_affairs/legal_co-operation/biological_safety_and_use_of_animals/Laboratory_animals/Revision%20of%20Appendix%20A.asp (2004).
53. Huerkamp MJ. Management of laboratory animals. https://www.msdvetmanual.com/exotic-and-laboratory-animals/laboratory-animals/management-of-laboratory-animals#top (2022).

Biosecurity and Gnotobiology

9

Marion Berard

Abstract

The management of the sanitary status of laboratory animals is essential both from an animal welfare and a scientific standpoint. Poor sanitary status may have clinical impact and lead to invalid and/or irreproducible scientific results. Most of the laboratory animals are bred for research under strict hygienic procedures in order to exclude microorganisms that can impact their health and the outcome of experimental procedures. In these circumstances, the microbiological component of the animal models is defined by an exclusion list, i.e. the animals are free of certain microorganisms. In certain fields of research, the microbiota carried by the animals (microorganisms present in the animal, at interfaces with the environment, i.e. skin, mouth, nose, respiratory tract, genital tract, digestive tract) needs to be defined, and therefore gnotobiotic animals need to be used. Indeed, the phenotype of an animal depends on both its genotype and the envirotype, and like the genome, the microbiota can be manipulated to investigate its impact on the biology of the host.

In this chapter, we will answer to practical questions to understand the procedures to put in place when building a standard biosecurity program, and the specific ones that need to be implemented to produce germ-free and gnotobiotic animals.

We will focus mainly on laboratory rodents, but the main principles may apply to other species used in research.

Keywords

Sanitary management · Health monitoring · Animal welfare · Validity and reproducibility of results

9.1 What Do We Mean by Biosecurity? What Is Specific to Gnotobiology?

Biosecurity refers to measures aimed at preventing the introduction (bioexclusion) and/or spread (biocontainment) of microorganisms (e.g., viruses, bacteria, parasites, fungi) in the environment of laboratory animals in order to minimize the risk of transmission to the animals that can impact the scientific results generated with them (and also prevent the transmission to the staff when the microorganisms are zoonotic). These measures can be technical (designing the facilities, writing the standard operating procedures (SOP), choosing the equipment) or non-technical

M. Berard (✉)
Centre for Gnotobiology, Institut Pasteur, Université Paris Cité, Paris, France
e-mail: marion.berard@pasteur.fr

J. Guillén, V. Galligioni (eds.), *Practical Management of Research Animal Care and Use Programs*, Laboratory Animal Science and Medicine 3, https://doi.org/10.1007/978-3-031-65414-5_9

(designing the program, the organization/organization chart of the program, training and evaluation of knowledge, evaluation of the program).

They also include the quality control of the efficacy of the program (environmental monitoring, animal health monitoring).

There is consensus on the main principles to follow when developing a standard biosecurity program [1, 2] but there are different ways to put them in practice that will depend, for instance, on the species, the health status chosen for the program, and the local constraints (e.g., prevalence of the microorganisms, availability of the technologies to prevent and monitor microbiological contaminations, economical constraints).

Developing gnotobiotic animal models relies on the same general principles but involves specific techniques to produce the animals (germ free, gnotobiotic status), protect and monitor their microbiological status (isolator technologies and related processes, bacteriological aerobic and anaerobic cultures, sequencing) during routine husbandry or while implementing experimental procedures or transfer/ship the animals [3–5].

9.2 What Different Sanitary Status Can Be Found, and How They Can Relate to Research Needs?

Laboratory animals can be produced under different sanitary status that may be chosen to meet different experimental needs (Table 9.1).

Germ free also known as axenic animals are free of all living microorganisms and are commonly used to compare to genetically identical animals carrying a microbiota to identify alterations of biological functions of the host in the absence of microbiota (comparing the biological functions before/after eliminating the microbiota). They can be produced using embryo transfer or cesarean section. The axenic status is also the basis to produce gnotobiotic animals, i.e., animals that will be generated by administrating a defined microbiological cocktail to germ-free animals, to study the impact of the component(s) of the defined microbiota on biological functions of the host (comparing the biological functions after/before the implantation of the flora).

Table 9.1 Different sanitary status and their applications

Sanitary status	Types/examples of applications
Conventional (undefined)	To be avoided (uncontrolled validity and reproducibility of results). For pilot studies when the animal model is not available under another controlled status.
Specific Pathogen Free	Most commonly used status, universal.
Specific and Opportunistic Pathogen Free	For immunofragilized animals models.
Germ-Free and Gnotobiotic	To study the interactions between microbiota and the host, their effects on each other. To study the interactions between microorganisms.

Specific Pathogen Free (SPF) animals are free of a limited number of microorganisms that can alter their health and/or scientific results that are generated with them. This term has been adopted by the community of laboratory animal users, and especially the animals' suppliers worldwide to define the most currently used animals to facilitate their supply and transfer between facilities. One should be aware of the purpose of this definition (commercial, facilitation of transfers) which does not correspond to a unique sanitary status that must be adopted in all circumstances. Lists of microorganisms that may have an impact on the animals' health and biological reactivity were established in the 1990s [6] and are regularly updated [7] with the increasing knowledge in this field (adding new microorganisms that are identified, eliminating microorganisms that have no more impact). Facility managers should define their own list to answer to scientific needs and adapt to the characteristics of the animal models kept in their units.

In some facilities, where the immune system of animal models is particularly fragilized or in which human cells have been transferred, facility managers might have to exclude additional microorganisms to create environments free of opportunistic agents (Specific and Opportunistic Free, SOPF) or free of human pathogens, where they can be kept.

Animals with undefined health status could be carrying undesired microorganisms. If this is the case, the animals are referred to as conventional and should be used with caution, because they represent a source of contamination for the rest of their conspecifics and a potential threat to human health if they carry zoonotic agents. When the use of such animals cannot be avoided to generate scientific data (e.g., wild life studies), and the validity and reproducibility of the results cannot be guaranteed, one should describe as precisely as possible their microbiological characteristics.

9.3 What Are the Resources and Constraints to Be Evaluated Prior to Setting Up a Biosecurity Program?

Planning a biosecurity program requires a preliminary evaluation of the context, the objective of the program, the means available, and the constraints. The analysis should be led by a competent person, and performed together with the main stakeholders, such as representatives of the animal facility staff, the animal users, and the support services.

First, the scientific needs have to be identified:

- The species and their origin will determine, for instance, if quarantine, or rederivation processes should be available (may be unnecessary if animals originate from reliable commercial suppliers).
- The type of projects (breeding/experimental, fields of research, short-/long-term studies, type of risks involved) will determine which sanitary status to choose and the type of management and monitoring to implement. Breeding and long-term studies will require some level of health monitoring, while short-term studies on commercial animals may not require systematic microbiological quality control. Health monitoring on live animals should be avoided when environmental monitoring is available, and may not be possible when some biological or chemical or radioactive risks are involved.
- The number of animals and projects also need to be taken into account to evaluate the cost of the program and optimize.

The resources to manage the sanitary status then need to be analyzed. The evaluation will differ if the animal facilities are already operating or not, and if new infrastructures can be built. The financial resources for investment and operating/running costs have to be identified. The human resources component is also essential, and needs to be defined both in terms of quantity and quality. The competences that are required will have to be identified before the needs for recruitment or/and for training are expressed. The technical means to manage the sanitary status include the infrastructures (space available and design), the equipment as well as the engineering competences required. Some services linked to the biosecurity program can be outsourced if the competence or infrastructures are not available in the unit (quarantine, embryo transfer/cryopreservation, health monitoring, but also specific engineering consultancy).

Once these data are collected, a biosecurity plan can be developed.

9.4 What Are the Main Principles to Follow When Designing the Biosecurity Program?

The biosecurity program aims at preventing microbiological contaminations in the unit. This involves identifying the sources of contaminations and implementing sufficient preventive measures to manage them efficiently. Crisis management is part of the biosecurity program. It is necessary to plan it pre-emptively and to take into account the return of experience once the crisis is over in order to improve the design of the program.

9.4.1 How Do We Identify the Risk Factors of Contaminations? How Should They Be Evaluated? How Should Preventive Measures Be Designed?

Most of the factors of contaminations are identical in all the types of animal facilities, but their risk of occurrence may differ. Basically, all the incoming flows are potential routes of contamination. Main principles regarding prevention of contamination involve basic hygiene (cleaning, disinfecting, sterilizing), infrastructures and equipment (designing the facilities and choosing the equipment to protect animals through bioexclusion, and in certain circumstances prevent the spread of contaminations through biocontainment) to build a barrier around the microbiological unit to protect (Fig. 9.1; the concept of microbiological unit is further discussed in Sect. 3.2). The number of measures to put in place to efficiently prevent contaminations will depend on the level of the risk that has been identified. In any case, at least two measures should be implemented for each risk of contamination, so that if one fails there still remains one protective measure. Financial resources will orientate towards affordable measures and should be spared not to waste money in unnecessary measures. The number of protective measures should also be kept at minimum since any measure means a new constraint for the staff (impedes the development of research projects, reduces the ergonomics of work, increases the exposure to harmful substances) and increases the carbon footprint of the activity.

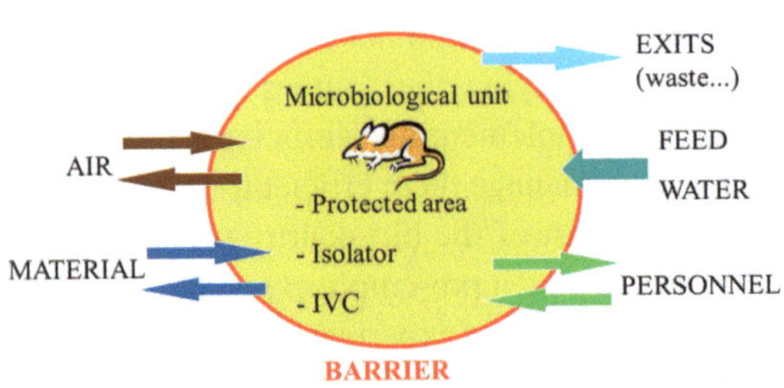

Fig. 9.1 The concept of microbiological unit and barrier

9.4.2 Animals: Which Ones Should Be Considered in the Context of the Biosecurity Program and How?

The experimental animals and the wild animals that can carry undesired microorganisms represent both reservoirs (where microorganisms survive or multiply between infections and from which contamination will spread) and vectors (intermediate carrying the microorganisms, from the reservoir to the unit/to the animals in the unit) of contamination. The contamination can be direct (the infected animals enter the facility) or indirect (the infected animals contaminate some material that will be introduced in the facility).

The entry of infected experimental animals can be avoided through quarantine and testing. When animals need to be introduced in the unit, the risk of contamination must be evaluated by collecting information about the facility from which they originate. The description of the health management and health monitoring program and the historical results of health monitoring must be provided and analyzed by a competent person, typically a veterinarian. The operating procedures of some commercial suppliers can be considered safe enough not to quarantine their animals. The decision not to quarantine these animals need to be based on a thorough analysis which should preferentially be complemented by auditing the supplier's production site, and be regularly updated. On the contrary, animals originating from non-commercial sources should always be considered as a potential risk of contamination, because of inherent characteristics of these institutions (e.g., number of staff coming inside the facility and heterogeneity of their experience in biosecurity, number of new animals introduced into the facility, experimental material used in the facility, limitations of the health monitoring program due to the containment of the animals and their heterogeneity/versatility). If a space where animals can be isolated is identified in the unit, it must be microbiologically totally independent from the rest of the facility, i.e. the animals need to be kept in a contained area (i.e., a sanctuary, optimally in isolators or isolator-cages) and flows coming out of the quarantine space must be identified and treated to eliminate any risk of spreading contamination (e.g., waste must be decontaminated without any breach of containment, staff working in this space must be aware of the risks and take all the hygienic necessary measures not to passively transfer contamination to the rest of the animals). In order to save time and identify rapidly the presence of contaminants, the sanitary status of the imported animals can be checked upon arrival (some samples can be taken on live animals or some of the animals can be sent to a diagnostic laboratory), but if the initial tests are negative the animals should still stay isolated for enough time to let a recent contamination develop at a level where it will be detectable. As far as the microorganisms affecting rodents are concerned, 4 weeks of quarantine are enough. At the end of the quarantine period, in order not to miss any contamination, the testing of imported animals should not exclusively be direct (the imported animals can get infected and resolve the infection during the quarantine period) but also rely on either contact sentinels (animals which initial status is controlled and compliant with the rest of the unit, and which should not resolve the infection during the exposure to the imported animals, e.g. immunodeficient animals can be used for sentinels) or environmental testing (sampling the environment with swabs or filters will allow for the detection of any undesired microorganism that will have been excreted during the quarantine period).

If the testing of animals reveals the presence of contaminants, the animals will have to be rederived through a cesarean section or an embryo transfer procedure.

If a quarantine space or competence in the rederivation procedures is not available in the unit, isolation, testing, and rederivation of imported animals can be outsourced to a third party.

Wild animals must not enter the unit. Surveillance of the wild rodents can be performed using baits around the units, and if necessary, items to trap or kill the animals will have to be installed. This aspect of the biosecurity program is often outsourced to professionals who update the use of traps and killing baits to avoid generating resistance in the wildlife population, and allow for the staff of the unit not to be in contact with potentially contaminated animals. It is important to consider daily checks of live traps to avoid animal suffering.

Animals of different species from the ones kept in the facilities should also be considered, if they can be the reservoir of the microorganisms that can infect the resident animals, or if they can passively transfer contaminants (e.g., crawling and flying insects). As far as insects are concerned, there are different measures that can be put in place to stop them from entering the facility, such as pressure cascade, interlocking doors, insectocutors, and insecticides. The choice of the preventive measures will have to be made after evaluating the level of risk, i.e. enough measures need to be implemented so as not to detect any insects in the unit.

9.4.3 Staff: Who Are They and How to Manage Them in Terms of Biosecurity?

Staff entering the facility represents one of the most difficult factors to manage. As far as their knowledge of biosecurity is concerned, they can be a very heterogeneous population (animal technicians, veterinarians, permanent scientists, students, support teams). Their training is one of the corner stones of the program. It should be performed before staff first enter the facility so that they are made aware of the risks at stake (factors of contaminations which they are part of, impact of contaminations on the research programs) and include an evaluation of the acquired knowledge. The applicable SOPs need to be clearly presented to the staff, available in written as reference documents but also sometimes in more accessible formats (videos, photos, and drawings). Continuous training should be planned to provide regular updates on the risks and their management.

Staff represent a risk because they may passively transfer contaminants from infected animals to the unit. The "infected animals" can be their pets, wild animals they may have direct or indirect contact with outside of the facility, but also other experimental animals (living experimental animals but also biological materials of animal origin that they keep in their laboratories).

Staff can also be a reservoir of zoonotic microorganisms. When sick, they should not enter the facility if their disease is zoonotic and can affect the resident animals.

In any case, staff should wear equipment to prevent contaminated particulates that they may carry, to transfer in the facility, such as cover shoes, lab coats or gowns, hair nets, gloves, surgical masks. These protective equipment should not replace basic hygiene, and staff should also be aware that they have to wash their hands and wear clean clothes when entering the facility.

One very frequently asked question is whether staff should be quarantined when they have contact with animals outside of the facility. Some commercial suppliers forbid their staff to have pets of the same species they care for. If staff are allowed to have pets at home, or work in two independent facilities, a quarantine may be impossible to implement. Therefore, they should be informed of the risk and of the preventive measures to take in order not to transfer potential contaminants to the unit (e.g., avoid taking care of the pets themselves, and if they do, take a shower and shampoo and change clothes before going to work).

Finally, staff should be aware they need to declare the biological material they will introduce in the facility, so that the risk of contamination can be evaluated. The detection of this risk can easily be implemented during the ethics evaluation process through which all the projects using animals are run. A question regarding this risk can be added to the general form to fill in and the collected information passed on the competent person who will decide the appropriate preventive measures to implement (e.g., antibodies still produced with animals can be filtered, cells can be tested easily using PCR).

Animal technicians as well as staff from the support teams also represent a risk and should be trained to understand the procedures they will have to follow to avoid contamination. They should organize their work so as not to enter different independent microbiological units on the same day or without taking necessary hygienic precautions. When possible, the activity of animal technicians should be restricted to the care and/or implementation of procedures on animals, and the waste management as well as the supply of material to them should be performed by an independent team, to avoid having the same staff handling potentially contaminated materials and live animals. Technical services should plan their intervention in the facilities to allow enough time for their tools and equipment to be sanitized before they are introduced into the unit. Toolboxes could also be designed together with them to be left in the facilities to be used in case of emergency. Another way to limit the entry of technical services into the facilities is to train animal technicians for certain operations (e.g., how to change filters in ventilated unit, how to change light bulbs, how to repair frequently observed failure of computers or printers).

9.4.4 Structural Components (Facility, Equipment): How to Design and Choose Them to Facilitate and Strengthen the Biosecurity Program?

Obviously, the ideal situation when designing a biosecurity program is to simultaneously design the structure of the unit and choose the equipment that will be used for sanitization or to house the animals. When possible, the facility should be designed to avoid clean and dirty flows crossing each other. If this is not possible, operating procedures should be put in place to decrease the risk of cross contaminations, e.g., cleaning and disinfecting the common corridors frequently, separating the timing of "dirty" operations such as waste management from the implementation of procedures on animals. The choice of efficient sanitizing equipment (washing machines, autoclaves, chemical vaporizers) and of their location is also essential and should facilitate the separation of clean and dirty flows. The detergents and disinfectants should be active against the microorganisms to exclude from the unit. The staff responsible for the cleaning and disinfection should be trained to understand the processes and use their equipment efficiently.

Equipment where animals are kept should be adapted to the risks to manage. The more isolated the animals the more protected they are, but also the more expensive and less ergonomic the procedures. The use of isolators or isolator-cages should be restricted to potentially contaminated animals (to avoid contamination spreading from them) or to germ free/gnotobiotic or immunofragilized animals (to protect them from a contamination which would alter their microbiological characteristics or impact their health). SPF animals can be maintained in open cages if the barrier at the level of the room is sufficient, as it is the case for commercial animal production (separation of staff working in contact with animals and staff managing waste or supply of material, full change of clothes after wet shower when entering the room, sanitization of all the materials that go through the barrier by autoclave or chemical disinfection, HEPA filtration of the air supply). In experimental facility, SPF animals are kept most of the time in individually ventilated cages, which offer a better protection since the barrier at the level of the room and in the room cannot be as efficiently controlled (frequent introduction of animals, numerous members of staff with heterogeneous biosecurity competences, biological risks related to experimental material). The use of laminar flow hoods can help maintain a barrier around the animals when they are handled outside of their cages. The treatment of the air supply to the room should be consistent with the sanitary status of the animals, and the choice of filtration made accordingly.

Scientific equipment, especially for imaging or behavioral monitoring, might be installed in the facility. Their operating procedures as well as their maintenance should be developed together with the biosecurity manager to avoid (cross-) contaminations.

Some other scientific equipment (e.g., imaging, irradiation) might not be available in the facility and the animals may have to be transferred outside of the facility and kept alive after the procedure. If the animals are not protected during the process (through containment or sanitization of the equipment they will be in contact with), they should be considered as potentially contaminated and then be kept isolated from the rest of the animals (their isolation could be shortened if their sanitary status is checked and compliant after 4 weeks of quarantine).

Cleaning and disinfection also apply to the rooms and their large equipment. Ideally, there should be some space available to regularly empty each room, clean and disinfect them and their equipment before populating them again with animals.

9.4.5 How Should Materials Necessary for the Husbandry (Food, Bedding, Water, Environmental Enrichment, and Husbandry Procedures) Be Chosen and Sanitized?

Food, bedding, water, and environmental enrichment will be used for husbandry and in direct contact with the animals. Their microbiological quality should therefore be consistent with the sanitary status of the animals.

The same logic applies to the suppliers of these materials as to the animal suppliers: their choice should be based on the evaluation of their operating procedures including the auditing of their production site, and be regularly updated. In order to maintain a controlled sanitary status, the materials should be free of the live microorganisms excluded from the unit. This can be achieved either through autoclaving in the unit, or irradiation by the supplier. If autoclaving is chosen, the unit should be able to ensure the reproducible efficiency of the process through calibration and microbiological validation. The procedure used to autoclave food should not alter its nutritive and physical characteristics. Technical services should be readily available to repair and maintain the autoclaves that will be a vital part of the biosecurity program. If autoclaving is not available or not reliable, the materials can be irradiated by the supplier. There are different levels of irradiation, which guarantee different microbiological qualities. Commonly, 10 kGys irradiation is used for

SPF animals, 25 kGys for SOPF animals, and 45 kGys for germ-free and gnotobiotic animals.

As far as environmental enrichment is concerned, autoclavable items should be preferred to non-autoclavable ones since the sterilization process is easier to control and does not leave any residues that could be in contact with the animals if chemical disinfection was used. The frequency and the procedure of cleaning and disinfecting the reusable items should be determined to ensure they do not become a source of contamination.

Water does not have to be necessarily sterilized. The decision to decontaminate tap water should be based on the analysis of its microbiological quality and of the robustness and stability of the results. If needed (i.e., when the quality of water is poor, or because of the high sanitary status of the animals), the water can be filtered, UV treated, acidified, chlorinated (for SOPF animals), or autoclaved (for germ-free and gnotobiotic animals). The efficiency of each process will also have to be validated with microbiological tests. Mineral water bottles for human consumption are sometimes used, but these habits may not survive the analysis of sustainability of the animal facility processes.

9.4.6 What Procedures Should Be Considered When Handling Animals?

The SOPs of the facility will have to be decided while designing the structure, and choosing the equipment and the materials that will be used. Some procedures might contain information regarding biosecurity (e.g., husbandry of animals), but the biosecurity program should also be fully described in a dedicated procedure which will refer to the documents that allow for its implementation, and be accessible to all the stakeholders. The following procedures/policies should be considered:

- For the animals:
  - the sanitary status chosen for the facility
  - the policy on which animals are allowed to enter the facility and how
  - the list of suppliers from which the animals can be introduced without quarantine
  - the process to evaluate the risk linked to non-commercial animals (including the documents to be collected, i.e. health management and monitoring programs, health monitoring results)
  - the policy to orientate non-commercial animals towards quarantine or cesarean/embryo transfer rederivation and the duration of each process
  - how the husbandry of animals should be conducted; the pest control program
  - who is managing these processes and how to contact them.
- For the staff:
  - who is allowed to enter the facility and which processes they have to follow to be authorized
  - the trainings to take
  - the documents to provide (training and professional experience in the field) to the animal facility manager
  - the recommendations regarding contact with non-experimental animals
  - the protective equipment to wear
  - what materials can be introduced into the facility and how
  - who is managing these processes and how to contact them.
- For the experimental procedures:
  - the procedure describing how to introduce experimental material in the unit
  - how to declare the use of biologicals of animal origin
  - the procedure to handle animals (this one could refer to specific procedures regarding husbandry, surgical procedures and asepsis, imaging or inside or outside the facility, behavioral tests or other experimental procedures)
  - who is managing these processes and how to contact them.
- For the technical services and outsourced maintenance of equipment:
  - how to access the facility for planned versus urgent operations including how to enter equipment

- toolboxes available in the unit
- who is managing these processes and how to contact them.
- For the cleaning-disinfection:
  - the procedure for each reusable material or piece of equipment as well as for the rooms and their large equipment
  - the frequency of cleaning and disinfection
  - the validation of the efficacy of the process
  - the storage conditions of the material before use
  - the microbiological validation of the efficacy of cleaning/disinfection/autoclaving as well as for the microbiological monitoring of the quality of water: the details of the tests to be performed for each process, the frequency of testing (routine testing, additional testing after incidents or following maintenance of the sanitizing equipment).
- For the waste management: The different types of waste and specific procedures for each type (with or without microbiological risk), i.e. contaminated waste should be contained and ideally decontaminated before disposal.
- Health monitoring of the animals/unit: The detailed procedure on how to perform them, record and communicate the results (cf. 3.2.).
- For the disaster planning: The main principles to follow when the presence of a contaminant is suspected or confirmed (cf 3.3.).
- For the responsibilities in the biosecurity program: An organizational chart describing who is in charge of the design and implementation, including the role of each stakeholder (animal technicians, scientific staff, support teams, biosecurity manager).

9.4.7 How Can Quality Control Measures Be Implemented?

The efficacy of the biosecurity program can be assessed at different levels. This work could be performed together with the institutional staff dedicated to quality. The following activities can be considered:

- One basic check should be done by visiting the facility regularly and verifying that there is no breach in the structure, that the maintenance of the equipment is up-to-date (washing machines, autoclaves, chemical vaporizers, laminar flow hoods, ventilated units of animals' caging systems); that the detergents, disinfectants, and all the protective equipment available are not expired; and that the procedures related to biosecurity are followed (e.g., the audit can be complemented by the analysis of the records of cleaning/disinfection, pest control, training records). A report of the visit should be sent to all the stakeholders, including the institutional official and should be associated with an action plan and a follow-up if some discrepancies have been observed.
- Calibration of the sanitizing equipment should be done by the supplier before their first use in the unit, and then at a defined frequency to detect and correct any non-compliance. The recording of each sanitizing cycle should be checked when available. Some tests can be performed to check the compliance of the cycles (e.g., verify adequate steam penetration into every pack/pouch by integrating three essential criteria for proper steam sterilization: time, temperature, and steam, evaluate the performance of the air removal (vacuum) system of pre-vacuum equipped steam sterilizers. Any incidents should be communicated to the staff in charge of biosecurity. The recordings and results of the tests should be archived and accessible.
- Microbiological validation of the efficacy of the sanitization processes should also be done when the equipment are first installed, and regularly afterwards. The unit can develop its own tests, but commercial kits are available and qualified for each process (Geobacillus *stearothermophilus* coated spore strips to test gas disinfection or inoculated vials to test solid and liquid autoclave loads).
- Health monitoring (a more complete description of health monitoring programs is available in Chap. 8): In the laboratory animals' vocabulary, health monitoring means testing animals or their environment for the presence

of microorganisms that should be excluded (i.e., the ones defined in the biosecurity program to answer to the scientific needs). In certain circumstances, the need for health monitoring can be questioned (e.g., in animal facilities, where studies are very short (less than a month), not overlapping (the rooms are sanitized between two studies) and performed with commercial animals.

When health monitoring has to be performed, it can be done at several steps of the biosecurity program:

- Testing a batch of imported animals kept in quarantine to decide whether they will be able to be transferred into the unit or be rederived
- Testing animals produced by embryo transfer or cesarean section to check if the rederivation is successful
- Testing sick animals, or regularly testing animals or the environment in the units to provide a quality certificate to the scientists regarding the animals they use in their project. It is indeed the final aim to provide them with the proof that the microbiological quality of their animals is compliant and cannot bias their results

Health monitoring of the unit and the animals is the final quality control of the biosecurity program, summarizing the results of all the preventive measures, checking if the goal to maintain a given sanitary status is reached.

In certain species, regulation requires that some agents be tested (e.g., brucellosis or Q fever in cattle). For the rest, there are widely followed recommendations [1, 7–9], which the person responsible for the health monitoring program needs to adapt by defining:

- First, the microbiological unit to be tested, i.e., the self-contained microbiological entity, with separate space and traffic for animals, personnel, and materials, that is going to be tested. This can be a batch of animals kept in quarantine in an isolator, most of the time a group of cages in a room. This definition is important since the results of the tests will only apply to the unit tested.
- Then the samples to be tested. They can be live colony animals representative of a population (this is the routine method used by breeders in their SPF barriers where thousands of animals of the same strain are kept in open cages), live animals exposed to the population to be tested either by direct contact (contact sentinels that can be used, for example, to test animals in quarantine) or by indirect contact through their dirty bedding (these sentinels are often used when testing heterogeneous population of animals kept in isolated ventilated cages) but also samples of the environment (swabs of the cages or the rooms, filters exposed to the air exhaust of the ventilated cages where the animals are kept).
- The frequency of the tests that should take into account the needs of the scientists to have regular update of the quality certificate of their animals, the risks of contamination (the more open the barrier is, the more frequent the tests should be, e.g. large numbers of introduction of animals/staff/materials, minimal bioexclusion measures), and the impact of a contamination (e.g., breeders test their units more often than what is recommended by FELASA, since a contamination of their production can impact many units receiving their animals).
- The duration of exposure of the sentinels or of the filters to the environment: This can be linked to the frequency of testing if health monitoring is a continuous process (i.e., for animal rooms continuously populated, sentinels or filters are continuously present in the room, and the duration of exposure is the time between 2 tests) or to be defined for other processes (e.g., when testing for the efficiency of a rederivation, the foster mother is the animal exposed and cannot be sent to a diagnostic lab before the weaning of its pups, so that the duration of exposure in this case will be at least 6 weeks).
- The laboratory that will perform the tests: They can be done in-house if the technology is available, or outsourced. The choice of the laboratory should be based on the robustness of the diagnostic methods they use. Like any supplier, the diagnostic laboratory should be audited regularly to verify the quality of its production.

The results should be communicated and easily accessible by the facility manager and the scientists. The report can follow the format recommended by FELASA, to facilitate the communication inside the unit but also with collaborators when animals need to be shipped to them. When undesired microorganisms are detected, the internal communication should be clear and open (avoid emails, prefer in-person communication that allows for question & answer sessions), and the written results reports should be enriched with comments/interpretation and the follow-up actions led in the unit.

9.4.8 How Should a Crisis Due to Contamination Be Managed?

The main principles to manage a contamination are:

- To prepare the disaster plan while designing the biosecurity program (before detecting an undesired microorganism) and communicate it to the stakeholders so that when the situation occurs, they are already aware of the consequences and of their roles in the action plan. This is essential to avoid panic and also will facilitate the implementation of the plan. For instance, when breeding of animals is involved, the lines should be cryopreserved to be able to recycle the colony easily if a contamination occurs.
- To confirm the results: Like any biological data the result could be a false positive. The confirmation is easy to be done with environmental samples such as filters placed on the exhaust airflow of ventilated units. In this case, a duplicate of the filter that was sent to the diagnostic lab should always be produced (by cutting the filter in two, or placing 2 filters side by side during the exposure time) and ready to be sent for confirmation. It is also easy when colony animals are used for health monitoring and if a new group of animals are available and can be readily sent for confirmation. When using sentinel animals, planning for immediate confirmation means using additional animals exposed together with the first animals sent for diagnostic. These extra animals will be ready to be sent in case of a suspicious result on the first animals, which is ethically questionable and not consistent with a 3R approach.
- To define a security perimeter around the suspicious microbiological unit. Before confirming the result, but also during all the procedure that will follow the confirmation to manage the contamination, measures must be taken to avoid the spread of the contamination to other units. It is especially in this circumstance that the definition of the microbiological unit takes sense. The components of the unit are defined (animals, staff, material, equipment, waste) and should not exit the microbiological unit outside of a containment and without prior sanitization:
- all the stakeholders should be informed to adopt the appropriate measures if they have to enter the unit. Units where animals or materials from the suspicious one have been transferred to since the last health monitoring results should also be identified and their facility manager alerted so that they can take the necessary biosecurity measures on their side
- animals should not exit the unit (and ideally no new animal should be introduced in the unit)
- the number of staff should be reduced to the essential and should wear additional protective equipment dedicated to the microbiological unit
- when possible, staff taking care of the suspicious unit should not work in another unit and if not possible, they should enter the suspicious unit the latest in the day and a minimal number of times
- materials and equipment should stay in the suspicious unit and be sanitized (disinfected or sterilized) if they have to get out (e.g., waste should be contained, for instance, in double bags, and autoclaved before elimination).

- To resolve the contamination if the result is confirmed. The process applies again to all the components of the microbiological unit, but will differ depending on the nature of the microorganism detected and the context:
- all the stakeholders should be informed of the confirmation of the contamination. The communication should be adapted to the severity of the contamination and the need to co-construct the action plan (e.g., detection of opportunistic agents in a SPF facility can be communicated by email with no further corrective action; detection of a major interfering contaminant such as Mouse Parvovirus may require an in-person meeting with at least one representative of each stakeholder group)
- in case of detection of a major interfering agent that requires the elimination of the animals and sanitization of the room, the scientists should be asked to provide the list of ongoing studies mentioning the identification of the cages, the end date of the studies, and the possibility to stop the experiments/eliminate the animals. Depending on the number of animals that need to be kept, the duration of the studies, and the availability of a quarantine area, different decisions can be made. For example, isolation of animals in a quarantine area (on site or outsourced) until the end of the studies or stop the studies earlier can be considered. Once the microbiological unit will be depopulated, the materials and equipment will have to be either eliminated (if single use) or disinfected/sterilized
- certain major interfering agents do not require the elimination of all the animals [8]. For example, this is the case with pinworms that can be managed with an antiparasitic treatment of the animals and strict hygienic measures in the room; with Mouse Hepatitis Virus in a colony of immunocompetent animals where "burn-out" or "herd-immunity" strategies can be used; or with certain contaminants that are not highly contagious where contaminated cages can be identified with further monitoring and eliminated. In these cases, materials and equipment in the room can be vectors of re-contamination and should therefore be treated (e.g., single use material can be eliminated, reusable material and equipment will have to be sanitized with some procedure that can be applied in the presence of animals such as steam sanitization).
- To search for the cause: All the protective measures that are part of the biosecurity plan need to be audited to identify if one is defective (e.g., autoclave dysfunction, staff not following the procedures) and if this is the case necessary corrective measures will have to be taken (repair the equipment, sanction/retrain staff). If all the protective measures are compliant with the biosecurity plan, this means that the risks of contamination have been undervalued and additional measures need to be put in place.
- To finally communicate on the actions taken to resolve the crisis, and the change in the biosecurity plan if necessary (sharing the updated procedures in this case).

9.5 What Specificities of the Biosecurity Program Can Be Adopted for Germ-Free and Gnotobiotic Animals?

The same biosecurity principles apply to gnotobiotic production but there are some specificities:

- Financial resources: Biosecurity measures are more expensive than for non-gnotobiotic activities because of the containments that are necessary to maintain and transfer the animals, and also the type and frequency of quality controls that need to be performed on the sanitization processes and the animals. Doing an experiment with gnotobiotic animals also takes more time than with SOPF or SPF animals.
- Animals: They must be kept either in isolators or in isolator-cages (Fig. 9.2), and therefore the experiments will be performed either in isolators or in a biosafety cabinet with very strict hygienic procedure. The transfer of animals between different units will be performed under containment either in isolators, in isolator-cages or equivalent (Fig. 9.3).

- Staff: Their training takes longer and is more specific especially to the technology (isolator and isolator-cages handling) and to the management of risk (people working in this field consider that "paranoia" is an asset since one microorganism is enough to lose a breeding/an experiment, and so they need to be constantly focused on the implementation of strict biosecurity techniques).
- Materials: Everything needs to be sterile. When irradiation is used, it must be at higher levels (45 kGys) than for SOPF and SPF productions [3–5]. When autoclave is used, pretreatment of some equipment at high degrees with dry heat might be needed, and autoclave cycles need to be even more controlled than for the other types of productions (monitoring the microbiological inactivation in each cycle is recommended prior to using the material). Ethylene oxide can also be used for materials that do not resist to heat/steam treatment (to be outsourced in most countries where this chemical is considered highly toxic, and its use is forbidden in building open to the public).

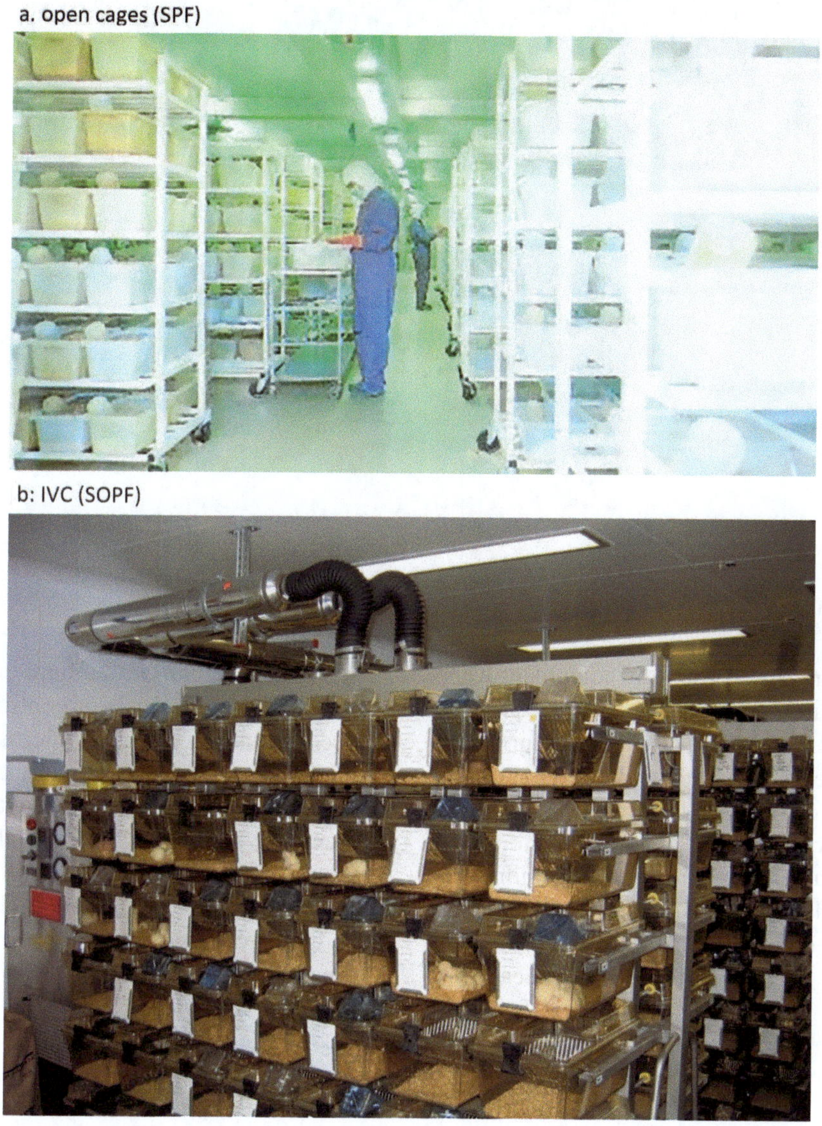

Fig. 9.2 Different type of containment adapted to different sanitary status. (**a**) Open cages (SPF), (**b**) IVC (SOPF), (**c**) isolators or isolator-cages (Germ Free and Gnotobiotic)

c: isolators or isolator-cages (Germ Free and Gnotobiotic)

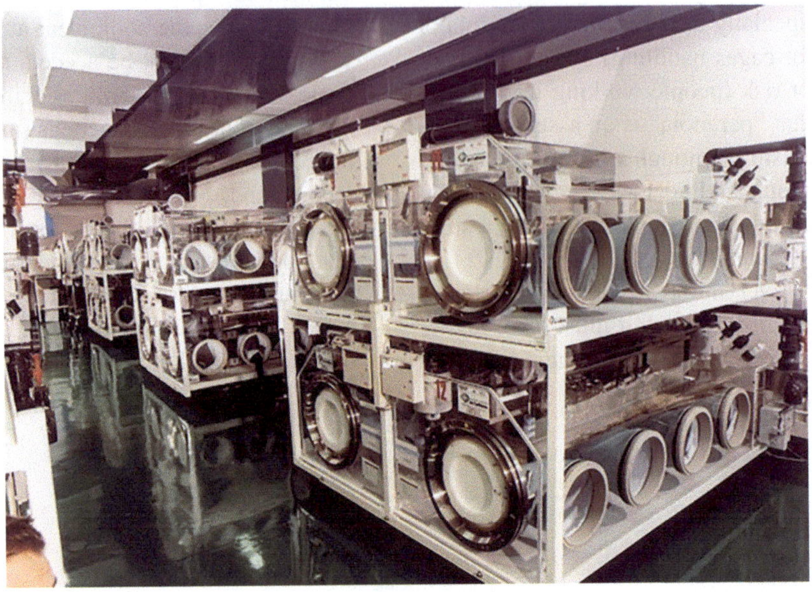

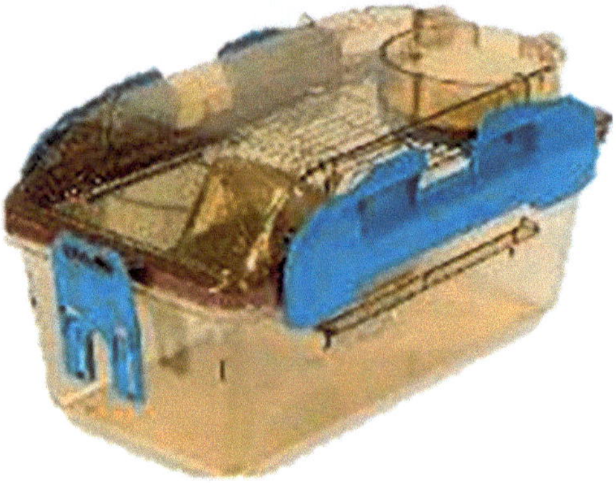

Fig. 9.2 (continued)

- Equipment: Aside from the equipment where animals are housed, experimental equipment will need to be adapted to the biosecurity constraints (e.g., miniaturizing behavioral tests so that they can fit in an isolator).
- Quality control: One isolator is one microbiological unit and needs to be monitored independently. As far as isolator-cages are concerned, it is difficult to perform dirty bedding exposure of sentinels because of the risk of cross-contamination. Protocols may vary, but the basis of controlling germ-free animals is a direct microscopic fecal examination complemented by cultures that should be able to grow both aerobic and anaerobic bacteria [5]. Molecular methods should be used to monitor gnotobiotic animals (in-house or outsourced sequencing is easily available nowadays, but still expensive).

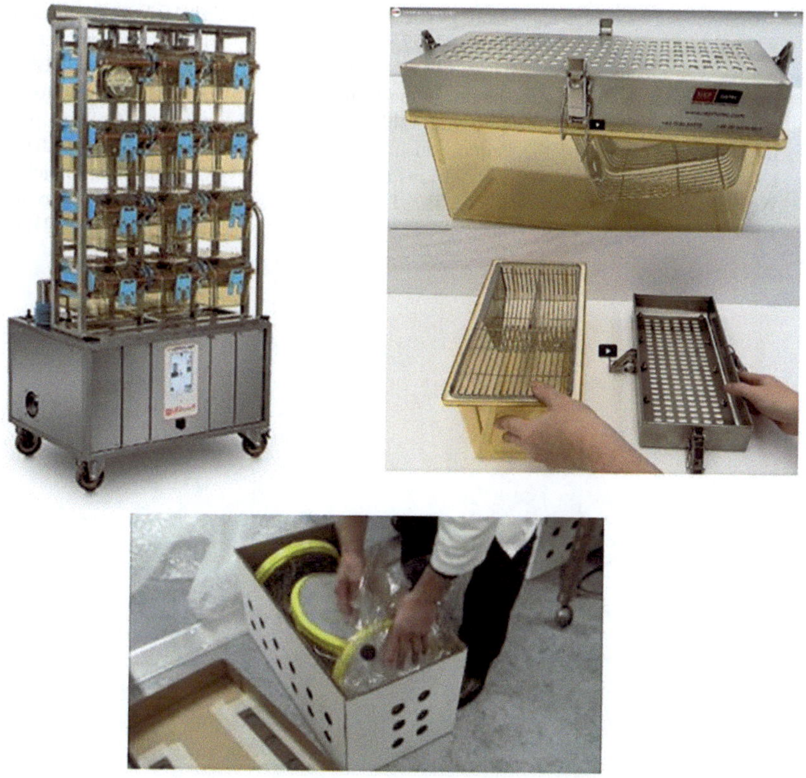

Fig. 9.3 Transport systems to control the gnotobiotic sanitary status

9.6 Conclusion

Prior to its implementation, the biosecurity program will have to be presented to the stakeholders for approval. The cost of each process should also be evaluated and provided to the staff in charge of managing financial resources. Because of all the constraints linked to biosecurity, to emphasize the importance to comply with it the program will also have to be sponsored by upper management (scientific and administrative/financial and technical) to develop a culture of biosecurity at all levels of the organization.

The biosecurity plan will have to be audited regularly to adapt to new constraints, like any other continuously improving process.

References

1. Mähler M, Berard M, Feinstein R, et al. FELASA recommendations for the health monitoring of mouse, rat, hamster, guinea pig and rabbit colonies in breeding and experimental units. Lab Anim. 2014;48:178–92.
2. Committee for the Update of the Guide for the Care and Use of Laboratory Animals, National Research Council US. Guide for the Care and Use of Laboratory Animals. 8th ed. Washington, DC: National Academies Press US; 2011.
3. Trenton, et al. Gnotobiotics. In: Fox JG, Anderson LC, Otto G, et al., editors. Laboratory animal medicine, American College of Laboratory Animal Medicine Series. 3rd ed. Academic; 2015.
4. Vowles CJ, Anderson NE, Eaton KA. Gnotobiotic mouse technology: an illustrated guide. 1st ed. CRC Press; 2015.
5. Schroeb TR, Eaton KA, editors. Gnotobiotics. A volume in American College of Laboratory Animal

Medicine Series. American College of Laboratory Animal Medicine Series. Academic; 2017.
6. Kraft V, Deeny AA, Blanchet HM, et al. Recommendations for the health monitoring of mouse, rat, hamster, guineapig and rabbit breeding colonies: Report of the Federation of European Laboratory Animal Science Associations (FELASA) Working Group on Animal Health. Lab Anim. 1994;28:279–80.
7. FELASA Guidelines and Recommendations. https://felasa.eu/working-groups/recommendations/id/32
8. Whary MT, et al. Biology and diseases of mice. In: Fox JG, et al., editors. Laboratory animal medicine, American College of Laboratory Animal Medicine Series. 3rd ed. Academic Press; 2015.
9. Buchheister S, Bleich A. Health monitoring of laboratory rodent colonies-talking about (r)evolution. Animals-Basel. 2021;11:1410–41.

Colony Management (Genetics) 10

Belén Pintado, Jan Parker-Thornburg,
and James Bussell

Abstract

Genetically altered animals have entered most animal facilities during the past 50 years. They provide refined models to study different biological issues, but their use requires specific management and more resources when compared with their wild-type counterparts. Housing these models requires facilities to adapt old and implement new procedures. Resources, including assisted reproductive technology, genotyping, and genetic quality diagnosis are used daily when dealing with such colonies. As such, animal resource personnel must have a deep understanding of them in order to offer support to animal researchers. This chapter offers recommendations and strategies for managing Genetically Altered (GA) and wild-type (WT) animals, including breeding and handling and methods for preservation of their genetic integrity, all of which consider and implement the 3Rs.

B. Pintado (✉)
Transgenesis and Genetic Edition Service CNB-CBMSO, CSIC, Madrid, Spain
e-mail: bpintado@cnb.csic.es

J. Parker-Thornburg
Department of Genetics, MD Anderson Cancer Center, Houston, TX, USA

J. Bussell
University of Oxford, Oxford, UK
e-mail: James.Bussell@BMS.ox.ac.uk

Keywords

Genetically altered · Transgenic, gene editing · Gene targeting · Genotyping · Genetic drift · Speed congenics · Assisted reproductive techniques · Rodents · Zebrafish

10.1 Introduction

A new director, brought into manage the animal colonies of a facility, can face two different scenarios. The more favourable one is when a new facility is being planned and it is possible to start from scratch. However, this is generally not the usual situation. In most cases, the facility has been running for a number of years and there are existing approaches and standard procedures that require reviewing and updating. This chapter will focus on current best practices to set up, plan and manage colonies of rodents and zebrafish, the most frequent species housed in animal facilities around the world. The chapter is based on the premise that taking good care of animals, balancing good management, scientific reliability and animal welfare will save money in the end. We will provide recommendations for managing wild type and genetically altered animals, focusing on methods to establish and maintain animal models that implement 3Rs without compromising experimental results. Different technologies will be explored that can help in identifying and

J. Guillén, V. Galligioni (eds.), *Practical Management of Research Animal Care and Use Programs*, Laboratory Animal Science and Medicine 3, https://doi.org/10.1007/978-3-031-65414-5_10

troubleshooting specific problems such as genetic contamination and drift, cage and population management and health status whilst maintaining business continuity.

10.2 The Basics

10.2.1 How Do I Start?

With a new appointment to manage an animal facility, the first step is to become acquainted with the capabilities and resources available to define what services can be reliably delivered. Setting the baseline; finding the balance between resources and expectations when making major procedural changes is essential. These have to be agreed upon with the institute and the staff to ensure a shared understanding by both parties. To change protocols that have been running for years requires a deft hand, strong support from the administrative authority and a demonstration that the change will return a benefit for the users and the animals housed. It is always a mistake to offer impossible goals or unrealistic milestones. When implementing changes that apply to animal welfare, care must be taken to avoid having staff effort or funding becoming limiting factors.

The species to be housed should be evaluated and agreed upon early in the process, as housing and environmental standards will be driven by this decision. When deciding on the colonies to be housed, a review of legacy breeding should be undertaken to determine if they can be replaced by external or commercially available species. These two evaluations will allow accurate planning of size and occupancy of the new facility. Tailoring the facility to the animals and procedural needs will save resources and effort that can then be redirected to other tasks.

A second important consideration with serious implications for a facility is the health status to be maintained. Trying to maintain a specific pathogen-free (SPF) health status whilst lacking the technical resources, appropriate equipment, or manpower will result in failure in the long run, regardless of good intention and effort.

Thirdly, another crucial point is space availability. Sometimes, for historical reasons some infrastructures are placed inside the animal facility when they could easily be located outside. If this is the case, the best strategy is to move them out. This would reduce the number of people entering the animal facility reducing health risk implications and saving precious square metres for other activities that really need to be inside. One good example is the cryopreservation unit. Embryo or sperm recovery can be performed in any standard laboratory, the same for any other procedure that takes place with animals that will not return back to the animal facility. A limitation to this strategy is when access to very specialised equipment is shared amongst users that require different health status levels. In such cases, preference has to be given to the stricter needs, but a pragmatic evaluation needs to be done case by case, before using precious animal holding space to house equipment that could be located elsewhere or procedures that could be performed outside the facility.

10.2.2 When Is the Best Time to Schedule Major Changes?

The best time for major procedural changes is when an external factor forces adaptation, whether it be legal regulation, infection, change of personnel or facility renovation. These major changes, whilst challenging, afford an opportunity to make things work better.

How Do I Approach Monetary Expectations Amongst Stakeholders? (See also Chapter 2 on Financial Matters)

Important aspects to address and clarify are the underlying monetary expectations, whilst providing transparency over the full economic costing (FEC). These factors will allow the development of any charges and ultimately assist the investigator in applying for grants. Private facilities have very defined financial expectations, cost-benefit studies have been carefully performed and the cost of animal maintenance is well established. As users are charged the actual cost, this is possibly the best system to maintain the number of animals at the essential minimum. Public-based institutions may have different approaches to funding. In Europe, animals maintained for research grants are subsidised by the host institution, outsourcing only part of the real expenses to the cage fees applied [1]. In some extreme situations, even a complete cage fee waiver is given, which may result in the maintenance of unnecessary cages and animals unless other limiting factors are applied.

10.2.2.1 What Should Be the Basic Requirements for Setting Cage Fees?

The best practice is to establish a transparent method for calculating cage fees that include all the costs needed to run the basic functions of the facility. These would include not only staff, utilities, food, and bedding, but also enrichment, security equipment, expenses for cleaning, autoclaving and disinfection and costs of health monitoring. In general, all expenses required for facility operations should be included. Often forgotten or ignored are the costs of preventive maintenance and repairs and equipment replacement costs [2], which should also be factored into cage fees. Extra fees may be restricted to procedures or equipment that are for the exclusive use of individual groups or protocols, e.g. irradiators, metabolic cages, rederivations and shipments.

10.2.2.2 Are Fees Managed Better via Centralisation or User-Based Management?

Another monetary consideration is the type of colony management system used. A centralised system reduces the number of personnel in the facility by having all animal care and procedures performed by dedicated staff. Centralisation is the most cost-effective approach as it reduces competition for room use and equipment, allows better use of resources, reduces the number of external personnel in the facility and optimises costs for both equipment and staff. However, each facility may have its own drivers and requirements. Whilst centralisation may be more efficient, one will find a myriad of approaches to managing animal facilities; from those where each investigator has his/her own animal room where animal facility staff only perform cage changes, animal shipments and health checks, to those where all procedures are performed by the animal facility staff with only a virtual interface between staff and users. Once the management system and financial expectations are set, one can begin to address specific colony management needs.

10.2.3 What Is the Best Way to Set Performance Expectations Amongst the Stakeholders?

A critical step in colony management is to establish good communication with the users. This can be easier in pharmaceutical companies, CROs or facilities managed as business-like institutions. By their very nature, these types of businesses have very clear goals, where decisions are made by the administrative manager or scientific director. Public research institutions generally have a less defined decision-making structure. In these, the administrative manager usually does not want to, does not have the background, or does not have the authority to be involved in setting scientific priorities.

10.2.3.1 What Is the Best Way to Establish Reliable Communication with Skateholders?

To solve everyday problems, the interaction is between the animal facility manager and/or care staff and multiple investigators, each with his/her own scientific requirements, needs and preferences. In the best-case scenario, there are active, involved principal investigators (PIs) who closely manage the colonies used in their research. In the worst-case scenario, there is no real direct interaction with the PIs; communication is only with trainees and technicians. The first step in such multiuser facilities is to establish who the decision maker is for each laboratory and to use that contact to establish a strong and proactive communication link with each laboratory and PI. This link should include a questionnaire to get a very clear idea of their needs, expectations and resources. The questionnaire should be completed by the assigned point person whether that is the PI or is assigned to an authorised person (one the PI has delegated to represent the needs of the laboratory). A written questionnaire is optimal. However, if setting expectations is a result of a face-to-face conversation, a written summary should be made and shared after the meeting with both entities approving the agreement. Such documentation can be seen as the basis of a Service Level Agreement (SLA).

The participation and agreement to the plan by all of the stakeholders is essential. This strategy can only be successful if it is fully supported and enforced by the administrative manager, if the action plan is designed with the support and collaboration of the animal facility personnel, and if it is produced, agreed upon and shared with all users. Input from the scientists, the technicians and the colony managers is critical, but decisions cannot rely solely on them.

10.2.4 What Strategies Can I Use to Minimise Surplus Animals?

Most research animal facilities will have many different genetically altered (GA) lines of animals. The breeding and maintenance of GA colonies often produce more animals than needed for the overall needs of the intended research. This is generally due to the by-product of breeding between the experimental animal and its wild-type control (i.e. heterozygous offspring). Careful consideration should be given to all the phases of colony progression and timely decision-making to facilitate good management at all stages. Initially, backcrossing and subsequent intercrossing to obtain lines of experimental animals should aim to use the minimal number of offspring (e.g. 2–3 pairs) to allow for littering failure, number of pups born and any pre-weaning mortality. Key milestones should be established for close monitoring of the progress. These include likely dates of birth and tissue sampling for genotyping prior to weaning (with timely analysis of genotypes to allow consolidation of caging). Mating should occur as the required animals reach sexual maturity. During the initial phases of colony development, one should perform the first round of intercrossing and phenotype analysis to identify any potential factors that may affect the final experimental cohort production.

Before expanding the line for experimental use, the experimental design should account for any deleterious phenotypes that may impact the experimental hypothesis or that may alter the projections for colony size or statistical relevance of an experiment. The harder it is to show statistical significance the larger the likely breeding schema will need to be.

Investigators often require homozygous lines for their research, and should be made aware of some pitfalls that are associated with these. Care should be taken when generating homozygous colonies, considering the control animals required and avoiding any potential drift in the background. Due to genetic drift with inbred colonies, regular resetting of the strain background is required. In rodents, this should be done before reaching the tenth generation [3] using animals that themselves come from a correctly maintained background. Whilst this is often a consideration with rodent colonies, it is also important to keep in mind that zebrafish are very sensitive to inbreeding depression; even in the case of a viable homozygous mutation, alternating homozygous and heterozygous generations is the recommended approach.

When breeding complex crosses of mutations, the normal 1 in 4 ratio for a single mutant will become even rarer. For example, if there are two mutations, crosses will only yield double homozygotes from 1 in 16 pups on average. To allow some savings of animal numbers, consideration should be given to fixing one part of the intercross (i.e. generate a line with one mutation homozygous and the second mutation heterozygous that can then be used for a second backcross to generate homozygotes for both mutations).

This will then return the line to a 1 in 4. However, noting the above concerns of managing homozygous colonies, closer monitoring and resetting of backgrounds will need to be factored in. When publishing your data, be clear about the decisions made so that researchers utilising a line will have a good awareness of how the colony was developed.

Finally, where possible, consider sharing commonly used mouse models amongst researchers at your institution. Animal numbers for many models (e.g. Cre expressing lines, ROSA26-LoxP models and background colonies) can be more efficiently managed if they are shared amongst groups. This ensures that breeding strategies can be matched to demand and allows surplus animals to be used effectively. Allowing such access will also reduce the overall number of animals used and will help prevent groups from duplicating animal lines already available at the institution.

10.2.5 What Solutions Are Available for Obtaining and Maintaining Animal and Colony Records?

When managing genetically modified colonies avoid paper records whenever possible. There are a number of suppliers of computerised colony management systems. Depending on the origin of their development, they can range from simple spreadsheets to complex integrated software that manages not only the genetic modification but also other relevant aspects such as European Union (EU) statistical and severity reporting.

10.2.5.1 What Information Should I Record?

The breadth of information gathered should be appropriate to the user's needs. However, systems are growing ever more complex, and integration through solutions such as application programming interfaces (API) are allowing seamless information sharing. Such integration increases the power of the data and challenges how we interpret and use such information. Below is a list of information that should be maintained for each animal:

- A unique identifier—usually an alphanumeric combination that can be traced back to a particular genetic modification.
- Pairing identification—sire and dam's genotypes and dates of birth. For each litter, the date of birth, the number of animals born, and a date of weaning and/or death provide information about the breeding performance of a colony.
- Individual animals—a unique permanent identity such as an earmark, species, sex or observable characteristics, e.g. coat colour. Cage and room location allow ease of locating an animal.
- Legally required information—experimental experience (e.g. a list of procedures performed on the animal throughout its life), the fate of the animal and an assessment of the actual severity experience (e.g. the animal's peak or cumulative suffering).
- Phenotype and welfare—to assist in understanding the experience of the animal, any record should provide a link to the phenotype(s) exhibited by the animal with a clear description of the effect. Additionally, any welfare conditions should be stated in a defined vocabulary and assigned to either the modification, background or environmental factor (e.g. health status).
- Genetic modification and genotype—clear reference to the origin of the modification and genotyping strategy will codify analysis of the colony and provide information for subsequent publications and distribution.
- Background information—numbers of backcrosses, pedigree charts.

10.2.5.2 What Is the Information that Needs to Be Reported to the European Union?

Since the entry into force of Directive 2010/63/EU, specific data regarding creation and maintenance of genetically altered lines have to be provided. Data gathered through databases should allow the researcher to supply a clear overview of the number of animals produced, species and if they have been used in an experimental procedure or not. Surplus animals also need to be reported via a separate mechanism. Genetically modified lines are subdivided into either newly created or established animals carrying either a harmful phenotype or non-harmful phenotype. Other information required for the statistics are the place of birth, research area, category of procedure, genetic status, genotyping procedure and the actual severity experienced (classified as being mild, moderate, severe or non-recovery). Collection of these data is time consuming and processing requires precision. To assure accuracy, it should be integrated into the colony management system whenever possible.

After basic questions about overall facility management and general colony considerations have been met, one can then identify and address the needs of the individual investigator. Regardless of animal type, some very basic questions apply, including maintaining strains and stocks commonly used, generating and identifying genetically altered (GA) animals or managing established GA colonies. Each animal type will require colonies for maintenance, subsequent breeding, genotyping, tracking and health management. In the next sections, we will attempt to address these to suggest best practices.

10.3 Colony Management

10.3.1 Breeding In-House or Outsourcing?

There are multiple reasons to avoid in-house breeding of commercially available animals, as one is duplicating efforts already made by animal vendors. However, there are also situations that require it, and the decision can only be made after knowing the needs of the users. Amongst the reasons to *avoid* in-house breeding are the required resources needed to do it properly. If breeding in-house, there must be a consistent plan to avoid inbreeding of outbred lines or genetic drift of the inbred lines, both of which will require frequent renewal of the breeding colony using vendor-sourced animals. One needs to consider not only the cost involved, but also the space limitation and the added problem of generating surplus animals. If an accurate cost-benefit study is performed that accounts for all factors (not only those that usually are included in the user's fee), the cost of in-house breeding can be equivalent or even higher than buying the animals from commercial vendors [4]. However, one caveat is that any entry of external animals introduces the potential for health contamination. As well, certain lines are not commercially available, or the investigator may require the use of wild-type animals with the exact microbiota and environmental conditions. A further consideration for breeding in-house is the age at which the animals would be needed. For any experiment starting during pregnancy, lactation or weaning, in-house breeding is unavoidable.

10.3.1.1 How Do I Breed Outbred Stocks as Wild-Type Animals?

Investigators generally request outbred stocks due to their better reproductive performance and their perceived increased genetic variability that supposedly more closely mimics the human condition. Whether or not this is truly the case is debatable [5], maintenance of an outbred stock requires strict attention to the pairs being mated, such that inadvertent inbreeding is avoided.

In general, the costs of maintaining the number of animals required to sustain a robust genetic diversity of outbred stocks are prohibitive. Thus, for these animals, it is truly more cost-effective to purchase them from a vendor. The major drawback of this strategy, however, is that vendor stocks may contain prohibited pathogens, in which case, breeding may be required.

Mice: Most of the major mice vendors will sell outbred stocks that are pathogen free. If the outbred stock required cannot safely be imported, or pre-weaning ages are required, then in-house breeding should be established keeping in mind the need to ensure genetic variability [6], as explained in the next section.

Fish: Wild-type strains (both AB and TU) are available from the Zebrafish International Resource Center (ZIRC) https://zebrafish.org/home/guide.php), or from other zebrafish laboratories. These strains may also be used for in-house breeding using much the same strategy as that used for mice–multiple breeding tanks where progeny are not mated to closely related fish. Again, it is critical to maintain accurate breeding records that are easily shared with users.

10.3.1.2 How Do I Maximise Genetic Variability of Outbred Stocks?

When in-house breeding is required, it is critical to pay careful attention to detail. It will require a careful manager who can keep detailed electronic records and make them available to any investigators using the stock.

Mice: In order to ensure outbred genetic variability, at least 25 mating pairs are required to achieve maximum diversity. Each time a new mating cage is set up, members of the pair must not be related. For example, if cage 1 mates male A with female A, the next mating cage could be set up using pup AA1 and be mated to an animal weaned from an unrelated pair (say pup MM-1). In the subsequent generation pup AM-1 could be mated to pup BN-1, etc. Obviously, very careful pedigree records are required to ensure maximum genetic variability over time.

It may be possible to set up a smaller colony. However, in such a scenario it would be critical to perform frequent matings using animals imported from a vendor to maintain diversity and avoid accidental inbreeding. Such animals may need to undergo a period of quarantine prior to introducing them into the colony.

Fish: In general, outbred stocks of fish are not maintained in the lab. Collection of native strains from the wild has been proposed to represent true diversity and genetic variability. Practically, most labs will purchase outbred fish to introduce new wild-type laboratory strains to increase genetic variability. AB and TU are the most commonly used outbred fish stocks in North America and Europe, respectively.

10.3.2 How Do I Maintain Inbred, Non-GA Animals Used as Wild-Type Mice/Controls?

If the animal facility houses GA animals, then it is likely that investigators will rely on inbred animals of the same strain as controls. These could be sibling animals that have the same generation status as well as the same microbiotic flora, or they could be unrelated inbred animals of the same strain that could arise in house or be ordered from a vendor. Below are critical concerns for generating the wild-type controls if the wild-type is an inbred strain (mixed or hybrid strains require a different strategy).

Mice: A "wild-type" colony is often the non-GA inbred background strain of mice. In most instances, it is preferable to have a *breeding contract/plan* where the outcomes are stated in advance. Critical points include:

- Is this a maintenance colony or breeding to produce experimental controls?
- How many animals are needed?
- What is the background strain of these animals (using precise nomenclature to avoid problems; e.g. C57BL/6N is not C57BL/6J, and "black" or "C57" could mean C57BL/10)?
- If the animals are for experimental control, how old do the animals need to be? Can the age vary by a week or two?
- What sex do the animals need to be?
- When are the animals needed?

10.3.2.1 What Is the Best Approach to Maintain a Colony of Inbred Mice?

When breeding a maintenance colony of inbred strains, the mouse numbers can be kept quite low (depending on their fertility and fecundity). With average fertility/fecundity, a strain can be successfully maintained using 3–5 breeding cages. The number of pair matings that meet the required demand can then be set up, understanding that the animals typically have a prime mating age range of 3–8 months. Mating cages should be set up on a rotation basis (e.g. Month 1: Pair 1,

Month 3: Pair 2, Month 6: Pair 3. In Month 6, also remove pair 1 and start pair 4 using a male obtained from an outside vendor to reduce genetic drift, or use a male from the same genetic line but an unrelated pair). Thus, new mating pairs are set up every 3 months to ensure continuous production. Each pair mating will only be on the shelf for 6 months, taking advantage of optimal breeding ages. If pairs are unusually productive, the matings can be spaced out farther, or the males removed from the pair until pups are weaned thereby bypassing the post-partum mating.

As discussed in Sect. 10.2.6, careful records should be maintained to track pedigree/parentage.

10.3.2.2 How Do I Plan a Short-Term Breeding Scheme to Produce Wild-Type Control Mice on Demand?

Investigators will often set up experiments requiring a large cohort of wild-type siblings of their inbred strain to serve as experimental controls. By advance planning, the animal facility can accommodate those needs. Again, one should use a defined plan of action as follows:

- How many animals are needed over what period of time? For example, an investigator may want to have 10 age-matched, inbred, non-GA mice of the same sex (females) for an experiment taking place 8 months from now when the experimental GA females will be 6 months old. The keys here are:
  - Inbred strain—You should know the average pup number per female for this particular inbred strain.
  - 10 Females—You will need at least 20 pups born at that time (and likely more, to ensure having 10 females).
  - 6 months of age—You will need animals birthed in 2 months.

If, for example, the average pup number is 6, and the sex ratio (M:F) is 60% male, for any female mated, 3–4 of the animals will be male, and only 2–3 will be female. Thus, to get 10 females, a minimum of five females should be mated. Six mated females would be optimum.

- The next consideration is the type of mating scheme to use; *pair mating* (1 male × 1 female), *trio mating* (1 male × 2 females) or *harem mating* (1 male × up to 5 females—after regulatory approval). One can use fewer males by rotating the males. Two males of prime mating age (3–8 months of age) can be paired with 2 females (Trio mating). The females are checked daily for copulation plugs. Plugged females are removed for gestation and replaced with naive females.
- If using a non-littermate wildtype control it is essential to state this in any subsequent publication along with the measures used to ensure the animals remain suitable controls (e.g. the GA colony has been genetically monitored to ensure it is true to the wildtype background other than the intended mutation).

Fish: Many standard operating procedures (SOPs) consider optimal breeding age between 6 months to 1 year. These are set up in pairwise matings for experiments requiring timed breeding. Generation of wild-type siblings can generally be done in a single tank due to the large numbers of fry produced in a single mating. For large-scale egg production to generate wild-type fish, a continuous breeding approach is commonly used.

10.3.3 How Do I Generate Wild-Type Controls for Mixed Background GA Lines?

Mice: There are often occasions where GA mice are produced in a mixed strain of mice—often 129xC57BL/6 or B6D2F1s. Generating genetically matched controls in this instance is problematic, since the chromosomes undergo crossing-over and reassortment in every mouse with each generation. Thus, even if strain typing has been done, each animal will have different ratios of chromosome contribution from one strain to the other. An exact genetic control is impossible even with siblings from the same litter. One possible solution is to keep a colony where the strain is outcrossed to one or the other inbred strains with each generation. Doing so will at least allow for a 50:50 strain type in the progeny. However, the investigator should be aware that the "control" is not an exact genetic match, and never can be as long as the strain is mixed.

Fish: As controls, it is common practice to use siblings that are not carrying the mutation/transgene (based on genotyping) as controls. Again, one needs to be cognizant that not all of the siblings will have the exact same strain background.

10.4 Colony Management: Genetically Altered Animals

Regarding Genetically altered animals there are two major scenarios. The most usual one is when any user wants to obtain an already created genetically altered line from another laboratory or an international repository. However sometimes it is necessary to create a new one, this can be done in-house, but most of the time, a core facility, public or private is used. In the second case, it is always critical to determine if the needed animal already exists, or if it can be created by mating existing animals, as this reduces animal use overall.

10.4.1 How Do I Manage Already Existing GA Strains?

10.4.1.1 What Information Do I Need to Obtain Them?

If the necessary animal line already exists, the investigator will need assistance in obtaining the line and often with maintaining the line as well. The following information is essential to understand the origins of or the subsequent dissemination of GA animal colonies:

- Correct designation of a line—if registered, a line should contain the correct nomenclature which provides an unambiguous description of the model, including Institute Laboratory Animal Research code designation [7]. At a minimum, the gene and nature of the mutation should be provided. The origin of the model, background strain and the numbers of backcrosses should be included in the nomenclature designation.
- General Information—This can include Information such as expected coat colour, housing conditions, diet, offspring numbers, the housing system and environmental conditions and any publications that may exist.
- Specific information whether the line has been established according to the guidelines of the EU [8]. This requires that transmission of the mutation can be predicted (Mendelian, sex-linked) and that a preliminary welfare study has been performed. Unless the line is established and no harmful phenotype has been reported, in EU countries, a project authorisation will be needed to house the line.
- Phenotypic abnormalities and observable traits—these allow the recipient to understand what is expected from the model and what they may need to provide if the trait exhibits any condition that has welfare implications.
- Breeding—specifics about the background and breeding strategies should be stated.
- Availability of the line—this should include whether live or cryopreserved stocks are available.
- Genotyping—A clear and reproducible genotyping protocol to be used to identify modified animals.
- Contact details—an up-to-date contact (e.g. email or archive details) ensures support can be provided to those not familiar with the model's history.

10.4.1.2 Where Can I Find and Get Established GA Lines of Mice, Rats or Fish?

There are international repositories that scan publications for new GA animal lines of rodents and fish (and other animals as well—e.g. *Drosophila*) and annotate them for public use. One can search the relevant database, obtain information about the particular line required, and acquire ordering details. Below are the commonly used resources for mice, rats and zebrafish, these and others are listed in table 10.1.

Table 10.1 International useful resources for the location, characterisation and management of genetically altered mouse, rat and zebrafish models

Species	Organisation	Link
Mouse	CMMR Canadian Mouse Mutant Repository	http://www.cmmr.ca/
Mouse	CARD Center for animal resources and development	http://card.medic.kumamoto-u.ac.jp/card/english/
Mouse	EMMA European Mouse Mutant Archive	https://www.infrafrontier.eu/resources-and-services/deposit-mice-emma-repository
Mouse	IMSR International Mouse Strain Resource	http://www.findmice.org/index.jsp
Mouse	IMPC International Mouse Phenotypic Consortium	https://www.mousephenotype.org/
Mouse	MGI Mouse Genome Informatics	http://www.informatics.jax.org
Mouse	MMRRC	https://www.mmrrc.org/catalog/StrainCatalogSearchForm.php?SourceCollection=KOMP
Mouse	RIKEN	https://mus.brc.riken.jp/en/search_for_mouse_strain
Mouse	TIGM	https://www.tigm.org/
Rat	RRRC Rat Resource and Research Center	https://www.rrrc.us/
Zebrafish	ZFIN Zebrafish Information Network	https://zfin.org/
Zebrafish	ZIRC Zebrafish International Resource Center	https://zebrafish.org/home/guide.php

MICE: The easiest way to search for a mouse line is to use the website www.findmice.org (a website run by the international mouse strain resource). Alternatively, mouse strains that are published are annotated in the mouse informatics website hosted by the Jackson Laboratory—www.informatics.jax.org . The latter site includes a vast amount of additional information that can give valuable information about homologies, DNA sources, phenotypes etc.

RATS: The Medical College of Wisconsin hosts a database listing various rat models—https://rgd.mcw.edu/rgdweb/models/allModels.html, as does the Rat Resource and Research Center: https://www.rrrc.us/. This site also has additional information that will be useful for rat studies.

FISH: The Zebrafish International Resource Center (ZIRC—https://zebrafish.org/home/guide.php) is a centralised repository that houses live and frozen stocks, and distributes transgenic/mutant lines of interest to the community. The lines distributed are linked to specific genes and associated information in the ZFIN database.

10.4.1.3 What Is the Best Genotyping Strategy?

Genotyping of genetically modified lines should be carried out as early as possible so that timely decisions on the development of a model can be made. Regardless of the type of mutation that has been created, the investigator must develop a genotyping strategy that will unambiguously validate the presence and structure of the mutation. One could genotype using contributing components of the targeting strategy such as the neomycin cassette (used in many ES cell-based targeting projects). Whilst this is, in theory, a useful way to screen animals, it should be noted that one could miss structural anomalies generated during the creation of the model that may confound results (e.g. partial recombination of the targeting vector). Thus, genotyping strategies must verify the successful integration of all required sequences into the animal's genome. This would normally require a series of assays spanning the integration sites both 5′ and 3′ of the desired mutation for targeted mutations, and assays that span a unique junction site for standard transgenic mutations.

Once the line has been fully characterised during development, routine genotyping can be based on a standard PCR that amplifies a specific sequence of the mutation. However, a robust PCR strategy should be set. Timely genotyping is better for colony management. In the specific case of fish, it is important to keep in mind that larvae genotyped and discharged before day 5 post-hatching would not be counted as animals used in experiments according to Directive 2010/63/EU.

10.4.1.3.1 What Requirements Are Needed for a Robust PCR?

Correct genotyping is crucial for a correct GA mouse management; it should combine 2 characteristics, (1) it has to be specific for each line housed in the facility and (2) it can be performed quickly. If assays are used that only identify a single, commonly used gene even if unique to that organism (e.g. those that target Green Fluorescent Protein (GFP) or Cre-recombinase), cross-contamination between different lines that have the same gene would be impossible to detect.

PCR genotyping should always rely on the appearance of a band corresponding to the amplification of the target DNA sequence, never on the absence of a band. In a targeted mutation line, whenever possible, the same reaction should amplify the wt and the mutated allele. In all cases, reliable controls should include a known positive, a known negative and a reaction sample without DNA to ensure lack of DNA contaminations of reagents.

In terms of colony management, it is advised that a suitable method of identification and genotyping is applied at a time point before weaning. Rapid turn round of results before weaning allows key decisions regarding which mice are required for the continuation of the colony or experimental use. Animals can be consolidated, which assists when housing males to prevent future aggression and fighting. Animals that are no longer required can be removed. Outsourcing genotyping can contribute to centralisation of colony management. The use of a genotyping service within the institution or an external entity would reduce unnecessary maintenance of animals due to delayed results from the research group. From a financial perspective, this will allow better management of cage costs.

10.4.1.3.2 What Is the Best Method of Sample Collection for Rodent Genotyping?

When taking tissue samples for genotyping, the welfare of the animal should be paramount. The method that is least invasive and only causes transitory pain should be used [9]. If the sampling can be combined with permanent identification of the animal, then such methods should take precedence (e.g. ear clipping). The age of the animal is important in the context of how it interprets pain. Younger animals will have a less developed pain response and, as such, the transitory nature of the sampling is more strongly considered. In older animals with a more developed response, the sampling of the tail (especially where the cartilage has developed) should be avoided. Alternative methods such as buccal swab, faecal pellet and hair bulb can provide a genotype. However, each of these is prone to the real possibility of cross-contamination. As well, there is still the need to permanently identify the animal. In some situations, when mice have to be genotyped at a very young age (prior to 15 days of age), ear clipping is not feasible. In such situations, removal of the distal phalanx provides a suitable method for animals under the age of 10 days. Care should be taken to distinguish between this approach and toe clipping which removes a digit regardless of age and is not considered a suitable method [10].

10.4.1.3.3 How Do I Collect Tissue for Zebrafish Genotyping?

Along with rodents, the use of fish as a model organism adds to the bulk of GA animals used in research across Europe. As with mice, it is advisable to genotype fish at the earliest opportunity to allow good management of fish stocks. Unneeded animals can be culled to ensure the lowest possible stocking of tanks resulting in good financial management.

Whilst genotyping of mice can incorporate the identity of the mouse in the sampling method, there is currently no viable solution to identifying individual fish beyond visible distinguishable marks. Using zebrafish as the example, the most widely used identification method is the removal of a sample from the caudal fin, which requires immersion in a suitable anaesthetic (e.g. ethyl 3-aminobenzoate methanesulfonate [MS-222] buffered to pH 7.2 with sodium bicarbonate). This method will yield sufficient high-quality DNA for genotype confirmation by PCR. Collection of a sample can be performed on fry pre-5dpf, during this period, this manipulation is not considered a procedure requiring authorisation. However, it is recommended that the smallest possible caudal fin sample should be taken (under 3 mm) to limit any impact on the animal.

An alternative to fin clipping is swabbing of fish [11]. This procedure requires animals that are large enough to be handled and restrained and would preclude the use of pre-authority fish. Generally, this would be animals that exceed 20 mm in length.

To obtain a swab sample, individual fish are netted and placed on a wetted sponge and secured with thumb and forefinger (for zebrafish). Skin mucus samples are collected by gently stroking with the tip of a sterile rayon-tipped swab five times along the flank of each fish, from the operculum to the caudal fin. It is important to follow the direction of the scales to avoid abrasion when swabbing.

A third method that supports the 3R is the use of microfluidic harmonic oscillation. The technique requires the purchase of equipment (Zebrafish Embryo Genotyper—ZEGTM) that provides a roughened glass surface that gently abrades the surface of embryos to obtain small amounts of tissue for genotyping by PCR. Embryos are loaded and unloaded from the equipment manually with a pipette; the system allows 24 embryos at a time to be loaded and sampled. Sensitivity of genotyping and survival of animals have been reported at greater than 90% with no apparent effects on body morphology, development, or motor behaviour tests [12].

10.4.1.4 How Do I Avoid Genetic Drift?

Genetic drift is the genetic variation within an inbred line over time caused by random fluctuations in the frequency of gene variants (alleles) within a population due to chance events. As a consequence, the genetic makeup of a population over time can change, particularly in small populations. Inhouse breeding of genetically altered lines is a perfect scenario for this situation. Brother-sister mating tends to maximise the chances of substantial genetic variations as random mutations become fixed. It is generally accepted that after inbreeding a line for more than 20 generations, a substrain is obtained. It is important to note that 10 generations are easily reached after 3–4 years. Thus, substrains are commonly achieved when breeding the same line in two different institutions in spite of having obtained it from a common source.

Genetic background can be a modulator of gene expression in many mutations [13] and a source of variation in certain studies [14]. In order to ensure the repeatability of experimental data, attention to genetic drift is essential for managing GA lines. Genetic drift is a natural process, and whilst complete prevention is impossible (especially in small populations), some tools can help to avoid or slow the process. In those lines where the mutation is either heterozygous or hemizygous, periodic breeding with wild-type (wt) animals from a commercial resource would consistently diminish genetic drift. This is a general husbandry protocol in zebrafish, but it is not that common in mice, where double and triple homozygous mutants are kept and sibling mating is often the rule. Care should be taken to monitor the breeding performance of a colony to monitor for signs of genetic drift. One common indication is inbreeding depression [15], which occurs when deleterious spontaneous mutations become homozygous during closed colony breeding. As a general recommendation, a backcross to the original genetic background should be performed before reaching the tenth generation. Unfortunately, at least a year may be required to recover the original genetic profile. A better option is to recover complex lines using embryos from a time period prior to when genetic drift was observed through the use of cryopreservation and periodic cryo-recovery. Embryos from early generations should be periodically cryopreserved and then recovered when reaching a designated generation; the breeding scheme would start again from the same genetic status present 3 or 4 years earlier. This strategy is followed by The Jackson Laboratory and is known as the Genetic Stability Program (GSP) to avoid genetic drift in their inbred strains (https://resources.jax.org/white-papers/whitepaper-gsp-2).

10.4.1.5 How Do I Stabilise the Genetic Background of My Mutant Mouse Line or Do I Need to Change It to a Different One?

When breeding GA models, a key requirement is to obtain and/or maintain the genetic background of the animal on the desired background of choice. After obtaining or creating the initial model there may be a need to move it to an inbred background (if in a mixed strain) or transfer the mutation to an entirely new strain via congenic backcrossing (e.g. moving the mutation from 129S6 to C57BL/6J). This is what it is called to make a strain congenic. The background strain can have significant effects on the gene of interest resulting in undesirable variations of the phenotype [16]. It is, therefore, important to backcross sufficiently to avoid any remaining contribution of the original background that might confound experimental data. Ten generations of backcrossing to the desired strain will leave approximately 0.09% of the original background. It is suggested that at least five generations of backcrossing be completed for all lines. This method of changing the background strain can take up to 2 years of careful backcrosses.

An alternative to standard backcrossing to make a congenic strain is the use of speed congenics [17]. This procedure uses single nucleotide polymorphisms (SNPs) to identify specific base positions to distinguish between the current and the desired background. The comparison between the backgrounds looks for base pairs spaced evenly across the chromosomes that can only be representative of the background of interest. Through each round of breeding a minimum of five (generally male) animals have their SNP profiles evaluated to allow the selection of those with the highest percentage of the desired background to be used in the next round of breeding. With this method, the time required to create a congenic model can be potentially halved from 10 to 5 generations. One point to note is that during any backcrossing, the X and Y chromosomes will need to be fixed. The best approach is to include chromosome Y as soon as possible, by mating a positive female to a wt male in the first or second backcrossing.

10.4.2 How Do I Manage a Newly Created GA Models?

10.4.2.1 What Are the Differences Between GA Models Generated in Different Ways?

Few current animal facilities have a unit to generate new GA animal models. Those that do exist were set up in the early days of animal transgenesis (1980s–1990s), but very seldom is this service implemented *de novo*. The infrastructure and know-how needed are only justified by the extremely high demand for new models found in a single research centre. The most sensible approach is to request an experienced core facility (public or private) to provide service to generate the specific model. This approach also represents a consistent reduction in the number of animals needed, due to their higher efficiency.

New GA animal lines could be of several types [18]. Transgenic animals are those where DNA is injected into a fertilised egg after which it is incorporated randomly into the genome. Gene-targeted animals are generated using embryonic stem cells (for mice) that are manipulated to obtain the genotype needed and then injected into mouse embryos to create chimaeras. Targeted animals can also be generated using new gene editing systems (ZFNs, TALENS, CRISPR/Cas9, or Prime Editing). This technology has a global scope, being successfully used in plants and animals, invertebrates and vertebrates. Models generated by gene editing could have both the desired mutation as well as unwanted insertions, deletions, and off-target mutations. It is essential to take this possibility into account when establishing a line.

GA animal models generated externally need to be imported for use. Management of the imported models depends on the type of model requested, as different GA models need to be managed in different ways. Thus, it is extremely important to have very clear information regarding the kind of model (e.g. transgenic, knock-out, knock-in and conditional), the genotype of animals received and the final model that will be needed for the experiments. In some cases, the final model needed may differ considerably from the original, which will require a careful breeding scheme.

10.4.2.2 How Do I Manage a Transgenic Founder?

Traditional transgenic models, those that carry a transgene in their genome, are designed to express a gene of interest under the control of a specific promoter. However, the method used for their generation can cause random insertion of one or more copies of the gene into the genome and result in different expression levels in lines derived from the F0 founder animals. As well, unexpected phenotypes can occur due to the insertion location. If the transgene integration disrupts an endogenous gene, the resulting animal may show the expected phenotype derived from the transgene mixed with the phenotype caused by the disruption. This is frequently seen if the transgene is bred to homozygosity (e.g. B6.Cg-*Edil3*$^{Tg(Sox2\text{-}cre)1Amc}$/J). For these reasons, core facilities generating transgenic models usually ship 2–3 potential founders to the research group. These founders would each be bred to wild-type animals to establish different lines, which have to be maintained and characterised separately.

The first step in generating a transgenic line is mating F0 animals individually with a wt animal/animals to establish transmission of the transgene. Not all positive animals may transmit to their progeny because the founders could be mosaic [19] (that is, they do not carry the same genetic information in all of their cells). It is also important to determine if transmission is sex-linked as well as the percentage of positive pups. As mating to wt animals should result in only a 50% expected transmission of the transgene, values of genotype-positive progeny that are statistically higher than 50% suggest that the transgene has been inserted in more than one place, and each insertion should be segregated before starting any further characterization.

Because the transgene is inserted randomly, the expected phenotype has to be determined for each line separately. If the phenotype seen is due to the transgene, one should expect that independent lines should exhibit the same phenotype. Once this is established, the line expressing the transgene at the appropriate level will be selected for experimentation. It should be recommended to freeze sperm of the non-selected lines because they may be useful in the future.

Insertion location in transgenic lines is unknown in many cases, and the genotyping procedure is usually based on unique internal sequences of the transgene. For this reason, it is impossible to use standard PCR technology to distinguish between different lines with the same transgene or to determine if the transgene is hemizygous (not heterozygous, since there is no complementary wt allele for the transgene) or homozygous. If the investigator requires a homozygous genotype of the transgenic line, either a quantitative PCR or test matings of putative homozygous animals to wild-type animals should be carried out. (Note: if the animal is homozygous, all offspring of the test mating will carry the transgene; a representative number of pups would need to be tested, a minimum of 8–10.)

As described previously a distinctive PCR should be always available for each line in the animal facility, typically one where the amplified DNA crosses a unique junction within the transgene. Management of transgenic lines requires not only caring about incorporation of the transgene, but also how it is affected by the genetic/strain background of the founder. Transgenes should be injected into embryos of inbred strains, as the resulting phenotype will be more likely due to the transgene. However, hybrid backgrounds are also used due to better superovulation responses and zygotes that survive injection at better rates, thereby requiring fewer animals for the injection process.

It is important to know the background that will be used in the experiments, as effects of the transgene can be amplified or reduced due to inherent genetic properties of the inbred strain (e.g. there is a greater propensity for tumorigenesis and retinal degradation in FVB mouse strains). Whilst the hybrid vigour with mixed strains can alleviate concerns about background mutations, it does present problems with obtaining exact experimental controls (see Sect. 10.3.3). In case of mixed backgrounds, the best controls would be littermates, and this has to be included in the breeding scheme to obtain the experimental animals. The second option, which requires more time, is to generate a congenic line. This will be a very lengthy (2 year) process, but the development of speed congenics has reduced the time required [20, 21].

10.4.2.3 How Do I Manage Targeted Mutations [Knock-In (KI) and Knock-Out (KO)] Obtained from ESC Lines?

Classical targeting technology using embryonic stem cells has been used for many years, as it was the only method that could modify an endogenous gene in mammalian systems. Now, it has been relegated to a secondary role by CRISPR/Cas9-based gene editing although it remains a valid alternative for mice when the DNA to be inserted is large or complex. The use of this technology was accelerated by the establishment of an international consortium [22] with a goal to provide gene knock-out cell lines for every gene in the mouse genome. Mice or ES cells are available for many mouse genes as a result of this effort. If obtained as cells, they are aggregated or injected into mouse morulae or blastocysts, and chimaeras are generated that require crossing to wild-type animals to establish germline transmission. The chimaeras obtained will carry all the genetic information needed to generate different models. Many of the ES cells distributed through the IMPC can be used to generate several different types of mutations. Animals containing the *tm1a* allele, known as "KO-first", will lack gene function. If crossed with an flp recombinase (flp) carrier line, the resulting animal will recover gene function, but the gene of interest will be "floxed" (i.e. surrounded by loxP sites). This is the allele *tm1c* or "conditional". If the *tm1a* mouse is bred to a Cre expressing line, then allele *tm1b* is obtained, a model that tags the gene with a LacZ reporter [23]. Thus, it is important to know exactly which animal (*tm1a, tm1b or tm1c*) is sent from the core facility and also very important to know exactly which final genotype is necessary for the intended experiments.

Generally, only chimaeras with a large contribution of the coat colour obtained from the ES cells are used for further analysis, as they are likely to contribute to the germline. However, one should be aware that these chimaeras may not transmit the mutation regardless of the high coat colour contribution. If chimaeras are received, they should be bred to wt animals and no less than 25 animals from the progeny should be analysed before concluding that germline transmission will not occur. At least 2–3 chimaeras should be tested, preferentially coming from different ES clones. The IMPC reports a success rate of 33% of their ES cell clones that result in germline transmission.

Transformation of allele *tm1a* into *tm1b* or *tm1c* can also be requested as a service. To obtain the conditional *tm1c* requires crossing animals carrying allele *tm1a* with a mouse line expressing flp recombinase at very early embryonic stages. Such a line may not be available in the investigator's colony, but if carried elsewhere in the animal facility, asking for such assistance with the crosses would save animals and time. Generation of allele *tm1b* can be done in vitro using permeable cre-recombinase, which reduces animal use with crossing to Cre lines [24].

Because each allele (*tm1a, tm1b* and *tm1c)* is genetically unique, it should be strongly recommended to freeze the sperm of each allele. In addition, those receiving ES cells from the IMPC are requested to contribute their modified mouse lines to the IMPC repository for archiving and to be made available for other researchers, thereby promoting reduction of animal use (since the line will not need to be generated again once it has been archived in the consortium repository).

Colony management of models generated with ES cell lines also requires paying attention to the genetic background. ES cell lines from the IMPC are C57BL6/N, and cre or flp expressing lines used should be of the same substrain to preserve genetic uniformity.

A substantial number of KO and KI lines are also generated using ES cell lines of mixed genetic background. Cell quality is very important to guarantee germ line transmission and hybrid ES cells have been widely used for such purposes. In these cases, the chimaera generated should be bred to a wt animal of the chosen genetic background and a line with a stable genetic background established before experiments are performed. Again, speed congenics can save animals and time.

10.4.2.4 How Do I Manage Gene Edited Animals Produced Using ZFNs, CRISPR, Prime Editing or TALENS?

Gene editing has completely changed the scenario of genetically modified animals. Not only is the procedure highly efficient, but it is technically easier and it can be applied widely, from plants to animals. As well, the technology can be used to generate different models–KO, KI or conditional. Insertions can vary from point mutations to large DNA sequences, and it can be applied to other goals, for example erasing methylation marks (hence modulating imprinting). Genome editing is achieved through a process of cut-and-repair mediated by endonucleases that are directed to specific target sequences in the genome by guides that, in theory, are specific to the target sequence. However, in practice, the process can generate off-target mutations. In addition, the repair process at the target locus can be inexact, since the process of cut and repair remains active for several cell cycles. As a result, the animal born from the editing process is often a mosaic animal that may carry multiple alleles for the gene of interest [25]. Thus, it is critical to breed the G0 founder mice with wt animals to segregate the various mutations; the definitive genotyping occurs in the next generation. As this generation is the founder generation, it will be termed F1. This process, then, requires more than one backcrossing as it is the F2 generation that will be used to establish stable lines. The advantages in this case are that: (1) segregation of the correct allele also often promotes segregation of potential off-targets and (2) multiple useful alleles can be generated from one mosaic G0 animal. When establishing a line generated by gene editing, careful sequencing of the targeted allele is essential to be completely sure that there is only one mutated allele and no accompanying insertions/deletions (indels) before starting any other characterisations.

With genome editing, conditional models can be obtained in a single step without using ES cells. This is a clear time advantage (animals are produced within 3–6 months rather than 12 months), but it can also be a challenging approach. When the donor sequence is double-stranded DNA, random insertion can be as frequent as in any traditional transgenic project. It is very important to have a genotyping strategy that allows one to discern between them and also to confirm that a KI insertion is not accompanied by a random one. Once the founder is confirmed, management of the line is similar to those obtained through ES cell targeting.

10.4.2.5 How Do I Manage a Conditional Model?

Conditional models are probably one of the best examples of refinements in animal experiments. The possibility to control gene expression in time and space offers a myriad of opportunities to characterise gene function. However, this strategy requires crossing two genetically unrelated lines to achieve the configuration required for experiments. This implies that at least two generations are required with a careful breeding scheme to reduce animals produced to the minimum. Of note, this breeding scheme is one source of surplus animals bred but not used registered in the EU statistics.

The most demanding model to obtain is the conditional KO, because of the requirement that the animal is homozygous for the floxed gene and hemizygous for the Cre transgene. This can be achieved by first crossing the Cre-containing line to the floxed line (which can be homozygous or heterozygous). In the next generation, a double heterozygote (heterozygous for both the floxed gene and Cre), is then backcrossed to the homozygous floxed line and subsequent progeny are genotyped for homozygosity of the floxed gene and hemizygosity of the Cre transgene. The floxed/floxed; Cre animal is then maintained by continually backcrossing to the floxed/floxed line and screening progeny for transmission of the Cre transgene, resulting in consistent production of the animals with the requested genotype. However, note that it will be impossible to obtain wt littermates as they are not produced using this mating scheme.

It is also important to avoid any breeding scheme that may lead to obtaining homozygous cre animals. Several cre lines in homozygous state have been reported to have a phenotype and this could confound characterisation of the conditional line.

It can be quite challenging to calculate the number of animals that will be used to generate the final model and to generate the cohort of animals used in an experiment. A simplistic approach based on Mendelian percentages may lead to an underestimation of the animals needed to be bred [26]. It is important to be aware that the probability of obtaining a minimum number of two populations of a given phenotype, for example flox/flox and wt/wt, breeding heterozygous parents should be calculated based on the probability of obtaining both groups at the same time, correspond to a binomial distribution A larger number of breeding pairs will be needed to ensure that the needed number of experimental animals is produced.

10.4.2.6 What Is the Basic Welfare Assessment to Perform in a Newly Created GA Line?

When new models are produced, a basic welfare assessment should be performed. This should account for the expected phenotype and a review of any additional phenotypes that could affect the viability of the model. The initial assessment can be performed cage side, most likely by an experienced research or animal technician. Several templates for welfare assessment of different species that can serve as guidance have been developed by an expert group organised by the European Union [8].

A strategy to observe key time points in the animal's development will allow verification that animals carrying the mutation are following the expected developmental pattern (e.g. the presence of colostrum, eyes closed at birth but open at day 11, pinnae thinned, lifting and fully extended by day 15).

Secondly, it is key to understand whether the normal ratio of homozygous, heterozygous and wild-type animals are represented across the breed. A ratio of 1:2:1 should be present and assessment of a minimum of 28 animals will give confidence that this ratio is met. If the ratio is not met, then factors such as reduced viability or lethality should be noted. The sex of the animal may also be a contributing factor, and thus, should be recorded. This phase of the colony progression also allows one to understand if the model is fecund, able to establish and maintain litters without issues and can produce normal-sized litters.

Finally, as good practice, a weight curve from birth to 24 weeks should be established and compared to the background of choice. Any variation, such as reduced growth patterns, will allow one to assess feeding capability and dentition. Failure to thrive can be related to many factors including craniofacial abnormalities and the animal's ability to move and seek food (e.g. onset of ataxia).

By performing and monitoring the welfare of the animal, strategies to support or provide early interventions to allow lines to remain viable, to ensure breeding performance (e.g.

B6.Cg-Tg(HDexon1)61Gpb/J) or to establish humane endpoints will support animal welfare and the 3Rs. All data should be maintained to allow comparison to expected background rates.

10.5 Reproductive Biotechnology Tools for Managing GA Lines

10.5.1 How Can Assisted Reproductive Technologies (ARTs) Help to Manage GA Colonies?

Assisted Reproductive Technologies (ARTs) are essential tools for colony management. For rodents, these technologies are embryo cryopreservation, sperm cryopreservation, in vitro fertilisation, rederivation and combinations of all of these. Zebrafish are also amenable to management and archiving using these ARTs.

GA lines, when generated, are typically one of a kind. When published, they must be shared amongst researchers, necessitating methods to insure they can be imported without jeopardising the health of the receiving facility. Additionally, if a line is genetically contaminated, infected, or stops breeding, the entire line may require extensive work to recover to its original status. In extreme cases, it may be lost entirely. Some GA lines are designed to recapitulate inherited diseases that worsen with each successive generation (generally due to expansion of repeat sequences that happen with each generation, e.g. Huntington's disease). By employing cryopreservation in an early generation of a GA line, lines can return to this earlier status and be compared to lines that start to differ in the number of repeat sequences found. In both cases, a line should be recoverable even if a catastrophe occurs.

Generally, a transgenic core facility will have training in ARTs and should be able to assist investigators. In the absence of this competency, the investigator can contact any of the large consortiums that are used for their species (MMRRC, NORCOM, EMMA, CARD, ZIRC, RRRC etc.) or work with a commercial entity that offers archiving services.

10.5.1.1 Cryopreservation: Should One Archive Sperm or Embryos?

Embryo cryopreservation has long been the standard method of archiving rodent lines, especially those where homozygosity of more than one gene needs to be maintained. Minimum numbers to archive will depend on the zygosity of the line. Projects, where both donor males and donor females are homozygous, will need fewer embryos to reconstitute than those where one or both animals are heterozygous or where one is wild type. Additionally, one needs to determine how many embryos are recoverable (i.e. what % of embryos will survive upon thaw and produce live pups), and how many mating pairs may be needed to recover a line.

Cost and/or space issues influence what type of cryopreservation to perform; the large number of animals required for embryo cryopreservation will incur a larger cage cost. To generate 4–5 mating pairs, one would generally need 6–8 homozygous males of prime mating age (3–8 months) and 6–8 homozygous females that are at the age best used for superovulation for their background strain [27]. Typically, one would want to isolate 20–30 embryos per female upon mating 1:1 with a primed stud male after superovulation. Such a scheme should result in enough cryopreserved embryos to allow for generation of up to 5 mating pairs whilst still maintaining a good stock of cryopreserved embryos.

For heterozygous lines, embryos can be produced by mating GA males to wt females. Since wild-type pups will also be produced, typically double the number of embryos is required, and thus, double the number of males and females are used to generate the embryos. However, if IVF can be performed, the embryos can be generated using sperm from only 1–2 GA males. Thus, the disadvantage of embryo cryopreservation is that larger numbers of animals are required for the procedure. However, the advantage of doing so is that the zygosity of the line is maintained. Recovery of cryopreserved embryos occurs by thawing and implanting the embryos, which is a fairly standard procedure, but is also critically dependent upon the freezing procedure used.

Whilst both mouse and rat lines can be cryopreserved as embryos, the freezing medium will vary between the two as a result of differences in embryo permeability.

Sperm cryopreservation is generally used for archiving rodent lines that are heterozygous or that have only one gene that is homozygous (and that may also have additional genes that are heterozygous). The advantage of sperm cryopreservation is that a line can be archived effectively using only 2–3 males. However, the disadvantage is that recovery requires in vitro fertilisation to produce fertilised embryos for implant. With two males that exhibit fertilisation rates of at least 20% (i.e. after a test IVF, 20% of oocytes are fertilised and will divide and/or generate pups), one can easily produce 4–5 mating pairs using only 5% of the archived sperm samples. Critical to the procedure is using males that have been primed to produce fresh sperm, usually by a short, standardised period of mating and then resting prior to the cryopreservation. Confirmation that the male will successfully transfer the mutation through the germline should be factored in.

One overlooked advantage of sperm cryopreservation is that sperm can maintain viability for up to 4 days after the death of a male, provided that the carcass is kept refrigerated. Thus, should one lose the last male of a line, viable sperm can generally be recovered and used in IVF to reconstitute the line.

10.5.1.2 When Should In Vitro Fertilisation Be Considered as an Alternative?

In vitro fertilisation (IVF) is used for many purposes: to recover a line frozen by sperm cryopreservation, to generate mating pairs from animals that may not easily breed, and even to generate large cohorts of age-matched animals for a study. IVF can also be used to generate embryos for embryo cryopreservation using only 1–2 males. For IVF, depending on the line's fecundity and the number of embryos required, between 4 and 20 females may be used to generate oocytes after superovulation. Because IVF can be affected by many variables, it is essential to adhere strictly to the chosen procedure. For all of the rodent technologies, proven protocols have been developed and disseminated by major archiving sites (The Jackson Laboratory, the Centre for Animal Resources and Development, and the European Mutant Mouse Archive).

10.5.1.3 Are Assisted Reproductive Techniques (ART) Possible in Fish?

ART technologies in fish are less well developed and reliable than those in rodents. As a result, most zebrafish investigators will send their lines to the Zebrafish International Resource Center (ZIRC) for archiving, storage and later distribution. ZIRC has developed effective methods of cryopreservation and in vitro fertilisation that are standardised for subsequent recovery.

10.5.2 Rederivation: When Should I Use It as an Alternative to Introduction of Live Animals in the Facility

Generating and characterising GA animal models requires a substantial number of animals, which has resulted in regulatory oversight to reduce animal numbers used. In compliance with the 3Rs principle, very few situations justify recreating a new line if it is already available. Even though international repositories are gaining prominence as suppliers of both common and unique GA lines, it is still very common that new lines are acquired from other institutions, often in the early stages of their creation and characterisation. As a first choice, importing archived sperm or embryos should be the strategy. But in some situations, cryopreserved samples are not available and only live animals can be obtained. When this happens, a major concern is that their health status may differ considerably from that maintained in the importing institution. Depending on the institutional health requirements, often even the cleanest health report is not accepted and the new line is imported into the new facility through a process known as rederivation.

10.5.2.1 How Do I Rederive Mice and Rats?

Rederivation is possibly the primary and most necessary ART to be incorporated within a rodent animal facility to maintain the requisite health status. Most animal diseases are spread into the host colony through imports/movement of live animals. Originally, rederivation was performed by transferring foetuses at term. In this process (caesarean transfer), the intact uterus of the donor female was dissected and passed through a disinfecting solution. After transfer to the clean area, the uterine horns were opened, the foetuses were extracted, revived, cleaned and placed with a foster mother. The health risks of this procedure were high, since tissue from a potentially infected animal had to enter into the clean part of the new facility. This system has been almost completely replaced with embryo transfer.

Rederivation by embryo transfer has two steps: the first step involves collecting embryos from animals provided by the donor facility, and the second requires implanting those embryos into clean recipients located inside the importing facility. An understanding of rodent embryo development is essential for success. Rodent embryos develop outside of the uterine horn for their first 4 days. The isolated embryos are surrounded by a natural "HEPA filter"—the zona pellucida that protects them from most infectious pathogens.

10.5.2.1.1 How Do I Obtain Rodent Embryos?

Embryos are easily isolated, handled and cultured. It is possible to collect them at different developmental stages from different parts of the reproductive tract. 1-cell embryos are collected from the ampulla of the oviduct, 2-cell embryos to compacted morula are isolated from the oviduct/fallopian tubes, and late morula and blastocysts are isolated from the uterine horn.

If embryo collection from potentially infected donors is to be performed at the importing venue, the procedure should be done in a laboratory away from the main facility or a quarantine zone within it. However, it would be optimal if collection were performed at the donor institution and the embryos transferred to the importing institution. This has the following advantages:

- It reduces the number of animals needed.
- It minimises health risks.
- It avoids transport of live animals with the potential welfare issues of shipping.

Per the standards adopted by the International Embryo Transfer Society (IETS), embryos collected from potentially infected donors have to be extensively washed, and subsequent studies indicate that this should be a minimum of five times in a new drop of media to minimise the risk of transferring any infectious agent [28]. Such media will have antibiotics such as penicillin and streptomycin added to further enhance their ability to minimise transferring pathogens into a facility. Surviving embryos should be carefully selected, removing those with any zona pellucida breaks, or that carry attached cellular debris. Whilst culturing the embryos can be helpful, if the collection and transfer are going to take place soon after isolation, it is not required.

10.5.2.1.2 How Do I Reimplant Rodent Embryos?

In order to establish a pregnancy with reimplanted embryos, the recipient females have to establish hormonal signals of pregnancy, a status that maintains active corpora lutea activity until day 10 post-mating. To avoid competition between endogenously fertilised embryos and implanted embryos, embryos are transferred into pseudopregnant females. Pseudopregnancy in rodents is activated via a neural signal triggered by intercourse with a male, who is either vasectomized or naturally sterile. In rats, pseudopregnancy can be induced by cervical stimulation. Pseudopregnancy allows the transferred embryos the chance to implant and send the endocrine signals required to maintain gestation to term.

For a successful embryo transfer, one should synchronise the pregnancy stage between the embryos and the recipient and implant the embryos in a location that matches their developmental stage. However, there are many instances when pseudopregnant females are not available at the time when they are most needed. Fortunately, the plasticity of the embryo at early stages of development allows for some leeway; progression of the embryo will pause until the developmental stage of the recipient matches that of the embryo. This means that pregnancy can also be achieved if later-stage embryos (2–8 cell, morulae or blastocysts) are transferred into day 0.5 recipients that would naturally be carrying 1-cell embryos, and that embryos can be implanted into the oviduct even though they would normally be located in the uterine horn.

Unfortunately, this plasticity does not work in the other direction (i.e. early-stage embryos cannot be placed into areas where later-stage embryos would normally be found). This is an important caveat when requiring non-surgical methods for embryo transfer—those that implant embryos into the uterus through a vaginal speculum. Non-surgical methods can only work with blastocyst-stage embryos, as those are naturally located in the uterus, the anatomical part that can be accessed non-surgically.

10.5.2.2 Do I Need to Rederive Fish?

The introduction of outside fish models into the importing facility proves to be much simpler than that required for rodents. Typically, live fish are imported that can either be bred in a quarantine facility onsite prior to introduction into the clean facility, or they can be introduced directly into the clean facility by passing them through a sanitisation process. This consists of the physical cleaning and chemical disinfection of the egg surface with different agents. Detailed recommendations on the best practices to introduce a new fish line have been published and should be followed to avoid the risk of contaminating the host facility [29]. Adult fish represent a higher risk than pre-hatching stages, where a sanitisation process can take place, preferentially prior to transport, because hatching may occur before arriving at the host institution. Alternatively, some lines can be exchanged in the form of frozen sperm or embryos, but it has to be noted that cryopreservation does not remove existing pathogens in the biological samples and that embryo cryopreservation in zebrafish is still a challenge [30].

Facilities located in EU countries are required to follow Directive 2010/63/EU, and hence are obliged to import zebrafish only from establishments authorised to supply purpose-bred *Danio rerio* for research. This is the only fish species currently included in the list of animals provided in this European Directive regarding acquisition.

10.5.2.3 What Are the Regulatory Aspects of Rederivation? Is Rederivation a Procedure?

Rederivation required steps, superovulation and embryo transfer (including non-surgical embryo transfer) are considered to be above the threshold of pain, and should be considered procedures subject to regulation according to Directive 2010/63/EU unless they are performed for animal health reasons and/or to protect the health status of the host colony. Many microbes, included in the FELASA Health profile [31], have minimal or no clinical impact on immunocompetent rodents, but can be devastating in immunocompromised ones. Also, some diseases clearly interfere with scientific studies (e.g. altering the immune response). This is why many facilities try to maintain a specific pathogen free (SPF) health status. Incorporating new live animals presents a substantial threat to the host colony. Directive 2010/63/EU clearly states that veterinary acts are not under its scope and in this context, it would not require a project authorisation. However, further interpretation released by the Commission [8] states that "when rederivation is not for the welfare benefit of the animals and is being done to retain animals/colonies of suitable quality and consistency for good science then it is done for scientific purposes and rederivation must comply with the Directive requirements including project authorization". The final decision for any project should rely on the Designated Veterinarian, and this decision has to be documented and performed under the relevant national veterinary legislation by a veterinarian or their legal delegate.

10.6 Best Practices for Sharing GA Animals

10.6.1 What Do I Need to Import a GA Line into My Facility?

Models obtained from other institutions will require various authorisations dependent on the country one is importing from or to. The first step is to request an agreement from the local institution, usually in the form of a Material Transfer Agreement (MTA) which includes intellectual property rights and authorises transfer of the animal model to the new institution. As this agreement will often involve legal representation from both sides, it could take some time. Additional legal requirements will be based on laws of the importing country. Many countries will have border control/customs requirements and require authorising paperwork to be completed. These will be linked to the control of disease within the country, country-based financial considerations and road and aviation requirements. When setting up animal imports/exports, institutions should contact their international shipping agent and the governmental body for cross-border environmental protection to seek appropriate advice.

10.6.2 What Additional Documents Should I Expect When Importing a New GA Model?

Basic information about the animal model should be sent prior to import and also accompany the transfer of a GA animal model. This is often referenced as a "Mouse Passport". With reference to the basic information required for the line, facilities should develop information sheets that outline the breeding strategies and performance of a model as well as a clear genotyping protocol. The concept of the mouse passport allows those sharing models to present useful and often critical information prior to the shipment of animals. Some examples of such documents can be found in these links:

- Mouse Passport RSPCA https://science.rspca.org.uk/documents/1494935/0/GA+passport+booklet.pdf/7050500f-4b6d-13ce-9a6d-93fb01743ca9?t=1552661824197
- Sample Mouse Passport (Oxford University Wellcome): https://www.well.ox.ac.uk/files-library/mouse-passport.pdf

10.6.3 How Can I Determine the Health Status of the Animals Being Imported?

When required to import an existing GA animal model, many facilities will ask for the health report of the supplying facility so that they know which pathogens the mouse may have as well as those that have not been tested for. In this way, they can make decisions about importation that protect the health status of the receiving facility. The designated veterinarian and the animal welfare officer can provide support in defining what is permitted in the facility. A good policy is to develop an institutional description of your animal facility, which would likely include the type of barrier, process for entry of new lines, any quarantine capability and rederivation screening etc. that is performed. A description of the screening report, accepted pathogens and those restricted from entry will provide insight into how the facility is operated. It is good practice to describe the screening methodology and state the provider of the screening services.

10.7 Concluding Remarks

Our goal throughout this chapter has been to provide the reader with information that would allow decision-making based on our experience in the management of genetically altered lines and their wild-type controls, from creation to phenotypic characterisation and establishment of the line. However, the intrinsic nature of genetic mutation makes it very difficult to cover all the potential scenarios. As a general and last recommendation, we would like to remind you that both the animal welfare officer and the designated veterinarian are the two experts set to uphold animal welfare and championing of the 3Rs in an animal facility. By working closely with these two individuals, excellent colony management underpinned by the 3Rs can be achieved, thus ensuring the welfare of the facility's animals is protected.

References

1. Hau J, Macy J, Preisig P. Comparison on university animal resources/research programmes in the European Union and the United States. In FELASA Congress 2019 Prague. Lab Anim. 2019;53(1S):110.
2. Leszczynski JK, Tackett J, Wallace-Fields M. Basic animal facility management. Chapter 26. In: Weichbrod RH, Thompson GAH, Norton JN, editors. Management of animal care and use programs in research, education, and testing. 2nd ed. Boca Raton, FL: CRC Press/Taylor & Francis; 2018. https://doi.org/10.1201/9781315152189-26.
3. The Jackson Laboratory, Breeding Strategies for Maintaining Colonies of Laboratory Mice, A Jackson Laboratory Resource Manual. 2007.
4. Elliott JJ, Miller CT, Hagarman JA, et al. Management of research animal breeding colonies. In: Weichbrod RH, Thompson GAH, Norton JN, editors. Management of animal care and use programs in research, education, and testing. CRC Press/Taylor & Francis; 2018. https://doi.org/10.1201/9781315152189-29.
5. Olson E and Graham D. Chapter 5: Animal models in pharmacogenomics. In: Handbook of pharmacogenomics and stratified medicine. 5.2.3-Outbred rodent stocks, pp 74–75. Pabmanabham S (ed); 2014 doi:https://doi.org/10.1016/C2010-0-67325-1
6. Chia R, Achilli F, Festing M, et al. The origins and uses of mouse outbred stocks. Nat Genet. 2005;37:1181–6. https://doi.org/10.1038/ng1665.
7. Brayton C. Laboratory codes in nomenclature and scientific communication (Advancing organism nomenclature in scientific communication to improve research reporting and reproducibility). ILAR J. 2021;62:295–309. https://doi.org/10.1093/ilar/ilac016.
8. European Commission, Directorate-General for Environment. Framework for the genetically altered animals under Directive 2010/63/EU on the protection of animals used for scientific purposes. Publications Office of the European Union; 2022. https://doi.org/10.2779/499108.
9. Bonaparte D, Cinelli P, Douni E, Hérault Y, Maas M, Pakarinen P, Poutanen M, Lafuente MS, Scavizzi F. FELASA guidelines for the refinement of methods for genotyping genetically-modified rodents: a report of the Federation of European Laboratory Animal Science Associations Working. Lab Anim. 2013;47 https://doi.org/10.1177/0023677212473918.
10. Dahlborn K, Bugnon P, Nevalainen T, Raspa M, Verbost P, Spangenberg E. Report of the Federation of European Laboratory Animal Science Associations Working Group on animal identification. Lab Anim. 2013;47(1):2–11. https://doi.org/10.1177/002367712473290.
11. Breacker C, Barber I, Norton WH, McDearmid JR, Tilley CA. A low-cost method of skin swabbing for the collection of DNA samples from small laboratory fish. Zebrafish. 2016;14:35–41. https://doi.org/10.1089/zeb.2016.1348.
12. Lambert et al. PLoS One. 2018;13(3):e0193180. doi: 10.1371/journal.pone.0193180. eCollection 2018 An automated system for rapid cellular extraction from live zebrafish embryos and larvae: Development and application to genotyping
13. Montagutelly X. Effect of the genetic background on the phenotype of mouse mutations. J Am Soc Nephrology. 2000;11(suppl_2):S101–5. https://doi.org/10.1681/ASN.V11suppl_2s101.
14. Bryant CD, Zhang NN, Sokoloff G, Fanselow MS, Ennes HS, Palmer AA, McRoberts JA. Behavioral differences among C57BL/6 substrains: implications for transgenic and knockout studies. J Neurogenet. 2008;22:315–31.
15. Charlesworth D, Willis J. The genetics of inbreeding depression. Nat Rev Genet. 2009;10:783–96. https://doi.org/10.1038/nrg2664.
16. Doetschman T. Influence of genetic background on genetically engineered mouse phenotypes. Meth Mol Biol. 2009;530:423–33.
17. Markel P, Shu P, Ebeling C, et al. Theoretical and empirical issues for marker-assisted breeding of congenic mouse strains. Nat Genet. 1997;17(3):280–4.
18. Parker-Thornburg J. Breeding strategies for genetically modified mice. In: Larson MA, editor. Transgenic mouse: methods and protocols, methods in molecular biology, vol. 2066. Springer Science and Bussiness Media LLC; 2020. p. 163–9.
19. Wilkie TM, Brinster RL, Palmiter RD. Germline and somatic mosaicism in transgenic mice. Dev Biol. 1986;118:9–18.
20. Gurumurthy CB, Joshi PS, Kurz SG, Ohtsuka M, Quadros RM, Harms DW, Lloyd KCK (2015) Validation of simple sequence length polymorphism regions of commonly used mouse strains for marker assisted speed congenics screening. Int J Genom, vol 2015, Article ID 735845, 17 pages. doi:https://doi.org/10.1155/2015/735845
21. Wong GT. Speed congenics: applications for transgenic and knock-out mouse strains. Neuropeptides. 2002;36(2-3):230–6.
22. International Mouse Knockout Consortium; Collins FS, Rossant J, Wurst W. A mouse for all reasons. Cell. 2007;128(1):9–13. https://doi.org/10.1016/j.cell.2006.12.018.

23. Skarnes WC, Rosen B, West AP, Koutsourakis M, Bushell W, Iyer V, et al. A conditional knockout resource for the genome-wide study of mouse gene function. Nature. 2011;474(7351):337–42. https://doi.org/10.1038/nature10163.
24. Ryder E, Doe B, Gleeson D, et al. Rapid conversion of EUCOMM/KOMP-CSD alleles in mouse embryos using a cell-permeable Cre recombinase. Transgenic Res. 2014;23:177–85. https://doi.org/10.1007/s11248-013-9764-x.
25. Yen ST, Zhang M, Deng JM, Usman SJ, Smith CN, Parker-Thornburg J, Swinton PG, Martin JF, Berhinger RB. Somatic mosaicism and allele complexity induced by CRISPR/Cas9 RNA injections in mouse zygotes. Dev Biol. 2014;393:3–9.
26. Milchevskaya V, Bugnon P, ten Buren EBJ, Brand F, Tresch A, Buch T. Group size planning for breedings of gene-modified mice and other organisms following Mendelian inheritance. Lab Anim. 2023;52:183–8. https://doi.org/10.1038/s41684-023-01213-1.
27. Luo C, Zuniga J, Edison E, Palla S, Dong W, Parker-Thornburg J. Superovulation strategies for 6 commonly used mouse strains. JAALAS. 2011;50:471–8.
28. Gardner D, Lane M. Culture of the mammalian preimplantation embryo. In: Gardner DK, Lane M, Watson AJ, editors. A laboratory guide to the mammalian embryo. New York, NY: Oxford University Press; 2004. p. 41–61.
29. Mocho JP, Collymoore C, Farmer SC, Leguay E, Murray KN, Pereira N. FELASA-AALAS recommendations for monitoring and reporting of laboratory fish diseases and health status, with an emphasis on zebrafish (Danio rerio). Comp Med. 2022;72(3):127–48.
30. Khosla K, Bischof J, Varga ZM. Sperm cryopreservation, in vitro fertilization, and embryo freezing. In Livia D'Angelo, Paolo de Girolamo (Eds.) Laboratory fish in biomedical research (pp 157–181). Academic; 2022. ISBN 9780128210994. doi:https://doi.org/10.1016/B978-0-12-821099-4.00007-9
31. Pritchett-Corning KR, Prins JB, Feinstein R, Goodwin J, Nicklas W, Riley L. AALAS/FELASA Working Group on Health Monitoring of rodents for animal transfer. Lab Anim Sci. 2014;53(6):633–40.

State-of-the-Art Surgery, Anaesthesia, and Analgesia: How to Set-Up Best Practices for Facility and Procedures?

11

Alessandra Bergadano, Delphine Bouard, Bertrand Lussier, and Eric Troncy

Abstract

State-of-the-art anaesthesia, analgesia, and surgery are **key for achieving excellent experimental results, their reproducibility**, for guaranteeing the **highest** standards of **animal welfare** and **honouring an ethical commitment**. They are the practical application of the **Culture of Care** of an institution in daily research activities.

Key for success is establishing an **optimal peri-anaesthetic and operative care program**:

- Surgical suites should be well organized and exclusively dedicated to surgery. Anaesthesia and monitoring equipment should be checked for functionality.
- *Pre-operative care:* Minimise stress (acclimatisation, quiet environment, handling, habituation, premedication) and start temperature support.
- *Intra-operative care:* Use balanced, multimodal anaesthesia, pertinent with the model. Provide oxygen, support ventilation, cardiovascular function, and normothermia. Protect their eyes. Closely monitor throughout.

Use aseptic, minimally invasive, and atraumatic surgical techniques with adapted instrumentation, prevent tissue desiccation, judiciously use sutures (appropriate size), avoiding tension upon closure.

- *Post-surgical care:* Keep animals under close monitoring and accelerate awakening through antagonisation. Support normothermia until complete recovery. Weigh and check animals on a daily basis for at least 3 days; provide critical care feed. Limit individual housing time.
- Use **preventive analgesia** and emphasise loco-regional anaesthesia. Continue analgesia

A. Bergadano (✉)
Experimental Animal Center, University of Bern, Bern, Switzerland
e-mail: alessandra.bergadano@unibe.ch

D. Bouard
Vetsalius, Lyon, France
e-mail: delphine.bouard@vetsalius.com

B. Lussier
Faculty of Veterinary Medicine, Department of Clinical Sciences, Université de Montréal, St-Hyacinthe, QC, Canada

Groupe de recherche en pharmacologie animale (GREPAQ), Université de Montréal, St-Hyacinthe, QC, Canada
e-mail: bertrand.lussier@umontreal.ca

E. Troncy
Groupe de recherche en pharmacologie animale (GREPAQ), Université de Montréal, St-Hyacinthe, QC, Canada

Faculty of Veterinary Medicine, Departement of Biomedical Sciences, Université de Montréal, St-Hyacinthe, QC, Canada
e-mail: eric.troncy@umontreal.ca

J. Guillén, V. Galligioni (eds.), *Practical Management of Research Animal Care and Use Programs*, Laboratory Animal Science and Medicine 3, https://doi.org/10.1007/978-3-031-65414-5_11

post-surgery as required, at the proper dose, frequency, and assess its efficacy.

Keywords

Anaesthesia · Analgesia · Surgical best practices · Animal welfare · Pre/peri/post-operative care · Reproducibility · Surgical suite

11.1 Preamble

State-of-the-art anaesthesia, analgesia, and surgical procedures are **key for achieving excellent experimental results and their reproducibility**, for guaranteeing the **highest** standards of **animal welfare**, and for **honouring an ethical commitment.**

They are the practical application of the **Culture of Care** of an institution in daily research activities.

To date, veterinary guidelines for **standards of care for clinical patients** have been published and they should be applied also to laboratory animals.

Paraphrasing a famous sentence of Gandhi, one could say that "the greatness of an institution and its moral progress can be judged by the way in which anaesthesia, analgesia and surgery are performed".

11.2 How Is a State-of-the-Art Surgical Facility Organised?

11.2.1 How Should an Ideal Surgery Suite Be Organised?

Ideally, surgical suites should:

- Be sized and equipped for the species used in the program.
- Exclusively be dedicated to surgery, to avoid potential environmental contamination from other activities.
- Allow to clearly separate non-aseptic (animal anaesthesia induction and preparation, post-operative care) and aseptic (surgery, some tissue sampling) activities.
- Be designed to minimise traffic flow in the surgery room, allowing surgeons to work in a clean, efficient, and quiet environment.
- Be equipped with high-quality lighting systems, to provide adequate illumination.
- Be well-ventilated (positive pressure) areas, avoiding direct ventilation on surgical tables.
- Ensure that anaesthetic gases will be correctly eliminated, avoiding exposure by personnel members.
- Be equipped with sufficient electric outlets, ideally placed underneath surgery benches to prevent the accumulation on the surgery area of electric cords or plugs.
- Be easy to clean or even fully disinfected (by fumigation): as empty as possible and made of easily cleanable surfaces and kept in good maintenance.
- If material must be stored in the surgery room, be equipped with closed cupboards, drawers, or closed carts.
- Include or be close to a clean surgical support area with equipment for surgeons' preparation (a properly equipped sink or hand gel distribution system, for hand disinfection) and material washing, sterilisation, and storage (Fig. 11.1).

Common problems classically encountered with laboratory animal surgical facilities that have to be avoided are:

- Overcrowded rooms, very uneasy to keep clean and not allowing to clearly separate aseptic and non-aseptic tasks.
- Surgery performed in "mixed" activity rooms including highly contaminating ones (necropsies, blood sampling, behavioural tests).
- Insufficient lighting and/or electric outlets.
- Insufficient ventilation.

The above-listed usual problems are associated with a high risk of failure, especially related to post-operative infection. If you feel like your surgical facilities organisation is suboptimal, please discuss it with your animal welfare body

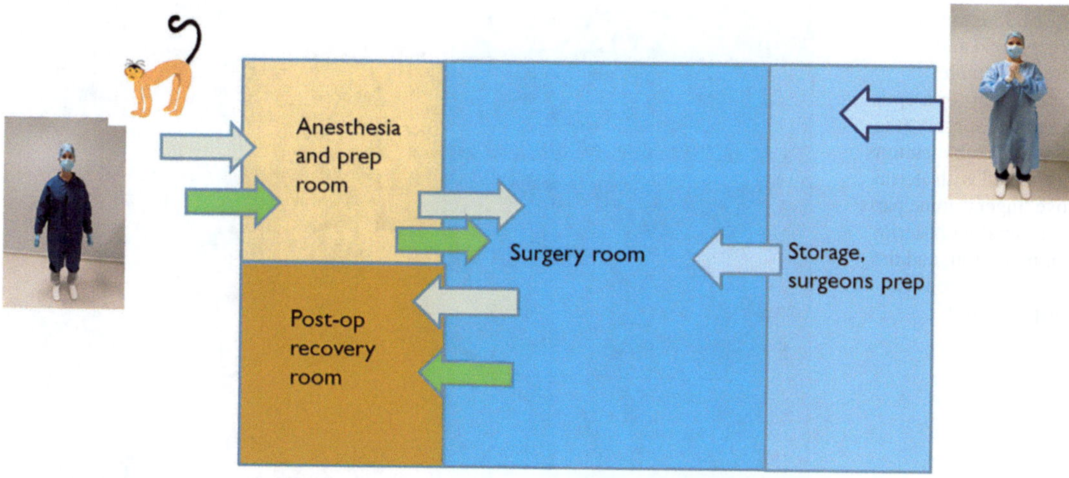

Fig. 11.1 Schematic representation of an ideal surgical suite organisation

(AWB) and/or management to plan and restructure the surgical suites as required.

11.2.2 What Are the Key Preparation Steps of a Surgery Session?

11.2.2.1 Material Preparation

Few days ahead of the session, make sure that all the requested material is available (a detailed and comprehensive list should have been built with an experienced trainer). Instruments and consumables requiring sterilisation should be sterilised on time. Most surgical items could be autoclaved but some specific consumables or equipment (brain cannula, microdialysis systems, telemetry implants, Hamilton syringes, for example) might need alternative sterilisation processes (cold sterilant or gamma irradiation, for example).

For rodent surgeries, many items that are close to the surgical field might not be sterile or sterilisable (light, binoculars). These items should be covered with sterile items. Many classical laboratory consumables (shoe cover, aluminium foil, caps) could be autoclaved and used as protection (see Figs. 11.2 and 11.3).

Define a strategy regarding instruments cleansing and re-sterilisation during the day whilst performing surgeries in series. Small autoclaves with short cycles duration are now available, they are very useful tools when surgeries must be performed in series.

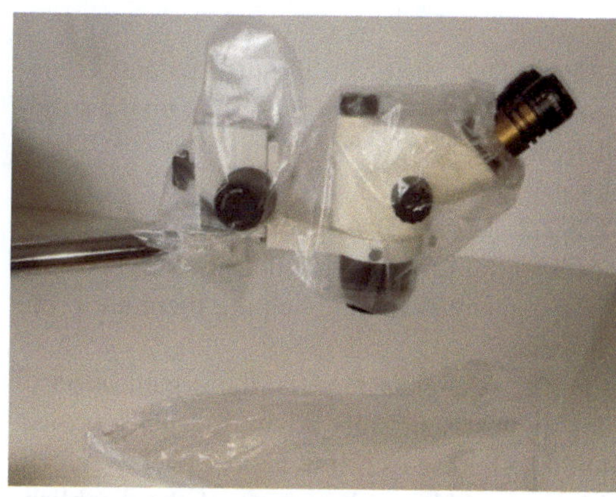

Fig. 11.2 Use of autoclavable plastic shoe covers to protect basic binoculars used for rodent surgeries

11.2.2.2 Surgery Room Preparation

If working in a centralised surgery room, check surgical facility availability.

On D-1 or D Day, install the material in the room and clearly identify "dirty" (dedicated to peri-operative care) and "clean" (dedicated to surgery) areas. Make sure that the clean area is as empty and clean as possible. Check all requested material functionality and position (microscopes, anaesthesia systems, chairs etc.)

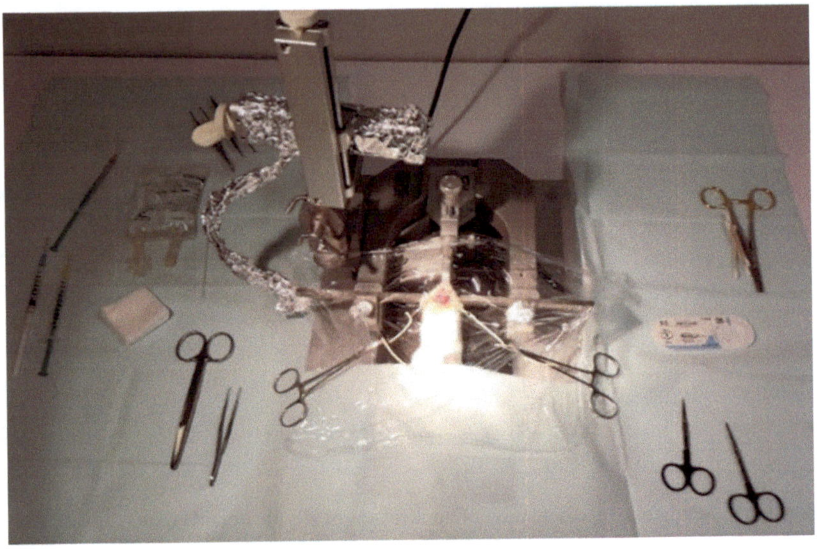

Fig. 11.3 Example of surgery field and stereotaxic table management for aseptic stereotaxic surgery (the stereotaxic table buttons are covered with sterile glove fingers, some parts are covered with sterile aluminium foil, and the animal is covered with a transparent foil

On D Day, disinfect all surfaces and equipment in the clean area before setting up the surgical area.

11.2.2.3 Team Preparation

It is essential to make sure that the surgeons but also the persons who are helping them are properly trained.

For new surgical models, the organisation of pilot studies is strongly advised. A pilot project should be realised several days or even weeks in advance to address all aspects of the establishment of a new model in your facility. Make sure that the post-operative period is long enough to identify complications, assess limit points, and refine the protocol.

For the experiment itself, if operating batches of animals, estimate the number of animals to be operated per day. Do not be overoptimistic! Especially during the first days, difficulties will be encountered, which will require fine-tuning.

Define team members' tasks: ideally, surgeries should be performed at least as a team of two persons, with one person dedicated to the non-aseptic tasks (animal anaesthesia induction, surgical site preparation, post-op care) and one surgeon dedicated to aseptic surgical techniques. Make sure that the persons in charge of the anaesthesia are experienced enough and that anaesthesia equipment is well adapted and functional.

On D Day, the person assigned to non-aseptic tasks should take care of anaesthesia induction, hair clipping and disinfection, eye gel application, per-operative rehydration, and monitoring equipment setting.

11.3 How Is a State-of-the-Art Veterinary Pharmacy Organised?

11.3.1 Location and Personnel

The pharmacy should be located in a room close to the surgical suite or within the vivarium and sized according to the program's needs. The room(s) should be organised with sufficient closable cupboards and at least one safe for storing regulated drugs. Light, temperature, and ventilation are controlled and recorded.

A temperature (T°)-controlled refrigerator should be available and T° checked weekly.

Its access should be strictly controlled (key, badges, other electronic means) to prevent unattended access to third parties.

A pharmacist or a veterinarian oversees all drug management; these persons are legally responsible and must have the appropriate education and titles. Deputies and all other persons who are authorised to access the pharmacy are listed in an organisational chart.

Veterinary pharmacies are inspected annually by the competent authorities or the institution responsible.

11.3.2 What Is the Flow of the Drugs and Which Rules Should I Follow?

11.3.2.1 Drug Flows

Anaesthetics, analgesics, and other medicines must be purchased, stored, used, recorded (in, out, use), and discarded according to national laws and regulations. Also, the regulations around the cascading of human drugs must be observed. All processes of the veterinary pharmacy should be described in a standard operating procedure and updated regularly.

Records of the income and outcome of the drugs must be kept on paper or electronically, indicating at least the product name, the active substance, the manufacturer, the concentration, the standard pack size, the batch number (or lot number), the expiration date and, if applicable, special storage conditions.

Stocks are sized to the use and a monthly and yearly inventory must be performed.

Special attention must be paid to addictive substances like ketamine, pentobarbital, and opioids to avoid misuse.

11.3.2.2 Timelines for Use

Medical grade drugs must be used according to manufacturer instructions. All anaesthetic, analgesic, adjuvants, and other drugs must be used within their validity date noted on the vial.

For broached vials, the shelf-life recommendations are listed in Table 11.1.

- Opened medicines and infusion solutions must be clearly labelled with the date and time of opening.
- Opened infusion solutions must be provided with a label stating that the solution may no longer be used for injections 24 h after opening.
- Drawn/filled syringes shall be labelled with details of the content.

11.3.2.3 Disposal

Medicines that are still stable by date but show untypical discolouration, turbidity, sedimentation, or precipitation should also be disposed. Expired drugs are to be returned to the veterinary pharmacy officer and disposed according to national laws and regulations. Diluted drugs can be discarded as chemicals, but opioids must be returned and sent to the local authorities for destruction as expired opioids.

11.3.3 Is the Use of Non-pharmaceutical Grade Substances Acceptable?

The use of non-pharmaceutical grade substances is to be avoided as they have undefined or higher levels of impurities, can have unexpected or even toxic effects, and introduce unwanted experimental variables. However, they can be used in live animals only when there is no pharmaceutical grade alternative available and there is a scientific justification approved by the regulatory body.

Table 11.1 Example of guidelines for broached drugs vials

Application type/ Type of medication	Shelf-life	Storage condition
Intravenous (i.v.)	24 h or according to manufacturer guidelines	According to manufacturer guidelines
Intramuscular (i.m.), intraperitoneal (i.p.)*	28 days or according to manufacturer guidelines	According to manufacturer guidelines
Orally/topically	According to manufacturer guidelines	According to manufacturer guidelines
Mixed/diluted medicines without preservatives	24 h [1] or according to manufacturer guidelines	Fridge
*Exception: Pentobarbital	3 months	In a safe, as a narcotic (undiluted)

Nowadays, in anaesthesia and analgesia this is limited mostly to the use of urethane and tribromoethanol in rodents. Both methods should only be used if there are no viable alternatives or if there is scientific justification for their use.

11.4 Which State-of-the-Art Anaesthesia Equipment Is Required?

11.4.1 Which Equipment Should Be Available?

11.4.1.1 Carrier Gases

Oxygen is always available and possibly also medical air; depending on the size of the program tanks, cylinders can be used for delivery. Tanks are intended for large volumes programs and are placed outside the facility. Cylinders are organised in manifolds. These must be housed in a safety cabinet in compliance with OSHA and NFPA standards. For smaller programs, single bottles can be sufficient; these are directly connected to the anaesthesia machine and must be safely secured to the wall or to a dedicated portable card. The medical gases are carried via pipelines to the anaesthetic machines. These must be inspected annually for leaks. Manometers indicate the pressure in the piping.

If oxygen generators are used, an oxygen cylinder must be available in case of an electricity breakdown as a contingency plan.

11.4.1.2 Anaesthesia Equipment

The anaesthesia set-up depends on the species which will be anaesthetised in the institution.

For rodents a non-rebreathing system is commonly used, the minimal assembly will include a flowmeter, the vaporiser, and a tubing connecting via a dual diverter the induction box and the non-rebreathing system. To date electronically controlled equipment is available from different providers, allowing for low flows and lesser environmental exposure.

A facility will need many replicates of the non-rebreathing anaesthesia units to accommodate the needs (surgical and imaging suites). Table tops can be moved easily and are a valuable option ensuring flexibility.

The vaporiser should be installed with a selectatec system [2], allowing for interchangeability when a different halogenate is required or for maintenance and repair.

For large animals, re-breathing circuits are used and machines for humans with integrated ventilators are used up to 100 kg. Above this weight, veterinary machines especially sized are to be used.

At least one mechanical ventilator for very small (piston ventilator), medium, and large animals depending on the animal species anaesthetised and the type of anaesthesia and surgeries should be available.

Species-specific instrumentation for intravenous access and endotracheal intubation is required.

Anaesthesia equipment must be kept clean, disinfected after use and kept in good working conditions, and checked yearly by the manufacturer. Modern vaporisers (TEC 7 and above) do not need yearly maintenance.

11.4.1.3 Monitoring Equipment

Reliable and relatively accessible monitoring systems exist and should be used in large animals' species.

Monitoring devices for small rodents do exist but are sometimes challenging to use because not compatible with, for example:

- Other required equipment such as stereotaxic frames.
- Animal's position changes during surgery such as for catheter implantation surgeries.

However, in most cases, at least pulse oximetry (HR and SpO_2) could easily and should ideally be measured, with the help of basic monitoring systems adapted to rodents. Some suppliers do offer specific accessories allowing to use of basic pulse oximetry devices in small animals (for example, Nonin® Transflectance Sensor Model 2000 T).

If monitoring devices are difficult to use, at least clinical observations including respiratory rate, mucosa colour, and signs of dehydration (skin pinch test) can and should regularly be made.

11.4.1.4 Scavenging

When halogenates are used for anaesthesia, these must be collected and removed from the surgical suite/procedure room to avoid pollution (and the consequent threat to occupational health). The efficient reduction of waste anaesthetic gases (WAGs) can be achieved by using low fresh gas flows (based on the species and anaesthesia circuit), use of the appropriate scavenger system, and adequate operating room ventilation. The latter should be at least 20 air changes/hour or determined based on risk assessment with halogenate concentration measures.

Scavenging may be active (suction applied via a vacuum system) or passive (WAGs proceed passively down corrugated tubing through the room ventilation exhaust or to a charcoal).

Both the decision on which driver gases, their delivery, and scavenging systems will be required in a research facility must be well evaluated and decided whilst planning new buildings based on the major impact on the construction.

11.4.2 What Are the Occupational Health and Safety Concerns Around Anaesthesia?

It is also part of the Culture of Care of an institution to take care of the health of the personnel whilst handling and administering anaesthesia. Some injection anaesthetics, i.e. urethane and all inhalational have toxic or cancerogenic properties and adequate policies including equipment, instruction, and vigilance should be in place to avoid personnel exposure.

For inhalant anaesthetics, it is a legal requirement to have an anaesthetic gas waste management system to protect the health of the personnel (https://www.osha.gov/waste-anesthetic-gases; https://www.issa.int/sites/default/files/documents/prevention/2%20-%20Consensus%20Paper%20Anaesthetic%20Gases-36710.pdf; http://www.sohf.ch/Themes/Operation/2869_29_D.pdf).

It is very important to endorse safe anaesthesia working measures such as avoiding leaks, minimising cage induction, using funnel fill systems for filling vaporisers, checking that masks are properly fitting and tight, and having adequate active or passive scavenging systems.

Waste management systems must be adapted to the species anesthetised and the gas turnover (hours*volumes used).

https://acvaa.org/wp-content/uploads/2019/05/Control-of-Waste-Anesthetic-Gas-Recommendations.pdf

Also, whilst performing anaesthesia the "no-recap" policy should be observed. Please refer to the occupational safety rules of your institution (see Chap. 16 OHS).

11.4.3 Which Basic Preparation Steps Are Required Before Starting with the Anaesthesia?

Before starting a procedure, the anaesthesia equipment must be checked to ensure the functionality and the safety of both animal and the personnel.

- The anaesthetic machine must be controlled for tightness (leak test) [3] and appropriate for the size of the patient. https://researchanimaltraining.com/elearning/
- The vaporiser and the pumps are calibrated, https://www.aaalac.org/accreditation-program/faqs/#D1 and the vaporiser is ready to be used.
- The exhaust and gas elimination devices are operational.
- The necessary equipment (intubation, drugs and fluids administration, monitoring, warming) is ready.
- The anaesthetic records are prepared, and anaesthetic plan has been revised for the corresponding procedure and patient. This includes verification of the anaesthetic and analgesic drugs, which are prepared.

- Emergency drugs are present in the theatre.
- The recovery cage and warming device are clean and safe.
- The approved experimental protocol and the telephone numbers of scientists and veterinarians are in the room.

11.5 What Are Best Practices in Preparing the Animals for Anaesthesia and Surgery?

Animals must be acclimatised to the facility (see Chap. 6 on Husbandry) and clinically healthy.

11.5.1 Acclimatisation

During the pre-operative period, the main objective is to reduce animals' stress as much as possible. Stress activates the neuro-endocrine system and increases peri-operative morbidity and mortality. For example, too short acclimatisation periods are frequently associated with higher post-operative self-mutilation rates (author's (DB) personal data 2021: in rats undergoing a bile duct ligation surgery, the occurrence of skin sutures self-mutilation was approximately 15% in animal batches acclimatised for 1 week and of less than 3% in similar animal batches acclimatised for 3 weeks).

If animals must be transferred from one unit to another (e.g. if they are ordered from a breeder), they should be allowed to rest during an adapted acclimatisation period. This acclimatisation period may vary on the transportation conditions, the animal strain, sex, and age range as well as the specific surgery to be performed in various experimental conditions. A relatively short acclimatisation period such as 1 week might be sufficient for young adult animals undergoing a short transportation and a basic surgery such as an Alzet pump implantation. However, much longer acclimatisation periods might be required (3 weeks or more), for example when the animals are known to be naturally stressed or physiologically impaired, when they have to be transported during long distances by plane, or when the next steps of the experiment and/or the surgery are known to be impaired by stress [4–6].

Additionally, high levels of adrenaline can induce arrhythmias but also decrease the effectiveness of alpha2 agonists-based protocols as adrenaline and noradrenaline are already occupying the postsynaptic receptors on the sympathetic noradrenergic nerves jeopardising the quality of the anaesthesia.

An adapted habituation program (regular gentle handling, pre-operative administration of post-op food to prevent neophobia, for example progressive exposure to outcome(s) assessment on five occasions over 2 weeks to decrease measurement variability) should be implemented on a case-by-case basis [7–9]. For instance, animals who will "carry" any specific post-operative devices such as harnesses to protect exteriorised catheters should be gradually habituated to the equipment pre-operatively.

11.5.2 Weighing

Knowledge of body weight (BW) allows for an accurate drug dosing and therefore action. This is most important in very small animals to avoid rough overdosing and in very sick animals where BW can change in the shortest time.

11.5.3 Health Check

According to the animal protection law, only healthy animals can be used for animal experimentation. Sick animals can introduce undesired variability in the scientific read out and peri-anaesthetic morbidity and mortality can increase. Special care must be taken to diagnose subclinical disease, especially at lung level i.e. infections with *P. carinii* in rodents. A full clinical examination should be performed before anaesthesia also for smaller animals; health reports should be reviewed. Specificities of the phenotype should be considered, i.e. diabetes or age or pregnancy.

11.5.4 Pre-operative Treatment

It can be administered, if needed, i.e. in the case of parathyroidectomies, animals should be provided with additional calcium in their drinking water as early as Day-1 pre-surgery, to prevent post-operative hypocalcaemia [10–12]. Providing the animals with calcium before the surgery is much more efficient than doing it post-operatively only. In rats of 250 g BW, 4 mg of calcium/mL can be added to drinking water (personal communication).

11.5.5 Pre-anaesthetic Fasting

Pre-anaesthetic fasting reduces anaesthesia-related vomiting and regurgitation and the risk of pneumonia secondary to aspiration; it also facilitates respiration by reducing the pressure of the gastrointestinal system on the lungs. The requirements for pre-anaesthetic fasting are species specific, ranging from no fasting in very small mammals like mice and rats to avoid metabolic failure to longer fasting times in ruminants to reduce regurgitation and associated risks. Recently, pre-anaesthetic fasting times have been reduced.

https://www.gv-solas.de/wp-content/uploads/2021/08/2020_10Food_withdrawal.pdf

In a laboratory setting, time is often influenced by the feeding times in the facility and excessively long fasting times should be avoided.

If animals are group housed, all animals in the cage or pen might need to be fasted. This raises an ethical question of balancing isolation stress and group fasting.

In some laboratory species as NHPs, aspiration of the gastric content after induction of anaesthesia can be valuable [13] to reduce silent regurgitation.

11.5.6 Dosing

If very small volumes are to be administered, it is very meaningful to prepare dilutions of the drugs with a chemically *compatible* solvent (aqua ad inj. or NaCl) to allow for accurate dosing.

Remember that syringes have a dead space volume and this must be taken into account when injecting small animals to guarantee that the whole calculated dose is administered (risk of under dosing) [14].

https://arc-w.nihr.ac.uk/research/projects/low-versus-high-dead-space-syringes-user-preferences-and-attitudes/

11.6 Which Are Surgical Best Practices?

11.6.1 Is Asepsis Necessary for Any Kind of Surgery and for Any Species?

Absolutely, as soon as you are performing non-terminal surgeries. All animal species, including rodents, are susceptible to develop post-operative infections. Post-operative infections do not necessarily lead to post-operative mortality but induce physiological bias that could significantly impact the results of experiments. It may also lead to a reduction of group size, thus resulting in decreased statistical power, invalidating results of the study.

Applying aseptic conditions is one of the basic principles of surgery, whatever species is operated.

Therefore, **aseptic conditions should always be used whatever species and surgical model you are working with**.

Preventing contamination from the usual microorganisms' sources is crucial. Therefore, good practices regarding protection against microorganisms coming from:

- Animals
- Surgeons
- Environment
- Instruments and consumables

should be applied (Table 11.2).

For rodent surgeries, the small size of the animals, the animal facilities organisation (for exam-

Table 11.2 Prevention strategies for the different sources of contamination with microorganisms

	Classical strategies applied for strict aseptic conditions compliance	Acceptable compromises for small animals (if classical strategies not applicable)	Not acceptable
Surgeon	• Proper surgeon hand washing (jewellery removed) • Sterile gloves, eventually doubled or changed on a very regular basis • Sterile gown changed in-between each animal	• Proper hand disinfection with hand gel (jewellery removed) • Sterile gloves changed on a regular basis • Sterile gown or sterile sleeves (for rodents' surgeries) changed on a regular basis	• No hand disinfection • Jewellery • Examination gloves • No forearm protection
Animals	• Hair clipping • Proper skin disinfection in several steps (cleansing with soap, rinsing with water, disinfectant application; amphibians/fish require special care) • Draping with sterile barrier drapes and/or films	No compromise	• No shaving • No skin disinfection • No draping or draping with nonsterile and/or non-barrier items
Environment	• Dedicated rooms for preparation, surgery, and recovery • Dedicated teams for animal peri-op care and clean team for surgery • Very clean and "empty" surgery room, sterilised or decontaminated on a regular basis	• Dedicated spaces with clear separation between « clean » and "dirty" areas • Dedicated teams for animal peri-op care and clean team for surgery • Room as empty and easily decontaminated as possible	• Animal preparation and surgery performed at the same station • Dirty and clean tasks performed by the same persons • "Busy" rooms with a lot of non-surgical equipment
Instruments Consumables Equipment	• One set of sterile instruments per animal • Sterile consumables • Non-sterile equipment close to the surgical field covered with sterile items	• One set or two sets of sterile instruments, decontaminated between each animal with a heat glass-bead steriliser or a cold sterilant • Sterile consumables only • Non-sterile equipment close to the surgical field covered with sterile items	• Non-sterile instruments or use of the same set for several animals without decontamination • Non-sterile consumables • Non-sterile equipment not covered and regularly touched by the surgeon, the consumables or the instruments during the surgery

ple, the absence of adapted sinks for proper surgeon's hand washing) and the requested material specificities (for example, non-sterile stereotaxic frames, non-sterile binoculars, and non-sterile light sources) make usual veterinary aseptic conditions practices sometimes difficult to be applied, *requesting specific strategies to be implemented.*

11.6.2 How Should a New Surgical Model Be Developed?

First, please do consider that **all surgical practices standards applying to pet animals also apply to laboratory animals** and surgical practices standards if available (for example, UK "Code of Professional Conduct for veterinary Surgeons"[1]) should be followed.

The very first steps of an experimental surgical model development are:

- Selecting a relevant model, answering your experimental question(s).
- Making sure that you have:

[1] https://www.rcvs.org.uk/setting-standards/advice-and-guidance/code-of-professional-conduct-for-veterinary-surgeons

- The authorisation from the institutional oversight body before starting the project.
- The necessary skills to implement this model in an efficient and reproducible manner (efficient means reaching its goal, i.e. getting patent vascular catheters or good quality signals for telemetry implants, surgeries performed without any major complication).

Regarding model selection, here are key points to be considered:

- What is the specific scientific question you wish to answer?
- Are there already published or validated models answering this question?
- If yes, are these models:
  - **Accessible?**
    In terms of animal model (for example, animals' actual availability in your country, ease to handle in the context of your experiments, compatibility with the equipment available in your lab)
    In terms of regulation
    In terms of requested expertise (surgical or non-surgical such as expertise requested for imaging techniques, for example)
    In terms of requested material/equipment.
  - **Reliable?**
    Do they have a translational value?
    Are they easily reproducible?
  - **Compliant with the 3Rs principles?**
    Replacement: can't they be replaced by inert models or less invasive in vivo models?
    Reduction: can the number of animals be reduced as much as possible, using previous studies' results or pilot studies and statistical analysis?
    Refinement: is the surgical technique and the peri-operative care program optimal, allowing to minimise animal potential distress as much as possible?
- If no,
  - Can you, with the help of experienced mentors, develop a new model consistent with the key points listed above?

If the primary analysis allows you to identify a relevant surgical model that is accessible, another key step is to check that the personnel is authorised to perform surgeries in laboratory animals. In some countries, in addition to initial statutory courses, a **specific surgery course** should be successfully completed before being allowed to practice surgery. Upon countries' regulations, this authorisation could be species specific. If you have any doubts, verify with the local authorities. The basic statutory surgery courses allow to acquire basic knowledge of general good practices.

However, **additional hands-on training** on your specific model(s) of interest is always required. Local or external experienced mentor(s) should be able to provide you with specific recommendations on:

- Animals' anatomy and physiology
- Aseptic technique implementation.
- Animal model selection (strain, sex, age, or weight range).
- Adapted pre- and post-op care, including anaesthesia and analgesia.
- Surgical approach.
- Material selection including suture material and technique.

Some of these challenging surgical models require intensive training including numerous repetitions of critical gestures. You are strongly advised to initially train on inert supports (such as suture pads for basic suturing technique training, MD-PVC rat ND model for vessel anastomosis, bone models such as SawBones® plastic bones, for example) or cadavers. The acquired technical expertise leads to standardisation of the surgical animal models, resulting in animal number reduction, decreased morbidity, and mortality [15, 16].

Surgeons with very limited experience and limited ability to train on a regular basis should consider alternative options for challenging surgical models, such as ordering pre-operated animals from vendors or getting the help of experienced surgeons for critical gestures.

Please also consider that apart from the initial training, some surgeries require to be performed on a regular basis to maintain surgeons' and assistants' skills and prevent technical bias (Table 11.3).

11.6.3 How Can the Surgical Technique Improve the Outcome and Wellbeing of the Operated Animals?

During the surgery, appropriate instruments should be used to minimise as much as possible tissue trauma. For example, suture material needles should be carefully chosen upon the tissue to be sutured. Fragile tissues such as bladder or intestine walls should be sutured with specific, atraumatic (taper) needles of adapted size and absorbable monofilament threads. The composition and diameter of sutures also have a significant impact on wound healing quality (Table 11.4).

For the skin, intradermal suture should be performed, if possible, to decrease wound tension, improve apposition, and decrease the risk of tearing the suture leading to wound dehiscence, especially in NHPs.

Specific needle holders, adapted to the needle size, should be used to manipulate the suture material. Similar selection criteria apply to all surgical instruments (forceps, scissors, retractors etc.).

The choice of appropriate consumables is also a key factor: for example, for some delicate surgeries, the use of unwoven gauze is much safer as compared to woven gauze.

Novice surgeons should get the help of experienced surgeons to select and learn how to properly use instruments for their specific surgical models.

When targeting a specific anatomical structure (for example, the ovaries for an ovariectomy), a proper and minimally invasive surgical approach techniques, should be used. Appropriate surgical approaches allow the surgeon to reach a specific organ, avoiding as much as possible critical structures such as vessels and nerves and creating as minimal damage as possible. *Please do not reinvent the wheel!* These approach techniques have been described in many different species and should be respected; they are associated with less morbidity.

Strategies regarding haemostasis should be defined. For some surgeries such as organ complete or partial excision, major risk of haemorrhage does exist. Upon the expected type of bleeding, some haemostatic devices or consumables might be of help such as electrocautery systems, bone wax, haemostatic sponges, or haemostatic powder. Please keep in mind that even minor bleeding could compromise postoperative recovery, as it enhances the infection risk and could compromise wound healing.

If major bleeding occurs, compensative administration of fluids should be implemented. Blood transfusion from donors could also be considered.

Table 11.4 Example of guidelines for skin suture material selection management in various species

Animal species	Suture size (USP)
Dogs/Pigs (10–30 kg)	3-0 (decimal 2)
Cats/Non-Human Primates (NHPs) (approx. 3–5 kg)	4-0 (decimal 1.5)
Rats (approx. 300 g)	5-0 to 6-0 (decimal 1)
Mice (approx. 30 g)	6-0 (decimal 0.7) to 8-0 (decimal 0.4)

Table 11.3 Examples of the required level of surgical experience

	Surgeries requiring basic surgical experience	Surgeries requiring advanced surgical experience	Surgeries requiring highly advanced surgical experience	Surgeries requiring surgical expertise
Example of surgeries	Castration Small devices' subcutaneous implantation	Ovariectomies Basic stereotaxic injection	Double vascular catheterisation or complex telemetry device implantation	Spine surgeries Organ graft Thoracic surgeries
Typical number of gesture repetitions needed for an initial training	5–10	10–20	10–30	50–200

Decreasing the total surgery and anaesthesia time is a major refinement. Experienced trainers should provide novice surgeons with information regarding optimal surgery duration. For some critical surgeries, intensive training on cadavers is a good way to step by step reduce total surgery time, until optimal timing is reached [17].

11.6.4 How Is the Surgical Technique Reviewed to Decide If Appropriate, or If It Requires Refinement?

Two major types of surgeries are performed in laboratory animals:

- Implantation of medical devices allows to ease measurements, administration, or sampling (e.g. vascular catheters, telemetry devices, infusion pumps, and brain cannula).
- Surgeries inducing physiological modifications/alterations (e.g. injection of tumour cells, exeresis, nerve ligation or central nervous system resections, and vascular ligations).

For implantation surgeries, upon the surgery duration and severity as well as upon animal species and strain specificity, complete recovery (wound healing, weight recovery or weight gain, normal behaviour) is expected within a few days, maximum of few weeks post-surgery.

For example, after a jugular vein catheterisation in rats, young adult rats should gain weight again as early as Day 1 or Day 2 post-operatively and get complete wound healing within 5 days.

Healthy and young adult dogs undergoing a blood pressure and ECG telemetry device implantation should maintain or gain weight again within 72 h post-op max and get complete wound healing within 15 days max.

For surgeries inducing physiological changes, discomfort or distress could be expected but every effort should be made to reduce it as much as possible, without compromising the scientific objectives. Quite high post-operative issued rates are sometimes considered as "normal" or "expected" but can in fact be reduced with appropriate care and refinement strategies.

Whatever the surgery type, post-operative problems such as anorexia, abnormal behaviour, self-mutilation, and healing issues should be registered, in a systematic way.

Any recorded post-operative issue should be analysed with the help of experienced persons (veterinarians, technicians, oversight body members).

For example, self-mutilation of surgical wounds could be related to:

- Suture issues (most classically: overtight sutures or staples, unappropriated suture material, inappropriate suture techniques).
- Infection related to aseptic conditions issues.
- Inappropriate environment (no enrichment, no social housing).
- Suboptimal analgesia, leading to difficulty in controlling pain.

Possible causes should be classified upon probability and an action plan should be defined. Its efficacy should be assessed by the working group.

Refinement plans relevance cannot be assessed based on "feelings" but rather on actual data analysis (weight curves, percentage, and severity assessment of self-mutilation etc.).

Other post-operative issues, apart from animal welfare, should lead to discussions and potential change or refinement of the protocol:

- Inefficiency in inducing the desired model or producing the excepted data.
- Lack of reproducibility, reflected by a variation in the expression of the desired model.

11.6.5 Additionally to the Surgical Technique Itself, What Can Improve the Outcome and Wellbeing of the Operated Animals?

Ocular issues: To prevent corneal dehydration resulting in exposure keratitis, animals may

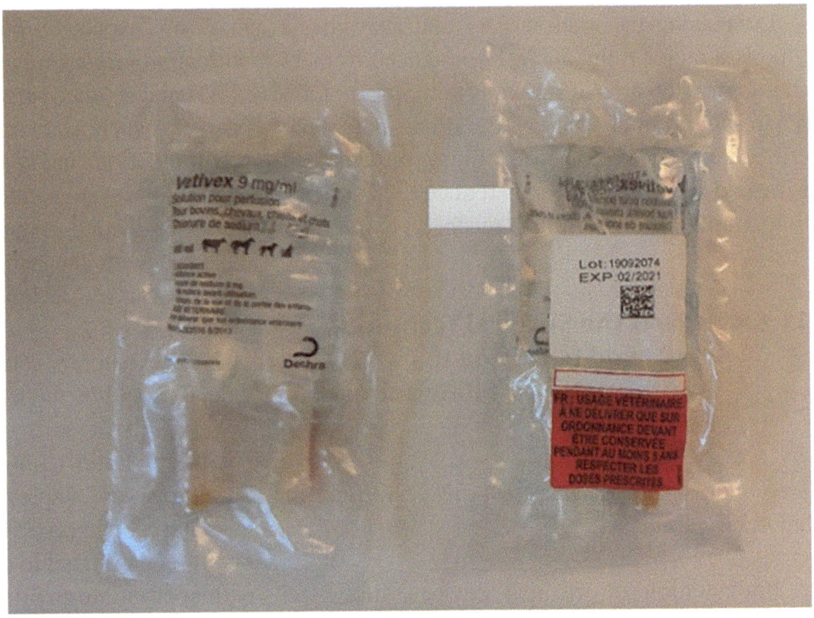

Fig. 11.4 100 mL infusion sterile pockets of NaCl 0.9%

experience during surgery, eye gel should be applied to animals' eyes as soon as the pre-op phase. Common remnant gels, often containing Vaseline, are preferred over water-based gels requiring more regular reapplication. Eye gels are mandatory with ketamine-based protocols.

Dehydration: animals undergoing anaesthesia for long time periods of time are highly susceptible to fluid loss, leading to dehydration and hypotension. In large animals, continuous intravenous infusion of sterile fluids is easily implemented and should be performed. The basic recommended flow rate is 6–10 mL/kg/h in large animals, to be adapted upon monitoring the cardiovascular parameters.

https://www.aaha.org/globalassets/02-guidelines/fluidtherapy/fluidtherapy_guidlines_toolkit.pdf

By contrast, implanting a peripheral catheter and performing a continuous infusion could be highly challenging in small animals (especially, rodents). Alternatively, an intraperitoneal or subcutaneous bolus of warm saline could be administered at pre-op. Boluses of 10–20 mL/kg (to be repeated every 2 hours) are recommended.

Local tissue dehydration: In addition to general rehydration, local tissue dehydration should be prevented. Warm sterile saline should be made available at every step of the surgery and used to regularly irrigate exposed tissues. The use of small sterile infusion pockets, continuously in contact with a heating pad lying underneath sterile drapes, is a convenient way to always have warm saline at your disposal (Fig. 11.4).

11.7 Which Are Anaesthesia Best Practices?

11.7.1 How Do I Choose the Adequate Anaesthetic Protocol for My Experimental Work?

The choice of the anaesthetic protocol depends on:

- The animal species and strain.
- The read outs of the experimental model.
- The available equipment.
- The knowledge of the personnel performing the anaesthesia.

The anaesthetic protocol chosen should guarantee optimal anaesthesia quality for the planned procedure: sufficient duration, adequate depth, and short recovery. If needed, it should provide sufficient analgesia.

Also, it should be safe for the target species, with low morbidity and mortality. It should minimally depress the physiology and homeostasis of the animal and minimally influence the experimental readouts.

It should endorse veterinary best practices, international guidelines and reflect the culture of care of the research institution.

Finally, it must be approved by the responsible authorities according to the national regulations.

11.7.2 Is a Veterinary Anaesthesiologist Required?

It is valuable to consult a veterinary anaesthesiologist (dipl. ECVAA, ACVAA) for selecting the most adapted anaesthesia machine, monitoring and support equipment required (warming blankets, volumetric and syringe pumps, filters etc.) for the planned procedures and building. Also, the veterinary anaesthesiologist can help establish the waste anaesthetic gas (WAG) program and instruct the involved personnel.

Whilst drafting the anaesthetic protocol, it is advisable to discuss with a specialised veterinary anaesthesiologist the choice of drugs, the level of instrumentation required, the peri-operative care, and the preventive analgesia.

Ideally, a veterinary anaesthetist should be present to support the anaesthesia and recovery, when a new protocol is performed for the first time, if large animals are anaesthetised, and in an ideal world should be considered as often as possible. For very complex anaesthetic procedures, an anaesthesiologist caring for the animal is mandatory.

A list of specialists in veterinary anaesthesia is available at https://acvaa.org/diplomate-dashboard/members/ and ECVAA website - Diplomates.

11.7.3 Which Are the Minimal Veterinary Anaesthesia Standards to Be Considered?

The ACVAA, the AAHA, and the ECVAA/AVA have produced standards and guidelines for the safe practice of anaesthesia in clinical veterinary medicine, analogue to the standards for providing safe anaesthesia in humans [18].

https://ava.eu.com/wp-content/uploads/2018/01/AVA-Safer-Anaesthesia-Guildlines-Booklet-VET-Web.pdf

https://acvaa.org/veterinarians/guidelines/

https://www.aaha.org/aaha-guidelines/2020-aaha-anesthesia-and-monitoring-guidelines-for-dogs-and-cats/anesthesia-and-monitoring-home/ [19]

By implementing these standards, the risk of peri-anaesthetic morbidity and mortality is significantly decreased and makes anaesthesia more qualitative and safer.

Despite the tighter regulatory frames for working with laboratory animals, no specific guidelines for anaesthesia exist. These “clinical” guidelines can and should be extrapolated to anaesthesia of animals in a laboratory setting.

11.7.4 What Is the Peri-anaesthetic Period?

The peri-anaesthetic period includes pre-anaesthesia, anaesthesia, and recovery.

The pre-anaesthesia involves the preparation of the equipment, drugs, records, and the animal(s).

11.7.5 To Premedicate or Not? This Is the Question

Premedication is the administration, prior to anaesthesia induction, of drugs aiming to decrease stress, ease anaesthesia induction (and maintenance), and/or prevent side effects of anaesthesia drugs. Phenothiazines, butyrophenones, benzodiazepines, and $\alpha 2$-adrenergic receptors agonists can be injected alone or in combinations with opioids “neuroleptanalgesia” or with hypnotics to induce calmness before and during anaesthesia induction, reduce the sympathetic response to surgical stimulation, reduce anaesthetic requirements and promoting smooth induction and recovery. Analgesia is a feature of some sedatives ($\alpha 2$-adrenergic receptors agonists, opioids), but not all.

Premedication plays an important role in the daily large animal laboratory veterinary practice whilst is less used in small laboratory animals alone because of the limited clinical relevance of the achieved sedation and the preponderant hypotensive and hypothermic side effects. It is mostly part of a multimodal and balanced anaesthesia and analgesia protocol.

Please discuss with the veterinary anaesthesiologist about the best option for your model.

11.7.6 Which Types of Anaesthesia Are Available? What Is Most Preferable?

Based on the animal species, requirements of the experimental model, the equipment available, and personal preference, one can choose between inhalation or injection anaesthesia or a combination of both. The anaesthetic should be "balanced." The concept of balanced anaesthesia was introduced by John Lundy in 1926 in which combinations of drugs are used to produce general anaesthesia, with each drug chosen for a specific effect. The broader goal is to achieve beneficial synergic effects to obtain optimal hypnosis, muscle relaxation, analgesia, and sympathetic stability with the lowest doses of each agent and therefore less undesired side effects.

Figure 11.5 illustrates the role of the different drugs within a balanced anaesthetic protocol in the peri-anaesthetic period [20].

11.7.7 Is It Acceptable to Perform Anaesthesia Without Analgesic Drugs?

This is acceptable for non-painful procedures (i.e. imaging) with short anaesthesia times. If painful procedures are performed, only for terminal experiments (non-recovery) with short anaesthesia times and if the activation of nociception has no impact on the measured parameters. Since the depth of anaesthesia is dose dependent, a correspondingly sufficient depth over a longer period of time can lead to severe respiratory and circulatory depression, especially with injectable mono-anaesthetics (e.g. propofol, alfaxalone, pentobarbital, and etomidate) because of the narrow therapeutic index; this can have a relevant influence on the scientific data obtained and is associated with a high attrition rate due to deaths.

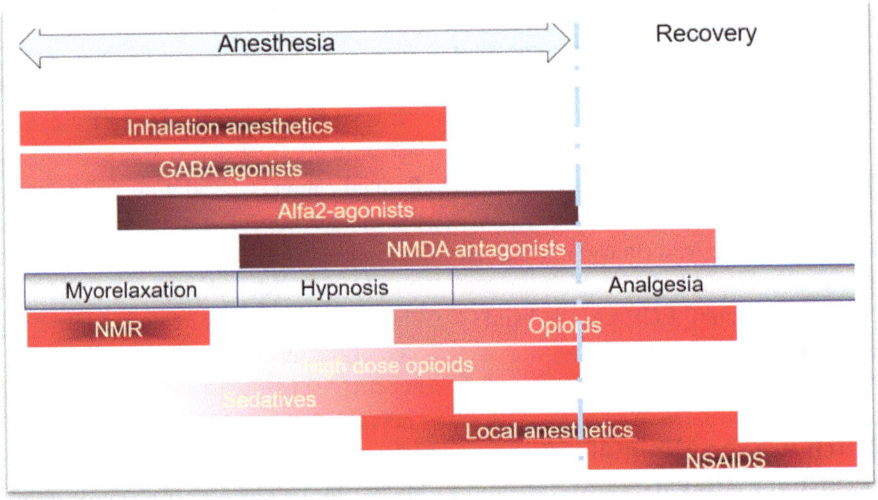

Fig. 11.5 Balanced anaesthesia and analgesia; possible associations over time

11.7.8 Which Is the Minimal Respiratory Support?

Oxygen ***must*** **ALWAYS** be supplemented during anaesthesia, independently of inhalation or injectable, to support tissue oxygenation and avoid hypoxia. As a rule of thumb, 100% O_2 can be used for short procedures, whilst for longer procedures (>2 h), it is strongly advised to use a mixture of air and at least 30% O_2. The recommended inspiratory fraction of oxygen (FiO_2) is 0.3 and should be increased according to the oxygen saturation of the animal measured by pulse oximetry (SpO_2).

Pre-oxygenation is an easy technique to augment the arterial partial pressure in oxygen (PaO_2) and therefore delay desaturation [21, 22] and should be applied as always feasible.

Ideally, endotracheal intubation should be performed for all anaesthetics to protect the airways from aspiration and to allow ventilation of the lungs to maintain normocapnia (End Tidal CO_2 35–45 mmHg). In very small animals (i.e. mice and rats) it can be technically challenging and is therefore not performed routinely. Oxygen and inhalation anaesthesia are administered via face masks in such small patients. Laryngeal masks can be valid alternatives, particularly for rabbits; "mini" devices for rodents are in development [23].

Ventilation can be manual or mechanical and should be used to keep normocapnia. An $ETCO_2$ above 50 mmHg, and associated acidosis, is impairing the normal functioning of Ca^{2+} channels at cellular level and therefore negatively affects cardiac activity and vascular tone. This should be imperatively corrected. Intubation and ventilatory support should be considered (mandatory) for any anaesthesia lasting longer than 60 min as respiratory fatigue and consequent hypercapnia are expected. It is mandatory for thorax surgery, if intracranial hypertension should be avoided or if muscular blocking agents are used.

11.7.9 Which Is the Minimal Cardiovascular Support?

The cardiovascular function must be supported to counteract anaesthetics-related hypotension, bradycardia, arrhythmias, or decreased contractility. These adversely affect organ perfusion and increase morbidity and mortality.

An intravenous catheter will allow the administration of fluids, inotrope, and anticholinergic drugs as needed. Even for the shortest anaesthesia, the placement of a venous access is recommended to administer drugs for anaesthesia but also for support. In the smallest laboratory animals, this is technically difficult and is not performed routinely; the intraperitoneal route is a surrogate alternative.

Before administering additional drugs, it is essential to check and correct excessive anaesthetic depth, hypothermia, and drug overdose, i.e. due to accumulation over time. Also, the selected anaesthetic protocol (total intravenous vs. inhalation anaesthesia vs. balanced) can help minimising the influence on the cardiovascular system and on the model.

11.7.10 Why Is It So Important to Achieve Normothermia?

Mammals need to maintain a nearly constant internal temperature (T°) for optimal enzymatic activity (homoeothermic). If the internal T° deviates substantially from normal, metabolic function generally deteriorates. Mild intraoperative hypothermia (1–2 °C) leads to numerous complications [24]:

1. Triples the risk of cardiac arrhythmias
2. Triples surgical wound infections
3. Prolongs hospitalisation by 20%
4. Increases surgical blood loss (coagulopathy)
5. Modulates pain perception

Hypothermia during anaesthesia is very common because of: (1) a dose-dependent inhibition of thermoregulation: ALL anaesthetics increase the hypothalamic cold threshold up to 20 times (from 0.2 to 2–4 °C) [25, 26] and inhibit vasoconstriction (acepromazine, halogenates, propofol etc.) [27] and shivering (opioids and alpha2 agonists). (2) Furthermore, there is an increased heat loss from the patient's exposure to a cool environment of the operating room, skin preparation and surgery and (3) decreased heat production.

Heat loss during anaesthesia follows a typical three phases pattern [25, 28].

The smaller animals are more prone to hypothermia as they have a high weight/body surface ratio.

11.7.11 What Is the Most Effective Treatment Against Hypothermia?

Animals should be protected against hypothermia *as soon as anaesthesia is induced* and until the animal's full recovery from anaesthesia via heat maintenance systems. Hypothermia leads to increased morbidity and mortality: peri-operative hypothermia increases the risk of bleeding, infection, wound dehiscence, and cardiovascular failure. Also, pain and distress are enhanced whilst being cold [29, 30]. Passive insulation reduces heat loss through the skin [31] but most patients require active warming to maintain a normal T°. Various surface warming systems prevent hypothermia from developing and provide effective warming. The most often used are closed-loop electrical mats in small rodents and forced air [32] or warm water circulation devices in rabbits and onward sizes. When large volumes of fluids must be infused intravenously [33], they must be warmed to body temperature to avoid heat loss. The same process could be used for disinfectant, too.

Monitoring of core temperatures amongst other vital parameters is advisable to detect T° changes, pathophysiologic effects and check the efficacy of measures to prevent or treat hypothermia. It should not be limited to the operative and immediate recovery periods.

Ideally, warming starts already before induction and continues for several hours up to several days after recovery, depending on the surgery and its physiological consequences.

Many different heating systems exist (heating pads, heating lamps, warming cabinets, and so forth) that should be carefully chosen in accordance with, for example the duration of the surgery, animals' size, the animals' position during the surgery. In large animals, beware of electrical heating pads as they often can induce dermal burn lesions. The use of water circulatory pads and forced air warmers is strongly recommended in large animal species.

11.7.12 What Do I Need to Monitor During an Anaesthesia?

The goals of monitoring under anaesthesia are to evaluate (1) the animal's response to anaesthesia, including anaesthetic depth and level of analgesia, (2) its physiologic condition (i.e. cardiovascular, respiratory, and metabolic systems), and (3) equipment function. This allows titrating anaesthesia, to detect early physiologic perturbations and allow intervention before the animal suffers harm, and to detect and correct equipment malfunction.

Ideally, monitoring is done by a person dedicated almost entirely to this task and using clinical skills as instrumental devices on a regular (every 5 min) interval.

Based on the recommendations of the ACVA https://acvaa.org/wp-content/uploads/2019/05/Small-Animal-Monitoring-Guidlines.pdfand AAHA [19], monitoring of the major physiological variables of (1) circulation, (2) oxygenation, (3) ventilation, (4) temperature, and (5) neuromuscular blockade under anaesthesia is mandatory.

Cardiovascular function

- **Mucous membrane colour (MMC)** and capillary refill time (CRT)
- Heart rate (HR)
- **Pulse rate (PR)**
- Electrocardiogram (ECG)
- Systemic arterial blood pressure (sABP)

Anaesthetic depth: The monitoring of different reflexes (mostly oculo-palpebral and pedal) is useful for determining adequate depth of anaesthesia.

- **Whiskers** movements
- **Palpebral** and corneal—stops blinking if too deep or dead
- **Pedal**—pulls away if light and is feeling pain

- Sympathetic stability
- Bispectral index (BIS)

Every precaution to ensure that anaesthetic depth is adapted to the ongoing procedure should be taken. Excessive anaesthesia depth could lead to respiratory depression, respiratory arrest, and eventually death. Most common causes of excessive depth are inadequate injectable doses when injectable drugs are used, or inadequate isoflurane management. When the same isoflurane evaporator is used for induction and maintenance, do not forget to decrease the isoflurane percentage after the induction phase, this is a very common source of incidents. Insufficient anaesthesia depth could lead to partial recovery during surgery, which is a major welfare and ethical concerns.

Oxygenation and respiratory function

- **SpO_2**
- MMC
- **Respiratory rate (RR)**
- Spirometry: Peak inspiratory pressure (PIP), minute volume (MV), Tidal volume (TV)

Temperature (T°)

Neuromuscular relaxation

Haematology and biochemistry (glycaemia, total solids)

Long-lasting procedures, especially in very small animals, may lead to major post-operative hypoglycaemia increasing mortality and morbidity risks. In these cases, glycaemia should be monitored, and species-based adapted methods of post-operative glucose administration should be identified and implemented [34].

Renal function

- Urine output

In **bold**, the minimal set of parameters to be monitored.

11.7.13 Why Is Anaesthetic Record Required?

In practice, the anaesthetic record helps to identify significant trends or unusual values for physiologic parameters and allows assessment of the response to intervention. Records are quite helpful for the retrospective evaluation of adverse events, to understand possible causes and planning of corrective actions. In a nutshell, the records should list all the drugs received by the animal over time and at least HR, sABP, RR, SpO_2, and T° every 5 min.

Please refer to https://acvaa.org/wp-content/uploads/2019/05/Small-Animal-Monitoring-Guidlines.pdf for the practical recommendations.

The records belong to the raw data of your experiments. https://www.aaalac.org/accreditation-program/faqs/#D1

11.7.14 What Are the Strategies to Recognise Anaesthetic Emergencies and Solutions?

Emergencies mostly result from a sum of small problems.

Accurate and regular monitoring (see above) help detect malfunction of equipment or physiologic deregulation and put in place corrective measures before it becomes a catastrophe.

If things still go weird, it is important not to panic, search for help (ideally from an anaesthesiologist or surgeon or senior veterinarian), so one person can care for the patient whilst the other person looks for the cause of the problem, be logical in the approach and apply causal treatment.

It is highly recommended to have an emergency drugs box with the doses (see Table 11.5 as example) and some action flow charts printed and emergency contact numbers in the surgical suite or in locations where anaesthesia is performed.

Preparedness is the best strategy: have a functioning and checked equipment, have a plan, have emergency drugs available.

11.7.15 How to Optimally Take Care of the Animals Post-operatively?

Recovery is an integral part of the peri-operative period and must be monitored and supported

Table 11.5 Emergency drugs for rodents with dose and volumes

Mice/Rat												
					ml / body weight in g							
Drug	Concentration/Dilution in ml NaCl	Route	Dosis	Unit	25	50	100	150	200	250	300	350
Adrenaline (ADRENALIN Sint 0.1 mg/ml)	0.01 mg/ml1 ml in 9 ml NaCl	i.v./i.p.	0.00001	mg/g	0.025	0.05	0.1	0.15	0.2	0.25	0.3	0.35
Amiodarone (AMIODARON Labatec Inj Lös 150 mg/3ml)	0.5 mg/ml0.1 ml in 9.9 ml NaCl	i.v./i.p.	0.005	mg/g	0.25	0.5	1	1.5	2	2.5	3	3.5
Atropine (Atropin sulphate 0.5 mg/l)	0.01 mg/ml0.2 ml in 9.8 ml NaCl	i.v./i.t./i.p./i.os	0.00005	mg/g	0.125	0.25	0.5	0.75	1	1.25	1.5	1.75
Bicarbonate 8.4% (1 mEq/ml)	0.1 mEq/ml1 ml in 9 ml NaCl	i.v./i.os/i.p.	0.001	mEq/g	0.25	0.5	1	1.5	2	2.5	3	3.5
Calcium gluconate 10%	10 mg/ml1 ml in 9 ml NaCl	i.v./i.os/i.p.	0.05	mg/g	0.125	0.25	0.5	0.75	1	1.25	1.5	1.75
Flumazenil (Flumazenil 0.5 mg/5 ml)	0.01 mg/ml1 ml in 9 ml NaCl	i.v./i.t/i.p./i.os	0.00002	mg/g	0.05	0.1	0.2	0.3	0.4	0.5	0.6	0.7
Furosemide (Lasix 20 mg/ml)	1 mg/ml1 ml in 9 ml NaCl	i.v./i.m.	0.005	mg/g	0.125	0.25	0.5	0.75	1	1.25	1.5	1.75
Lidocaine 2% (20 mg/ml)	0.2 mg/ml0.1 ml in 9.9 ml NaCl	i.v./i.t./i.p./i.os	0.002	mg/g	0.25	0.5	1	1.5	2	2.5	3	3.5
Mannitol 20% (MANNITOL Bichsel Inf Lös 20 g/100ml)	200 mg/ml	i.v./i.p./i.os	1	mg/g	0.125	0.25	0.5	0.75	1	1.25	1.5	1.75
Meth-Prednisolone (Solumedrol 40 mg/ml)	0.4 mg/ml0.1 ml in 9.9 ml NaCl	i.v./(i.m.)	0.002	mg/g	0.125	0.25	0.5	0.75	1	1.25	1.5	1.75
Naloxone (NALOXON OrPha Inj Lös 0.4 mg/ml)	0.04 mg/ml1 ml in 9 ml NaCl	i.v./i.t./i.p./i.os	0.00004	mg/g	0.025	0.05	0.1	0.15	0.2	0.25	0.3	0.35

until the animal is fully conscious, is able to maintain its normophysiology and expresses its species-specific behaviours. Depending on the species and the severity of the model, the first 24–48 h are crucial but can range from a few hours to one week. It is easy to do, does not require specialist knowledge or expensive technology, but is the key to a successful outcome.

Any sign of post-operative hypothermia, dehydration, hypoxia, and haemorrhage should be detected and treated accordingly.

Overarching recommendations are:

- Consider antagonisation if recovery is delayed. Remember antagonisation can antagonise analgesia.
- Empty the bladder for a quiet recovery, especially if a lot of fluids have been administered.
- Eye gel should eventually be applied again.
- Place the animal in its home cage with soft bedding and known smell. Social animals should, as much as possible, be group housed again as soon as completely awake. The presence of skin suture stitches or staples is not a valid reason to single housing animals, as congeners-mutilation is very rare. However, for some specific surgeries for which fragile items (e.g. brain cannula and catheter ports) are accessible to congeners, individual housing may have to be considered. In this case, large cages with mid-separation allowing at least some contacts between animals are preferred [35].
- Many surgeries lead to post-operative discomfort and anorexia that might not be fully compensated by the administration of analgesics. Therefore, strategies should be defined to help animals access to water and feed. For example:
  - Animals undergoing abdominal surgeries may have difficulties to climb and access food in cage grids = > few pellets can be placed in the bottom of the cage.
  - Animals undergoing long-run stereotaxic surgeries may experience difficulties in chewing hard pellets = > pellets can be moistened or of soft food can be delivered.
  - Different laboratory animals food suppliers are offering special post-operative flavour-enhanced, nutritionally fortified soft food. It could be of major interest to avoid post-operative anorexia. However, many animal species especially rodents and pigs tend to be neophobic and will not eat new food at first presentation. Therefore, when special post-operative food must be provided, a habituation of classically 3 days to 1 week is strongly advised, before surgery.
- Provide warmth and O_2 until the animal can maintain normothermia by placing the animals in a warm environment (warming cabinet, cages on heating pads, or cages under heating lamps "cave": NO direct exposure to infrared lamps!!) until complete recovery. Some surgeries may lead to long-run sensitivity to hypothermia (e.g. hypophysectomies). For these models, housing the animals in dedicated warm rooms or cabinets for several days post-surgery might be of interest.
  - For rodents 32 °C to 36 °C for 24 h–48 h.
  - Check body T° regularly with the use of non-invasive IR thermometers or microchips.
- Once the animals are fully awake, they should be checked on a very regular basis. They should be weighed daily for at least 3 days post-op (minor procedures) and their wound healing assessed at least daily, until complete healing. Food and water intake could also be followed.
- Post-operative animals' environment should allow animals to hide, build nests and chew. Absence of sufficient enrichment items is significantly increasing self-mutilation or congeners-mutilation risk.
- When animals are exposed to post-operative constraints (e.g. if animals must wear a collar or a jacket post-operatively, be continuously connected to a balanced arm), strategies to prevent discomfort as much as possible should be identified. For collars, for example many teams are reporting that removing collars 1 hour per day (with a close observation from animal caretakers) allows the animals normal grooming behaviour and significantly increases their comfort and wellbeing as compared to a situation where the collar is left in place 24 hours a day.

- Provide and monitor analgesia (see questions below).

11.7.16 What Is Terminal Anaesthesia?

Terminal anaesthesia can be:

- An anaesthetic which continues until the animal is euthanised at the termination of the experimental procedure.
- An anaesthesia is purposefully induced for performing euthanasia.

In all cases, anaesthesia must be sufficiently deep (surgical anaesthesia) and at no point during the procedure the animal is permitted to regain any level of conscious pain perception [36]. The choice of the drugs depends on their influence on the experimental readout.

As a rule of thumb, three times the anaesthetic dose or > MAC_{bar} is adequate for terminal anaesthesia.

Death occurs secondary to irreversible respiratory and cardiovascular depression for an overdose of pentobarbital or MS222 but a physical method should be used to confirm death. In other cases, i.e. overdose of xylazine/ketamine or inhalation anaesthesia, a secondary chemical (i.e. i.v. injection of K^+) or a physical method must be used to induce death.

Please refer to the question on performing anaesthesia without analgesics and to Chap. 12 on euthanasia for more detailed information.

11.8 Which Are the Best Practices for Peri-operative Analgesia?

11.8.1 What Is Preventive Analgesia?

In the case of surgical or painful procedures, **preventive** analgesia—which includes a) pre-emptive, b) intra-operative, and c) post-operative analgesia—must be planned, to effectively cover the chronological development of pain and the estimated intensity. This is regarded as an integral part of balanced anaesthesia and includes the post-operative phase.

Preventive analgesia is intended to prevent the wind-up phenomenon and the development of secondary hyperalgesia. This has a positive effect on the perception of pain following the return to consciousness and also reduces the development of chronic pain. The latter might be less relevant to laboratory animal medicine but important for long-term experiments or heavily instrumented large animals. It should be used in all experiments with recovery, whenever possible.

One size does not fit all … The analgesic protocol must be tailored to the species, the peculiarities of the model, the expected pain intensity, and very importantly, the influence on the experimental readouts.

Some systematic guidance is provided in https://www.gv-solas.de/wp-content/uploads/2021/08/2021-04_Pain_Management_for_laboratory_animals.pdf

11.8.2 Which Drugs Can I Use for Analgesia?

Analogue to anaesthesia, combined analgesic regimens (balanced analgesia) or multimodal approaches are state-of-the-art to prevent/treat post-operative pain [37]. Multimodal analgesia uses a combination of analgesic drugs from different classes along with analgesic techniques targeting different pain mechanisms (mechanistic analgesia). The goal is to maximise the quality of analgesia whilst decreasing the doses of the single analgesics and the related side effects. Saying this, post-operative pain being mostly inflammatory in nature, cornerstone analgesic (if you have to select one drug) must be an anti-inflammatory drug, such as NSAID.

According to the WHO Pain ladder [38] non-opioids drugs as NSAIDs or local anaesthetics (LA), weak and strong opioids, and adjuvants should be combined over time depending on the pain intensity. Local anaesthesia, or loco-regional anaesthesia, is the only analgesic procedure able to prevent any pain perception and to decrease drastically the anaesthetic needs. Opioids and adjuvants often present the advantage to decrease the anaesthetic needs, so the general anaesthetic depth, and in consequence the undesired side effects of general anaesthetics.

11.8.3 For How Long Should I Provide Analgesia?

Pain is a dynamic process and can vary chronologically in its severity. The pain should, therefore, be regularly and frequently assessed during the expected peaks of pain, e.g. in the first hours following an operation or in the later stage of painful, progressive diseases. These times are dependent on the species and the nature of the experimental procedure. Pain treatment should be continued until pain symptoms are present.

Classically, post-operative pain requires an analgesic cover by a minimum of 2 days, and in general 4 days. Depending on the surgical procedure, it could go up to 2 weeks (or, even more).

11.8.4 Is It Recommended to Perform a Local Anaesthesia?

Yes! Local anaesthetics (LA) are administered through various routes to desensitise-specific areas or regions of the body and provide effective and reliable analgesia throughout species without major side effects. They are increasingly used in laboratory animal anaesthesia for preventive pain treatment and contribute to balanced anaesthesia and analgesia.

Local anaesthetic can be administered topically on the intact skin or mucous membranes and implies that the drug penetrates the stratum corneum of the epidermis or the mucosal layers, respectively. For neuraxial use, including both intrathecal and epidural administrations, LA are often combined with other classes of analgesics, such as opioids, alpha2 adrenoreceptor agonists, and ketamine, which act synergistically with the LA agents enhancing the sensory block. Infiltrations of LA are commonly performed to provide peri-operative analgesia in laboratory animal species.

At the end of the procedure and before terminating general anaesthesia, do not hesitate to repeat local blocks.

11.8.5 Are Local Anaesthetics Safe?

The non-specific molecular targets of the LA are at the origin of some of their adverse and toxic effects in various organ systems [39]. Local anaesthetics interfere with the axonal voltage-gated Na^+ channels preferentially, which implies blockade of also voltage-dependent K^+, L-type Ca^{2+}, and Na^+ channels in the brain and heart; as a result, most of the clinically relevant adverse effects of LA are produced on the central nervous and cardiovascular systems.

If the dose is well calculated, they are very safe for use and they minimally interfere with the experimental read outs. They might have minimal anti-inflammatory action.

11.8.6 How Is Pain in Animals Undergoing Anaesthesia Assessed?

Under anaesthesia animals **cannot feel** pain as they are unconscious. Therefore, under anaesthesia we monitor nociception, that is the neural conduction and processing of noxious stimuli in the central nervous system [40]. Clinically we can observe sympathetic instability with increased systolic BP, HR, and RR, eventually arrhythmias and lightening of the anaesthetic depth, up to sudden movements. So far, there is no device that measures "nociception" to be used routinely in veterinary anaesthesia.

11.8.7 How Is Pain in Awake Animals Assessed?

Assessing pain in animals is problematic, as they are not able to express themselves verbally. Whilst it is difficult to investigate their emotional state directly, it is possible to draw indirect conclusions based on a combination of clinical symptoms, and physiological or behavioural changes "composite pain scores". In the recent past, major advances have been made in the development and validation of methods for the identification and quantification of pain in different animal species. One example is the development and validation of the Grimace Scale for acute, post-surgical pain for different species. Aside from classical bioindicators (clinical symptoms, physiological changes, and appearance), there are also various ethological indicators for pain and diminished wellbeing that have been introduced for different animal species. They are based on pain-induced changes (reduction or stimulation) of typical behaviour [41]. The indicators should be tested for their sensitivity (the ability to identify animals in pain correctly), particularly different intensities of pain, and their specificity (the ability to identify those that are not suffering pain), for example pain being confounded with persisting sedation affecting bioindicators [42].

It is possible to treat pain only when it is recognised and quantified.

11.8.8 Why the Compilation of a Post-intervention Score Sheet Is Required?

The use of score sheets allows for a structured and objective recording of clinical indicators of wellbeing and pain. Score sheets should be as simple as possible, but as detailed as needed, and tailored to the model. They help reduce inter-observer variability and allow the setting of actions and endpoints.

11.8.9 Why Is It Important to Treat Pain?

Pain in animals must be relieved for a series of interlinked reasons:

- To comply with an ethical must and to honour an ideal of preserving animal rights to integrity.
- To reduce scientific bias: the systemic effects of unrelieved pain represent a great scientific bias leading to greater data variability, increased numbers of animals, data that cannot be reproduced, missing data points … and finally with unpublishable data. This "waste of animals", of time, and resources is unethical and unacceptable.
- To comply with legal dispositions and accreditation, the main purpose being to prevent or, at least, minimise pain and distress.
- The public views pain and suffering in animal experiments as the major argument against research using animals. And many scientists share this concern.

11.8.10 What to Do in Case of a Disaster and Animals Are Under Anaesthesia?

The disaster plan of the Institution should include actions to be taken in case of emergencies or disasters, and animals are under anaesthesia/surgery [43].

If there is imminent danger to the surgical staff, the team should evacuate immediately. If time permits, the animal should be euthanised with an overdose of an appropriate injectable anaesthetic or euthanasia agent.

In case a surgical team evacuation is required, but there is not an immediate danger present, different actions can be taken, if the surgical incision has been/not been made at the time of the alarm.

Please refer to Chap. 17 on Emergency Plan and Disaster Planning for more details.

11.8.11 Is the Description of the Anaesthesia and Analgesia Protocols in the Manuscript Important?

Anaesthesia and analgesia protocols must be reported in published work to serve as guidance to the scientific community, increase the reproducibility of the performed research and support transparency.

Anaesthesia and analgesia reporting are included in the "ARRIVE Essential 10"; these ten items are the basic minimum that must be included in any manuscript describing animal research. Without this information, readers and reviewers cannot assess the reliability of the findings [44]. https://arriveguidelines.org/arrive-guidelines

11.9 Which Are the Key Strategies for Achieving State-of-the-Art Anaesthesia, Analgesia, and Surgery in an Animal Care and Use Program?

Key points are:

- Establishing an **optimal peri-anaesthetic and operative care program**

  Pre-operative care:

  Minimise stress as much as possible (tools: acclimatisation, environmental strategies, handling, habituation, premedication) and start temperature support.

  Intra-operative care:

  – Anaesthesia:

    Check and have the equipment ready. Use balanced, multimodal anaesthesia and analgesia, anaesthetise in a quiet environment, care for drug doses, and closely monitor throughout. Support ventilation if anaesthesia is lasting >1 h. Support cardiovascular function. Protect their eyes. Fill your protocol.

  – Surgery**:**

    Use aseptic, minimally invasive, and atraumatic techniques with adapted instrumentation, prevent tissue desiccation, judiciously use sutures (appropriate size), and avoiding tension upon closure.

- *Post-surgical care:*

  Keep animals under close monitoring and accelerate awakening if necessary (through antagonisation and rewarming). Support normothermia until complete recovery. Prolong analgesia administration for few days' post-surgery as required, at the proper dose and frequency. Weigh and check animals on a daily basis for at least 3 days; provide critical care feed. Limit individual housing time.
- Avoiding peri-operative hypothermia.
- Using **preventive analgesia** and local blocks with LAs and loco-regional techniques.

11.10 Some Nice Sentences

- Progress is impossible without change and those who cannot change their minds cannot change anything (GB Shaw).
- *Primum, non nocere.*
- There are no safe anaesthetic agents, there are no safe anaesthetic procedures, and there are only safe anaesthetists.
- Science sans conscience n'est que ruine de l'âme (Rabelais).
- Pharmacological treatment is the base of pain treatment (American Pain Society).

11.11 Legal Frames

Directive 2010/63/EU of the European Parliament and of the Council of 22 September 2010 on the protection of animals used for scientific purposes https://eur-lex.europa.eu/legal-content/EN/TXT/?uri=CELEX:32010L0063

Directive 89/391/EEC, Occupational Safety and Health (OSH) "Framework Directive" https://eur-lex.europa.eu/legal-content/EN/TXT/?uri=CELEX%3A31989L0391&qid=1615985898418

National Laws and Regulations

Resources (Recap')

https://acvaa.org/veterinarians/guidelines/

https://acvaa.org/wp-content/uploads/2019/05/Control-of-Waste-Anesthetic-Gas-Recommendations.pdf

https://acvaa.org/wp-content/uploads/2019/05/Small-Animal-Monitoring-Guidlines.pdf

https://www.aaalac.org/accreditation-program/faqs/#D1

https://www.aaha.org/aaha-guidelines/2020-aaha-anesthesia-and-monitoring-guidelines-for-dogs-and-cats/anesthesia-and-monitoring-home/ [19]

https://arc-w.nihr.ac.uk/research/projects/low-versus-high-dead-space-syringes-user-preferences-and-attitudes/

https://arriveguidelines.org/arrive-guidelines

https://ava.eu.com/wp-content/uploads/2018/01/AVA-Safer-Anaesthesia-Guildlines-Booklet-VET-Web.pdf

https://ccac.ca/en/guidelines-and-policies/

https://grants.nih.gov/grants/olaw/guide-for-the-care-and-use-of-laboratory-animals.pdf

https://www.gv-solas.de/wp-content/uploads/2021/08/2020_10Food_withdrawal.pdf

https://www.gv-solas.de/wp-content/uploads/2021/08/2021-04_Pain_Management_for_laboratory_animals.pdf

https://www.issa.int/sites/default/files/documents/prevention/2%20-%20Consensus%20Paper%20Anaesthetic%20Gases-36710.pdf

https://nc3rs.org.uk/e-learning-resources

https://www.osha.gov/waste-anesthetic-gases

https://researchanimaltraining.com/elearning/

http://www.sohf.ch/Themes/Operation/2869_29_D.pdf

Disclaimer The authors declare no conflict of interest.

Authorship All authors contributed in equal parts to this chapter.

References

1. Mike A. Assessing the shelf life of aseptically prepared injectables in ready to administer containers. Eur J Hosp Phar Sci Pract. 2012;19:277.
2. Chakravarti S, Basu S. Modern anaesthesia vapourisers. Indian J Anaesth. 2013;57:464–71.
3. Goneppanavar U, Prabhu M. Anaesthesia machine: checklist, hazards, scavenging. Indian J Anaesth. 2013;57:533–40.
4. Castelhano-Carlos MJ, Baumans V. The impact of light, noise, cage cleaning and in-house transport on welfare and stress of laboratory rats. Lab Anim. 2009;43:311–27.
5. Obernier JA, Baldwin RL. Establishing an appropriate period of acclimatization following transportation of laboratory animals. ILAR J. 2006;47:364–9.
6. Arts JW, Kramer K, Arndt SS, et al. The impact of transportation on physiological and behavioral parameters in Wistar rats: implications for acclimatization periods. ILAR J. 2012;53:E82–98.
7. Gouveia K, Hurst JL. Optimising reliability of mouse performance in behavioural testing: the major role of non-aversive handling. Sci Rep. 2017;7:44999.
8. Boxall J, Heath S, Bate S, et al. Modern concepts of socialisation for dogs: implications for their behaviour, welfare and use in scientific procedures. Altern Lab Anim. 2004;32(Suppl 2):81–93.
9. Otis C, Gervais J, Guillot M, et al. Concurrent validity of different functional and neuroproteomic pain assessment methods in the rat osteoarthritis monosodium iodoacetate (MIA) model. Arthritis Res Ther. 2016;18:150.
10. Alsafran S, Sherman SK, Dahdaleh FS, et al. Preoperative calcitriol reduces postoperative intravenous calcium requirements and length of stay in parathyroidectomy for renal-origin hyperparathyroidism. Surgery. 2019;165:151–7.
11. Milovancev M, Schmiedt CW. Preoperative factors associated with postoperative hypocalcemia in dogs with primary hyperparathyroidism that underwent parathyroidectomy: 62 cases (2004-2009). J Am Vet Med Assoc. 2013;242:507–15.
12. de Brito Galvao JF, Chew DJ. Metabolic complications of endocrine surgery in companion animals. Vet Clin North Am Small Anim Pract. 2011;41:847–68.
13. Van de Putte P, Perlas A. The link between gastric volume and aspiration risk. In search of the Holy Grail? Anaesthesia. 2018;73:274–9.
14. Cambruzzi M, Macfarlane P. Variation in syringes and needles dead space compared to the International Organization for Standardization standard 7886-1:2018. Vet Anaesth Analg. 2021;48:532–6.
15. Couceiro J, Castro R, Tien H, et al. Step by step: microsurgical training method combining two nonliving animal models. J Vis Exp. 2015:e52625.
16. Spain DA, Miller FB. Education and training of the future trauma surgeon in acute care surgery: trauma, critical care, and emergency surgery. Am J Surg. 2005;190:212–7.
17. Akalestou E, Genser L, Villa F, et al. Establishing a successful rat model of duodenal- jejunal bypass: a detailed guide. Lab Anim. 2019;53:362–71.
18. Gelb AW, Morriss WW, Johnson W, et al. World Health Organization-World Federation of Societies of Anaesthesiologists (WHO-WFSA) International Standards for a Safe Practice of Anesthesia. Anesth Analg. 2018;126:2047–55.
19. Grubb T, Sager J, Gaynor JS, et al. 2020 AAHA anesthesia and monitoring guidelines for dogs and cats. J Am Anim Hosp Assoc. 2020;56:59–82.
20. Fish RE. Anesthesia and analgesia in laboratory animals. 2nd ed. London: Elsevier/Academic Press; 2008.
21. Nimmagadda U, Salem MR, Crystal GJ. Preoxygenation: physiologic basis, benefits, and potential risks. Anesth Analg. 2017;124:507–17.

22. Azam Danish M. Preoxygenation and anesthesia: a detailed review. Cureus. 2021;13:e13240.
23. Cheong SH, Lee JH, Kim MH, et al. Airway management using a supraglottic airway device without endotracheal intubation for positive ventilation of anaesthetized rats. Lab Anim. 2013;47:89–93.
24. Kurz A, Sessler DI, Lenhardt R. Perioperative normothermia to reduce the incidence of surgical-wound infection and shorten hospitalization. Study of Wound Infection and Temperature Group. N Engl J Med. 1996;334:1209–15.
25. Sessler DI. Perioperative heat balance. Anesthesiology. 2000;92:578–96.
26. Armstrong S, Roberts B, Aronsohn M. Perioperative hypothermia. J Vet Emerg Crit Care. 2005;15:32–7.
27. Xiong J, Kurz A, Sessler DI, et al. Isoflurane produces marked and nonlinear decreases in the vasoconstriction and shivering thresholds. Anesthesiology. 1996;85:240–5.
28. Kurz A, Sessler DI, Christensen R, et al. Thermoregulatory vasoconstriction and perianesthetic heat transfer. Acta Anaesthesiol Scand Suppl. 1996;109:30–3.
29. Slotman GJ, Jed EH, Burchard KW. Adverse effects of hypothermia in postoperative patients. Am J Surg. 1985;149:495–501.
30. Frank SM, Fleisher LA, Breslow MJ, et al. Perioperative maintenance of normothermia reduces the incidence of morbid cardiac events. A randomized clinical trial. JAMA. 1997;277:1127–34.
31. Matsukawa T, Sessler DI, Sessler AM, et al. Heat flow and distribution during induction of general anesthesia. Anesthesiology. 1995;82:662–73.
32. Sessler DI, Moayeri A. Skin-surface warming: heat flux and central temperature. Anesthesiology. 1990;73:218–24.
33. Heimbach D, Jurkovich G, Gentiello L. Accidental hypothermia. 4th ed. WB Saunders; 2000.
34. Hsi ZY, Stewart LA, Lloyd KCK, et al. Hypoglycemia after bariatric surgery in mice and optimal dosage and efficacy of glucose supplementation. Comp Med. 2020;70:111–8.
35. Boggiano MM, Cavigelli SA, Dorsey JR, et al. Effect of a cage divider permitting social stimuli on stress and food intake in rats. Physiol Behav. 2008;95:222–8.
36. Silverman J. Terminal procedures: Should an IACUC require a literature review for less painful alternatives? Lab Anim. 2017;46:9–9.
37. Kehlet H, Dahl JB. The value of "multimodal" or "balanced analgesia" in postoperative pain treatment. Anesth Analg. 1993;77:1048–56.
38. Ventafridda V, Saita L, Ripamonti C, et al. WHO guidelines for the use of analgesics in cancer pain. Int J Tissue React. 1985;7:93–6.
39. Scholz A. Mechanisms of (local) anaesthetics on voltage-gated sodium and other ion channels. Br J Anaesth. 2002;89:52–61.
40. Ghanty I, Schraag S. The quantification and monitoring of intraoperative nociception levels in thoracic surgery: a review. J Thorac Dis. 2019;11:4059–71.
41. Tansley SN, Tuttle AH, Wu N, et al. Modulation of social behavior and dominance status by chronic pain in mice. Genes Brain Behav. 2019;18:e12514.
42. Golledge H, Jirkof P. Score sheets and analgesia. Lab Anim. 2016;50:411–3.
43. Kelly FE, Bailey CR, Aldridge P, et al. Fire safety and emergency evacuation guidelines for intensive care units and operating theatres: for use in the event of fire, flood, power cut, oxygen supply failure, noxious gas, structural collapse or other critical incidents. Anaesthesia. 2021;76:1377–91.
44. Percie du Sert N, Hurst V, Ahluwalia A, et al. The ARRIVE guidelines 2.0: updated guidelines for reporting animal research. PLoS Biol. 2020;18:e3000410.

Practical Aspects When Humanely Killing Different Species of Animals in Research

12

Susanne Rensing

Abstract

Most research animals being euthanized for research are rodents and fish, but also larger species (e.g., dogs and nonhuman primates) including agricultural animals. In the European Union, Directive 2010/63/EU is the legal framework, giving guidance on the selection of methods by species. This chapter offers responses to practical questions on the humane killing of animals in research including legal, ethical, competence, and safety aspects, as well as particularities by species. Euthanasia of animals shall be carried out as soon as possible, causing minimum pain and distress by applying humane endpoints. The procedure shall be performed in a dedicated room by trained personnel and the method shall be aligned with the purpose of the research. Safety of the research staff and animals must be ensured through all phases including discarding of the carcasses.

Keywords

Carbon dioxide · Chemical drugs · Equipment · Humane endpoint · Ethics · Chemical drug · Neonatal animals

S. Rensing (✉)
AbbVie Deutschland GmbH & Co KG, Ludwigshafen, Germany
e-mail: susanne.rensing@abbvie.com

12.1 Introduction

The *Guide for the Care and Use of Laboratory Animals* [1] is a widely accepted reference in the world of laboratory animal medicine and describes Euthanasia as the act of humanely killing animals by methods that induce rapid unconsciousness and death. Euthanizing laboratory animals is a sensitive and regulated procedure that must be carried out with the utmost care to minimize pain and distress, decision on euthanasia must be reached swiftly and appropriate actions taken promptly if suffering is to be prevented [2]. Identification and use of methods that offer a death with minimal suffering is a moral imperative [3]. Someone in the laboratory will have to carry out the procedure of euthanasia and actively killing the animal rather than leaving it to die, euthanasia is not necessarily the most difficult part of the procedure for the animal, but may be the most difficult part for the researcher. The specific methods and considerations can vary when euthanizing different species of laboratory animals. Paying attention to the logistics including tissue collection as some analytes, tissue quality may change rapidly within/after euthanasia, also to be consistent and data reproducibility. Stress may alter glucagon, gluconeogenesis, and blood glucose levels within seconds, and other parameters like insulin, B- and T-cells within minutes. Study needs should be taken into consideration when choosing the method and the

J. Guillén, V. Galligioni (eds.), *Practical Management of Research Animal Care and Use Programs*, Laboratory Animal Science and Medicine 3, https://doi.org/10.1007/978-3-031-65414-5_12

most recent literature consulted the impact on research [4].

12.2 What Is the Legal Framework?

Personnel performing euthanasia must ensure compliance with regulations, ethical guidelines, and institutional policies. This often involves obtaining approval from competent authorities and from an Institutional Animal Use and Care Committee (IACUC) or similar regulatory body (Oversight Body). The Directive 2010/63/EU lists in Appendix IV approved method of euthanasia by species. If based on scientific evidence the competent authorities may grant exemption from the requirements to allow the use of another method, which is considered at least as humane. The scientific justification must prove that the purpose of the procedure cannot be achieved using one of the killing methods listed in Appendix IV. The AVMA guidelines for the euthanasia of animals [5] are intended for the use by members of the veterinary profession who carry out or oversee the euthanasia of animals. As mentioned previously the sensitivity of euthanasia, it is critical to review the most recent research and literature on humane killing and ensure the training of personnel including continuous refinement of procedures. When reviewing Appendix IV of the Directive 2010/63/EU, the European Commission added more specific recommendations for cephalopods, zebrafish, and passerine birds [6]. The Directive 2010/63/EU indicates that the killing of animals shall be completed by one of the following methods: confirmation of permanent cessation of the circulation, destruction of the brain, dislocation of the neck, exsanguination, or confirmation of the onset of *rigor mortis*.

12.3 What Are the Ethical Considerations when Performing Euthanasia?

Experimental animals may need to be killed for numerous reasons, but mostly before their natural life expectations come to an end. The collection of usable data is essential since, without that, any suffering caused would be pointless and unethical, as the animal has been used without purpose or scientific input [2]. A decision to keep an animal alive at the end of a procedure shall be taken by a veterinarian. An animal shall be killed when it is likely to remain in moderate or severe pain, suffering and distress, or lasting harm (Directive 2010/63/EU, Art. 17). The welfare of the animals should be the top priority throughout the process. Euthanizing animals, especially in a research context, can be emotionally challenging for those involved, ensure that support mechanisms are in place to help personnel cope with the emotional aspects of the process. A Culture of Care Strategy is an important factor in how animal care and use programs operate considering both the staff and the animals used [7]. Personnel may prefer non-contact approaches (e.g., CO_2 Euthanasia) instead of physical methods. The goal of achieving an optimal killing method is multi-faceted, representing a balance between animal welfare outcomes, reliability, scientific integrity, operator safety, and the well-being of personnel [3].

12.4 Why Is the Implementation of Humane Endpoints So Important?

The idea behind humane endpoint is to define a set of intervention points that allow the collection of quality scientific data, but limits the amount of suffering, either contingent or direct [8]. Humane endpoints may not be identical to scientific endpoints. A detailed scoring sheet, specific for the research area and species may assist when humane endpoints are reached with clear instructions that euthanasia method must be used. The working group of the Berlin Animal Welfare officers published a guidance document on how to develop a scoring sheet including severity assessment [9]. The use of humane endpoints may be general or more specific, e.g., carcinogenicity studies considering tumor burden endpoints and in vaccine research.

12.5 What Are the Selection Criteria of Euthanasia Methods?

The appropriate euthanasia method should be chosen based on the species, size, and age of the animal. Rodents remain the most widely used species for scientific research. Common methods include overdose of anesthetics, injectable agents (e.g., pentobarbital), Carbon dioxide (CO_2) inhalation, and concussion by blunt force trauma, cervical dislocation, decapitation, and microwave irradiation. The selected method should cause minimal pain and distress. Animals should be handled and restrained to minimize stress and avoid injury during the euthanasia process. Animals should be handled in a gentle manner and maybe acclimatized to the procedure. Techniques will vary depending on the species. The location where the euthanasia takes place should also be taken into consideration as the animal may be frightened, when conscious and may show behavioral responses such as vocalization struggling, urination, or defecation. Any fear and distress may be communicated by sound or smell to other animals causing further distress. Animals should be monitored during the process when death occurs, and the animal does not recover consciousness. In some cases, confirmation of death may be necessary through methods like checking of absence of vital signs, lack of reflexes, the cessation of heartbeat, and the onset of rigor mortis. This becomes mandatory when using CO_2. Detailed records should be maintained of the euthanasia process, including the date, method, personnel involved, and any other observations made, proper documentation is essential for regulatory compliance and research purposes.

12.6 What Is to Be Considered for the Selection of the Euthanasia Equipment and Mechanical Methods?

Appropriate equipment and supplies, such as gas chamber for CO_2 euthanasia, sharp containers for discarding injectable agents, and instruments for cervical dislocation or decapitation must be available, well maintained, and regularly checked for proper functioning. The Occupational Health and Safety Officer should be involved in laying out the process for human safety. Regular servicing of the required equipment like vaporizers is recommended. Cleanliness is also important as blood or porphyrin staining are known stressors. Carbone et al. described that up to 25% of cervical dislocation was performed incorrectly [10]. Decapitation by guillotine avoids hypoxia, but hemolysis may be observed when collecting blood and aspiration of blood into the lungs. There is an ongoing discussion about retained awareness after decapitation. Increased EEG (electro-encephalogram) activity could be shown at least for 10–15 s after decapitation [11], visual evoked potential (VEP) decreased within 10–15 s. The exsanguination resulted within 2.7 s into hypoxia and loss of consciousness. Animals shall be anesthetized prior to cervical dislocation or decapitation when over 150 g of body weight.

Focused Microwave Beam Irradiation may be used for specific scientific questions to collect brain tissue but may decrease the level of RNA. The method is rapid, within 600–900 milliseconds (ms) in rats and 100–330 ms for mice. Cervical dislocation requires placing the finger (manual) or an instrument (mechanical) behind the base of the skull while pulling the tail firmly to achieve rapid separation of the cervical vertebrate [3]. This method may also not be feasible for neonatal animals. As a physical method it is often considered unpleasant. The accuracy and efficacy are crucial for the success rate and to be recognized as a reliable method. Studies have reported that 20–25% of mice exhibited thoracic rather than cervical fractures and 9.6% had no cervical dislocation at all. Therefore, regular checks of practical skills should be assessed. Concussion is a reversible procedure and must be followed immediately by another killing method.

12.7 What Is the Most Common Chemical Drug Used for Euthanasia?

When choosing a chemical method, Pentobarbital is the drug of choice, resulting first in respiratory depression, followed by hypoxia and death. It has a narrow safety margin, is potent and can be formulated as a concentrated solution so that relatively small volumes are needed and a rapid onset when given intravenously. Pentobarbital is a strong alkaline, and even dilution will not change the pH dramatically, a pH>10 may cause local tissue damage and decrease smooth muscle functions, especially in the spleen (engorgement with blood). A formulation with rhodamine dye may alter histology. Although the intravenous route is preferred, it is often impractical and will be administered intraperitoneal in rats and mice. Newer research showed that when given intraperitoneal in rodents, it causes pain before the onset of unconsciousness. Animals may vocalize or show writhing behavior. Combining with a local anesthetic may prevent the pain, following the veterinary practice of multi-modal anesthesia/analgesia. A higher dose (>100 mg/kg) results in a higher effect and faster onset of unconsciousness. Attention should be paid during intraperitoneal dosing not to mis-inject, e.g., into the cecum resulting also in a delayed onset of unconsciousness and may be seen as failed euthanasia if time to death exceeds 20 min [12]. Alternative intrahepatic injection is not recommended as it results in higher mis-injection in mice. The AVMA Guidelines describe ethanol as an alternative chemical agent, 100% of ethanol given at a dose of 15.3–15.8 g/kg in rats showed similar rates of onset of respiratory and cardiac arrest but also pain-related behavior such as vocalization or kicking at the needle but was also not effective in mice.

12.8 How Should Euthanasia by CO_2 Inhalation Be Performed?

Using the CO_2 for euthanasia is considered relatively safe for the user and the environment, cost–effective, and can be used to euthanize multiple rodents at the same time. The use of CO_2 for euthanasia is accepted "with Condition" [5], the flow rate must be set between 30 and 70% by using an empty chamber and to be cleaned between use to remove porphyrin or other staining from animals. The time to lose unconsciousness must be as short as possible and to produce death. CO_2 is known to build up carbon acid in the mucosal membranes and may cause pain and distress. Directive 2010/63/EU requires a controlled flow rate by using a flow meter or restriction valve. Recent literature indicates a strain-dependent difference in rodents in response to euthanasia methods such as CO_2 inhalation [4], in addition, sex, age, and disease state and handling techniques can impact the response. Inhalation of CO_2 causes rapid acidosis. When mixing animals of different ages and sexes, the CO_2 exposure time must be sufficient for the least-susceptible animal. Guinea pigs and rabbits can hold breath and alternative methods are preferable. Argon is also listed in Appendix IV of the Directive 2010/63/EU, inert gases can cause asphyxia while still conscious and are not considered a humane method as a sole agent. The Canadian Council on Animal Care [13] requires anesthesia (e.g., Isoflurane) before exposure to CO_2. Isoflurane is known to be averse to the animal when being exposed multiple times and bears the risk of recovering before exposure to CO_2 and causing possible harm. Animals that appear to be dead in the induction chamber (cyanotic, cold, unmoving) may revive after removing from the CO_2 or isoflurane exposure, death must be confirmed by a second method. Hickmann [14] mentioned that rats must be exposed at a minimum for 10,5 min to CO_2, mice at a minimum for an additional 2 min when 100% CO_2 has been reached.

12.9 What Should Be Considered Euthanasia of Large Groups of Rodents?

A disease outbreak or a disaster may require mass euthanasia should be part of the overall disaster plan. In breeding facilities routinely large numbers may be euthanized by CO_2, cervical dislocation [15]. The Canadian Guidelines on euthanasia (CCAC 2019) recommend using inhalant gas before CO_2 induction. Separation of animals during these euthanasia processes should be also considered as the Guide for the Care and Use of Laboratory indicates that animals should not be euthanized in front of other animals (NRC 2011); for sensitive species, it is desirable that other animals are not present [5]. Rats and mice have poor distance vision. Animals should be euthanized, when possible, in their home cage, minimizing social stress and overcrowding and considering how this may influence the CO_2 flow in the chamber and requiring longer exposure time. Larger animals may be euthanized by an overdose of barbiturates, requiring keeping larger amounts on the stock of a controlled drug and the involvement of more staff.

12.10 How Should Euthanasia of Neonatal Rats and Mice Be Performed?

Directive 2010/63/EU does not allow the euthanasia of neonates by carbon dioxide because of their resistance to hypoxia. This may require the use of inhalant gas, intraperitoneal injection of an overdose of anesthetics, or mechanical methods such as decapitation. Hickman [16] described the use of Carbon Monoxide for neonatal rats and mice to be effective after day 5, using 8% of CO with a replacement rate of 0.75 L/min. Exposure time was 5 min. Use of 100% CO_2 may be approved for neonates, but animals should be exposed for a minimum of 50–60 min to confirm death. When euthanizing pregnant females, anesthesia of the dam must be sufficient for euthanasia of the fetuses [4]. Fetuses may be unconscious for a prolonged time, if the fetuses are removed from the amniotic sac, they may start breathing (mouse, rat, and hamster >E15/ guinea pig > E35) and should be euthanized by an approved method [5, 17]. Such methods may include decapitation, cervical dislocation, hypothermia (by avoiding direct contact with ice or cold surfaces), rapid freezing in liquid nitrogen, or chemical anesthetic overdose.

12.11 How Should Euthanasia of Surplus Animals Be Considered?

Euthanasia of healthy research animals is a serious concern. Rehoming of animals should be considered whenever possible. The European Commission also requires the reporting of all animals bred for research but not used in procedures on a regular base. As many research projects are carried out under time pressure and/or with time-limited funding, breeders maintain a large stock of animals with diverse genetic backgrounds [18]. The production at breeding facilities should be optimized and requires good planning of experiments and the breeding of animals. Surplus animals may be used for training purposes, tissue collection for scientific purposes, or may be donated as food animals. The most common procedure to euthanize surplus rodents is by the induction of Carbon Dioxide.

12.12 Euthanasia of Other Species?

Larger species like cats, dogs, and ferrets are routinely euthanized by an overdose of anesthetics. These may be controlled substances (e.g., Barbiturates), depending on compound and legal requirements. Potassium chloride may be used to euthanize swine and cattle as it causes cardiac arrest after intravenous administration or directly into the heart but requires deep anesthesia before administration to prevent the distress associated with the cardiac arrest. Birds can be killed by thoracic compression. This seems to be more practical in a field setting as it does not require equipment or drugs. The AVMA Guidelines regard this method as unacceptable, also under anesthesia.

Captive bolt or electrocution may be used to euthanize livestock, rabbits, amphibia, reptiles, or fish, for other species only "with condition" depending on age and body weight [17].

Table 12.1 lists exemplary approved methods by different species from Directive 2010/63/EU.

Tricaine methane sulfonate (MS-222) is commonly used for the euthanasia of aquatic species.

Table 12.1 Approved methods of euthanasia for the most common species from Directive 2010/63/EU

	Fish	Amphibians	Reptiles	Birds	Rodents	Rabbits	Dogs, cats, ferrets	Large mammals	Nonhuman primates
Anesthetic overdose	+	+	+	+	+	+	+	+	+
Captive bolt			+			+		+	
Carbon dioxide				+	+				
Cervical dislocation				+	+	+			
Concussion	+	+	+	+	+	+	+		
Decapitation				+	+				
Electrical stunning	+	+		+	+	+	+	+	
Inert gas				+	+			+	
Shooting with bullets and appropriate rifles			+				+	+	

The solution must be buffered with sodium carbonate before animals are immersed. Alternatively, eugenol (clove oil) or hypothermic shock can be used. Immersing in Propofol has also been shown to be effective, animals must be exposed at minimum of 20 min to prevent recovery.

12.13 What Adjunctive Methods Can Be Considered?

Some research protocols require perfusion of tissue under deep anesthesia and analgesia, allowing to open the thoracic cavity and replacing blood with a fixative. Removing more than 25% of blood volume means exsanguination and results in animal death. Amphibians may be killed by pithing, inserting a sharp tool by destroying the brainstem. These methods require extensive training and skills and must be approved in the research protocol [19]. Electrical stunning requires specific equipment. The laboratory space for performing those procedures should be away from animal rooms to limit the stress for all animals requiring specific attention to logistics and the layout of the room, especially when done on larger species.

12.14 How Is Disposal of Carcasses to be Managed?

Animal carcasses are classified as clinical waste and as such must be disposed of correctly. The routine procedure is incineration. Temporary storage may be necessary until final disposition. Special attention including all legal obligations must be directed to the biosecurity level when performing infectious research and using genetically modified animals. Storage may be challenging when using larger species and agricultural animals. Transportation of carcasses, storage, and final disposition may be contracted out to a third party. Licenses according to federal law must be in place at the contractor and an audit of the outsourced process conducted.

12.15 What Is the Expected Training and Competencies to Perform Euthanasia?

Personnel involved in euthanasia must receive proper training and be competent in the chosen method. This involves the husbandry staff as well as the research team, the principal investigator, and the veterinary team. They should understand the anatomy and physiology of the specific species they are working with to ensure the procedure is carried out effectively. This training may be part of the education, competencies can also be gained by participating in a FELASA Course, function D. Species-specific training may be necessary, especially when euthanizing higher species such as sheep, dogs, or nonhuman primates. Personnel performing euthanasia should also be listed in the animal license. The training of the personnel should be regularly reviewed by the oversight body to ensure competency and continuous refinement of the procedure. Psychological support should be in place for all staffs involved in the euthanasia of research animals, not only for chronic studies to prevent compassion fatigue syndrome.

References

1. Guide for the Care and Use of Laboratory Animals, 8th edition, NRC, 2010.
2. Wolfensohn S. Euthanasia and other fates for laboratory animals. 2010;17:219–226. The Care and Management of Laboratory and other research animals. 8th ed. Wiley-Blackwell.
3. Clarkson JM, Martin JE, McKeegan DEF. Lab Anim. 2022;56:419–36.
4. Shomer NH, Allen-Worthington KH, Hickman DL, Jonnalagadda M, Newsome JT, Slate AR, Valentine H, Williams AM, Wilkison M. Review of rodent euthanasia methods. J Am Assoc Lab Anim Sci. 2020;59:242–53.
5. American Veterinary Medical Association, 2020: AVMA guidelines for the euthanasia of animals: www.avma.org/sites/default/files/2020-01/2020-Euthanasia-Final-1-17-20.pdf
6. Review of Annex III and IV of Directive 2010/63/EU on the protection of animals used for scientific purposes regarding accommodation parameters and methods of killing zebrafish, and accommodation parameters for Passerine birds.
7. Robinson S, Sparrow S, Williams B, Decelle T, Bertelsen T, Reid K, Chlebus M. The European Federation of the Pharmaceutical Industry and Associations' research and animal welfare group: assessing and benchmarking 'culture of care' in the context of using animals for scientific purpose. Lab Animals 0(0) 1–12, 2019.
8. Russel WMS, Burch RL. The principles of humane experimental technique. London: Methuen & Co. Limited; 1959.
9. Arbeitskreis Berliner Tierschutzbeauftragter; Empfehlungen zu Score Sheets, Belastungskategorien und Abbruchkriterien. 2023. https://www.ak-tierschutzbeauftragte.berlin/
10. Carbone L, Carbone ET, Yi EM, Bauer DB, Lindstrom KA, Parker JM, Austin JA, Seo Y, Ghandi AD, Wilkerson JD. Assessing cervical dislocation as a humane euthanasia method in mice. J Am Assoc Lan Anim Sci. 2012;51:352–6.
11. Turner MD. The most gentle of lethal methods: the question of retained consciousness following decapitation. Cureus. 2023;15(1):e33830. https://doi.org/10.7759/cureus.33830.
12. Laferriere CA, Pang DSJ. Review of intraperitoneal injection of sodium pentobarbital as a method of euthanasia in laboratory rodents. J Am Assoc Lab Anim Sci. 2020;59:254–63.
13. Canadian Council on Animal Care. Guidelines on euthanasia of animal used in science. 2010. http://www.cccac/documents/Standards/Guidelines/Euthanasia.pdf
14. Hickman DL. Minimal exposure time for irreversible euthanasia with carbon dioxide in mice and rats. Jam Assoc Lab Anim. 2022;61:283–6.
15. American Veterinary Medical Association, 2019: AVMA guidelines for the depopulation of animals: www.avma.org
16. Hickman DL. Euthanasia of neonatal rats and mice using carbon monoxide. J Am Assoc Lab Anim Sci. 2023;62:274–9.
17. European Parliament and the Council of the European Union. Directive 2010/63/EU of the European Parliament and of the Council of 22 September 2010 on the protection of animals used for scientific purposes. Off J Eur Communities. 2010;L276:33–79.
18. Wewetzer H, Wagenknecht T, Bert B, Schoenfelder G. The fate of surplus laboratory animals. EMBO Rep. 2023;24:e56551.
19. Weichbrod RH, Thompson GAH, Norton JN. Euthanasia - management of animal care and use programs in research and education, and testing. 2nd ed. CRC Press; 2018.

13 Education, Training, and Competence in Laboratory Animal Science

Rafael Frías and Paul A. Flecknell

Abstract

This chapter explores the concepts of education, training, and competence, particularly within the context of Laboratory Animal Science (LAS). Education and training encompass the acquisition of knowledge and skills through formal or informal means, while competence extends beyond knowledge and skills to include personal qualities and the ability to achieve desired outcomes. LAS competence standards emphasize adherence to the principles of the 3Rs and require advanced knowledge, skills, and professional conduct. The evolution and standards of LAS competence regulations, methods for knowledge acquisition and assessment, practical skill development, supervision duration, and continuous professional development are discussed. Future directions involve leveraging technology, global collaboration, and promoting non-technical and professional skills to enhance LAS standards.

R. Frías (✉)
Department of Comparative Medicine, Karolinska University Hospital, Solna, Sweden

Laboratory Medicine, Karolinska Institutet, Huddinge, Sweden
e-mail: rafael.frias@ki.se

P. A. Flecknell
Newcastle University and Flaire Consultants Ltd., Newcastle, UK

Keywords

Laboratory animal science (LAS) · Education · Training · Competence · Knowledge · Skills · Supervision · Assessment

13.1 What Are the Definitions and Differences Among the Terms Education, Training, and Competence?

Education is a broad term that refers to the process of acquiring knowledge and skills through formal or informal learning experiences. Formal education includes attending courses, while informal education involves learning from personal experiences and observing others. Education includes diverse activities, ranging from attending university to reading books or papers to participating in meaningful conversations with others. Training is a more specific form of education that is focused on developing the skills and applied knowledge necessary to perform a particular role or task. Training is typically more hands-on than education, and it often involves practical exercises and simulations [1, 2].

Competence is the ability to apply knowledge, skills, and attitudes to achieve a specific outcome to the expected levels. It is a broader concept than education or training, and it also encompasses

J. Guillén, V. Galligioni (eds.), *Practical Management of Research Animal Care and Use Programs*, Laboratory Animal Science and Medicine 3, https://doi.org/10.1007/978-3-031-65414-5_13

Table 13.1 Key difference between education, training, and competence

Feature	Education	Training	Competence
Focus	Broad knowledge and skills	Specific skills and applied knowledge	Application of knowledge, skills, and attitudes
Approach	Formal and informal learning	Hands-on learning	Engaged, empathy, creativity, and problem-solving
Outcome	Acquisition of knowledge and skills	Development of task-specific skills	Ability to perform tasks and roles

personal qualities such as motivation, communication, empathy, and problem-solving skills [3, 4] (Table 13.1).

13.2 What Is the Definition of Competence in the Context of Laboratory Animal Science (LAS)?

Laboratory Animal Science (LAS) is a multidisciplinary scientific field that addresses societal, legal, ethical, and optimal standards of care and use of animals for scientific purposes. This field of science is strongly influenced by the Three Rs of Replacement, Reduction, and Refinement (3Rs). The 3Rs, initially introduced by William Russel and Rex Burch in 1959 in their book "The Principles of Humane Experimental Technique," have become a cornerstone in promoting humane and responsible animal use in research, education, and testing. Their concept provides a framework for balancing animal welfare and research quality. The principles of the 3Rs have been universally adopted in legal frameworks worldwide for the protection of animals used in scientific endeavors [5, 6].

In the field of LAS in the European Union, the competence of the personnel involved in the care and use of animals used in science is defined by their ability to perform specific roles, referred to as "functions," related to the scientific or academic use of animals. These functions consist of "function a" (carrying out scientific procedures on animals), "function b" (designing procedures and projects), "function c" (taking care of animals), and "function d" (killing animals). Competence standards for all these functions require that personnel are able to demonstrate advanced levels of knowledge, skills, and professional conduct, in line with the principles of the 3Rs. This ensures adherence to the highest standards of legality, ethics, science, and veterinary practices [7, 8] (Table 13.2).

Table 13.2 Overview of the requirements for development of competence set out in the Directive 2010/63/EU

Location	Description
Recital	
15	(…) the **level of competence** is important.
28	(…) the welfare of the animals used in procedures is highly dependent on the **quality** and **professional competence** of the personnel (…).
	staff are **supervised** until they have **obtained** and **demonstrated** the requisite **competence**
Article	
23	(…) have **species-specific knowledge**.
	(…) be adequately **educated and trained**.
	(…) be **supervised** in the performance of their tasks until they have **demonstrated** the requisite **competence**.
	(…) **obtain, maintain** and **demonstrate** the requisite **competence**.
	(…) **maintain** the requisite **competence**.
24	(…) be **continuously trained, supervised** and have **demonstrated** the requisite **competence**.
Annex	
VI	(…) **Competence** of persons involved in the project.

13.3 How Have LAS Competence Regulations Changed over Time, and What Are the Current Rules and Recommendations?

In the European Union, from 1986 to 2010, the Directive 86/609/EEC and the Council of Europe (Convention ETS 123) established standards for staff competence, requiring appropriate education and training for roles involving laboratory animals [9, 10]. Between 1995 and 2000, the Federation of European Laboratory Animal Science Associations (FELASA) introduced a categorization system for personnel, defining four distinct roles: "Category A" for animal care [11], "Category B" for performing experiments [12], "Category C" for conducting animal experiments [11], and "Category D" for specialists in laboratory animal science [13]. Each category had a recommended curriculum emphasizing theory, practice, and assessment. From 1986 to 2010, completing a formal course, most likely based on FELASA's curriculum, was considered adequate for acquiring competence in undertaking these roles with laboratory animals.

However, in 2010 the Directive 2010/63/EU broadened the approach to competence. Post-2010, the updated standards required not only completion of a general course for any laboratory animal species but also the acquisition of species-specific knowledge. Personnel were also required to undertake supervised work to obtain and demonstrate competence, and continuing education for different functions and roles, including functions (a) Carrying out procedures on animals; (b) Designing scientific procedures and projects; (c) Taking care of animals; and (d) Killing animals [7].

In 2014, the Directorate-General for Environment at the European Commission introduced specific guidelines outlined in the Working Document (2014) on the Development of a Common Education and Training Framework to Fulfill the Requirements under Directive 2010/63/EU. Since 2014, there has been a notable shift in the learning process, with a renewed focus on attaining competence in Laboratory Animal Science (LAS) through prescribed learning outcomes using a modular approach. These recommendations received endorsement from all national competent authorities of Member States. The guidelines underscored a crucial point: competence cannot be exclusively achieved through education and training and must be species specific. Following the release of these guidelines, it became increasingly evident that the traditional notion of "course contents" from the previous period (1986–2010) underwent a transformation or upgrade into "learning outcomes." These outcomes delineate what trainees should know, understand, and be capable of doing by the conclusion of the learning period [8].

13.4 How Can One Obtain and Facilitate Formal Knowledge in LAS?

Personnel who intend to perform procedures or specific tasks involving laboratory animals must acquire species-specific knowledge for functions (a–d). This knowledge is typically obtained by successfully completing modules aligned with predefined theoretical learning objectives [8]. Knowledge in laboratory animal science and medicine can be acquired through synchronous or asynchronous learning methods, using either in-person or online formats.

Synchronous learning means that students and teachers interact in real time, for example, in live classes or webinars, where everyone is involved at the same time. On the other hand, asynchronous learning allows students to learn at their own speed and convenience, without the need for simultaneous participation or having to be online at the same time as others. This can include online courses or modules where students work through materials on their own, watch pre-recorded videos, view recorded demonstrations, or take part in discussion forums. Synchronous learning promotes immediate engagement and interaction, while asynchronous learning provides flexibility and accessibility. The choice between the two depends on the educational goals, learner preferences, institutional' possibilities, and the nature of the content being delivered. Synchronous learning methods, conducted in real time, include live virtual lectures, interactive webinars, and virtual laboratory simulations. These approaches facilitate immediate interaction, Q&A sessions, and live demonstrations, mimicking traditional classroom experiences and ensuring real-time engagement. Group projects and live practicals encourage collaborative learning, fostering teamwork and problem-solving skills. Asynchronous methods include pre-recorded online lectures, e-learning platforms, and discussion forums, allowing students to learn at their own pace and engage in reflective discussions. Self-paced modules, recorded demonstrations, and e-learning platforms are widely available and affordable, and provide flexibility and accessibility, which are objectives of the EU Education and Training Framework. Hybrid approaches, such as the flipped classroom model and asynchronous pre-work followed by synchronous sessions, strike a balance between flexibility and real-time interaction. These methods leverage the benefits of both approaches, combining the advantages of self-paced learning with the richness of live engagement. Additionally, online office hours provide personalized support and clarification of doubts, addressing individual needs [14–19].

By adopting a diverse range of teaching methods, educators can create a dynamic and comprehensive learning environment. This approach accommodates various learning styles, promotes flexibility, and ensures a well-rounded educational experience in laboratory animal science and medicine, whether delivered in traditional classroom settings or online.

13.5 What Are the Specific Training Requirements for Practical Skills in LAS?

In terms of practical skills, individuals assigned specific roles or tasks for particular species must also acquire species-specific skills. This includes mastering the art of handling and restraint animals with calmness, confidence, empathy, and an appropriate level of care and skill (module 3.2). They should be capable of conducting humane and proficient animal euthanasia (module 6.2), and they may need to demonstrate proficiency in performing specific procedures, either with anesthesia, analgesia, or surgery (modules 20, 21, and 22) or without anesthesia (module 8). Practical learning outcomes play a crucial role in gaining applied knowledge and specific skills for these procedures. Initial education and training, upon course completion, aim to provide basic knowledge and facilitate the initial development of task-specific skills.

Staff members must undergo sufficient training to acquire skills for functions (a), (c), and (d). Practical training sessions should be conducted by qualified trainers, and the training should distinguish between minor procedures without anesthesia (as outlined in EU modules 3.2, 6.2, 8) and major procedures involving anesthesia, analgesia, and/or surgical techniques (as outlined in EU modules 20–22). The differentiation should be based on the trainee's eventual role and the specific tasks they will be performing on animals [8].

13.5.1 Should Live Animals Be Used for Hands-on Skill Training?

Another important consideration is the use of live animals for educational and training purposes. It is important to note that regulatory approval of the use of animals for this purpose varies widely among countries. Some member states permit the use of live animals for acquisition of a range of practical skills, whereas others permit such use only under very specific circumstances. Directive

2010/63/EU deems it acceptable to use animals for higher education and training to acquire, maintain, or improve vocational skills within the EU. Only those individuals who are at a stage in their career development where animal use is considered necessary should be offered the possibility to use animals in procedures for training purposes [7, 8].

Practical training for procedures can be accomplished through various methods and tools designed for the purpose, including synthetic animal models and cadavers, which should be the preferred initial approach, especially in skills training [20].

Given the differing opinions on animal use in training, scientists from a Member State restricting such use may attend courses in other states. The use of live animals for training, which may cause them pain, suffering, distress, or lasting harm, always requires appropriate regulatory approval. Before using live animals for training, alternative strategies should be thoroughly explored, and specific objectives with defined benefits must be presented in any request for animal use. If the use of live animals is justified and project authorization is obtained, additional limitations, such as limiting severity to mild or reusing animals under non-recovery anesthesia, are often included to minimize the number of animals used and to reduce suffering.

13.6 What Are the Various Assessment Methods That Can Be Used to Evaluate Theoretical Knowledge, and How Could They Be Applied in the Context of Laboratory Animal Science and Medicine?

The methods used to evaluate knowledge and skills should be valid (measuring what they intend to measure), reliable (yielding stable and consistent results), and feasible (practical in application). Assessing knowledge in learning involves diverse methods such as quizzes, exams, participation, observations, portfolios, self-assessment, peer assessment, performance-based tasks, rubrics, technology-based tools, concept mapping, and open-ended questions. Formative assessments like quizzes and homework provide ongoing feedback, while summative assessments like exams and projects evaluate overall comprehension. Participation, self-assessment, and peer assessment encourage engagement and reflection. Technology and visual tools enhance assessment variety, fostering a comprehensive understanding of student knowledge and skills. Constructive feedback is crucial across these methods to guide improvement in the learning process [14, 21, 22] (Table 13.3).

Table 13.3 Assessment methods for theoretical knowledge with examples in the context of Laboratory Animal Science and Medicine

Assessment method	Description	Examples in Laboratory Animal Science and Medicine
Written exams	Comprehensive tests covering theoretical concepts in Laboratory Animal Science	Design an exam covering principles of anesthesia in laboratory animals
Research papers	In-depth exploration of specific laboratory animal science topics through research papers	Write a paper on the ethical considerations of using genetically modified animals in research
Concept maps	Visual representation illustrating connections between theoretical ideas in the field	Create a concept map depicting the relationships between different animal welfare standards
Critical essays	Evaluation of analytical skills in discussing theoretical frameworks in animal research	Critically analyze the impact of environmental enrichment on the behavior of research rodents

(continued)

Table 13.3 (continued)

Assessment method	Description	Examples in Laboratory Animal Science and Medicine
Case studies	Application of theoretical knowledge to real-world scenarios within laboratory settings	Analyze a case study involving the implementation of a new housing system for laboratory rabbits
Multiple-choice questions	Testing broad understanding across various laboratory animal science topics	Select the correct option: What is the optimal temperature range for housing laboratory rabbits? (a) 10–15 °C (b) 18–22 °C (c) 25–27 °C (d) 28–30 °C
Extended matching questions	Questions where students match items in one column to items in another	Match the anesthesia method with the appropriate laboratory animal: (A) Isoflurane (B) Ketamine (C) Etomidate (1) Mice (2) Rabbits (3) Zebrafish
Short-answer questions	Questions requiring concise written responses	Explain the three Rs in the context of laboratory animal research
Pick-list questions	Questions where students select items from a list to match a given prompt	Choose the appropriate handling method for mice: (A) Tail (B) Cupping (C) Tunnel (D) Ladder
Oral presentations	Verbal expression of theoretical knowledge, focusing on laboratory animal science topics	Present a summary of the principles of the 3Rs and their application in laboratory animal research
Debates	Engaging in discussions to defend or challenge theoretical perspectives in laboratory animal science	Debate the pros and cons of using non-human primates in neuroscience research
Peer reviews	Evaluation of peers' theoretical work, fostering collaboration in laboratory settings	Review and provide feedback on a peer's proposal for an animal behavior study
Socratic seminars	Group discussions led by student questions, promoting critical thinking in animal research	Facilitate a seminar discussing the ethical considerations of using transgenic animals in research
Problem-solving scenarios	Application of theoretical knowledge to solve complex problems in laboratory settings	Solve a scenario involving unexpected complications during a surgical procedure on laboratory rodents
Simulations	Role-playing activities simulating theoretical situations in Laboratory Animal Science	Simulate a scenario where researchers need to adapt protocols for unexpected changes in animal behavior
Online forums	Virtual discussions on platforms to exchange theoretical ideas in the field	Participate in an online forum discussing recent advancements in animal welfare standards for laboratory animals
Portfolio assessment	Compilation of work showcasing diverse theoretical understanding in laboratory science	Develop a portfolio containing reports, essays, and reflections on various aspects of laboratory animal science
Interactive workshops	Collaborative sessions for applying and discussing theoretical concepts in animal research	Participate in a workshop exploring the practical implementation of the 3Rs in laboratory animal care
Open-book exams	Assessing the ability to apply theoretical knowledge with resources in laboratory science	Take an open-book exam on the ethical guidelines and regulations governing the use of animals in research
Reflection journals	Personal reflections on the understanding and application of theories in animal science	Maintain a journal reflecting on the challenges and ethical dilemmas encountered during laboratory animal research
Mind maps	Visual representation of the interconnections between theories in Laboratory Animal Science	Create a mind map illustrating the relationships between different animal research methodologies

(continued)

Table 13.3 (continued)

Assessment method	Description	Examples in Laboratory Animal Science and Medicine
Collaborative projects	Team-based projects integrating theoretical knowledge in the laboratory animal field	Collaborate on a project developing a set of best practices for the humane handling of laboratory rodents
Assessment method	Description	Examples in Laboratory Animal Science and Medicine
Literature reviews	Synthesis and analysis of existing theoretical literature in Laboratory Animal Science	Conduct a literature review on the use of analgesics in laboratory animals post-surgery

13.7 What Practical Skill Assessments Are Valuable for Ensuring Competence?

Assessment involves gathering information from candidates about their performance or competence. For learned skills, assessment in a course primarily involves providing feedback to help the trainee enhance their skills. On the other hand, assessment of learned skills occurs at the end of the supervision period, certifying, and recording the trainee's achievements. During a course, evaluating learning outcomes for practical skills is crucial. It determines the level of supervision needed and ensures that the trainee can transition to working under supervision in a real environment without increasing risks to animal welfare. A qualified assessor should use valid, reliable, and feasible methods to assess the acquisition of skills. Examples include Direct Observation of Practical Skills (DOPS) and Objective Structured Clinical Examination (OSCE) [8, 23, 24].

In a formative environment, assessing skills offers benefits such as increased engagement, personalized learning, skill development, and reflective thinking. The level of supervision should align with the skillset, with higher skills requiring less supervision. Only those assessed as competent can work without direct or indirect supervision. At this stage, a deeper understanding of the knowledge base and proficiency in functions (a), (c), and (d) should have developed. Assessing adequate skill levels, as in Step 4, is best done in the trainee's normal working environment. Additional assessment methods may include mini-clinical evaluation exercises, mini-peer assessment tools, multi-source feedback, portfolios, and workplace-based assessments. In a summative environment, competence assessment gauges a trainee's progress, laying the groundwork for certification where no supervision is needed to work with animals [8, 23–26] (Table 13.4).

Table 13.4 Example of Direct Observation of Practical Skills (DOPS), with permission and courtesy extended by ETPLAS

EU 3.2. Basic and Appropriate Biology – Species-specific (Skills)

Objective: To assess the individual's ability to handle animals skillfully, carefully, and empathetically, ensuring no distress or harm is caused to the animals.

Instructions: You will be observed performing specific tasks, and your actions will be assessed based on various criteria. The assessor should be competent in the process of assessment. This assessment evaluates your ability to handle and restrain animals with care and skill.

Details:

Trainee:	Assessor:
Species:	Date:

Assessment of practical competence: This table aims to rate the trainee's performance with the assessment criteria. Each criterion is rated on a scale from (-) to (+++), where (-) is the lowest and (+++) is the highest.

Criteria	Descriptor	Rating scale *(encircle the correct option)*			
Calm and confident	Approaches and handles animals with care, using safe and gentle techniques.	-	+	++	+++
Empathy	Adjusts handling techniques to the animal's reactions to reduce stress and focus on well-being.	-	+	++	+++
Skillful handling	Handles and restraints animals carefully, minimizing harm and stress, and checking animal behavior post-handling.	-	+	++	+++

Example situation:
[+]: The trainee handles animals well, but there was an incident of overscruffing that caused distress. The assessor notes the trainee's overall skillful handling but emphasizes the need for more consistent handling.
[++]: After training with habituated animals, the trainee handles them skillfully and with minimal stress. The assessor notes the need for further training with diverse strains and real scenarios, such as handling jumpy young mice.
[+++]: The trainee has completed multiple training sessions and is now able to work independently and competently in real scenarios..

Global rate (EU module 3.2): This section provides an overall rating of your expertise and the level of supervision required. Your performance in individual criteria will contribute to this global rating.

PRACTICAL COMPETENCE: ☐ Novice; ☐ Intermediate; ☐ Competent		
Novice: [-] Handles animals with care but needs more practice to improve calmness and confidence; primarily trained or assessed with simulators such as dummies or cadavers.	**Intermediate:** [+, ++] Generally handles animals well with occasional lapses; primarily trained or assessed in a single scenario or with habituated animals.	**Competent:** [+++] Handles animals consistently with skill and empathy, demonstrating experience across various phenotypes and scenarios.

(contined)

Table 13.4 (continued)

LEVEL OF SUPERVISION: ☐ Hands-on; ☐ Hands-off; ☐ No supervision		
Hands-on supervision: [-, +] Needs more training and close, direct supervision.	**Hands-off supervision:** [++] Needs occasional supervision; can independently perform some tasks.	**No supervision:** [+++] Capable of working independently.

Observations/Feedback: The assessor may provide specific feedback, noting strengths and areas for improvement. This section helps in tracking progress and identifying training needs.

13.8 What Factors Affect Trainee Supervision Duration and Transition to Independent Work?

Following initial practical training, it is likely that working under supervision will be necessary to facilitate a deeper understanding of the knowledge base and proficiency in skills related to functions (a), (c), and (d). The duration of the supervision period and the time taken to achieve competence will vary among trainees. Supervised training provides an opportunity for the application of learned skill sets in the local environment. Trainees possessing only cognitive skills (knowledge or know-how to carry out a procedure) should operate under "hands-on" supervision. Meanwhile, those capable of demonstrating or explaining how to perform a procedure but still unable to do it independently should continue under "hands-off" supervision. Only individuals assessed as competent should work without supervision [3, 4, 8, 24, 27, 28].

13.9 How Often Should Competence Be Reviewed?

Competence almost invariably declines if it is not adequately maintained. This underscores the importance of continuous review and the necessity of quality assurance oversight. Within an establishment, a system should be implemented to identify and report instances of poor practice among staff, enabling appropriate corrective actions. Quality assurance oversight methods encompass regular reviews of competence, unannounced spot checks, targeted assessments following internal audits, or in response to findings from retrospective reviews and incident reports [8, 24].

13.10 What Is Continuing Professional Development (CPD), and how Should Competence Be Maintained?

Competence in all functions (a)–(d) should be viewed as an ongoing process that can be maintained and further developed through a process of continuing professional development (CPD). CPD encompasses the systematic maintenance, improvement, and broadening of knowledge, skills, and personal qualities necessary for executing professional and technical duties throughout one's career. It is imperative that the majority of CPD activities directly align with Laboratory Animal Science (LAS), focusing on educational and training elements aimed at enhancing knowledge and skills for all functions (a)–(d). The Federation of European Laboratory Animal Science Associations (FELASA) has established guidelines for ongoing education in LAS, emphasizing the use of credits or the number of hours of education as a benchmark. Furthermore, ETPLAS has appointed a Working Group to develop updated guidelines on continued professional development in the field of Laboratory Animal Science [8, 28, 29].

13.11 What Is Next in Evaluating and Maintaining Competence?

Competence in LAS is essential for the implementation of optimal standards for the care and use of animals in scientific research. It is our duty to ensure the best possible health and welfare for animals, to generate high-quality scientific results from animal studies, and to foster trust in animal research among the general public.

Online learning platforms tailored to individual progress are key to providing a more customized education. Embracing cutting-edge technologies like virtual reality and augmented reality for hands-on training could significantly contribute to providing enhanced knowledge and skills in LAS using a more ethical and modern approach.

Encouraging global collaboration can help harmonize training standards and competence assessment while ensuring education remains current and increasing student engagement in this field.

Non-technical and soft skills such as respect, gentleness, and empathy are also important when assessing competence, promoting a well-rounded approach to animal welfare and scientific integrity.

Flexible Continuing Professional Development (CPD) programs using online resources for ongoing learning in the field should be encouraged.

Regular competence reviews prevent skill decline, and transparent, fair assessments maintain accountability in the field.

Collectively, all these efforts should contribute to enhance the standards in LAS education, training, and competence assessment.

References

1. European Commission. Key competences and basic skills. European Commission. 2006. https://education.ec.europa.eu/education-levels/school-education/key-competences-and-basic-skills.
2. Council of the European Union. Council Recommendation of 22 May 2018 on key competences for lifelong learning. Official Journal of the European Union, L 189/1. 2018. https://doi.org/10.2873/20180522-EN.
3. Eraut M. Concepts of competence. J Interprof Care. 1998;12(2):127–39.
4. Miller GE. The assessment of clinical skills/competence/performance. Acad Med. 1990;65(9):63–7.
5. Hau J, Schapiro SJ, editors. Handbook of laboratory animal science: essential principles and practices. 3rd ed. Boca Raton: CRC Press; 2011. ISBN:978-1-4200-8455-9 (vol.1)
6. Russell W, Burch R. The principles of humane experimental technique. London: Methuen & Co. Limited; 1959.
7. European Directive. Directive 2010/63/EU on the Protection of Animals Used for Scientific Purposes. OJ L 2010;276, 20.10.2010.
8. European Commission, Directorate-General for Environment. Caring for animals aiming for better science – Directive 2010/63/EU on protection of animals used for scientific purposes – Education and training framework. Publications Office; 2018. https://doi.org/10.2779/311480.
9. Council Directive 86/609/EEC. Council Directive 86/609/EEC of 24 November 1986 on the approximation of laws, regulations and administrative provisions of the Member States regarding the protection of animals used for experimental and other scientific purposes. OJ L 1986;358 18.12.1986, p. 1. CELEX: 31986L0609.
10. European Convention for the Protection of Vertebrate Animals used for Experimental and other Scientific Purposes. ETS No. 123. Strasbourg; 1986.
11. FELASA. FELASA recommendations on the education and training of persons working with laboratory animals: Categories A and C. Lab Anim. 1995;29:121–31.
12. FELASA. FELASA recommendations for the education and training of persons carrying out animal experiments (Category B). Lab Anim. 2000;34:229–35.
13. FELASA. FELASA guidelines for education of specialists in laboratory animal science (Category D). Lab Anim. 1999;33(1):1–15. https://doi.org/10.1258/002367799780578561.
14. Biggs J, Tang C. Teaching for quality learning at university. Open University Press; 2011.
15. Marton F, Hounsell D, Entwistle N, editors. The experience of learning: implications for teaching and studying in higher education. 3rd ed. Edinburgh: University of Edinburgh, Centre for Teaching, Learning and Assessment; 2005.

16. Harden RM, Crosby J. AMEE Guide No 20: The good teacher is more than a lecturer - the twelve roles of the teacher. Med Teach. 2000;22(4):334–47.
17. Kugel P. How professors develop as teachers. Stud High Educ. 1993;18(3):315–28.
18. Richardson J. Students' approaches to learning and teachers' approaches to teaching in higher education. Educ Psychol. 2005;25(6):673–80.
19. Peisachovich EH, Murtha S, Phillips A, Messinger G. Flipping the classroom: a pedagogical approach to applying clinical judgment by engaging, interacting, and collaborating with nursing students. Int J High Educ. 2016;5(4):114–21. http://files.eric.ed.gov/fulltext/EJ1116856.pdf
20. Ormandy E, Schwab JC, Suiter S, Green N, Oakley J, Osenkowski P, Sumner C. Animal dissection vs. non-animal teaching methods: a systematic review of pedagogical value. Am Biol Teach. 2022;84(7):399–404. https://doi.org/10.1525/abt.2022.84.7.399.
21. Brown G. Assessment: A Guide for Lecturers. Assessment Series. York: LTSN; 2001.
22. National Forum for the Enhancement of T&L in HE. Principles of Assessment OF/FOR/AS Learning. 2017.
23. Norcini J, Anderson B, Bollela V, Burch V, Costa MJ, Duvivier R, Galbraith R, Hays R, Kent A, Perrott V, Roberts T. Criteria for good assessment: consensus statement and recommendations from the Ottawa 2010 conference. Med Teach. 2011;33(3):206–14. https://doi.org/10.3109/0142159X.2011.551559.
24. Jennings M, Berdoy M (editors) LASA 2016 guiding principles for supervision and assessment of competence as required under EU and UK legislation. 2nd ed. A report by the LASA Education, Training and Ethics Section; 2016.
25. Smith E, Gorard S. They don't give us our marks': the role of formative feedback in student progress. Assessment Educ. 2005;12(1):21–38.
26. Dreyfus SE. The five-stage model of adult skill acquisition. Bull Sci Technol Soc. 2004;24:177.
27. Pastor Campos A, de la Cueva Bueno E, Martín Zúñiga J, Frias R, Muñoz Mediavilla C (2018) SECAL Working Group Report - guidelines for persons working under supervision in laboratory animal facilities. J Spanish Soc Lab Anim Sci Assoc (JSECAL).
28. Frias R. Let's do it right: 8 steps to competence in laboratory animal science in the European Union. Lab Anim. 2023;
29. FELASA. Guidelines for Continuing Education for Persons Involved in Animal Experiments—Recommendations of the FELASA Working Group; 2010.

The Concept of Culture of Care: Internal Program Communication

14

Thomas Bertelsen, Dorte Bratbo Sørensen, Helena Paradell, and Pascalle L. P. Van Loo

Abstract

By now we have all heard about Culture of Care in relation to the use of laboratory animals, but do we all have the same understanding of what it is?—not very likely, and this is probably good as "one size fits all" does not sit well when we are talking about culture. However, it is important to have a common understanding of some key features of Culture of Care, and this chapter on Culture of Care will take you through some selected key features and also outline a frame for roles and responsibilities.

T. Bertelsen
Novo Nordisk, Maaloev, Denmark
e-mail: TSBT@novonordisk.com

D. B. Sørensen
University of Copenhagen, Department of Veterinary and Animal Sciences, Copenhagen, Denmark
e-mail: brat@sund.ku.dk

H. Paradell
Zoetis Manufacturing and Research Spain S.L., Girona, Spain
e-mail: helena.paradell@zoetis.com

P. L. P. Van Loo (✉)
Animal Welfare Body Utrecht, Utrecht, The Netherlands
e-mail: p.l.p.vanloo@uu.nl

Does Culture of Care have a place in relation to management of animal care and use programs? The authors of this chapter strongly believe that it has! Our culture—what we think, what we say and what we do—is such a strong enabler of putting the written word into action. Your strategy, vision, policies and SOPs may look excellent on paper, but if the culture in the user establishment does not accept and adopt the good intentions in these documents, the likelihood of not succeeding will be high.

Working with Culture of Care can be a challenging task, as the concept of culture is much more elusive and fuzzy than the topics we typically deal with in the biomedical field, using live animals. Consequently, we have tried to structure this chapter by addressing relevant topics as Q&As, and we have included some hints on where and how to get started. This chapter is therefore not a chapter that needs to be read front to back. Instead, you can pick and choose topics for inspiration, depending on your current needs or interest.

Keywords

Culture of care · Performance standards · Ethics · Animal welfare · Animal experiment chain responsibility · Staff empowerment · Communication · Empathy · Compliance · Challenge

J. Guillén, V. Galligioni (eds.), *Practical Management of Research Animal Care and Use Programs*, Laboratory Animal Science and Medicine 3, https://doi.org/10.1007/978-3-031-65414-5_14

14.1 Culture of Care

For the past 40–50 years, the concept of a Culture of Care has existed in nursing and health professions where it has been widely used. However, the concept of a Culture of Care within laboratory animal science has received much attention since it was stated in recital 31 in the EU Directive 2010/63/EU on the protection of animals used for scientific purposes [1] that "*The [animal welfare] body should … foster a climate of care …* ." Even though it is stated as a "climate of care," the idea is the same as a culture of care. In the European Union (EU) Commission Guidance document "Animal Welfare Bodies and National Committees" [2], the concept of Culture of Care is exemplified in statements such as "appropriate behaviour and attitude towards animal research," "staff who work diligently, accept individual responsibility" and "an attitude that is not based on complying with the rules alone but on an individual's positive and proactive mindset and approach to animal welfare and humane science."

14.1.1 The Concept of a Culture of Care. Do we Have a Clear Definition?

Even though the name "Culture of Care" is increasingly used, there is no official or generally agreed upon definition of a Culture of Care in the context of research animal care and use.

In the EU guidance document "Animal Welfare Bodies and National Committees" it is stated that "*Simply having animal facilities and resources which meet the requirements of the legislation will not ensure that appropriate animal welfare, care and use practices will automatically follow. All those involved in the care and use of animals should be committed to the* 3Rs *principles and demonstrate a caring and respectful attitude towards the animals bred or used for scientific procedures. Without an appropriate Culture of Care*…." [2]. This paragraph clearly indicates that a Culture of Care is going beyond the minimum standards of the law and the basic principles of the 3Rs. A Culture of Care is based on care and respect for and toward the animals. In this aspect, a Culture of Care is in accordance with intentions of the legislation as stated in, e.g., recital 12: "Animals have an intrinsic value which must be respected" [1]. Obviously, compliance with relevant legislation is compulsory, but for the Culture of Care to be successfully implemented, there is also a need to acquire an animal-centric approach [3].

A working concept of the Culture of Care has been published by Penny Hawkins and Maggy Jennings [4]. This paper includes elements relating to appropriate attitudes, behaviors, mindsets, and mutual respect between staff with different roles.

Various suggestions for a working concept have been presented by the International Culture of Care Network [5] summarizing what has been presented both in the EU Guidance document on Animal Welfare Bodies and National Committees [2] and in Guiding Principles on Good Practice for Animal Welfare and Ethical Review Bodies [6].

In summary, the concept of a Culture of Care should include two main focus points.

First, a good Culture of Care demonstrates a respectful and caring attitude toward the animals; an attitude that goes beyond what is required as a minimum by the legislation. A Culture of Care is hence a culture in which people interact with the experimental animals with care, respect and a positive, proactive mindset, always aiming to improve animal welfare as much as possible. Such a culture is of course depending on senior staff taking the lead and supporting any animal welfare promoting initiatives explicitly and by supplying the necessary resources. In short, improving animal welfare to the highest possible extent (as stated in recital 31 of the EU directive) is a key component of a Culture of Care [1].

The second focus point is the respectful attitude between colleagues and different staff groups and a shared responsibility for continuously enhancing animal welfare. Care staff and veterinarians should be respected and listened to and good interaction and communication between animal care staff and animal users should be encouraged. This includes using a respectful and considerate language when talking about and to colleagues. Also, a respectful and emphatic language should be used when talking about the animals. In contrast to the first point, this point does not directly refer to animal welfare, but rather to the interactions and relations between staff members and the attitude toward the animals both on a vertical and horizontal management level.

Hence, the concept of a Culture of Care entails both the human–animal and the human–human relations. It is thus a very wide concept embracing both animal and human welfare and the Culture of Care in any given facility should benefit both animal welfare, staff morale as well as human welfare and science.

In recent years, a number of papers were published that may help organizations to assess [7, 8] and hence further develop [9] or benchmark [10, 11] the level of culture of care in your establishment.

What you can do:

- Investigate your Culture of Care with focus on animal welfare.
- Investigate your Culture of Care with focus on human welfare including human–human interactions.
- Investigate your Culture of Care with focus on human–animal interactions.

14.1.2 What Are the Key Concepts of Culture of Care?

One of the major concepts of a Culture of Care is, as previously stated, to go beyond and above the minimum legislative requirements. This means that you should understand the intentions, thoughts, and ambitions behind the legislative texts. To be in compliance with existing laws and legislation is to *do things right*; you simply do things the way the legislation stipulates, and your actions are—from a legal perspective—right. On the other hand, you can act in in accordance with the intention of the legislation, aiming for the most animal welfare enhancing interpretation of the "letter of the law," including also a consideration of the ethics of your actions—and then *do the right things*. This section of the chapter will give you an idea on how to *do the right things*—to live your Culture of Care.

A working concept of Culture of Care has been suggested with the following key aspects (modified from Hawkins and Jennings) [4]:

- Appropriate behavior and attitude toward animal research from all key personnel.
- A corporate expectation of high standards with respect to the legal, welfare, 3Rs and ethical aspects of the use of animals, operated and endorsed at all levels throughout the establishment.
- Shared responsibility (without loss of individual responsibility) toward animal care, welfare, and use.
- A proactive approach toward improving standards relating to both animal welfare, scientific quality and welfare of staff, rather than merely reacting to problems when they arise.
- Effective communication throughout the establishment on animal welfare, care and use issues, and the relation of these to good science.
- The importance of compliance with Directive articles and national legislation is understood and effected. This item addresses the balance between a Culture of Compliance, which you *must* have and a Culture of Care, which you *should* have.
- Those with specified roles know their responsibility and tasks.
- Care staff and veterinarians are respected and listened to and their roles and work are supported throughout the establishment. Dialogues must balance scientific objectives as well as animal welfare.
- All voices and concerns at all levels throughout the organization are heard and dealt with positively.

RSPCA and LASA published a helpful document back in 2015 (RSPCA and LASA, 2015) which in Chap. 11 offers a detailed list of potential features of Culture of Care within three main headers:

- Structural elements.
- Behavioral elements.
- Activities that can help in developing the culture.

14.1.3 Who Is Responsible for Fostering a Culture of Care at the Institutional Level?

The EU guidance document "Animal Welfare Bodies and National Committees" [2] describes the role of the Animal Welfare Body in relation to Culture of Care. See also 3.1, which addresses the key roles.

However, fostering a Culture of Care is a joint effort involving many different contributors placed in different places in the hierarchy of a user establishment.

The individual—you and I: each of us is responsible for working in compliance with legislative requirements. To foster a Culture of Care, you can also contribute to animal welfare through collaboration with others, raise a concern related to an animal welfare problem, support and listen to your colleagues' animal welfare initiatives.

The group—a group of animal technicians, a group of scientists, a group of veterinarians, or an interdisciplinary group: the group can discuss and agree on how much of our working hours should be spent on animal welfare, discuss common goals in terms of animal welfare, share knowledge on animal welfare within the group and with other groups, listen to others' ideas about animal welfare.

The leadership—local management as well as top management: Culture of Care should be visibly endorsed on appropriate management levels. When animal welfare or Culture of Care initiatives are agreed upon by relevant parties, local management must allocate resources and time for the training and implementation as well as ensure that the learnings and new procedures are embedded in the daily routines and practices.

The oversight body (OB): the Animal Welfare Body (AWB), the Animal Welfare and Ethical Review Body (AWERB), Institutional Animal Care and Use Committee (IACUC), etc.: The OB have a unique opportunity to promote and facilitate the development of a good Culture of Care. Together with the local management they have the ability to demonstrate effective leadership in this relation. The OB also has the role to ensure that outcomes and goals are achieved.

What you can do:

- Encourage and facilitate scientists and animal care staff to work together, and acknowledge each other's different competencies and contributions; an example could be duo-talks at symposia where a researcher and animal technician can present research both from scientific and from technical point of view [12].
- Arrange pre- and intra and post-study reviews, where relevant staff is represented.
- Provide information on the role and functions of the staff having key positions in the efforts of driving Culture of Care for new staff and encourage their contributions.
- Provide the opportunity and encouragement for any staff member to raise issues with animal welfare and Culture of Care in a safe environment.
- Communicate with all staff (using for example meetings, 3R Award ceremonies, presentations, newsletters and intranet) and spread the word about the 3Rs, Culture of Care, welfare improvements, policy changes, roles of care staff, training persons and veterinarians, and the AWB.

14.1.4 Which Resources Are Needed to Build a Culture of Care Spirit in an Organization?

Culture of Care is, as the name states, a culture and in this case, it is a Corporate or Institutional Culture. Strong and unambiguous statements from the management are, therefore, needed on all levels. The management must signal both by example and by clear announcements which behaviors (both toward animals and toward colleagues) are preferred and which behaviors are unwanted. Such statements must be followed by the monetary resources needed to create the time needed to nurture the caring and respectful environment between colleagues and peers and between animals on the one side and caretakers, technicians, and researchers on the other side.

Obviously, several resources are needed to build a Culture of Care spirit in an organization, and the common denominator is financial support. The economic resources will be the limiting factor when it comes to, e.g., the time the caretakers have for each animal to ensure optimal handling/care of animals.

Hence, the support from the management must come both in word and in deed. The financial resources needed to ensure positive animal–human interactions and preferably animal–human bonding should be available. It is important that time for animal training and socialization is made a mandatory and highly prioritized part of the daily work with the animals—not just something you can do if time allows. Also, resources to enhance cage complexity and enrichment should be prioritized.

Creating and supporting a good working environment (physical as well as mental) including good office facilities also requires financial commitment from the management. The importance of good facilities for the staff should not be underestimated; it is important that staff caring for the animals feels a sincere appreciation from the facility management and not just empty words in the vision/mission statement of the company. The management must provide the economic resources for additional staff, if needed; time for talking to and supporting colleagues who are not feeling comfortable for some reasons and resources for initiatives such as a yearly institutional 3Rs award for testing/implementation of new ideas for improving Animal Welfare or paying tribute to animals and staff [13].

Hence, most resources—including time—are fundamentally just a matter of money. However, staff and researcher attitude, commitment, and motivation, when it comes to showing empathy and solicitude toward animals and colleagues are also depending on the culture in the facility; a culture that is initiated, formed, and maintained by the facility management. In addition to having visions and policies in place and providing the financial support necessary, the management must acknowledge that the development and maintenance of Culture of Care is driven by dedicated and empathic pioneers and entrepreneurs at all organizational levels, who "walk the talk." An important step is therefore for the management to identify, hire, and unmistakeably support caretakers, technicians, and researchers, who in their actions and attitude are expressing the culture that the management wants.

What you can do:

- Consider various ways of making Culture of Care initiatives visible. This could for example be by establishing a yearly award for Best Refinement in a study or a biyearly award for best animal welfare improvement, or award a technician who openly lives a culture of care (Fig. 14.1).
- Put up a box for Ideas on animal welfare improvements and hold a small seminar every third month to discuss and choose one idea to be tested.
- Make for example "nudging-mugs" with fun Culture of Care prints such as "I love my CoC – Cup of Coffee," which implicitly reminds people of CoC—Culture of Care (Fig. 14.1).

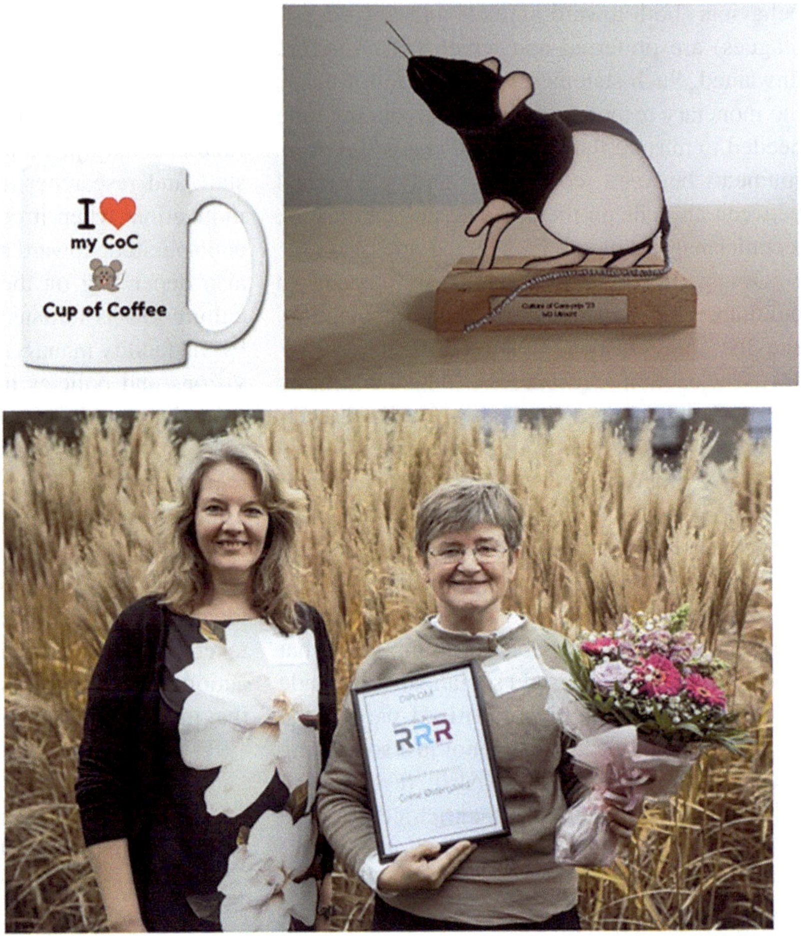

Fig. 14.1 Examples of Culture of Care initiatives: Nudging mugs (upper left; design/photograph courtesy Dorte Bratbo Sørensen), 3Rs award (below; photograph courtesy Kim Granli, DK) and Culture of Care award (upper right; photograph courtesy Lidewij Jansen van Galen, NL)

14.2 Establishment Values and Vision

As Culture of Care is about going beyond and above the minimum legislative requirements, the bar for setting values and visions in terms of animal welfare should be set high. Values and visions must be endorsed by top and local management as the support from these is essential and it gives legitimacy. Values and visions also facilitate that everyone in the user establishment who works with laboratory animals directs their efforts toward the same goals.

14.2.1 What Is the Added Value of Establishment Values and Policies?

Policies and corporate statements including mission and vision regarding Culture of Care are valuable as they show the direction for the establishment's animal welfare goals as well as demonstrating commitment. However, these statements must never stand alone as empty phrases, but should be inspirational and must be substantiated by actions.

Senior management must be seen to endorse and encourage a Culture of Care [14, 15]. This includes that supportive structures (e.g., an internal 3R Award, Refinement discussion groups, study meetings where relevant staff functions are invited and listened to) are developed and that Culture of Care has a legitimacy for the establishment. Qualities like responsibility, empathy, and compassion are not easily made operational in laws, regulations, and standard operating procedures (SOPs), and consequently the communication of these by leadership is essential and requires continuous attention. Working to find the right balance between *doing things right* (e.g., an SOP) and *doing the right things* (e.g., performance standards) is also an important task for management, see also 1.4 [16].

What you can do:

- As an individual, you must understand exactly what the animal welfare policies and values mean in your daily work.
- A group of, e.g., animal technicians can discuss and agree on how they—as a group—proactively will work with animal welfare.
- Local management can clarify the meaning of the policies and values and set out expectations for staff behavior according to this.
- Local management must ensure that staff competencies and skills are in place and that it actually is possible for the staff to work according to the expectations by allocating time and providing necessary tools when relevant.
- The AWB, AWERB, IACUC, or similar must facilitate the interpretation of the policies and values and assist in the practical implementation of these.

14.2.2 What Is the Benefit of an Animal Welfare and Culture of Care Vision?

An animal welfare vision describes the desired state of the establishment in the future and what it ultimately wants to achieve in terms of animal welfare. The benefit of such a vision is that it offers the possibility to go beyond and above a Culture of Compliance. To be in compliance is an absolute must; the EU Commission Guidance document on Animal Welfare Bodies and National Committees (2018) states "Simply having animal facilities and resources which meet the requirements of the legislation will not ensure that appropriate animal welfare, care and use practices will automatically follow"; this means, for example, that simply having a cage with the required dimensions does not by itself mean good animal welfare.

The vision helps staff involved in working with animals to focus on matters that will have the strongest impact on animal welfare. It also promotes a Culture of Challenge which encourages new ways, e.g., of housing and caring for animals. A Culture of Challenge represents a proactive willingness to see if there are more optimal solutions instead of choosing the existing solutions by default. A statement such as "*We have always done it in this way*" should automatically elicit a response to see if better alternatives are implementable. Visions can often seem "impossible" to reach, e.g., "our vision is that our animals do not experience pain, suffering or distress," "the use of every single animal must have a positive impact on the harm/benefit equation," or "the way we work with animals is an inspiration for other similar establishments." However, improving animal welfare often takes place in incremental steps, and it is a continuous process because new knowledge and new technologies mean that you can always do better. Recognizing and celebrating these small steps turn a seemingly unachievable animal welfare vision into an inspirational vision.

Absence of a vision may lead to a state of status quo and complacency, where procedures become outdated, and the staff may lose the sense of purpose and meaning in their work. On the other hand, changing long-established practices may be a challenge as some staff members will feel that their previous work and their professional knowledge are now being questioned or they may be afraid that their competencies and skills do not match the new way to do things. Consequently, changes must be dealt with professionally by management and colleagues.

A vision does not describe specific outcomes and consequently short-term goals must be identified to ensure continuous improvement.

What you can do:

- Arrange sessions with different staff groups and ask them to describe their "ideal" state of animal welfare.
- Invite external stakeholders (e.g., NGOs, laypersons, and authorities) to give input and to challenge your vision.
- Identify obstacles that prevent you from reaching your vision, and search for solutions to overcome these.
- Design a roadmap that step-by-step leads you toward your vision.

14.2.3 How Can Business Ethics and Animal Ethics Be Connected?

The purpose of Business Ethics is to make sure that you and the rest of the institution or company are acting in alignment with the stated values but naturally also in compliance with current laws and legislation. Furthermore, prevailing public perception should be taken into account.

Business Ethics is a very broad term and it tells you what are the "rights and wrongs," very often linking into the Triple Bottom Line (TBL) principle [17]. This sustainable business approach meant to positively impact the environment, society, and at the same time also benefiting shareholders or similar to guide the individual employee in hers or his decisions. Animal ethics belongs to the environmental bottom line. Corporate Social Responsibility (CSR) is another term that encompasses Animal Ethics.

It is a requirement that the individual employees act in accordance with the Business Ethics and consequently also with the Animal Ethics.

What you can do:

- Animal ethics practices should be visibly stated and include clear and visible roles and responsibilities for all those involved in animal research within the establishment.
- Understand and act in accordance with your role and responsibilities and with those of your colleagues.
- Make continuous professional training program an integral part of the yearly staff performance review.
- Share good practice and learning points within and across establishments.
- Ensure a safe environment where concerns can openly be raised. This is a task that requires a constructive dialogue between the AWB/AWERB/IACUC and management.

14.2.4 How Can Engineering Standards and Performance Standards Be Applied in Your Culture of Care Work?

Both engineering and performance standards aim to improve animal welfare and quality. Engineering standards describe the technical standards needed to ensure good welfare and quality, while performance standards describe the desirable outcome. As an example, an engineering standard could be that a cage must have a surface of X cm^2 as exemplified in Annex III of the EU Directive [1]. The equivalent performance standard could be that cage size should enable species-specific behavior. Engineering standards are often used in legislation, since they are easier to adhere to and do not lead to discussion on what is right. However, they do not necessarily lead to the desired outcome of good welfare and quality. After all, the welfare of animals in a large cage with minimal enrichment may be more compromised than in a smaller cage with ample enrichment, hiding places, social interaction, and exploration areas.

Both types of standards may provoke a different attitude toward being compliant. Engineering standards may lead to staff adhering to these because the law or the SOP says so. The "why" is not questioned, and consequently, engineering standards do not support continuous improvement. However, each engineering standard, e.g., cage size, is the result of experts' assessment of minimum requirements, whereas performance standards address the intentions behind these requirements and can thus be used to support a culture of continuous improvement [18].

What you can do:

- Ask yourself what the intended purpose of a particular engineering standard is and how this impacts animal welfare. For example, if the engineering standard requires environmental enrichment, then ask which environmental enrichment is best for a specific behavioral need of the animal in question.
- Add performance standards that impacts animal welfare to existing engineering standards.
- Review and update internal standards on a regular basis. Translate your animal welfare vision into operational engineering and performance standards which will explain the impact they will have. For example, "we believe that doing xxx (e.g. tunnel handling) will result in yyy (e.g. less stressed animals) which we can measure by zzz (e.g. observing their behaviour/better scientific results) and this standard consequently supports our animal welfare vision."

14.3 Culture of Care in an Animal Care and Use Program (ACUP)

An Animal Care and Use Program can be considered as an overall collective designation that encompasses the "activities conducted by and at an institution that have a direct impact on the well-being of the experimental animals. These activities and actions include animal and veterinary care, policies and procedures, personnel and program management and oversight, occupational health and safety, OB (AWB, AWERB, IACUC etc.) functions, and animal facility design and management" ([19], Chap. 2).

In an institution housing an animal facility, whether in academia or industry, several key roles within the ACUP are essential for establishing a Culture of Care with a strong foundation and an ability to reach any given employee whose work and attitude will affect the welfare of the animals [10].

In this section, we will discuss the obligations of the different key roles in an institution in relation to a Culture of Care and the importance of the technical staff. Suggestions for the responsibilities of these key roles in the animal experiment chain (the course of the project/animal study) and the resources needed to fulfil these obligations—including introduction of new employees to the working procedures and culture—are presented.

Incorporating the 3Rs and animal welfare goals in corporate vision or policies may not be the easiest, yet is a fundamental part of implementing a Culture of Care [10]. We all have a clear grasp of what is meant by replacement, reduction, and refinement, and animal welfare with regard to animals in our care is a well-defined term.

Setting animal welfare goals is also a joint exercise in which expert input from management, animal technicians, researchers, veterinarians, and the oversight body is of equal importance. Hence, when managed in the right way, will be a strong incentive for promoting a Culture of Care.

14.3.1 How Do the Different Key Roles in an ACUP Contribute to Culture of Care?

During the planning, performing, and evaluation of animal studies, various persons holding different roles and responsibilities relating to animal welfare are involved at different levels. These key roles may in various ways have both opportunity and an obligation to promote a Culture of Care [10].

The management of an animal facility will be responsible for the administration, availability, and quality of material and physical resources. Moreover, one of the roles of management is to select and appoint staff and decide how large the staffing should be in the animal facility. Also, the management is responsible for making sure that everyone can state any concerns in an open and safe environment, which can include for example an efficient and confidence-inspiring whistle-blower arrangement. Hence, the importance of the facility management cannot be overestimated. To facilitate a Culture of Care, the management must employ staff with the potential for empathy and genuine care and through the distribution of financial resources support as well as empower these employees, allowing for time to handle, train and care for the animals sufficiently.

The management also has the possibility to empower the animal caretaker staff by allowing staff to be in charge of planning and exercise control over their working conditions and animal care routines. The next step is to assign animal caretaker staff to be an integral partner, when researchers are planning and executing of procedures and protocols involving live animals. Researchers also hold a key role as they are planning and designing the studies and are thus responsible for including potential refinement strategies relating to their protocols.

The designated veterinarian (DV) holds a key role as she/he can plan and communicate, e.g., optimal pain treatment protocols by listening to and include information and concerns from the animal care staff throughout and between study periods. In the same way, the OB, holds a responsibility to consider concerns relating to 3Rs, advice on how to improve animal welfare and ensure the sharing of best practices on animal housing and handling.

The key element of a Culture of Care is to ensure that all these key functions; management, animal staff, researchers, designated veterinarian, and oversight body show a respectful attitude acknowledging each other's competences and knowledge.

What you can do:

- Ensure that policies are in place that enables those working with the animals to perform their job in an open, animal-friendly environment.
- Ensure open and easy access communication lines between different key roles.
- Contribute to the communication of a clear vision on Culture of Care that is embraced by all key roles. If no such strategy is in place, ask for one.

14.3.2 Why Are Animal Technicians and Caretakers' Empowerment So Important for Animals' Welfare?

To ensure a Culture of Care and a high level of animal welfare, it is vital that the animal staff (including animal technicians, care takers, and others working directly with animal husbandry and/or experimental procedures involving animals) is first sufficiently educated to evaluate the animals' normal behavior in order to detect, e.g., pain, fear, or frustration in the animals.

Second, the staff should be assigned responsibility for animal welfare combined with psychological empowerment of the staff, i.e., by ensuring that the staff feels a sense of meaning with their tasks; that they feel competent and experience that their efforts do have an impact and that their opinion matters. These experiences will add to self-determination and increased task motivation. Also, the management must ensure that the staff has opportunities, relevant information, support and resources available to reach their work goals, which will result in structural empowerment of the staff [20]. When animal staff experience power and control in their daily work, such empowerment will most likely increase mental health and social functioning. Disempowerment, on the other hand, may lead to increased anxiety and even depression, which may result in a reduced level of empathy ([21]; AALAS [22]; [23, 24]). It seems fair to suggest that a reduced level of empathy will negatively affect the way the person interacts with colleagues as well as animals. Also, if caretaker staffs do not feel empowered and comfortable in the daily work they will most likely lack the mental surplus that is needed to care for others.

Animal care staff and technicians can be empowered by giving the staff control and power over the planning and execution of procedures and protocols involving live animals. Such empowerment, however, demands that the animal staff shows a high level of sense of responsibility, due diligence and professional competences to ensure animal welfare. Moreover, the staff must share their ideas, thoughts and practices with, e.g., researchers, OB, and the DV with an including attitude. This is of course a two-way street and the researchers, OB, and the DV must—for their part—show a similar respectful and including attitude to ensure a productive and fruitful collaboration.

Such empowerment will most likely result in a higher level of job satisfaction as especially animal caretakers have chosen their job because they care for animals [22]. Being given responsibility and a safe and caring working environment will make it more acceptable to demonstrate a high level of empathy toward the experimental animals undergoing procedures [25]. Such a culture most likely will encourage animal staff to go that extra mile that may make the difference between noticing small signs of discomfort and not recognizing that there is an animal welfare problem.

What you can do:

- Actively involve animal care staff in decisions regarding execution of animal procedures, e.g., read and approve work protocols and discuss procedures and responsibilities before the study commences (see PREPARE guidelines [26] and ARRIVE guidelines [27]).
- All those involved in the study should give feedback on the execution at the study end and, when relevant, suggest ways to Refine the protocol.
- Ensure involvement of staff in improvement of for example housing, updates of SOPs, and facility audits.

14.3.3 How Do Different Levels of Responsibility in the Animal Experiment Chain Affect Culture of Care?

The animal experiment chain consists of all parties involved in the experiment from start to end including, e.g., the Competent authority issuing the license for the experiment, additional local approval committees, subcontractors or contract research organizations (CROs), OB, breeder facilities, transporter, and the persons responsible for and/or carrying out housing and husbandry routines before, during and after the experimental procedures, the experimental procedures and, finally, rehoming or euthanasia.

The actions and attitudes of all the above actors (companies, committees, and individual persons) will have an impact on the Culture of Care. For example, it is important to thoroughly and detailed give forward and conscientiously receive details on the history of the animal; both from the vendor (details on, e.g., health, socialization, and handling methods), from animal staff to research staff prior to study (information on, e.g., socialization, training, animals' personality, stress-reducing procedures, and handling methods based on animals' characteristics); and from researchers to animal staff and DV (e.g., post-surgery and/or if the animals are to be rehomed after the study).

What you can do:

- Consider making or asking for an animal history file, which follows the animal or animals from birth to end of study.

14.3.4 Which Elements Relating to a Caring Culture Should the Induction of New Staff Include?

New staff on all organizational levels should be presented with the management's chosen definition of Culture of Care and the management visions for the impact on animal and staff welfare.

When establishing a Culture, it is very important that all the statements in such a vision are followed by obvious actions. For example, in the case of new employees the management must make sure that new staff member feels welcome (e.g., their personal locker/desk is ready and with a small welcome token on it; work pc is ready and so on). This would clearly demonstrate what the management means when they state, for example, that "In our culture, new employees must feel welcome and included." It could be advisable to have a few dedicated persons assigned to be "a welcome committee." By doing this, the management sends a clear signal that they care about the new employee. Moreover, it is important to introduce the staff to the persons who they can contact if they have ideas for animal welfare improvements, ideas to increase job satisfaction or issues that have given cause for concern. Obviously, such requests must be taken seriously and the person assigned to this job must be both empathic and proactive. In many cases it will be better not just to assign a person, but to ask for a volunteer in the staff to fulfil this task.

What you can do:

- Clearly communicate the institutional standards commitment to animal care and welfare to the entire staff.
- Make new staff feel welcome and appreciated.
- Take an interest in the experience of new staff from their previous jobs and use all relevant knowledge to improve upon your management.

14.3.5 What Are the Animal Welfare Objectives in a Culture of Care?

An animal is in a good state of welfare if they are free from *hunger or thirst*, free from *discomfort*, free from *pain, injury or disease*, free to *express normal behavior* and free from *fear and distress* (The Five Freedoms, [28]).

In a laboratory environment, the freedom to express normal behavior as much as possible and the freedom from fear and distress are the most challenging, and give room for continuous improvement. In a Culture of Care, the animal staff should work dedicated both on enriching the environment to promote preferred, natural species specific behavior and on reducing fear and distress by socialization, correct handling, refinement of procedures, and training of the animals.

Therefore, the focus points of the animal welfare objectives are:

- Improvement of housing and husbandry conditions to meet the animals' behavioral needs and preferences.
- Reduction of distress in experimental and routine husbandry procedures through socialization, habituation, and various forms of training.

What you can do:

- Review housing and husbandry procedures in relation to the animals' behavioral needs. Identify gaps and set goals to overcome them.
- Build trust between animal and caretaker/technician by positive reinforcement training and/or the use of rewards (food or non-food) during or after stressful procedures.
- Review the full life span of the animal and consider what you can do to give them a better start (e.g., through agreements with the breeder) and a better end (e.g., rehoming).

14.3.6 How Do Culture of Care Initiatives Benefit the Quality of Animal Experiments?

A Culture of Care aims to improve animal welfare and beneficial communication between animal staff and researchers and an improvement in animal welfare will most likely have a positive effect on the quality of the study. When the animals' behavioral needs are met, their behavior and physiology are within normal ranges. Trevor Poole [29] already argued that this is a prerequisite for reliable research results: "Happy animals make good science." Although concern exists that changes in housing and husbandry may affect variability in experimental results, there are clear arguments that behavioral, immunological, and other physiological measurements will be more trustworthy, when the animals are not stressed, fearful, or in pain [30]. The researchers and the animal staff should join forces to evaluate and coordinate the animal welfare improvements suggested by the animal staff or the veterinarian.

In a Culture of Care, emphasis should be on providing housing and enrichment that allows the animal to perform as wide a range of natural behaviors as possible. Providing for social needs, shelter, and exploration and foraging opportunities is important.

Positive reinforcement training or other kinds of training, socialization, or habituation ensures that experimental procedures can be carried out with less or no stress for the animal [31]. It thus helps to get more reliable data. It will make procedures possible that could not have been performed on a stressed animal or would otherwise have required sedation (Ref: [32, 33]). Depending on the species, most impact can be gained when animals are socialized as early as possible in their life, whereas training based on operant conditioning such as positive reinforcement training can be initialized at all times in an animals' life. However, training presupposes that the animal is comfortable around humans and feels safe enough to accept, e.g., food treats offered by the trainer. This fact makes socialization and habituation an important part of animal management [34].

What you can do:

- Scientists, veterinarians, and animal caretakers regularly review the housing and enrichment provided, taking into account the natural behavior and behavioral needs of the species involved.
- Introduce gentle handling techniques with as little restraint as possible.
- Develop training programs for specific procedures and ask your breeder to cooperate by preparing the animals.
- Review the validity of your animal model after the changes.
- Facilitate education on animal welfare as well as interdisciplinary exchange of ideas and discussions regarding implementation, e.g., enrichment and training of animals.

14.3.7 Do Animal Welfare Goals/Policies Impact Staff Morale and Business Productivity?

Changes in housing, husbandry, and procedure routines are not always easy. They require investment from management, animal technicians, and researchers in terms of time and money. However, evidence suggests that changes in routine that are profitable for the animals, lead to higher staff morale, even if it means that they have to invest time [21]. A good example is changing from tail to tunnel or cup handling in mice. An increasing number of institutes is making this change. It takes effort to convince management and staff and it takes time to make the change fully, but once the change is made, both management and staff are positive. Mice become more docile and the time needed for routine procedures does not increase [35].

Empowerment of staff by involving them in setting animal welfare goals is also a strong incentive to increase work pleasure. Animal technicians, who in general are fond of animals, can share and execute their ideas on how to improve animal welfare and interact with the animals in a positive way. Evidence suggests that empowerment of staff in this way is linked to less long-term absenteeism caused by compassion fatigue or burn-out [21].

What you can do:

- Ensure that setting animal welfare goals is a joint effort that involves all staff.
- Monitor staff commitment and check for early signs of compassion fatigue.
- Share inspirational examples of AW goals that have succeeded within and outside your institution.

14.3.8 How to Acquire Resources to Support Culture of Care Initiatives?

Budget constraints are a factor that most, if not all, institutes have to deal with. It is, therefore, important to involve management early in the process of implementing animal welfare initiatives. Visualizing costs and benefits, as well as other drivers and barriers, of proposed initiatives enables you to set short- or long-term goals with regard to these initiatives. If statements regarding culture of care and animal welfare are clear in the company or institutional goals and visions, any suggestions should refer to these statements. For initiatives that are costly, or otherwise difficult to implement, a stepwise implementation plan including budget reservations is important. But not everything is costly. With some creativity, you may actually be able to implement several low budget Culture of Care or animal welfare initiatives. Finally, you may be able to request funding or be eligible for a prize for specific animal welfare initiatives.

What you can do:

- Reserve a yearly budget for culture of care initiatives.
- Use "old" inventory in a new way, such as transforming old water bottles into tubes for mouse handling, or old rabbit cages to enriched rat housing.
- Include a budget for animal welfare initiatives in your research grant.

14.4 The Impact of Internal Program Communications in Culture of Care

Internal program communications play a fundamental role in establishing and nurturing a culture of care within an institution. By fostering understanding, trust, collaboration, and a supportive environment, communication enables individuals to work cohesively toward a common goal.

A chapter by Weichbrod et al. in the book "Management of Animal Use and Care Programs in Research" [36] describes how to work with this collaborative approach.

Effective communication facilitates a clear understanding of each individual's roles and responsibilities within the institution. Open and transparent communication is vital for establishing trusting relationships within an institution. Understanding each individual's roles and responsibilities prevents misunderstandings, conflicts, and duplication of work, ultimately ensuring the highest standards of animal care and use.

14.4.1 What Are the Expectations of Communication between the Principal Program Key Roles?

Communication between the principal ACUP key roles is essential for Culture of Care.

Transparent and engaging communication, across different levels of expertise is important to facilitate a broader perspective analysis. Effective communication is the key to ensure that the institutional team, administration, the OB, animal technicians, veterinarian(s), researchers, the environmental health and safety (EHS) office, facilities maintenance staff, and others are working in a coordinated manner and have a common goal of a high-quality program.

Management should be both well informed about and engaged in the program and should provide sustained and visible support. The OB should clearly articulate institutional governance documents so that everyone understands the institutional vision and expectations.

The veterinarian and animal technicians should work in concert and as a partner with the OB and investigators/researchers, should ensure adequate care of the animals, and should exercise professional judgment to facilitate the science in the context of animal welfare. There should also be interaction between the animal program and other key institutional components such as the EHS office.

All key staff should be listened to and respected in their roles, ensuring a working environment that continuously stimulates the mindset and proactive participation of all involved in animal procedures.

Special attention should be given to communication between scientists and animal technicians, who may have different objectives and very different expertise. It is important to share common goals and to have shared and aligned expectations. The closer the working relationship between scientists and animal technicians and care staff, the better the communication and mutual respect.

What you can do:

- Identify the type of working relationship between technicians and researchers.
- Identify the types of formal and informal communication lines between the different key roles.
- In your institute or personal role, identify which communication is valuable and which is missing.

14.4.2 Why Are Well-Established Communication Channels within the ACUP Key Roles Important?

In an institution, processes for communications need to be facilitated, supported and nurtured by management. Consistent good leadership from senior management, and having the time and resources to facilitate good communication, are key.

The principal communication channels between the program key roles can be summarized (by two-way arrows) as follows (Fig. 14.2):

However, we cannot forget other important roles with which communication is essential in ongoing animal care and use program such as EHS, Maintenance, and the Quality Unit (in GMP and GLP environments).

Effective communication channels include regular scheduled or refresher two-way meetings involving scientists, animal technicians, veterinarians, unit managers, and OB members. These meetings serve as platforms for open dialogue, information sharing, and addressing any concerns or questions. Additionally, unit managers may conduct regular catch-up meetings with EHS teams and the maintenance team to ensure the smooth operation of the facility. These communication channels foster transparency, collaboration, and a sense of shared responsibility, ultimately contributing to the overall Culture of Care within the institution.

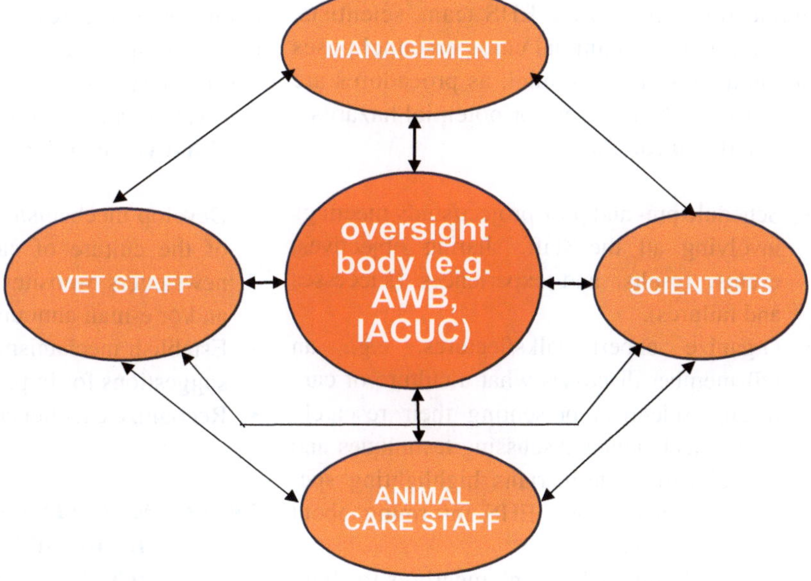

Fig. 14.2 The principal communication channels between program key roles (Original diagram: Javier Guillén)

On the other hand, internal miscommunications within an institution can have significant consequences leading to impaired animal welfare and bad quality of science. Such miscommunications include a lack of communication between management, the OB, and the veterinarian, resulting in unclear institutional standards and a lack of resources to address program issues. For example, coordination gaps between the OB and the veterinarian lead to a failure in communicating veterinary-related matters concerning approved animal protocols, or to the absence of consultation with the veterinarian in internal policies, such as humane endpoints and restrictions. And when lack of communication affects animal care personnel, this may have an effect in not reporting sick animals or not being aware of potential adverse events, also leading to delays in veterinary care. Additionally, insufficient information and training provided to animal care personnel regarding ongoing projects result in potential errors in biosecurity measures. And furthermore, the absence of communication between the EHS team, scientists, veterinarians, and animal care personnel poses potential risks to personnel, as procedures are not adequately assessed for potential hazards.

What you can do:

- Schedule pre- and post-project/study meetings involving all the staff, sharing objectives, events, results, and experiences (successes and failures).
- Organize expert talks/lectures, e.g., an OB member discusses what a culture of care means, scientists presenting their research, animal technicians discussing techniques and animal care, veterinarians highlighting specific veterinary care, EHS informing about personnel safety, etc.
- Informal "lunch & learn" meetings to share project/studies progress or to discuss topics related to animal use, e.g., research, techniques, animal welfare, equipment, and staff.
- Newsletter and/or updated website from OB.

14.4.3 How Do we Ensure That New Standards Are Communicated and Made Available Throughout the Program?

Communication begins with ensuring the visibility of the Culture of Care program throughout the institution. The concept and goals of a Culture of Care should be shared throughout the organization.

Expectations of the institution with regard to welfare and care practices should be communicated to all personnel, not just those directly involved with animal care and use. Cross-disciplinary communication and exchange of expert information, and professional standards of care are to be the same for everyone [37].

Promoting educational tools for better caring of animals and staff welfare remains at the core of best institutional Culture of Care [38, 39], and must be reinforced and protected. Personnel training programs should include topics central to a culture of care that impact attitudes, such as understanding why animals are used in research, the ethics of such use, and animal welfare. Every employee is a representative of the institution in the public sphere and is thus in a position to convey the institution's strong commitment to animal welfare and a Culture of Care.

What you can do:

- Develop mechanisms to communicate details of the culture of care internally: meetings, newsletters, websites, bulletin boards, posters, and/or e-mail announcements.
- Establish mechanisms to report concerns and suggestions for improvement.
- Recognize excellence within the daily work.

14.4.4 How to Foster Openness on Animal Welfare Concerns Within the Establishment?

The institution must provide space for expressing failure and/or reflecting on challenging circumstances, with a positive constructive approach and avoiding any negative consideration [40].

It is the responsibility of everyone associated with the animal care and use program to ensure animal welfare. In some instances, this may involve having to make a formal report regarding a welfare concern.

It is important that the focus is on *what happened* instead of *who did it* to avoid a blame culture, which is not helpful to foster openness. Concerns should be raised by objectively describing facts.

The institution should provide a method, supported by management, where animal welfare concerns can be raised, such reports can be made anonymously and without fear of reprisal, and enhancing staff awareness of the importance and means of reporting animal welfare concerns through training, the posting of signage on the website or in the facilities, and other communication modalities.

The system should be clear and accessible for all staff. It is crucial to guarantee that all voices and concerns are heard. Personnel at all levels throughout the organization should be encouraged to raise issues of concern.

Concerns should be investigated by the appropriate key staff and any necessary corrective actions taken.

Moreover, a system should be in place that regularly reviews all incidents reported in order to consider re-appearing concerns and also to evaluate potential changes in your Program.

What you can do:

- Treat any voice of concern with respect and if necessary, with confidentiality.
- Appoint a fiduciary and communicate on how to raise concerns anonymously.
- Organize workshops on (fictional) ethical concerns and other experiences.
- For a guideline, read "Care-full stories: Innovating a new resource for teaching a culture of care in animal facilities" [41].

14.4.5 How Do We Ensure That We Use Respectful Language?

Using respectful and considerate language when talking about colleagues or animals has several benefits. First, it makes communication more effective as misunderstandings may be reduced. A respectful language is the most effective way to play the ball and not the man. Moreover, if everybody is always being respectful in their mentioning of others, no one needs to fear being a victim of slander or bad mouthing. Hence, more honest communication can be promoted. Last, being respectful when talking about the animals indicates having an empathic attitude. It will increase the overall feeling that the animals have a right to be treated with care and consideration. In general, using proper language shows respect to both animals and colleagues.

Ensuring the use of a respectful language is part of the Culture of Care. The management must communicate clearly the rules for communication, and everyone must take a joint responsibility for making it happen. Disrespectful language is often related to not being comfortable and safe in daily work. The general well-being at work is crucial for creating a respectful language and a respectful language is an important contributor to the general well-being at work. Hence, these two factors must work together to reach the goal.

What you can do:

The mnemonic below sums up some of the features and benefits of respectful language.

- R—Responsibility. Take full responsibility for how you refer to animals and your colleagues. You are the one talking; you decide which words you use.
- E—Empathy. Do not be afraid to show empathy for animals and colleagues through our language.
- S—Sensitivity—Be sensitive; your words may have a great impact on other people. Think before you speak.
- P—Presence. Be present, attentive, and considerate if a colleague is approaching you with a difficult topic. Put your cell phone away.
- E—Examination. Examine your own assumptions, perceptions, and biases, before you speak. You could be wrong.
- C—Care—Care for your colleagues and the animals. Consider your wording, when speaking.

- T—Tolerance—Be tolerant, when colleagues state opinions different from yours. Present your views in a respectful language.

14.4.6 How Do We Work with a Shared Responsibility without Losing the Individual Accountability?

The excellence of research and teaching produced by higher education institutions (e.g., universities and research centers) is inherently linked to the integrity and professional attitude of their staff. Institutions have a collective responsibility in developing and implementing a research and educational environment which supports such professional integrity, thereby maintaining and strengthening confidence in their staff' work. Undoubtedly, this also translates to all the staff working with laboratory animals, reinforcing the institutional responsibility to establish a Culture of Care.

The culture of an organization relates to the beliefs, values, and attitudes of its staff and the development of processes that determine how they behave and work together. A Culture of Care is one that demonstrates caring and respectful attitudes and behavior toward animals and encourages acceptance of responsibility and accountability in all aspects of animal care and uses. This should go beyond simply having animal facilities and resources that meet the minimum requirements of the legislation.

In such skilled and multidisciplinary environment, it is important that staff across all different professional categories have the appropriate behavior and attitude toward animal research; operate and endorse a corporate expectation of high standards with respect to the legal, welfare, 3Rs and ethical aspects of the use of animals; Share responsibility (without loss of individual responsibility) toward animal care, welfare, and use; have a proactive approach toward improving standards, rather than merely reacting to problems when they arise; have an effective communication on animal welfare, care and use issues; are aware of their individual role and the importance and responsibility associated with this; conduct their duties with integrity and under compliance; are respected, listened, and supported in their work; have a voice and their concerns are heard and dealt with positively.

What you can do:

- Develop a continuous education program for all staff.
- Set up a 3Rs Awards Program: projects developed by the teams promoting the 3Rs principles are recognized and presented to the rest of the staff.
- Organize "out of the box" events, where anyone can submit "out of the box" ideas to improve practice.
- Perform workplace surveys, to hear the employee's voices, elicit information and pinpoint improvement.

14.4.7 How Can We Recognize Employees for a Job Well Done in Terms of Animal Welfare?

A program of recognition within an organization that has a strong culture of care should daily recognize staff who demonstrate caring by providing ideas for improvements to animal care and use, creating solutions to problems, going "above and beyond" their job description to enhance animal welfare, advancing the implementation of the 3Rs, or serving as role models in exemplifying the behaviors and characteristics consistent with a Culture of Care.

While some employees may be motivated by tangible rewards, others may find the act of being recognized and appreciated, particularly when done in a group setting by someone high up in the organization, to be even more rewarding.

Programs to recognize individual or team exceptional contributions are an extremely powerful employee motivational tool.

Some institutions have regular awards programs, for example, recognizing work done in the promotion and implementation of the 3Rs, celebrating "Animal Technician Day or week" or the "Lab Animal Day" in which recognition is given to staff responsible for the daily care and use of animals. Many examples of these programs can be found on the AALAS website for the International Animal Technician Week.

On the other hand, examples of tangible awards that have been used by some research organizations include special objects (coins, mugs, bags, etc.), gift cards, recognition certificates (paper or virtual), and monetary awards (see also paragraph 1.4).

There are also organizations having external awards programs that recognize excellence in animal welfare, laboratory animal science and medicine, and the 3Rs.

What you can do:

- When you have a colleague who goes that extra mile, do not just appreciate it in words; instead go and see what they are doing. Actions are often more powerful than words.
- Encourage your colleague to present the initiatives, for example, at 3Rs symposia.
- If you, as a leader or manager, present animal welfare/culture of care initiatives at your company or in your facility, be sure to credit the staff involved in any practical work.

14.5 Conclusion: "One Size Does Not Fit All"

From this chapter, it should be evident that Culture of Care will take many different forms according to the individual user establishment, and the authors emphasize that an effective and efficient culture of care in terms of animal welfare is based on an active ownership in each of these user establishments. The authors recommend this individual and adaptable approach rather than a prescriptive regulatory approach.

References

1. European Commission. Directive 2010/63/EU of the European Parliament and of the Council of 22 September 2010 on the protection of animals used for scientific purposes. Off J Eur Union. 2010;276:33–79. EUR-Lex - 32010L0063 - EN - EUR-Lex (europa.eu).
2. European Commission. Directorate-General for environment, caring for animals aiming for better science: Directive 2010/63/EU on protection of animals used for scientific purposes: animal welfare bodies and national committees. Publications Office; 2018. https://data.europa.eu/doi/10.2779/059998.
3. Sørensen DB, Cloutier S, Gaskill BN. Preface in animal-centric care and management. In: Sørensen DB, Cloutier S, Gaskill BN, editors. Enhancing refinement in biomedical research. Boca Raton: CRC Press Taylor and Francis Group; 2021. p. vii–x.
4. Hawkins P, Jennings M. The Culture of Care - a working concept. n.d. Available via NORECOPA https://norecopa.no/media/7711/culture-of-care-working-concept.pdf.
5. International Culture of Care Network. Available at NORECOPA. n.d. https://norecopa.no/more-resources/culture-of-care/.
6. Jennings M, editor. Guiding principles on good practice for animal welfare and ethical review bodies. A report by the RSPCA Research Animals Department and LASA Education, Training and Ethics Section; 2015. Available at https://www.lasa.co.uk/PDF/AWERB_Guiding_Principles_2015_final.pdf.
7. Bertelsen T, Øvlisen K. Assessment of the culture of care working with laboratory animals by using a comprehensive survey tool. Lab Anim. 2021;55(5):453–62. https://doi.org/10.1177/00236772211014433.
8. Hawkins P, Bertelsen T. 3Rs-related and objective indicators to help assess the culture of care. Animals. 2019;9(11):969. https://doi.org/10.3390/ani9110969.
9. Amarasekara DS, Rathnadiwakara H, Ratnayake K, Gunatilake M, Singh VP, Poosala S. The capability maturity model as a measure of culture of care in laboratory animal science. Altern Lab Anim. 2022;50(6):437–46. https://journals.sagepub.com/doi/10.1177/02611929221131313.
10. Robinson S, Sparrow S, Williams B, Decelle T, Bertelsen T, Reid K, Chlebus M. The European Federation of the Pharmaceutical Industry and Associations' research and animal welfare group: assessing and benchmarking 'culture of care' in the context of using animals for scientific purpose. Lab Anim. 2020;54(5):421–32. https://doi.org/10.1177/0023677219887998.
11. Turkménian O, Rocua A, Decelle T. Scoring the culture of care as økey performance indicator in a global pharmaceutical company. Lab Anim. 2023;57(4):432–42. https://doi.org/10.1177/00236772231151516.
12. RSPCA. Communication and a Culture of Care. 2018. Available at NORECOPA. https://norecopa.no/more-resources/culture-of-care/.
13. Narver HL, Hoogstraten-Miller S, Linkenhoker J, Weichbrod RH. Tributes for animals and the dedicated people entrusted with their care: a practical how-to guide. Lab Anim. 2017;46:369–72. https://doi.org/10.1038/laban.1346.

14. Robinson S, Kerton A. Contributing to your culture of care (practical advice for animal care staff). Anim Technol Welfare Dec. 2021;2021:211–4.
15. Robinson S, Kerton A. What does a culture of care look like? Lessons learnt from a workshop survey. Lab Anim. 2021;50:263–71.
16. Klein HJ, Bayne KA. Establishing a culture of care, conscience, and responsibility: addressing the improvement of scientific discovery and animal welfare through science-based performance standards. ILAR J. 2007;43(1):3–11. https://doi.org/10.1093/ilar.48.1.3.
17. Harvard Business School. The Triple Bottom Line: what it is and why it's important. 2023. https://online.hbs.edu/blog/post/what-is-the-triple-bottom-line.
18. Guillén J, Borkowski GL. Evaluation of ethical review and oversight. Processes by AAALAC international. J Appl Anim Ethics Res. 2020:1–22. https://doi.org/10.1163/25889567-bja10005.
19. National Research Council. Guide for the care and use of laboratory animals. 8th ed. Washington, DC: The National Academies Press; 2011.
20. Monje Amor A, Xanthopoulou D, Calvo N, Abeal Vázquez JP. Structural empowerment, psychological empowerment, and work engagement: a cross-country study. Eur Manag J. 2021;39:779–89. https://doi.org/10.1016/j.emj.2021.01.005.
21. LaFollette MR, Riley MC, Cloutier S, Brady CM, O'Haire ME, Gaskill BN. Laboratory animal welfare meets human welfare: a cross-sectional study of professional quality of life, including compassion fatigue in laboratory animal personnel. Front Vet Sci. 2020;7:114. https://doi.org/10.3389/fvets.2020.00114. PMID: 32195275; PMCID: PMC7066073
22. AALAS. Compassion Fatigue: The Cost of Caring - Human emotions in the care of laboratory animals. 2023. Available via AALAS https://wwwaalasorg/education/educational-resources/cost-of-caring. Accessed 9 June 2023.
23. Greasley K, Bryman A, Dainty A, Price A, Naismith N, Soetanto R. Understanding empowerment from an employee perspective what does it mean and do they want it? Team Perform Manage. 2008;14(1/2):39–55. https://doi.org/10.1108/13527590810860195.
24. Prilleltensky I, Nelson G, Peirson L. The role of power and control in children's lives: an ecological analysis of pathways toward wellness, resilience and problems. J Community Appl Soc Psychol. 2001;11:143–58. https://doi.org/10.1002/casp.616.
25. Herzog H. Ethical aspects of relationships between humans and research animals. ILAR J. 2002;43:27–32. https://doi.org/10.1093/ilar.43.1.27.
26. Smith AJ. Guidelines for planning and conducting high-quality research and testing on animals. Lab Anim Res. 2020;36:21. https://doi.org/10.1186/s42826-020-00054-0.
27. Percie du Sert N, Hurst V, Ahluwalia A, Alam S, Avey MT, Baker M, Browne WJ, Clark A, Cuthill IC, Dirnagl U, Emerson M, Garner P, Holgate ST, Howells DW, Karp NA, Lazic SE, Lidster K, MacCallum CJ, Macleod M, Pearl EJ, Petersen O, Rawle F, Peynolds P, Rooney K, Sena ES, Silberberg SD, Steckler T, Wurbel H. The ARRIVE guidelines 2.0: updated guidelines for reporting animal research. PLoS Biol. 2020; https://doi.org/10.1371/journal.pbio.3000410.
28. Brambell R. Report of the technical committee to enquire into the welfare of animals kept under intensive livestock husbandry systems, Cmd, (Great Britain. Parliament). HM Stationery Office; 1965. p. 1–84.
29. Poole T. Happy animals make good science. Lab Anim. 1997;31(2):116–24. https://doi.org/10.1258/002367797780600198.
30. Bayne K, Würbel H. The impact of environmental enrichment on the outcome variability and scientific validity of laboratory animal studies. Rev Sci Tech. 2014;33(1):273–80. https://core.ac.uk/download/pdf/33085907.pdf
31. Laule G, Desmond T. Positive reinforcement training as an enrichment strategy. In: Shepherdson D, Mellen J, Hutchins M, editors. Second nature: environmental enrichment for captive animals. Washington, DC: Smithsonian Institution Press; 1998. p. 302–12.
32. Sørensen DB. Never wrestle with a pig. Lab Anim. 2010;44(2):159–61. https://doi.org/10.1258/la.2010.009100.
33. Sørensen KE, Nielsen OL, Birck MM, Sørensen DB, Leifsson PS, Jensen HE, Aalbaek B, Kristensen AT, Wiinberg B, Kjelgaard-Hansen M, Heegaard PMH, Iburg TM. The use of sequential organ failure assessment parameters in an awake porcine model of severe *Staphylococcus aureus* sepsis. APMIS. 2012;120:909–21.
34. Sørensen DB, Pedersen A, Bailey REB. Animal training: the practical approach. In animal-centric care and management. In: Sørensen DB, Cloutier S, Gaskill BN, editors. Enhancing refinement in biomedical research. Boca Raton: CRC Press Taylor and Francis Group; 2021b. p. 73–90.
35. Hurst JL, West RS. Taming anxiety in laboratory mice. Nat Methods. 2010;7:825–6. https://doi.org/10.1038/nmeth.1500.
36. Weichbrod RH, Thompson GA, Norton JN. Developing a collaborative culture of caring. In: Weichbrod RH, Thompson GA, Norton JN, editors. Management of Animal use and care programs in research, education and testing. 2nd ed. Boca Raton (FL): CRC Press/Taylor & Francis; 2018. ISBN-13: 9781315152189.

37. Boden T, Hawkins P. Communicating the culture of care - how to win friends and influence people. Anim Technol Welf. 2016;15(3):151–6.
38. Tremoleda JL, Kerton A, Mazhary H, Greenhough B. New perspectives for teaching culture of care and their strengths and challenges. Lab Anim. 2023;57(2):170–81. https://doi.org/10.1177/00236772221127352.
39. Tremoleda JL, Kerton A. Teaching a culture of care: why it matters. Rev Bio y Der. 2021;51:43–60. https://doi.org/10.1344/rbd2021.51.31130.
40. Robinson S, White W, Wilkes J, Wilkinson C. Improving culture of care through maximising learning from observations and events: addressing what is at fault. Lab Anim. 2022;56(2):135–46. https://doi.org/10.1177/00236772211037177.
41. Greenhough B, Mazhary H. Carefull stories: innovating a new resource for teaching a culture of care in animal facilities. 2021. Available via Animal Research Nexus. https://animalresearchnexus.org/publications/care-full-stories-innovating-new-resource-teaching-culture-care-animal-research.

Other Resources

Bertelsen T. Measuring Culture of Care. A power point presented at the 10th World Congress on Alternatives and Animal Use in the Life Sciences, Seattle; 2017, [August 2017]. Available at NORECOPA https://norecopa.no/media/7939/bertelsen-measuring-culture-of-care.pdf.

Bertelsen T, Hawkins P. A culture of care. In: Sørensen DB, Cloutier S, Gaskill BN, editors. Enhancing refinement in biomedical research. Boca Raton: CRC Press Taylor and Francis Group; 2020. p. 15–29.

Brown M. Creating a Culture of Care. BLOG available at 3RNC3Rs. 2014. https://www.3rnc3rs.org.uk/news/creating-culture-care.

Franco N. The win-win-win-win scenario of a Culture of Care for animal research. Webinar available at YouTube; 2021. https://www.youtube.com/watch?v=6AuR20SBt18.

ILAR Journal. Special issue: Implications of Human-Animal Interactions in the Laboratory. 2002;43(1). ISSN 1084-2020. Available at Oxford Academic https://academic.oup.com/ilarjournal/issue/43/1.

National Animal Ethics Advisory Committee of New Zealand. A Culture of Care: A guide for people working with animals in research, testing and teaching. 2002. Available at https://www.mpi.govt.nz/dmsdocument/1473.

Research Institutes of Sweden 3R - Refinement in focus at RISE I RISE

Robinson S, Wilkinson C. Maintaining a culture of care during a research animal facility closure. Anim Technol Welf. 2022:11–6. https://www.atwjournal.com/_files/ugd/a30180_c5c159563b154d189a9537c31369848b.pdf

RSPCA. Assessing the Culture of Care: a survey of network members. 2017. https://www.rspca.org.uk/webContent/staticImages/Downloads/CultureOfCareNetworkSurveyReportFinal17.pdf.

Smith A. Ethics, Animal Welfare and the 3R3Rs: An Effective Culture of Care. A power point presented at the ESLAV Summer School, Stockholm; 2018 [June 2018].. Available at NORECOPA https://norecopa.no/media/8106/smith-eslav2018.pdf

White A. The importance of a culture of care. 2018. Poster available at NORECOPA https://norecopa.no/media/klepp411/culture-of-care-poster-gsk-uk.pdf.

Wolters Kluwer. The Culture of Caring in Nursing: 2019 Macrotrends in Nursing -- Reimagining the Future. Short presentation available at YouTube. 2019. https://www.youtube.com/watch?v=9J9rYbEvHA0.

Biosafety

15

Xavier Abad, Guillermo Cantero, and David Solanes

Abstract

The purpose of this chapter is to provide basic but also practical information currently no available on biosafety's books. To this end, the issue has been split into 23 questions and their corresponding answers, with the basic aim of providing all the details and aspects of biosafety applied in the daily work of public and private centers and institutions handling laboratory (or farm) animals, where experts and professionals in the field carry out their work. This feature allows to establish a virtual dialogue and complicity between the authors themselves, who try to reach some consensus in their replies and, hopefully, the readers. The aim of the chapter was never to present itself as a treatise on biosafety, but simply to discuss relevant issues, as considered by the authors: culture of biosafety, staff training and education, accident management, quality in biosafety, user's needs, supplies, animal welfare, waste disposal, and more. The final aim? To achieve, together, the maximum control of all the elements involved in biosafety.

X. Abad · G. Cantero
Bellaterra, Barcelona, Spain
e-mail: xavier.abad@irta.cat; juanguillermo.cantero@zoetis.com

D. Solanes (✉)
Vall de Bianya, Girona, Spain
e-mail: david.solanes@zoetis.com

Keywords

Biosafety · Biocontainment · Biorisk · Infection · Pathogen · Biosafety management

15.1 Why Do We Need Biosafety, Biocontainment, and Biosecurity Measures?

Biosafety, biocontainment, and biosecurity issues are not always fully understood by members of the scientific community, including those working inside such facilities, although useful and extensive guidelines have been published by several sources and are periodically updated [1–3].

Biosafety is closely related to the set-up and execution of procedures for non-risk (or, realistically, very low risk, as zero risk is unattainable) use, manipulation, and handling of pathogenic (for animal, plants, or humans) microorganisms, and it is definitively linked to the internal activities of a given research or production center. Therefore, biosafety practices and procedures depend on factors linked to the microbial agent (its pathogenicity, host range, stability, and transmission route, for instance) and to the activity (volume and infectious titter handled, kind of procedures involved, animal experimentation, etc.). Biosafety focuses on reducing exposure to and the release of biological materials and countering their accidental release.

J. Guillén, V. Galligioni (eds.), *Practical Management of Research Animal Care and Use Programs*, Laboratory Animal Science and Medicine 3, https://doi.org/10.1007/978-3-031-65414-5_15

Biocontainment is, in our opinion, more closely related to the physical and construction-related factors associated with the design of the facility and thus belongs to the realms of architects, engineers, and construction teams. Finally, biosecurity is strongly related to the enforcement of security measures established for the installation to prevent the external (but also internal) activities of some people (luckily, few) who may compromise pathogen containment. Biosecurity refers to ensuring the security of biological materials to prevent their theft or illicit use and to counter their deliberate release. Therefore, biosecurity tries to prevent the potential proliferation of bioweapons whereas the goal of biosafety is to try and mitigate biohazard [4]. In no case should we forget the national regulations and international guidance documents that establish the framework for any activity in which pathogens are used, although many of them are quite country dependent.

We must therefore keep in mind that safety cannot be expressed in absolute terms. It is a relative concept defined in terms of tolerability, acceptability, and feasibility limits; it implies a risk analysis between the cost of biosafety measures and the potential benefits of the work for all of society [5].

Do conflicts arise in achieving the goals of biosafety, biocontainment, and biosecurity? This is not often the case although it must be ensured that narrow biosecurity does not impinge upon or prevent well-thoughtout biosafety activities and programs. Nonetheless, biosafety, biocontainment, and biosecurity must always be considered as words with complementary meanings to describe a general environment of responsible work in the handling of highly pathogenic microorganisms.

15.2 We Need Biosafety for Our Expected Work. At Which Level?

Emerging and re-emerging pathogens represent a constant threat to the health of people and animals. In fact, 75% of emerging diseases in the human species originate in animals, and more than 60% of infectious diseases in people are transmitted from animals themselves, whether domestic or wild.

In recent decades, clinical trials have saved and improved the lives of many people. They are essential for the development of new forms of diagnosis and treatment of diseases and help to check possible side effects of drugs or therapies.

In low- and middle-income countries, where the technology is too expensive, are they doomed not to do research on dangerous pathogens? Do they have fewer rights? Do they have fewer duties? Should their Biosafety be "lower" because they cannot afford the latest technological improvements [6, 7] while others continue to do them? Designing, building, and maintaining complex facilities can take away already limited resources from daily laboratory operations, and impede proper training and education of personnel [8].

Biosafety must be proportional to the pathogenic agent that is handled and sustainable in the environment where it is handled. For a basic description of biosafety levels and hazard groups of microorganisms, we address you to Chapter 1, General Principles of the LBM, WHO, 2004. Is a high-biocontainment facility, biosafety level 3, necessary to handle diagnostic samples of a risk group 3 pathogen? What if we know that the electricity supply is far from guaranteed? What if we do not know if we will have technical personnel to carry out the repair of the HVAC system that allows us to maintain negative pressure? Is a high containment facility necessary to work with infected or uninfected arthropod vectors that have no ecological chance of establishing themselves in the surrounding geographic area?

The risk of handling a pathogen (or samples that may contain it) is multifactorial. It depends on the quantity (volume) and potency (infectious titer, concentration), the agent being handled, its infectious dose and pathogenicity, the route of infection and the ability of transmission, the severity of the infection (from benign to fatal), the endemicity of the pathogen, the susceptibility of the surrounding human or animal population to the activity, the activity we do with the pathogen (diagnosis, propagation, infection in animal models, etc.) and the competence or training of laboratory personnel. And we probably leave factors to be cited.

Many of the aforementioned factors that contribute to the biological risk cannot be managed solely based on the most advanced technology, also require a specific risk assessment, which will be dependent on location and legislation. We cannot stand biosafety and biocontainment on technology alone because we will lose sight of the ecological factor and, more importantly, the human factor. A risk assessment must be carried out that puts the activity at the center and selects the combination of biosafety elements and practices that best suit a reasoned and reasonable set or combination of technological elements (biological safety cabinets, specific PPEs, or engineering safety solutions).

In summary, In front of each sample or group of samples in which we want to isolate a specific pathogen, we do not have to use a checklist, assuming that the pathogen will always be present, and at high concentrations.... Instead, it is necessary to base it on the available evidence, and the measurable risks, and on the history of previous samples or origins. In short, perhaps what needs to be put at the center are the procedures and the personnel, their qualifications, training, and competence.

15.3 What Is the Financial Implication of Biosafety/Biocontainment Implementation?

Europe has the highest biosafety, biosecurity, and biocontainment standards in the world, on a par with the USA, Australia, and New Zealand. Financing these high standards is not an easy task. A very high level of investment is needed to keep these large infrastructures working with pathogens for humans, animals, and/or plants in optimal working order. In developed countries, there is enough funding to be able to cope with this.

The answer to the approach proposed by the question in the paragraph itself is clearly yes, not only it is possible, but it is vitally important for countries to maintain the necessary investments in the short and long term. Failure to do so can lead to a decline in the country's own research, weakening it in relation to the other countries in its own neighborhood. It is necessary to invest in research!

In a research center, whether public or private, it is necessary to consider a maintenance cost of the biosafety facility of approximately 10% of the total budget of the center itself.

This 10% maintenance cost cannot be reduced because doing so could jeopardize the control of all the critical elements on which the biosafety of the facility itself is based.

As an example, we could give a research center with a level 3 biocontainment unit of about 4500 square meters for experimental studies with farm animals, with a total number of working staff of approximately 100 people between technical and research staff, with an annual budget of approximately 6 million euros. The expenditure on maintenance of the center would be around 600,000 euros, including the minimum amount of critical material to keep the level 3 biosafety facility in operation at all times, 24 hours a day, 365 days a year.

Therefore, it is necessary, as already indicated, to invest in research and development in biosafety and biocontainment facilities. These facilities allow progress to be made in the development of new strategies for combating pathogens that cause diseases with devastating effects on humans, animals, plants, and others that have a major impact on the environment. For this reason, if a country is considering the construction, operation, and maintenance of a large infrastructure of this type, it must make provision for its financing in the short and long term. If it fails to do so, it will be putting the environment, flora, and fauna, as well as its own society at risk, not to mention the surrounding countries, in the face of new attacks by the different microorganisms that threaten humanity and biodiversity day in and day out.

15.4 Why the Biosafety in a Facility Where Animals Are Handled Must Be Considered?

At present, in biomedical research, whether in the field of human medicine or in the field of veterinary medicine, it is necessary to be able to have animal models that will help us to carry out the necessary research. This would make it possible to achieve great medical advances or face unexpected threats.

These animal models can only provide significant scientific results if they are maintained and cared for in the best possible conditions. However, we must not forget that, depending on the field of research, it will be necessary (i) to set up barriers for the protection of experimental animals against external elements or (ii) barriers for the protection of the environment regarding such experimental animals. An example of the latter is research which aims to investigate the different pathological alterations of living beings when suffering from an infection by microorganisms.

In the first case, it will be necessary to set up the necessary biological safety barriers to always avoid the pathogenic microorganisms present in the environment can make them sick, causing a serious impact on the welfare of these animals. This will also avoid that experimental outcomes are themselves affected and therefore, not accepted as reproducible.

To protect animals, biosafety zones labelled as specific pathogens free (SPF) have been established in which everything that surrounds the central core of the facility, the area in which the animals to be used will be housed, will be thought, and designed to avoid as far as possible that no pathogen can penetrate and make sick the animals present in the facility.

The barriers considered to be protection are related to the control of the accesses of the people (change of clothes and shower at the entrance) and the control of the materials' accesses (airlock or Sterilized Air Systems—SAS—and double door autoclaves to allow the sterilization of all thermostable materials) prior to access to the area to be preserved from external pathogens. In addition, we will avoid the entry of pathogenic microorganisms from the environment by maintaining a positive pressure, i.e., a flow of air from the inside to the outside of the facility.

On the other hand, if the research to be carried out is based on the challenge of the animals with known pathogens to reproduce a specific pathology or to test a pharmacological product against a disease caused by a microorganism, these animals must be confined to an area surrounded by biocontainment and biosafety mechanisms that prevent leakage of these pathogens to the outside of the confined area. In this case, the barriers considered to be protective will be related to the entrances and exits of people (change of clothes and shower at the exit of the facility) and the control of the exits of potentially or likely contaminated materials (again airlocks or Sterilized Air Systems—SAS—provided with nebulizers or sprayers and double door autoclaves which allow the exit of all thermostable materials through sterilization cycles). In addition, we will avoid the exit of pathogenic microorganisms by keeping a constant (365/24) negative pressure, i.e., a flow of air from the outside to the inside of the facility.

In short, we must keep our facilities under constant surveillance, always ensuring that the biocontainment and biosafety conditions established according to the activity to be carried out in our research are being met and kept (Fig. 15.1).

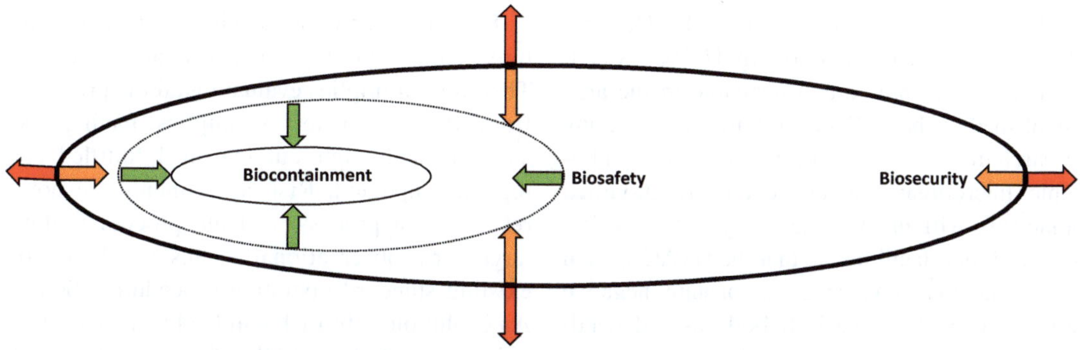

Fig. 15.1 Visual relationship among biocontainment, biosafety, and biosecurity concepts. Arrows (green for biosafety, and orange or red for biosecurity) indicate the main way each concept operates

15.5 Which Are the Basic Elements to Consider When Designing and Building a Facility Under Biocontainment and/or SPF Conditions?

Given the need to design and build a Biocontainment Unit, the Management of the company/university/research institute must set up a multidisciplinary working group in which all the involved Departments should participate, as their needs could be different, even contradictory and a common and agreed design must be reached within minimum technical criteria.

Initially, it will be advisable to propose this design based on the needs of the different lines of research, or stakeholders that will carry out their research, or experimental work, in the facility. Depending on the area in which the research will be conducted, the animal species to be used as preclinical models will be determined. The establishment of the main species to be worked with will be a key element in the process as it will initially determine the characteristics of the design and the materials with which the facility will be built.

"Therefore, it will be key in the decision-making process to determine whether or not to work with genetically modified laboratory animal models (Mouse, Rat, Hamster), or to work with farm animals (Poultry, Pigs, Ruminants), or with animal species considered as companion animals (Dog, Cat), or with Non-Human Primates, or with Fish (Zebrafish, Production Fish). All these fields have specific approaches and challenges. However, in most cases, the center/institute will want to cover more than one of these options which will lead to generating sections in the installation, with different demands.

Each species will need specific environmental (room) characteristics to be used. Depending on it, we will determine a robust material (concrete plus epoxy painting) for the construction of the walls, or we will consider the use of sandwich panels, for the finishing of the rooms. In addition, choosing the species to work with will determine the type of material washing room to be designed and built, although one single-use disposable cages are available. Laboratory animals will be housed in cages (of several sizes) and therefore large washing and sterilization equipment will need to be provided. If space limitations are very strong, the option of single-use cages should be considered but also its sustainability. In the case of other species, except fish—mainly Zebrafish—a large amount of equipment (drinkers, feeders, fences, doors, etc.) will be washed in the same facilities where the animals are housed. How to do it, and its washing circuit should be thought at this stage. In all cases, special attention should be paid to the storing areas.

On another hand, research based on working with GMO lines and immunodeficient animal models will require the design of the Heating, Ventilation, and Air Conditioning (HVAC) system so that positive pressure is available in the area established as the SPF area. On the contrary, any research that involves working with either pathogenic microorganisms or genetically modified organisms will involve the design of biosafety level 2, 3, or 4 facilities, so that the HVAC system allows the maintenance of a constant negative pressure, on a 365/24 basis. In both cases, depending on the number of rooms and their function, a cascade of differential pressures will be necessary, and this will again have repercussions on the initial design and maintenance costs.

15.6 Which Are the Main Elements to Assure Biosafety?

Biosafety is not an absolute concept. It is space dependent, it is time dependent, and it is device/technology dependent. The same problem can be faced with different approaches and different solutions and most of them will be correct.

The two main elements to ensure Biosafety in a facility are the firm commitment of the (executive) Management and a clear hierarchical chain with correctly assigned and implemented roles, and, secondly, promoting and establishing a culture of biosafety among staff. On this last point, continuous training will play an important role, as will the establishment of clear channels to convey all suggestions or criticisms of the personnel regarding the processes or equipment from the point of view of biosafety.

The WHO "Laboratory Biosafety Manual," in its 2020 edition, indicates that the factors that have led to more confirmed or potential exposures to biological agents include: inadequate or ignored risk assessments; lack of standard operating procedures (SOPs); an absence or improper use of personal protective equipment (PPE) and/or insufficiently trained personnel, among others. It can be argued, therefore, that the best-designed and most well-engineered laboratory is only as good as its least competent worker. This is a concept that will appear other times in this chapter.

Promoting and establishing a biosafety culture implies putting biosafety at the center. Therefore, it implies evaluating all the processes from this parameter, it implies having risk assessments thought out, reasoned, fulfilled, and regularly updated. Risk assessments are not a result, but a process, and the process is done largely by observational means but based on existing standard operating procedures (SOPs). An evolution of biorisk will lead to a continuous refinement of these SOPs, for example, of all those that involve the description and operation of critical systems such as autoclaves, airlock or passthrough, disinfection of facilities, effluent treatment, absolute air filtration, etc., but also the use, maintenance, and disposal of personal protective equipment. This will send an indirect signal to the workers about the importance given to the concept, which in turn will reinforce the message of the culture of biosafety, which must be participatory.

The culture of biosafety has one of its levers in the training, already mentioned above, an appropriate introductory, refresher, and mentoring training of personnel. An investigation of reported incidents and accidents. Reports that should always be promoted and never punished, that generate measured and fully explained corrective actions, are another action that sends a signal to the staff.

The technical means, the engineering solutions, the redundancy in the critical elements, the existence of double barriers, are elements that collaborate in biosafety and biocontainment. However, they may not exist, because they are unnecessary, for example, in many facilities that work with pathogens of hazard group 2. The biosafety of these facilities is based on good microbiological practice, good training, and making systems and devices work efficiently and within specifications. In high or maximum biocontainment facilities, handling dangerous group 3 and 4 pathogens, respectively, these technical means are added as a third element of importance to the two previously indicated, High Management commitment and building a biosafety culture (affecting both technical and maintenance staff).

15.7 Which Phases Should Be Considered When Starting Operation to Guarantee Compliance with Biosafety Requirements?

Before starting any activity in the facility, commissioning is mandatory. By commissioning, we should consider testing and validating the performance of the facility components, systems, and integrated systems in sequential methods. In fact, the goal is to check all the relevant elements of the facility working alone and, more importantly, in combination.

Containment laboratories must ensure their operating performances both in normal and, more importantly, emergency situations to avoid compromise the protection of workers, and environment. And environment implies not only humans, also animal beings and crops, plants.

Commissioning of the facility allows prove to regulatory authorities that the facility has taken the necessary precautions to work safely with hazardous infectious agents. In brief, check in advance what could be wrong and try to assure facility could cope with it.

Commissioning should be performed or lead by a third party with no interest in the further running of the facility or with the designer or building contractor to assure independence. The design of the project and its specifications will condition the commissioning of the facility. It is along commissioning that the specifications, the quality of the materials used and their finishings must also be checked.

Commissioning is as "unique" as containment facilities are unique. Two facilities could have different equipment, so give different outputs. Two facilities could have the same equipment, different quality, or differently arranged, so give different outputs. Two facilities could have different staff, so give different outputs. Final aim: all elements work together cohesively to ensure biocontainment, biosafety, and biosecurity which are site specific.

Ideally, all tests should have at least two sequential iterative successful test results. So, do it one time and if success do it a second time with success again. And the testing should be done for both normal and emergency operations.

Commissioning is, so, a comprehensive process that includes all systems. The following list, not exclusive, of tested elements are required: room integrity, tightness, and seals; impermeability; components' compatibility; pressure decay Test; barrier penetrations sealing; door interlocks for airlocks and anteroom; access control and security devices (CCTV and passive and active detection); communication devices; efficiency of HEPA filters; primary containment (BSC); autoclave and disinfection systems; backflow preventers on water and air systems; emergency generators; effluent treatment systems for environmental and biological parameters; solid inactivation systems (incineration, autoclaving, tissue digestion); tightness of containment ductwork (air supply and air exhaust); tightness of HEPA housing; normal power and emergency power supply; UPS; and building control systems.

In addition is good to prepare, in the final steps of the commissioning, emergency response plans, training plans, security plans, and fire response plans and the corresponding related SOPs taking profit from the lessons learned in such process.

If commissioning is OK, certification or permit will be issued but there will be the need to perform recertification sometime in the future in case of any major renovation or big structural change.

During recertification, certain main tests (directly related to biocontainment issues) should be repeated: room integrity-tightness and seals, Communication devices, Door interlocks for airlocks and anteroom, Efficiency of HEPA filters, Primary containment (BSC), Backflow preventers on water and air systems.

And when the activity in the facility finally ends, one day, it will be necessary to consider the decommissioning. But this is another story.

15.8 How Can We Plan a Flexible Facility to Cope with the Actual Needs of Users?

Nobody knows the distant future, but they do know the present and the near future. When designing a facility where biosafety is a key criterion, the basic columns to meet the future needs of internal and external users should be flexibility and redundancy. But these concepts are applied to a basic idea, and this is the intended use of the installation in the next 10 or 15 years.

A building may not be too flexible, but the circuits that are generated in it can be, either in space or in time.

It must be assumed, at the design stage, that critical systems are not exempt from scheduled maintenance needs, or failures, and that options must be considered so that they can be eventually disconnected without totally affecting the operation of the installation.

In all the elements or circuits that are considered critical, we should establish redundant systems (a main system and a secondary system) to deal with scheduled breaks but also with problems or eventualities. The existence of redundant elements in waste management, in air filtration, in the controlled entry of materials or reagents, can allow the maintenance of the facility's activity in the event of punctual or prolonged failures of any of the main systems; the installation is flexible to absorb the incidence.

The redundancy allows to be more flexible also, in the operational procedures.

The flexibility that was initially thought in the face of a specific worst case may be necessary not for this one but to face an unexpected need or request from a user in the future.

In the initial design, it is convenient to run various pre-installations that can be left non-operational but can be quickly activated and validated when the time comes. If they have not been thought of beforehand, the "de novo" installation may mean having to stop the activity of the entire installation or part of it, which makes the installation rigid to incidents or updates.

In the design, it is also convenient to establish sectors that can be punctually isolated from the general operating area of the installation. At this stage, it is convenient to establish alternative circuits without the affected area to verify that they are viable and operational.

Finally, even considering its cost due to inactivity, the existence of redundant spaces or rooms in Biocontainment facilities, or in which experimental animals are handled, can increase flexibility both to deal with an unexpected increase in existing activity and to face a new, urgent activity, but antagonistic to those already underway. The existence of some of these rooms from the very beginning of the design should be seriously valued, especially if we are talking about research or development centers.

15.9 Which Are the Critical Elements of the Facility and How Can We Control Them?

To plan the control of the critical elements of the installation, these critical elements must first be listed. In a biocontainment facility, but also in other scenarios, the following would be a non-exhaustive list:

- Negative pressure gradient, levels between areas and to the outer environment.
- Absolute (HEPA) filtration of exhaust air.
- HVAC system, including environmental conditions (temperature and relative humidity).
- Liquid effluent system (microbiological monitoring, decontamination systems).
- Sterilization equipment (autoclaves).
- Pass-through systems (airlocks, SAS, deep tanks).
- Disinfection program of surfaces (floors, walls, ceilings).
- Lighting system (intensity levels, on/off), mainly in animal boxes.
- Cage washing equipment.

In the second step, we must make a division between collective, general elements of the installation or individual elements, those that affect specific areas or spaces, which can be the object of maintenance decoupled from the installation in general. Within these non-general elements, we could mention anesthesia equipment, Biological Safety cabinets, air-tight centrifuges, housing systems (e.g., ventilated racks), and laboratory research equipment (balances, dispensers, micropipettes, incubators, ELISA readers, thermocyclers, etc.).

For all critical elements, a series of preventive control actions must be scheduled during the year, with a known schedule that must be recorded, and which will also depend on the frequency of use and a previous historical record of incidents (if available). For example, the surface disinfection program (a generic issue) must include the number of times (per week, per month) that floors, walls, and ceilings will be disinfected, which disinfectant will be used, how the disinfectant will be applied, at what concentration, the contact time, if disinfectants will be rotated, under what premises additional disinfections will be carried out, etc. For instance, the proper performance of Biological Safety Cabinets (an individual device issue) can be monitored monthly with some microbiological procedure, to confirm that sterility is maintained by the device when in operation.

These preventive actions may include verifications (which ensures correct operation according to its stated operating specifications) or calibrations (which ensures measurement accuracy compared to a known Standard), and validations. These actions are very frequent for all laboratory equipment, and mandatory if the facility and its procedures are under GLP certification or accreditation of technical competence under ISO17025, among other quality frameworks, such as AAALAC, and must be formally recorded to allow internal and external audits, with dates and responsible person, and may involve the use of stickers directly applied on equipment to show clearly to all if the action has been passed.

If the facility adopts a policy of annual technical shutdowns, many of these scheduled operations, which are usually annual, can be concentrated in that period (2 or 3 weeks). After a general disinfection or decontamination of the installation and according to the planning that was done, it is possible to act on generic critical elements (such as HEPA filtration systems, autoclaves, airlocks, and decontamination tanks) that at that moment have no demand for use, when safe access of external technical assistance personnel can be allowed to carry out calibrations or verification of the functioning of laboratory equipment, without all the restrictions and limitations that this activity implies when the facility is fully operational.

15.10 How Can We Apply a "Culture of Biosafety"?

The culture of biosafety is a set of ways of doing things and ways of thinking that are widely shared by the people who make up an organization in terms of controlling the main risks of its activities.

It is not possible to change biosafety behaviors in a lasting way without changing the way biosafety is viewed and its importance by all members of the organization.

It is not possible to change the way of thinking without evolving the specific messages issued by the Directorate. The culture of biosafety is built through the interaction of different stakeholders within the organization, which must adapt to the constantly changing environment while always ensuring the integration of all its members.

In short, the culture of biosafety reflects the importance that organizational culture in general must give to biosafety in every one of its decisions, departments, jobs, and at all hierarchical levels.

The main aim of a biosafety culture perspective should focus on the most serious risks, those that pose the greatest threat to the organization's survival, that is, serious and fatal accidents. In fact, when a very serious or serious accident occurs, it will almost certainly be due to a systemic failure of many barriers. In this sense, it should be noted that the different families of risks (minor, serious, or very serious accidents) do not fall into the same type of preventive actions: Failures at the organizational level play a much more important role in very serious, or serious accidents than in the case of minor accidents. This approach will be more likely to be successful in terms of consensus, involving all people and even being able to act, secondarily on less serious risks, but not otherwise.

Shared awareness of the most important risks becomes the cornerstone of a company's biosafety culture. They may vary in activity, location, and function, but they need to be known and shared by all organization's staff.

The approach to the most important risks must be based on those that affect the group of selfemployed workers, but also the staff of subcontracted companies and the staff of customer's companies, the environment, the facilities. and the continuity of the company's operations.

In short, acting on the culture of biosafety requires a comprehensive perspective on biosafety, taking coherent action on the technical issues, management of biosafety, and human and organizational factors.

It should be borne in mind that the culture of biosafety will require coherent actions on three pillars: Biosafety based on technical elements, the biosafety management system, and human and organizational factors.

It will be important to focus most of our attention on the organizational and human factors needed to develop and maintain optimal biosafety strategies.

In the end, however, it all boils down to a short, clear message. That the High Management is effectively and visibly involved in biosafety, in its continuous training and that it demonstrates it over time. Biosafety is a long run that only ends when one retires.

15.11 Regarding Biosafety, Which Are the Relevant Positions and Responsibilities to Consider?

As explained before, all staff is needed and it is important to keep proper biosafety in the facility. All individual roles should be involved to ensure success although some positions are more physically related to the concept than others.

So, the first level would be constituted by animal care staff, veterinary staff, and lab technicians handling the samples obtained in the animal facility. At this level, but aside from experimental staff, maintenance service is paramount as its performance can impact the biocontainment and so, the biosafety of the facility. In a secondary, and intermediate layer, we should account with animal facility manager, laboratory facility manager, the biosafety officer, or person assessing biosafety (in small facilities this activity could be performed by one of the previous positions). The Quality Assurance Unit and the person in charge of it are also allocated at this intermediate level. The upper level, which has the more relevant responsibility in keeping biosafety in the facility, giving resources and applying previously communicated policies, is constituted by the senior institutional management.

A Biosafety committee constituted by positions from the three levels is also a tool that should be implemented. It is not a relevant tool and, if affordable, the chairman of this committee can act as a Biosafety Officer, or person appointed to perform an advisory function regarding biosafety.

In the year 2008, it was drafted by European Committee for Standardization (CEN) the Workshop Agreement, the CWA 15793 [9]. In this document, it was proposed a Laboratory biorisk management standard.

A pdf of the document is downloadable at: https://biosecuritycentral.org/resource/requirements-and-protocols/cwa-15793/

The following biosecurity roles have been defined:

Top Management

Top management shall take ultimate responsibility for the organization's biorisk management system.

Top management shall ensure that roles, responsibilities, and authorities related to biorisk management are defined, documented, and communicated to those who manage, perform, and verify work associated with the control of biological agents and toxins.

Top management shall demonstrate its commitment by ensuring the availability of resources to establish, implement, maintain, and improve the biorisk management system.

Senior Management

A senior manager shall be designated with operational responsibility for overseeing the system for management of biorisk.

Functions of the system for the management of biorisk shall include:

(a) Providing appropriate resources to ensure adequate provision of personnel, facilities, and other resources deemed necessary for the safe and secure operation of the facility.
(b) Reporting to top management on the performance of the biorisk management system and any need for improvement.
(c) Ensuring promotion of the biorisk management system throughout the organization.
(d) Instituting review, audit, and reporting measures to provide assurance that the requirements of this standard are being implemented and maintained effectively.

Biorisk Management Committee

A biorisk management committee shall be constituted to act as an independent review group for biorisk issues.

Reporting to senior management, the committee shall:

(a) Have documented terms of reference.
(b) Include a representative cross-section of expertise, appropriate to the nature, and scale of the activities undertaken.
(c) Ensure issues addressed are formally recorded, actions allocated, tracked, and closed out effectively.
(d) Be chaired by a senior individual.
(e) Meet at a defined and appropriate frequency, and when otherwise required.

Functions of the committee should include:

(a) Contributing to the development of institutional biorisk policies and codes of practice.
(b) Approving proposals for new work or significant modifications to the potential risk associated with existing activities.
(c) Reviewing and approving protocols and risk assessments for work involving biological agents and toxins.
(d) Reviewing information relating to significant accidents/incidents, data trends, associated local / organizational actions, and associated communication needs.

Biorisk Management Advisor

A competent individual(s) shall be designated to provide advice and guidance on biorisk management issues.

This individual shall report directly to the responsible senior manager and have delegated authority to stop work in the event that it is considered necessary to do so.

This role shall be independent of those responsible for implementing the program of work.

Functions of the biorisk management advisor should include:

(a) Verifying, in conjunction with other relevant personnel, that all relevant biorisk considerations have been addressed.
(b) Advising or participating in the reporting, investigation, and follow-up of accidents/ incidents, and where appropriate referring these to management / biorisk management Committee.
(c) Ensuring that relevant and up-to-date information and advice on biorisk management is made available to scientific and other personnel as necessary.
(d) Advising on biorisk management issues within the organization (e.g., management, biorisk management committee, occupational health department, and security).
(e) Contributing to the development and / or delivery of biorisk training activities.
(f) Ensuring that all relevant activities are performed in compliance with biorisk regulations and that required biorisk authorizations for work are in place.

Scientific Management

An individual(s) with responsibility for the scientific program within the facility shall be designated with responsibilities relevant to biorisk management.

Functions shall include:

(a) Ensuring that all work is conducted in accordance with established policies and guidelines described in this Standard.
(b) Supervising workers, including ensuring only competent and authorized personnel can enter and work in the facility.
(c) Planning and conducting work activities, and ensuring adequate staffing levels, time, space, and equipment are available.
(d) Ensuring required authorizations for work are in place.
(e) Ensuring laboratory biosafety and laboratory biosecurity risk assessments have been performed, reviewed, and approved, and that the required control measures are in place.
(f) Ensuring that all at-risk employees have been informed of risk assessments and/or provisions for any recommended precautionary medical practices (e.g., vaccinations or serum collections).

Occupational Health
The organization shall have access to appropriate occupational health expertise and establish an occupational health program commensurate with the activities and risks of the facility.

The role should include providing input into risk assessment from a worker health perspective, advising on first aid / emergency treatment measures and follow-up, liaising with external healthcare providers, and coordinating medical examinations, surveillance, and vaccination programs. Roles and responsibilities of the occupational health professional should be determined considering requirements set out in this standard.

Facility Management
Facilities manager(s) shall be appointed with responsibilities relevant to facilities and equipment determined in accordance with requirements set out in this standard.

Security Management
A security manager shall be designated with responsibilities determined in accordance with requirements set out in this standard.

Animal Handling
In laboratories where animals are maintained, an animal care manager shall be designated with responsibilities determined in accordance with requirements set out in this standard.

At present, the CEN's scheme of work roles is still valid. We could only consider that the Biorisk management advisor is nowadays called Biosafety Officer.

15.12 How Should the Technical Staff of the Facility be Managed?

The most important resource of any animal facility is a competent and motivated staff. The organization of the technical support staff in a high-biocontainment unit is extremely important because they will oversee carrying out everything that is defined in the experimental procedures designed by the study directors but also will be involved in the day-to-day solving of technical challenges of biocontainment maintenance of the facility.

The technical staff must be highly skilled, and continuously trained regarding the different areas they are involved and the different studies in which they must participate. A non-exhaustive list of issues is shown.

In the first place, the training, updating, and life-long education of all the people in charge of the different tasks within the Unit. The technical personnel must understand and remember the basic principles/concepts of biosafety/biocontainment, in such a way as to give them the paramount importance required to properly carry out the work.

The staff receives specific instructions in the handling of pathogenic and sometimes potentially lethal agents and is supervised by competent professionals with experience in working with these agents. These instructions should be refreshed regularly.

Clear delimitation of working areas within the Unit and assignment of clear responsibilities, and persons in charge by defined areas.

Establish the number of people needed to cover the different experimental activities that are expected to be carried out in each of the aforementioned areas. In addition, it is important to consider weekends, holidays, pregnancy, and sick leaves.

Review and evaluation of the schedule of the different experimental procedures by the people in charge of the Unit together with the people acting as Study Director, to discuss the viability of the experimental procedures and in turn organize and assign a technical staff responsible for organizing all issues and materials required by the study. It is important that all relevant staff are involved at the very first moment to make them participate from the beginning.

A person acts as the person in charge of the Unit and is responsible for organizing all the experimental activities in a monthly operations table. This table is openly shared with the technical staff of the Unit, to visualize all the operations to be carried out throughout the month and its possible interactions and/or incompatibilities.

Weekly meetings with all the members of the Biocontainment Unit will be scheduled to update, discuss, and assign the tasks for the week. Open and constant communication by any means, either presential, by telephone, by walkie, or by email between the members of the team and those responsible for the Biocontainment Unit.

Staff should be encouraged to be fully autonomous but at the same time exercise continuous gentle monitoring of activities with on-site visits, joint work, review of recorded actions, etc.

15.13 How Can We Deal with The User's Needs/Requests?

A facility under Biocontainment must allow that all activities can be carried out without compromising the quality of work or the safety of personnel. But how do we respond in a timely manner to the needs of users?

In the first place, we must define who will be the people responsible for the organization of all the activities that will be carried out within the facility; this "committee" will oversee establishing the rules to be followed by all the users, responding to their needs under several biosafety and ethical requests.

Work in biocontainment implies a strict protocolization of the activities to be done. And one of the first things to be decided is the timetable booking of the experimental boxes. All the requests should be addressed to the person responsible for the Biocontainment facility or delegated person, registering and coding in strict order of entry, always prevailing the order of the request, first come first served. But the request should be accompanied by an own calendar of activities, sampling, and necropsies and, if possible, a complete protocol. The non-confidential information will always be public and kept open in the intranet through an "occupation calendar" so that all users can have access to book remaining time slots or discuss among them to insert additional activities. This calendar is open and active on a yearly basis, that is, the current year; however, for long, time consuming or strategical experiments (to be decided by Direction) a pre-booking could be made in the following year, but not beyond this established period. In the case of cancellation of the booking by the Study Director, by own reasons, and non-related with suppliers, or costumers, an economic penalty according to the existing internal regulations could be issued.

But all this is purely mechanical… How deal with the requests or expectations of the users?

Their expectations can be rocketed, in any case, can be hard to satisfy, due to the demands of their competitive projects and/or contracts. We must count on it, and be prepared. The idea of success and quality, however, lies in facing constructively to those expectations, surprisingly favorably.

One single word will be invoked. Communication. Simply, maintaining a constant and open communication channel between the person leading the Biocontainment Unit, and this functional committee with the final user. It does mean giving an adequate, complete, fast, and reliable response, which adds additional value to what would be a process solution. To be fully aware of the needs of the users, to advice quite in advance is some of the requests are unachievable or against animal welfare regulations, to be flexible to accept further changes in the protocol (only if previously accepted by the Ethical Committee). This is the only way to cover almost all known but also some unknown needs of the users. On the other hand, discussing with the researcher about the capabilities of the facility and the experimental boxes will increase, year by year, the understanding from the facility users, and achieve the greatest possible participation and involvement of all the personnel in the philosophy of excellence in service to the user personnel.

15.14 How Can We Manage the Experimental Procedures to be Done?

The continuous search for alternatives or new approaches is always necessary since as time and technology advance, the methodology by which experiments can be carried out can be surely improved. What is now the "Top," in a few years may be partially obsolete so you must review the techniques and update, avoiding inertia (staying the same). This also applies to the biosafety of the facility, although an update may be achieved by improving procedures and not by large changes and renovations. Improving the conditions of the animals, giving the utmost importance to animal welfare apart from favoring their lives, will be also very beneficial for the study since the results obtained are usually more accurate, reproducible, and publishable.

The best way to deal with an experimental procedure is through a specific and coded folder that contains all the subfolders or partitions to be fulfilled with different files. Experimental protocol, Deviations and amendments, Communications and emails, Ethical Committee evaluation, Biosafety Committee evaluation, calendar, etc.

The person who acts as Study Director or research responsible will send the details of the study protocol to the people responsible for the Biocontainment Facility (or the committee acting as a single person); this information being analyzed by the people who hold the positions of Animal Welfare Advisor, Designated Veterinarian, Biosafety Officer, responsible for the animal Unit. If there is any doubt, or gap, a fast meeting will be agreed with this person to discuss the controversial aspects. A record of the discussion and decisions will be issued and filed in the folder. Once the different controversial aspects have been polished, the study will be incorporated into the monthly Animal Facility's calendar, publishing it in the daily operations table together with the rest of the experimental procedures, to visualize all the daily activities of the current month. This incorporation of the study in the calendar with all the associated information will allow the technical animal facility staff to organize and prepare all the actions of the study (forecast of feed, supplements, preparation of sampling material, label printing, etc.).

At this point, it is highly recommended that the person who best knows the possible response of the animals during the study train the technical staff that will be involved in it so that this staff is familiar with the likely reactions that will appear during the study. All the information provided during this training course will be posted on the intranet, in the corresponding folder so that it can be consulted whenever there is a need.

Once the study in question begins, if the person who holds the position of Study Director requests any amendment from the agreed initial experimental procedure (for example, extra sampling), an assessment of the request will be internally made again. Any change can have ethical but also biosafety outputs, and both should be assessed. If, when evaluating the request, the conclusion reached is that this change is a relevant modification, the Ethical Committee should be urgently informed to get final permission.

Throughout the study, the data obtained, and the information handled will be duly filed in the corresponding electronic subfolders (data, consumables, deviations, photos, etc.). This information will be totally available both to the technical animal facility staff who provide the support service throughout the study, and to the research staff responsible for it.

Once the study ends, the file folders will be closed, conveniently kept in the secure space of the computer server. From that moment, files are available and can be downloaded but are not modifiable.

A common template, which organizes the necessary files and reduces subjectivity or mistakes when archiving them, is a good starting tool. Training staff in the proper use of office tools and in clear recording and archiving is a crucial improvement, too.

15.15 How Should the Supplies be Organized?

Supplies are essential in any complex technical activity. They must be received on time and in an adequate and balanced amount to allow an optimal execution of the activity. Installation supplies are basically energy sources (electricity, gas, diesel, etc.) and those derived from the functional maintenance of critical elements (absolute filters and other filtration elements, chemicals for decontamination, disinfectants, decontaminants), those involved in the safety of people (clothing, personal protective equipment, spare parts or consumable elements of primary barriers such as biological safety cabinets) or associated with experimental activities (feed, supplements, antibiotics, sedatives, reagents, molecular or serological diagnostic kits, single-use plastic, etc.).

There must be a list of these materials to be supplied, with their main and secondary supplier, contact information, and prices, which must be updated on a regular basis, at most annually. This review can coincide with an annual evaluation of the suppliers, in which their diligence, quality, price evolution, after-sales service, or attention to the resolution of incidents that have occurred, are analyzed. The evaluation must be, at least, semiquantitative, and kept in a written form, and must have consequences (search for alternative suppliers) if a minimum score established before starting the evaluation is not exceeded. At this point, collaboration with the Quality Unit is essential.

There must be a person responsible for each area (laboratories, stables, general maintenance) who oversees stock management and the purchase of the necessary references. Depending on the dimensions of the facility and the volume of purchases, all areas may depend on a single person.

Purchases must always be made assuming "worst case" scenarios, which are in a certain way the opposite of "just in time," because it implies that many supplies will have a storage stay of weeks or months. In a biocontainment facility or in which biosafety is a fundamental pillar of the activity, it is not admissible not to have supplies available when they are necessary; there can be no out of stock. There must always be a critical limit of units, kilograms, or liters that, when reached, activates the mechanism for a new purchase to reach an optimal level of availability. It is very risky to activate purchases with zero storage. This leads, as a corollary, to the need to have a storage space, outside biocontainment (the more storage space there is inside biocontainment, the better, but there are cost limitations in this approach), which acts as a nursery for installation. In a certain way, the previously mentioned concepts of redundancy are applied again.

The entries of a good part of the supplies in the facility must be by slots, through the enabled points (airlocks, SAS) and preferably at fixed times, and the aforementioned entries must be registered; intermediate storage points must be fixed and known to all.

The lack of supplies can lead to a partial or total stoppage of the installation. Therefore, supply management must guarantee that if a critical primary supply (such as electricity, which is not easily storable) fails, there is an abundant and secured alternative primary supply (generator in good condition, more than enough diesel, full reserve tank, replenishment agreement of daily diesel levels). That, if a feed supplier fails, there is a second known and evaluated supplier on the list that can fill the gap.

If the installation executes an annual technical shutdown, it may be a good policy to make, a few weeks in advance, a large purchase of supplies to make replacements and assistance in said technical shutdown (see Section 21 of this chapter).

15.16 How Should the Animals be Managed?

To scientifically address present and future public health challenges, it is necessary to have professionals trained in different aspects within the fields of medicine, veterinary science, and ecology/biology. The comprehensive approach to zoonotic diseases requires knowledge of their origin, trying to act at this first level to avoid the zoonotic leap, but also preparing to eventually counteract the effect of infectious agents on potential intermediate hosts and, of course, develop products to be able to prevent and treat infection or disease in the same animals and people. Hence the interest in having animal models of infection with zoonotic agents, ideally capable of recapitulating most or some of the clinical symptoms suffered by humans. Small laboratory animals, moreover, offer the possibility to work with pure human infectious diseases, and with human metabolic disorders; if the approach implies the use of genetically modified microorganisms, biosafety should be brought to the front.

These models contribute to generating knowledge about the pathogenesis of the disease and, very importantly, being able to test the efficacy of existing or newly developed products in the field of pre-clinical research. Infection models in animals represent one of the essences of translational medicine, since they allow disciplines, resources, knowledge, and techniques to be combined to promote improvements in the prevention, diagnosis, and treatment of diseases in people. These improvements should be done in a strong quality framework that also encompasses the handling and care of animal models (small or farm animals); the ways and standards to achieve this quality are diverse.

However, recapitulating the clinical and pathological features of a human disease caused by a zoonotic infectious agent in an animal model is not an easy task. All models have their limitations, since they usually reproduce some aspects of the disease (clinical signs, biochemical or metabolic parameters, pathology, etc.), but rarely all of it. Likely reproducing a human disease completely in an animal model is an impossible task, given that in addition to the conditioning factors of the species, there are those related to genetic variability within the same species, the epidemiology of the infection/disease itself, animal behavior, and the existence of co-morbidities. Based on these limitations, and paraphrasing Dr. David B. Weiner (Univ. Pennsylvania, USA) in his famous phrase "*mice lie and monkeys exaggerate*," the challenge for the pre-clinical researcher but also the technical animal staff of a Biocontainment facility is to find the best model (or even better, various animal models) that allow the maximum reproducibility of the symptoms and lesions of human diseases, including their variability. And that these animal models can be run in proper animal welfare and biosafety standards in the facility. However, it must be said that sometimes the objective is not to develop a preventive product for people, but for the animals themselves, and that possible zoonotic transmission can be limited. In both cases, however, the biosafety approach and the training should be the same as the source of hazard, the pathogen, is invariable.

Once the animal model has been chosen and the experimental protocol has been approved, the animals are received into the Biocontainment Unit, from which different protocols are established, always ensuring the welfare of the animals. They will be housed and distributed according to the study protocol and then the adaptation period.

Prior to the start of an experimental research study using animals, the researcher must submit a project evaluation form to be assessed by the Ethics Committee on Animal Experimentation. This project evaluation form must include an animal welfare monitoring protocol (which will depend on the pathogen and the disease), with very well-established qualitative and quantitative endpoint criteria (supervision protocol). Once the experimental study has been initiated, based on the established supervision protocol, the researcher, the technical staff, and the designated Veterinarian follow up the animals with the frequency established in the protocol. Once the first symptoms have been detected, direct and rapid communication between the personnel involved (researcher, technical staff, and designated veterinarian) should be paramount to proceed, if such symptoms progress, to euthanasia of the animal. The monitoring techniques include daily body temperature, body weight control, and the sampling of blood and swaps at the pre-established protocolized time points.

Equally, the kind of pathogen involved, the way this is excreted or secreted by the animal model, the expected viral loads, its transmissibility in the animal model used should always be considered prior the experimental start to implement the biosafety, biocontainment (cleaning and decontamination of the experimental box in which animals were housed) and mitigation measures (PPE) until the end of the experimental procedure (including cleaning and decontamination of the experimental box in which the animals participating in the experimental study have been housed).

It is also important to consider the ethological needs of the different species, which implies, currently, social housing, ad libitum feeding, and environmental enrichment. The social housing will be applied always for all species, with the sole exception of problems of hierarchism, in case of male mice; then, the males are individually housed and are provided with pipes to chew, cellulose paper, and paper rolls to use as hiding places. Always it must be considered the ad libitum feeding; however, depending on the experimental objectives, animals can be kept in fasting conditions, only after approval by the competent body. Finally, species-related environmental enrichment must be considered. For rodents, examples are pipes to chew, cellulose paper to build the nest, and paper rolls to use as hiding places. For rabbits can use wooden elements to gnaw, small amounts of hay that allow them to ingest long fiber with a clear entertainment function. For ferrets tubes to connect two cages will be used by the animal as a tunnel; also platform inside the cage and cloth rags that allow them to snuggle are useful. For pigs good environmental enrichment examples are hanging chains with multiple ropes resting horizontally on the ground, allowing the pig to bite and stretch them; yellow hard plastic balls that can move and soft plastic elements so they can bite and entertain. Cattle, goats, and sheep could use feed supplementation blocks to be licked by the animals, and plastic flanges that they can bite. For poultry, useful enrichments are the strips of red paper between the chips so that they entertain pecking.

In this complex set-up, animal management should always consider the elements all together and their interactions: the animal itself, feeding, welfare, and the pathogen. It is important that all different human actors establish crystal clear communication, particularly with extra attention to the biothreats resulting from these interactions.

15.17 How Can We Manage the Waste in a Safe Manner?

The correct waste management in a facility that handles laboratory animals, whether small or large, and pathogens is crucial and challenging since it usually includes a parameter that is not frequent in many laboratories: the load, the amount of waste, which is currently high.

By waste, we understand everything that cannot be recovered or properly reused and that is generated in the daily experimental activity. The air in the facility is a waste, which must be absolutely filtered (HEPA filters); all the solid materials that are discarded are waste (single-use plastic material, gloves, masks, work clothes, animal bedding, the animals themselves after a necropsy, etc.); and all liquids or effluents from the activity are waste (water from personnel showers; autoclave condensates; liquids discarded in laboratory sinks; water with detergent or disinfectant used to disinfect wall, floor or ceiling surfaces; or used in cleaning cages, for small animals, or experimental boxes, for large animals).

The waste must be taken by the shortest route possible to the point of inactivation or treatment. During their journey, it must be ensured that their insulation or tightness (this affects gaseous or liquid fluids) is maintained and that they do not transfer risk to the surroundings.

The circuits for waste disposal must be clear, with specific appointed persons in charge and a detailed record of the actions (material that is discarded, origin, person responsible for the treatment, optimal waste treatment parameters). These records, which must be integrated into the center's quality records, must be accessible only to personnel trained and involved in the activity, and to personnel concerned, as would be the case of the Biosafety Officer.

There are types of non-processable or manageable waste at the facility (for example, cytostatic waste and radioactive waste). For these, a safe exit circuit must be established, which does not compromise the facility operation or the environment, in a closed, watertight, and easy-to-disinfect container.

Below we provide examples of records to be kept. Please note this list is not exhaustive:

- Elimination of waste by autoclave.
- Disposal of animal waste by incineration.
- Disposal of animal waste by digester.
- Transfer of unprocessed waste to an external treatment company.
- Record of operation and critical parameters of the absolute air filtration system (coupled with a record of change of pre-filters and absolute filters).

15.18 How Could Maintenance and Repairs Impact Biosafety? How to Deal with Such Impact?

Scheduled maintenance operations should never affect biosafety or biocontainment if they are properly managed. Nor does it have to generate an impact on the general operation of the activity (research, diagnosis) if it is programed. One way to do this is through the annual technical shutdown tool that allows, once the entire facility has been decontaminated, to carry out maintenance operations safely for both internal and external assistance personnel (reviewed in Section 21 of this chapter). Another way to do it is by dividing the area in which the element to be maintained is located (within the schedule established in the year), decontaminating the area if the element may contain microbiological hazard, prohibiting access to all personnel not involved and signalling and warning of this prohibition, and intervening with the minimum necessary staff. This prohibition of access to the rest of the personnel will be maintained not until the end of the intervention, but until it is confirmed that the maintenance has been successfully completed and the element or device works correctly.

The case of repairs is different, as they are corrective. In principle, they cannot be planned, and maybe the consequence of preventive maintenance that has not covered all the weak points, or could follow unsafe or directly incorrect actions of the personnel on the equipment. In this case, the impact is double: on one hand, an activity is interrupted, without being completed, and, on the other, we have a non-operating element, device, or area with potential biological risks.

The direct impact of the activity can be solved using the two concepts indicated at the beginning of this chapter: flexibility and redundancy. If another biological safety cabinet, or centrifuge, or ELISA reader, or incubator, or deep freezer is available, the activity is safely diverted to the new item, after running a fast risk assessment. It is good practice to have assumed on paper a good number of contingencies or breakdowns and to have evaluated potential solutions from the biosafety point of view. Having thought about the contingency beforehand makes the resolution quicker and automatic afterward.

The indirect impact on the activity is the need for corrective action in uncontrolled circumstances, in a limited area that is out of use. The first step is to mark the area or element; the second is to decontaminate the space or inspect the element to be fixed, provided with the necessary PPEs. Thirdly, organize the corrective action and its duration (we must try to return to the initial situation in the shortest time possible since redundancy and flexibility are not unlimited), which requires having spare parts or being able to obtain them in a short time; then execute the corrective action, check the correct operation of the element, safely remove elements or parts out of service, considered as waste, and return to normal operation, formally notifying the personnel concerned.

All these activities must be carried out by facility personnel, preferably contracted for facility management tasks, with training in biosafety and knowledge of the equipment, who work side by side with trained maintenance personnel. It is good policy to minimize rotations among these responders who will function better as a cohesive team if they have faced equivalent operations together in the past.

15.19 Biosafety on the Road: How Can We Organize Safe Shipment of Infectious Samples from a Biocontainment Unit? (*)

A biological sample can reach the outside of a high or maximum Biocontainment (BSL3 and BSL4, respectively) area in two ways: either without inactivation (infectious) if it must be transferred to another equivalent Biocontainment facility, or after undergoing an inactivation process to render the biological sample non-infectious. For Biosafety Level 2 facilities, the exiting of samples with previous inactivation is not currently needed as most of the samples and pathogens handled can be assigned to Category B, UN 3373, Biological Substance.

15.19.1 Transferring Non-Infectious Samples

This is an important issue with further human and livestock health implications as well as economic impacts if inactivation is not properly performed. In this way, we can distinguish two main types of inactivation procedures. Firstly, in-house procedures, following internal protocols, many of which may have been previously reported in the scientific literature. Several procedures have been used for many years with seemingly good safety records (although difficult to quantify in terms of log10 reduction of viral infectious titers). These include thermal procedures, inactivation by solvent or detergents [13], use of chaotropic agents, phenol: chloroform extraction procedures, desiccation on specially treated papers (Flinders Technology Associates cards aka FTA cards), as well as inactivation by fixation for pathology purposes [10, 11, 12, 14, 15]. The choice of inactivation treatment (or step) should be closely related to the destination of the sample (pathology, molecular biology, immunological techniques, biochemistry, etc.), should be validated and records should be kept for further audit.

15.19.2 Transferring Infectious Samples

Researchers commonly refer to specific guidelines [Laboratory biosafety manual from WHO, PHAC, BMBL, or NIH-CDC], which distinguish between Category A and B infectious substances [16] and their methods of shipping. However, specific regulations within each country should also be considered. In this case, the danger exists in the transportation of the biological specimen between facilities (biosecurity issues may also play an important role), but not necessarily in their further handling as those materials will be used, propagated, and tested in a facility of equivalent biosafety level (either BSL3 or BSL4 facilities).

A restricted file to record all commercial kits, inactivation mixtures, protein extraction reagents, and viruses and bacteria assayed in such internal validation tests should be created. Moreover, it is necessary to set a follow-up of all inactivated samples, with an electronic file kept updated all the time with the following information: recording number of vials, volume, identification, animal, or human origin, bacterial or viral pathogen involved, inactivation treatment applied, contact time, person in charge, responsible of the exit through the airlock, and final destination of the samples.

15.20 Accidents Under Biocontainment; How to Deal with Them? Can We Take Advantage from Them?

Any human activity involves the possibility of errors. If the activity is very repetitive, the frequency of these potential errors, even if it is low, ends up emerging and manifesting itself. When handling biologically hazardous material, or being in an environment with various biological hazards, the accident, an event or circumstance that is not planned or intended and that causes injury, can have intense and long-lasting consequences.

How to manage incidents, events, or circumstances that are not planned or intended and that cause damage or non-desirable effects on processes, and accidents in a biocontainment and biosafety environment? The answer is in three basic words: transparency, actions, and communication, the TAC.

If healthy culture of biosafety has been generated in the facility, it will be guaranteed that all accidents are reported; this is, in principle, possible, since an accident generates personal consequences or consequences for the facilities. But it is also important that all incidents are reported so that they can be analyzed and reviewed. Incidents are frequent and are the prelude to minor accidents and these, in turn, to serious ones. Communication of incidents (a reagent that has expired, or is not located where it should be; a key that is not where it should be; misplaced IT of a device or equipment; systematic failure to record an action; repetitive repairs in a device or apparatus, etc., small hits suffered from different people in a specific action or location) implies keeping the personnel alert with regard to the operation of the facility; Moreover, one can allow to guess a possible future accident by mentally taking the incident further, or stronger and try to implement measures to avoid undesirable consequences.

In addition, analysis and review of incidents demonstrate the involvement of the management team with biosafety and biocontainment. This always reinforces the culture of biosafety. And, in turn, it can reveal gaps in staff training or understanding of written procedures. Both facts can be corrected, with more training and with a new wording of said procedures. The monitoring of these changes allows also a continuous improvement of the system, which will reduce the frequency of incidents, and, indirectly, of accidents with serious consequences.

Once the accident occurs, an investigation must be carried out both horizontally and vertically to analyze, i.e., if this action has been previously reported with one or more incidents; if the same person has been involved in similar accidents; if the person was properly educated and trained and updated with such training; the possible presence of concurrent causes; is these causes are present in other areas of the facility; whether devices or appliance alarms were bypassed or silenced, etc. The investigation and its conclusions must be public, accessible, and explained to the technical staff of the facility's management team, which is the one that accompanies and supervises the research team.

The analysis over the years of incidents or accidents occurred in various high and maximum biocontainment laboratories confirms that most of the accidents are due to human error, with more than 65% (see [17]). By categories, the category that represents a higher rate of incidents (between 60 and 70%) is incidents due to lack of competence when performing the tasks associated with the activity. For example, skin exposures to hazardous elements or possible spills, and/or generation of aerosols when pipetting. Between 20% and 30% are due to errors in the application of existing standards or protocols. Lastly, far behind, between 3 and 4%, incidents due to lack of knowledge or experience: for example, ineffective virus inactivation in a high-biocontainment facility prior to shipment to a lower biosafety facility.

Therefore, investigation of incidents and accidents helps us to reduce them, visibly applying the continuous improvement tools within the facility so that they can serve as an example for other areas within the company.

15.21 Is Periodical Scheduled Technical Shutdown Needed?

Biocontainment facilities cannot be shut down while ongoing experiments with dangerous pathogens are performed. Whenever these are handled, or experiments with infected animals are in progress, all critical parameters must be maintained: negative pressure, active barrier systems, outlet showers, effluent management, and absolute air filtration. During the usual experimental activities, small preventive, and corrective maintenance works can be carried out, but these do not cover the entire installation (e.g., accessing and manipulating the electricity supply panels and the ability to open the emergency doors).

A biocontainment facility also has many equipment and devices that must be verified, preventively maintained, and updated by technical personnel from external companies. The risk assumed by the managers of the facility with the entry of these personnel in periods of normal operations is greatly reduced if said personnel enters in a controlled manner in a limited period in which the installation has been placed on standby, without activity. This scheme would not apply, obviously, to urgent repairs, but it does reduce the overall risk.

The drawback of any "technical stop" lies in the loss of time, and therefore of efficiency of the facility. Devoting 2–3 weeks to a general review of the building and its systems, and allowing access to all the external technical assistance services that are necessary to maintain, verify, calibrate, update facilities and laboratory equipment, can initially look like wasted time, but it is, in fact, an investment.

The technical shutdown must imply the cessation of activity with any pathogen and any infected animal. An intense cleaning of the installation is then carried out and its subsequent decontamination (aerial disinfection) of all its volumes. The general decontamination equalizes the spaces that have different assigned protocols during the year, which facilitates the movement of people and materials in the maintenance work during this technical stop. The only thing that remains, for safety reasons, is the mandatory nature of the exit shower to exit the facility.

With the facility in standby, at minimal risk, it is possible to adjust general and sectorial electrical panels; check the operation of compressed air systems and their resilience; cut-off electricity and confirm operation, and response times, of the UPS system and diesel generator; activate emergency doors; carry out evacuation or emergency drills that involve the use of the above; schedule "general" changes of pre-filters or absolute HEPA systems, etc. In short, the standby allows to test and challenge the main control and security systems to adjust them, if necessary. Therefore, when the facility is reactivated, we are reasonably sure that it will be able to reach the next technical shutdown without the need for relevant corrective measures.

In small facilities with systems that are not very complex and easy to control or overview, a technical stop is still useful but perhaps not essential. In facilities with thousands of square meters, with a multitude of interconnected systems, and where a very diverse danger accumulates throughout the year, a scheduled technical stop, with an intense and detailed work program on critical systems and accessories, not only is useful, but it would also be essential.

15.22 How Can We Implement an Effective Training to Ensure the Necessary Competence of the Staff?

In BSL3 facilities, Basic Biosafety Training is achieved by reading the general Biosafety level 3 manual (Biosafety operational manuals are needed from BSL2 to BSL4, see Laboratory Biosafety Manual, WHO [18]) and accompanying SOPs detailing safety practices and procedures and common procedures (way of entry and exit, chemical and hazardous waste handling, transfer of infectious substances, emergency contact information). There are computers available in each laboratory, which enable electronic access to these various SOPs and protocols. Each principal investigator is also responsible for ensuring his/her personnel follow all procedures as outlined in the approved biosafety manual. Nevertheless, Biosafety Officer and Management Biosafety Staff conduct post-training monitoring to ensure full compliance with SOPs. Retraining is mandated for individuals who deviate from approved protocols and could imply total restriction of access to biosafety facilities (temporarily or permanently).

15.22.1 Specific Biosafety Training

This training must include information about the infectious agents to be used, routes of exposure, symptoms, medical surveillance, appropriate PPEs, incident response, post-incident response, post-exposure medical surveillance, how to report such exposures and incidents, and follow-up procedures. In a specific experiment, personnel should be trained on facility-specific equipment, and how this equipment interact with samples and modify (increase or decrease) the hazard.

Any change in an experimental procedure reported to the Biosafety Officer will lead to a new risk assessment analysis and, if it proceeds, additional training should be provided.

As part of the initial and refresher training, all personnel must review and sign laboratory manuals to acknowledge their existence and location as needed for consultation of procedural or safety concerns, and for review of any updated materials from the last reading. By signing, personnel acknowledge that they have been advised of the hazards associated with this research, that they have been properly trained in the handling of the biological agent following biosafety guidelines (irrespectively the biosafety level, from 2 to 4), and that they agree to adhere to these regulations.

So, as a general conclusion of biosafety training programs, they must be designed with people, facilities, and processes in mind. Three legs support the successful management and implementation of such a large and complex training effort: (1) proper implementation, (2) continuous assessment and refinement, and (3) development of a self-supporting culture of compliance (the staff is prone to communicate all incidents and ways to achieve improvements), which is strongly related to a successful implementation of a culture of biosafety.

15.23 How Can the Achieved Biosafety Level be Maintained in Time?

A competent risk assessment of the activity "ex ante" indicates at any time the level of biosafety and the necessary biocontainment elements. In an existing facility, the biocontainment constructive elements may not be modifiable, but practices and training, some updates of installations or circuits, and the use of new or different personal protective equipment (PPE) may allow to achieve higher biosafety standards than the initial ones.

The maintenance of biosafety standards implies, in the first place, a commitment from the Senior Institutional management on these issues. The level of biosafety that is acquired with education and training, and with an investment in the maintenance of biocontainment elements, can only be maintained over time if the Senior Management commits to maintaining biosafety as a critical parameter in the management of the facility, and devotes sufficient investment to it, in a sustained manner over the years.

Secondly, a culture of biosafety must be generated among the staff, who must be involved in the maintenance and continuous improvement of their skills and training. This implies, at a minimum, designing a training system that is not repetitive and that adds value to successive training sessions. In this aspect, the involvement of the Biosafety Committee and specifically, the Biosafety Officer, in the generation and management of contents is important. The culture of biosafety should also favor suggestions and proposals for improvements by the staff. There must be a clear and marked circuit for these inputs; all must receive an appropriate response, and even a bonus established in advance if it allows a relevant improvement.

In third place, openness. The center must be open to new trends, or approaches, or devices, or experiences. This implies the need for personnel directly involved in biosafety to visit and exchange experiences with other similar facilities. This exchange must be promoted by the respective Directorates. If there are no exchanges and new contributions, perhaps biosafety will be maintained in absolute terms IN the facility itself, but not in relative terms since the environment will have evolved.

The clear and marked circuits, and the training system, must be included in the quality program of the installation, they must be registered, there must be version control, and they must be updated periodically.

If the facility keeps operational its initial containment or barrier systems, the level of biosafety acquired is and will be a very human matter, in which training will play a capital role. And training always has a cost. *"A chain is only as strong as its weakest link"* (Thomas Reid, 1786). It is necessary to make sure that this link is never a human being.

References

From Section 1

1. PHAC. Canadian biosafety handbook. 2nd ed. Public Health Agency of Canada; Minister of Health and the Minister of Agriculture and Agri-Food; 2016.
2. USDHHS, CDC, NIH. Biosafety in microbiological and Biomedical Laboratories (BMBL). 6th ed. USA: US Department of Health and Human Services, Centres for Disease Control and Prevention and National Institute of Health; 2020.
3. WHO. Laboratory biosafety manual. 4th ed. Geneva: World Health Organization; 2020.
4. Cook-Deegan RM, Berkelman R, Megan Davidson E, et al. Issues in biosecurity and biosafety. Science. 2005;308:1867–8.
5. Kimman TG, Smit E, Klein MR. Evidence-based biosafety: a review of the principles and effectiveness of microbiological containment measures. Clin Microbiol Rev. 2008;21:403–25.

From Section 2

6. CReSA & City: La bioseguridad es sostenible y proporcionada o no será. 2018.
7. Abad FX, Solanes D, Domingo M. Reflections on biosafety: do we really know what biosafety, biocontainment, ¿and biosecurity mean? Contribut Sci. 2010;6:1.
8. Kojima K, Makison C, Summermatter K, Bennett A, Heisz M, Blacksell SD, McKinney M. Risk-based reboot for global lab biosafety. Science. 2018;360(6386):260–2.

From Section 11

9. CEN Workshop Agreement 15793: Laboratory Biorisk Management Standard, [CWA 15793], European Committee for Standardization (CEN). From: https://biosecuritycentral.org/resource/requirements-and-protocols/cwa-15793/

From Section 19

10. Blow JA, Dohm DJ, Negley DL, Mores CN. Virus inactivation by nucleic acid extraction reagents. J Virol Methods. 2004;119(2004):195–8.
11. Darnell ME, Subbarao K, Feinstone SM, Taylor DR. Inactivation of the coronavirus that induces severe acute respiratory syndrome, SARS-CoV. J Virol Methods. 2004;121:85–91.
12. Kraus AA, Priemer C, Heider H, Kruger DH, Ulrich R. Inactivation of Hantaan virus-containing samples for subsequent investigations outside biosafety level 3 facilities. Intervirology. 2005;48:255–61.
13. Mayo DR, Beckwith WH 3rd. Inactivation of West Nile virus during serologic testing and transport. J Clin Microbiol. 2002;40:3044–6.
14. Pastorino B, Touret F, Gilles M, Luciani L, de Lamballerie X, Charrel RN. Evaluation of chemical protocols for inactivating SARS-CoV-2 infectious samples. Viruses. 2020;2020(12):624. https://doi.org/10.3390/v12060624.
15. Rabenau HF, Cinatl J, Morgenstern B, Bauer G, Preiser W, et al. Stability and inactivation of SARS coronavirus. Med Microbiol Immunol. 2005;194:1–6.
16. Zaki AN. Biosafety and biosecurity measures: management of biosafety level 3 facilities. Int J Antimicrob Agents. 2010;1:S70–4.

From Section 20

17. Klotz L. Human error in high-biocontainment labs: a likely pandemic threat. Bulletin of the Atomic Scientist; 2019. Link at: https://thebulletin.org/2019/02/human-error-in-high-biocontainment-labs-a-likely-pandemic-threat/
18. From section 21 WHO. Laboratory biosafety manual. 4th ed. Geneva: World Health Organization; 2020.

Health and Safety

16

Tanusha Singh, Jan A. M. Langermans, and Viola Galligioni

Abstract

The aim of Health and Safety (H&S) programs is to provide guidance and set up guidelines to promote health, workplace safety, and environmental protection in animal research programs. Important parts of H&S are development of safety programs, systems, procedures, and adequate training, based on the risk associated with each hazard.

H&S is a right and responsibility of each individual in the organization. Individual and organizational attitudes regarding safety will influence all aspects of safe practice, including willingness to report concerns, response to incidents, and communication of risk.

Each country has its own Regulations or code of practice related to H&S, so in this chapter we discuss some main concepts that would help the animal facility director, manager, or H&S officer to develop and monitor the H&S program, with in-depth details on Laboratory Animals Allergy development and monitoring.

Keywords

Health and safety · Risk assessment · Occupational health · Laboratory animal allergy · Compassion fatigue

16.1 Which Are the Hazards to Consider in Animal Programs?

Hazard is any potential source of injury or damage to health, coming from exposure or use of that agent/process. In the animal research facility, exposure to risk depends on the individual role and, therefore, different personnel have different risks. Technicians, animal caretakers, veterinarians, and researchers are all exposed to the same environment and animals, but, for example, risk of chronic musculoskeletal disease is higher in animal caretakers (e.g., cage change and dumping of bedding) and in technicians (e.g., lifting of large animals) than in researchers.

T. Singh
University of Johannesburg, Department of Environmental Health, Faculty of Health Sciences, Johannesburg, South Africa
e-mail: TanushaS@uj.ac.za

J. A. M. Langermans
Animal Science Department, Biomedical Primate Research Centre, Rijswijk, The Netherlands

Department Population Health Sciences, Unit Animals in Science and Society, Veterinary Faculty, Utrecht University, Utrecht, The Netherlands
e-mail: langermans@bprc.nl

V. Galligioni (✉)
Netherlands Institute for Neuroscience, Royal Netherlands Academy of Arts and Sciences, Amsterdam, The Netherlands
e-mail: v.galligioni@nin.knaw.nl

J. Guillén, V. Galligioni (eds.), *Practical Management of Research Animal Care and Use Programs*, Laboratory Animal Science and Medicine 3, https://doi.org/10.1007/978-3-031-65414-5_16

The range of hazards present in the animal facility can be categorized according to the activities: physical/mechanical (i.e., musculoskeletal injury, fall due to slippery surfaces, injury due to high or low temperature, bites, and stretches), biological and chemical hazards; their origin can be environmental, animal related or research related. Table 16.1 lists the main potential occupational hazards and risks that can be encountered in a laboratory animal facility, categorized based on the source of the risk (environment, animal, and research related) (Table 16.1).

Regarding manual handling and repetitive actions, facilities should consider the importance of ergonomics training and courses provided by specialists. In daily operations, an effective strategy is to diversify tasks as much as possible, mitigating the risk of prolonged repetition of a single action. A generic infographic on work-related musculoskeletal disorders and how to prevent them can be found on the website of the European Agency for Safety and Health at Work, under the section infographics (https://osha.europa.eu/en/tools-and-publications/infographics/work-related-musculoskeletal-disorders).

With regard to biological agents, we refer to Chaps. 9 (Biosecurity and gnotobiology) and 15 (Biosafety). In the European Union, requirements for the health and safety of workers exposed to biological agents are detailed in the Directive 2000/54/EC [3]. In general, infectious

Table 16.1 Main potential occupational hazards and risks in animal facilities, based on the source of activity

Hazards in laboratory animal facilities		
Environment and husbandry related	Animal related	Research related
Slip or trip hazards, poor housekeeping: can lead to falls and musculoskeletal apparatus injury	**Animals infected with biological agents potentially pathogenic for humans**: microbiological agents used or not for experimental purposes can be source of zoonoses (e.g., pasteurellosis, salmonellosis, influenza viruses, Q fever, *Giardia* spp., and *Mycobacterium* spp.). Transportation procedures and/or use of infectious biological samples and carcasses, as well as their disposal, must also be considered a hazard[a]	
High and low Temperature: injuries and burns by using heat or steam to sanitize and sterilize equipment and instruments (cage washers, autoclaves); burns due to use of cryogens (e.g., liquid nitrogen and dry ice)	**Handling of animals**: musculoskeletal strain from lifting and handling large animals; bites or scratches	**Surgical set-ups**: use of a microscope (e.g., screening of fish embryos, surgical procedures) can cause musculoskeletal disorders
Chemicals: CO_2, cleaning agents and disinfectants. Can cause fires, explosions, injuries (skin/eye irritation), and diseases related to their use, but also to handling and storage (e.g., gas cylinders)	**Allergens**: sensitization to allergens from saliva, hair, urine, and dander allergens**.** Respiratory distress can further develop in asthma	**Sharps**: tissue injuries due to inappropriate use of surgical instruments, syringes, broken glass, needles, scalpels, guillotine, and other sharp equipment
Erroneous manual handling: repetitive activities (e.g., bending, lifting, twisting water bottle caps, cage cleaning, dumping of bedding, manipulation of higher/lower rows of IVCs) or use of (heavy duty) cleaning equipment (e.g., high-pressure cleaning in large animal facilities) can cause acute or chronic musculoskeletal disorders, pain (e.g., in lower back, knees, and legs), discomfort, or injuries	**Aerosolized endotoxin, volatile organic compounds, and ammonia** [1]: may be aerosolized during work with rodents and other species	**Chemicals**: anesthetic gases, CO_2, compressed gases, chemicals used in perfusion, surgical disinfectants. Can cause fires, explosions, injuries (skin/eye irritation), and diseases related to their use, but also to handling and storage (e.g., gas cylinders)

(continued)

Table 16.1 (continued)

Hazards in laboratory animal facilities		
Environment and husbandry related	Animal related	Research related
Machinery and Equipment: moving parts and/or poor maintenance can cause injuries to operators. In aquatic facilities the use of electrical equipment in a wet environment can cause electrical shock if no appropriate shoes and outfit are provided	**Erroneous manual handling**: repetitive activities (e.g., squeezing of bottles for Artemia feeding, pushing button feeders, moving of cages or tanks) can cause musculoskeletal disorders (arthritis, tennis elbow), pain, discomfort or injuries	**Drugs or chemicals exposure**: development of diverse clinical symptoms due to the use of detergents and disinfectants to decontaminate surfaces, sterilize equipment and clean cages, anesthesia, and euthanasia agents. Chemotherapeutics, cytotoxic, and carcinogenic drugs used in experiments can cause various symptoms, from irritation to ill health and serious injuries Route of exposure to chemicals may vary: inhalation, ingestion, mucocutaneous contact or percutaneous inoculation
Noises: elevated noise levels-generating equipment (e.g., cage washers, pressure washers, etc) can cause hearing loss	**Noises**: vocalization of some species (e.g., dogs) can cause hearing loss	**Radioactive material**: handling and use of medical diagnostic imaging equipment, irradiators, electron microscopes; use, storage, and disposal of radioactive materials
		Electrical and electromagnetic equipment: laser and UV light eye and skin injuries; electromagnetic hazards due to magnetic resonance imaging (MRI) (e.g life-threatening for people with implanted pacemakers or stents)
Psychosocial hazards: impact of working with animals, performing procedures, humane killing and euthanasia on mental health of personnel. Emotional distress related to developing emotional bonding with animals		

[a]For a thorough analysis of zoonosis in laboratory animals units, please refer to The Laboratory Animal Medicine book [2]

agents are categorized into risk groups based on different factors:

- Pathogenicity of the organism
- Mode of transmission and host range
- Availability of effective preventive measures (e.g., vaccines)
- Availability of effective treatment (e.g., antibiotics)

Updated information on the category risk for each microbiological agent can, e.g., be found on the webpage of the American Biological Safety Association [4].

16.2 How to Develop a Risk Assessment and Who Are the Key Players in That Process?

Any risk, whether existing or potential, to the H&S of an employee, resulting from any activity in the workplace, should be assessed in terms of nature, degree, and duration. The risk assessment (RA) is the process in which the risks arising from working with a hazard are evaluated. The resulting information is used to determine whether risk control measures can be applied to reduce those risks to acceptable levels. Risk is the combination of the probability that a hazard will cause harm and the severity of harm that may arise from contact with that hazard [5]. By performing a risk assessment, information is gathered, evaluated, and used to justify implementation of processes, procedures, and technologies to control the risks present. Analysis of this information will provide a deeper understanding of the associated risks and it will help to develop behaviors that will maintain a culture of safety in the workplace.

The typical risk assessment process is made of five different steps or principles (Fig. 16.1): (1) identify the hazards; (2) identify who might be harmed and how; (3) evaluate the risks and develop a risk control strategy; (4) record your findings and implement the risk control measures; and (5) review your risk assessment and update if necessary.

The information gathered during the first two phases would help to establish how much risk a specific situation presents, i.e., how likely and how severe. To visualize and quantify the overall risk of exposure (likelihood multiplied by consequence) a risk assessment matrix is a valuable tool (Fig. 16.2).

The matrix helps to identify the different categories of risk, from low to high, and which prevention and risk reduction measures should be implemented.

The risk assessment should be reviewed as necessary (e.g., change in procedures or change in equipment and biological agent) and be amended or updated.

The employer has the responsibility to take appropriate measures to ensure that each employee receives sufficient information and appropriate training related to: potential risks to health; precautions to be taken to prevent exposure; hygiene requirements; use of suitable work clothing, and personal protective equipment (PPE); and steps to be taken by employees to prevent incidents and in the case of incidents. The training should be reviewed and adapted to consider new or changed risks and should be repeated as often as necessary. For example, if the activity with a specific agent is not continuous, it would be good practice to repeat the training every time the activity with that agent would start again.

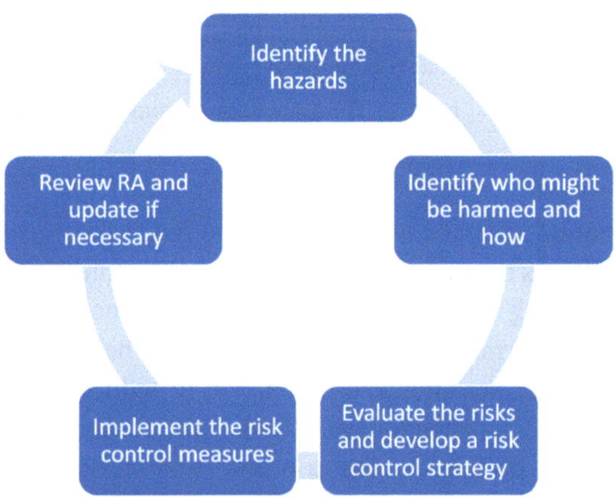

Fig. 16.1 Five steps to develop risk assessment

The employer should also indicate the procedure to be followed in case of an incident and make sure that the information regarding the incident is communicated to the employees and the appropriate measures are taken to protect the other employees and to rectify the situation.

As an *illustrative example*, we will now explore biological agents and their associated risk assessment.

The employer should take the appropriate measures to ensure that: employees do not eat or drink in any location where there is a risk of contamination by a biological agent; appropriate washing and toilet facilities, as well as eye washes and skin antiseptics are provided; procedures on handling and processing samples of human or animal origin are specified; suitable work clothing, special PPEs that might be contaminated, are removed on leaving the working area, are checked before and after each use, and cleaned and decontaminated or destroyed if necessary.

Fig. 16.2 Risk assessment matrix: likelihood multiplied by consequence

Likelihood that hazardous event will occur	**5 very likely**	5	10	15	20	25
	4 likely	4	8	12	16	20
	3 fairly likely	3	6	9	12	15
	2 unlikely	2	4	6	8	10
	1 very unlikely	1	2	3	4	5
		1	**2**	**3**	**4**	**5**
		Consequence of hazardous event (severity)				

The risk assessment for biological agents is an integrated process and it would include:

1. *Hazard identification and characterization*: Identification and classification of the biological agent and its potential adverse effects (hazards) to human health or the environment. The adverse effects include information on diseases, potential allergenic or toxigenic effects that are the result of the work of the employee. In this phase, it is important also to include any recommendations which have been made by the national authority indicating that a particular biological agent should be controlled in order to protect the employees and the environment.
2. *Exposure characterization*: the evaluation of the likelihood of the occurrence of each identified potential adverse effect. The risk assessment for biohazards must take into account also the worker's health status and the environment [6].
3. *Risk characterization*: which is an estimation of the risk posed by each identified characteristic of the biological agent that has the potential to cause adverse effects. It is important to consider that when working with animals, additional risks from the animals and the experimental activities must be considered.
4. Application of *management strategies* to reduce potential identified risks associated with the biological agent to a level of no concern, and to address the uncertainties.
5. Determination of the *overall risk* of the biological agent, taking into account the results of the risk assessment and associated levels of uncertainty and the risk management strategies proposed.

16.3 Which Are the Strategies to Minimize the Risk?

It is important to consider that the risk cannot always be determined with sufficient certainty. In this case, the precautionary principle can be used, since prevention is a response to a known risk. According to the European Commission [7], the precautionary principle can be invoked when the potentially dangerous effects deriving from a phenomenon, product, or process have been identified through scientific and objective evaluation, but this evaluation does not allow the risk to be determined with sufficient certainty. Resorting to the precautionary principle therefore sits within the general framework of risk analysis but is particularly relevant to risk management. Resorting to the precautionary principle is only justified when three preliminary conditions have been met: the identification of potentially negative effects, the assessment of available scientific data, and the degree of scientific uncertainty.

For each hazard, it is possible to apply control measures. From the most effective to the least effective, these are: Elimination >> Substitution >> Engineering controls >> Administrative controls >> PPE (Fig. 16.3) [8].

When it is not technically possible to prevent exposure to the hazard, all prevention and risk reduction measures must be implemented, to ensure that the level of exposure of employees is reduced to the lowest level and adequately protect the employees concerned. Examples of risk reduction measures are reported below:

1. Keep as low as possible the number of workers exposed or likely to be exposed to the hazard.
2. Design work processes and engineering control measures so as to avoid or minimize the release of the hazard into the place of work.
3. Use both collective protection measures and individual protection measures where exposure cannot be avoided by other means.
4. In case of biological or chemical hazards, use hygiene measures compatible with the aim of preventing or reducing the accidental transfer or release of the hazard from the place of work.
5. Use of the hazard pictograms (examples in Fig. 16.4) according to the Globally Harmonized System of Classification and labelling of Chemicals (GHS) [9] and other relevant warning signs.
6. Drawing up of plans to deal with incidents involving the hazard.

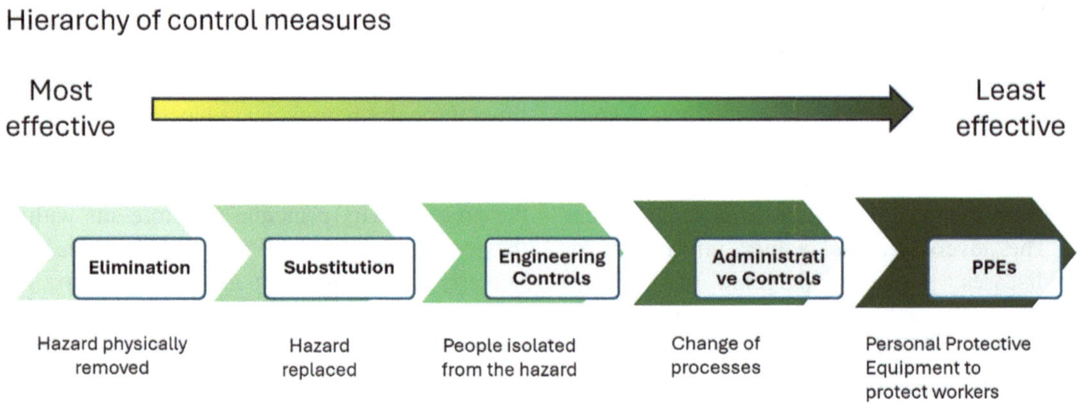

Fig. 16.3 Hierarchy of control for hazards management

Fig. 16.4 Example of biohazard pictogram (left), corrosive (center), and skin irritant (right) signs

7. Testing, where necessary and technically possible, for the presence, outside the primary physical confinement, of a biological and chemical agent used at work.
8. Use of means for the safe collection, storage, and disposal of waste by employees, including the use of secure and identifiable containers, after suitable treatment where appropriate.
9. Making arrangements for the safe handling and transport of a biological and chemical agent within the place of work.

16.3.1 Substitution

To decrease allergens in the environment, choosing absorbent and less dusty bedding could help. For disinfectants and gases, the use of less toxic agents would minimize the chemical hazard. Proper selection of floor and material would help to contain slips and falls. For repetitive motion injury, if no elimination (automation) is possible, modification of the task or distribution of the task to more personnel or during a longer time would help.

16.3.2 Engineering Control

By engineering control measures, we mean equipment or engineering devices that help to contain exposure to the hazard. To address allergies and zoonosis, engineering control would include the use of ventilated cage racks, High Efficiency Particulate Air (HEPA) filters, adequate ventilation, biological safety cabinets, and cage changing stations. Proper design of tools and equipment to minimize ergonomic risks would address the repetitive motion injury. Emergency shut-off of washers and sterilizers would minimize the hazards related to heat. It is important to highlight that engineering control measures are the primary means to minimize personnel exposure when the hazard cannot be replaced (e.g., allergens). PPEs should be only a secondary adjunct measure.

16.3.3 Administrative Control

- Sharing of information and development of Standard Operating Procedures (SOPs), are also part of the hazard mitigation strategies.
- Training is crucial for the safety of animal facility staff and researchers. The training should meet the needs of persons working with animals, depending on their role, and educational level. Researchers should be trained on the general health and safety, care and use of the specific laboratory animal species being used, and specific experimental protocol-related hazards. Animal care staff should also be trained for additional chemical and physical hazards they could encounter in their work (e.g., manual handling, use of disinfectants, and heavy-duty equipment).

Once fully trained, workers are accountable and responsible for their own H&S.

The International Federation of Biosafety Associations provides an example of SOP on training required to safely work with biological agents [10].

Proper signage is also part of the administrative control. The hazard identification should be present at the room level (identification on the door), at the container/cage level and bottle level (when needed). In the case of biohazards, stickers with biohazard symbols could be placed both on the door and on the cage, with identification of the substance, date of initial dosing/injection, required PPE or protective measures, contact information, and any other special instructions. This will make the husbandry staff aware of the special cage change, cleaning, and handling procedures. Those signs must be removed when the hazard period has been completed.

For non-aquatic species, there are some labels that can be washed off by a sponge or can completely disintegrate in water, so no residues are left on the container/cage (WashOffLabelBrochure.pdf (viratekinc.com)).

16.3.4 Personal Protective Equipment

Personal Protective Equipment (PPE) is important also to avoid that allergens or pathogens are brought to the external environment through clothes and therefore to avoid that other people (public transport, family, etc.) are exposed to them. Personal protective equipment varies based on the species and the hazards workers are exposed to. Usually, gloves, dedicated gowns/clothing, head covering, dedicated shoes, and respiratory protection (e.g., FFP2 masks, and respirators) are the norm in laboratory animal facilities. In case of chemical exposure, goggles or facial protection must be added for splash exposures. Hearing protection should also be considered for some species (e.g., dogs) (Table 16.2).

Examples of hazards and how to minimize the risk are reported in below table.

In case of exposure to biological agents, the employer should also make sure that vaccines (when developed) are available to those employees who are not already immune to them. However, while vaccination may provide an additional element of personal protection, the benefits and risks should be considered with equal rigor and the decision on vaccination should be made because of a clearly defined, recognized risk. Vaccination shall be carried out in accordance with any current best medical practice and employees should be informed of the benefits and drawbacks of both vaccination and non-vaccination.

Appropriate health surveillance programs should be developed for employees whose risk assessment reveals a risk to health as a result of the exposure. When appropriate, health surveillance should be made available prior to exposure and at intervals as necessary. In case an employee is found to be suffering from an infection and/or illness, suspected to be the result of exposure, health surveillance is made available to all other employees who have been similarly exposed. Moreover, the risk assessment must be reviewed and amended as necessary.

Table 16.2 Examples of hazards and how to minimize the risk are reported in below table

Risk	Strategies to minimize the risk
Allergens	Please refer to Sect. 16.7.9
Exposure to infected animals (biohazard)	Engineering control: proper ventilation, HEPA (high-efficiency particulate air) filter, pressurized rooms or cages, biosafety hoods, biocontainment systems, pest control program
	Administrative control: Personal hygiene (fomites), hand washing before and/or after working with animals, or shower procedures depending on risk level. Validation of inactivation methods (e.g., autoclave). Proper signage
	PPEs: Respirators, facial covers, arm protections, based on the risk level
Mechanical hazard/ slippery floor	Substitution: Floor resistant to biological materials and chemicals, impervious to liquids
	Engineering control: When drains are present on floor, floors should be sloped and drain traps kept filled with liquid and disinfectant to prevent migration contaminants. When drains are not in use for long periods, they should be capped and sealed to prevent backflow of sewer gases, vermin, and other contaminants; lockable drain covers may be advisable for this purpose in some circumstances
	Administrative control:Training and proper signage
	PPE: Use adquate footwear
Accidental escape of animals	Engineering control: Doors should be self-closing, door partitions, or trenches can be installed and floor drains and vents can be covered with a suitable grill
Ergonomics: e.g., twisting water bottle caps, fill in bedding in clean cages, fill supplies	Substitution: Investment in equipment that could automatize the action. This would save down time of personnel with wrists/ligament problems, e.g., use bottle machines that would decap, dump,wash, fill, and recap; solutions to automatize bedding refill
	Engineering control: Vendors of such equipment in the field are also open to discussions on tools to make the work easier (e.g., tools to remove bottle caps or simply jar openers) and can provide customization of equipment
	Administrative control: Spread the workload among different teams, so that, for example, not the same people have to cap and uncap the bottles. Or spread the workload on different days, if a number of people is limited. This would decrease the ergonomic risk

16.4 How to Develop a Safe Environment?

H&S needs a collaborative approach, with inputs from several sources within the organization. The Culture of Safety can be developed only with both individual and organizational attitudes. Not only development of procedures and risk assessment are necessary, but willingness to report concerns, response to incidents, and communication of risk will influence all aspects of safe practice. Each organization should strive to develop a Culture of Safety that is open and non-punitive. Each staff member has both the responsibility and the right to report and express concerns without any fear. Higher management has the responsibility to address concerns [11].

Safety assessment is an ongoing process that involves also addressing competencies at different levels, to make sure everybody is aware of the issues. Therefore, competence assessment is developed on four skill domains [11]:

- Recognize and understand the potential hazard.
- Understand what (tools, processes) are available to control the hazards.
- Communicate the hazard signage, guidelines, safety program, medical surveillance.
- Set up emergency preparedness and response plans

Competences will vary based on experience, but education and training should be available to understand and apply principles of safety to the specific field of work. For example, an experienced technician competent in Biosafety Level (BSL)-2 agents would begin again at the entry level to build competences when starting to work with BSL-3 agents. The technician would need to become competent in all four above-mentioned domains. As staff gain more knowledge over time concerning how to recognize and control hazards, the level of risk that is considered acceptable should become smaller, with the goal of moving continuously to eliminate or reduce risk to the lowest reasonably achievable level.

16.5 How to Manage Incident Reports?

Incidents are unforeseen occurrences that result in, or have the potential to result in, loss, injury, illness, unsafe conditions, or disruptions to normal procedures [11].

The employer has the responsibility to develop and maintain an environment that is safe. At the same time, the employee has the duty to report immediately to the H&S officer or to the employer, any incident he or she becomes aware of. That would include exposure, risk of exposure, or release of a biological agent that could involve or likely to involve, a risk to the health or safety of an employee.

By reporting, analyzing, and learning from incidents, it is possible to implement corrective actions and prevent, to some degree, future occurrences.

Near misses that did not result in an injury or damage but have the potential to do so should be also reported and investigated.

The International Federation of Biosafety Associations provides an example of SOP on incident reporting [10]. The report should include a description of what happened; why the situation occurred; why it was not prevented or detected before; the root causes of the problem and all causal factors (e.g., were work procedures available and being followed? Was there an equipment failure? Was the personnel trained and assessed competent?).

It is important that an H&S Emergency response is set up in case of disaster or hazardous material release/threatened release. The H&S emergency team should include personnel with specific requirements, able to address the critical situation.

16.6 How to Develop a Comprehensive Occupational Health and Safety Program?

Laboratory safety is a collaborative effort that, to be successful, should include participation of all persons involved at different levels. Internal groups necessary for collaboration might include human resources, facility engineering, occupational and environmental health and safety, biosafety, security, occupational medicine, risk management, and emergency preparedness personnel. External collaborators should include first responders (e.g., fire, police, and emergency medical personnel) and hospitals or other healthcare facilities that receive patients. Based on all these factors, the employer should develop a program that includes pre-employment medical evaluations (if allowed), vaccines, periodic medical evaluations, training required, medical support for occupational illnesses and injuries, and management for work restriction and accommodations upon return to work. A H&S program should address also specific categories of workers, such as pregnant and immunocompromised workers, in which exposure to allergens, anesthetic gases, and exposure to biological agents could be a higher risk. In these cases, the H&S program should always refer to physicians for counseling and advice.

The H&S program should consider:

- Strong presence on the ground by conducting laboratory surveys, diligently ensuring that required remedial actions are taken, and facilitating such changes in laboratory settings and activities, as necessary.
- Field-based outreach and education to promote best practices for non-regulated activities such as biological materials inventory, effective tissue culture practices, and hand hygiene.
- Certification programs for the equipment involved (e.g., biological safety cabinets) by performing annual certification checks.
- Written program policies, SOPs, newsletters, and training materials for safety programs,

including biological hazards (e.g., blood-borne pathogen program, biological materials shipping, and regulated medical waste tracking), chemical hazards (carcinogenic or cytotoxic drugs use and disposal, gas cylinders handling, validation of anesthetic/CO_2 machines), and ergonomics (loads lifting, pulling, or carrying).
- Risk assessments through review of in vivo and in vitro proposals to identify procedures and controls to ensure safe conduct of such activities not only in terms of biological safety but also in relation to other institutional policies, regulatory obligations, and best practices.
- Consultations about biological and other hazardous material shipping/importation with faculty, laboratory personnel, clinicians, and others on technical and regulatory matters by providing field-based consults on packaging, labeling and documentation, and ensuring compliance by surveying improper package preparation or drop-off.
- Response to emergency situations involving infectious materials and other hazards. Assist in investigations of indoor air quality, mold, and other workplace biological safety concerns.
- Investigation of incidents and implement corrective action plans. Maintenance of an incident database.
- Consultation on the design of new and renovated laboratories.
- Coordination of compliance activities for the use of controlled substances in research.
- Usually, the H&S program has also a representative at the Institutional Biosafety Committee and can participate in areas where H&S programs overlap with those related to animal research.

16.7 How to Deal with Laboratory Animal Allergy?

This section focuses on work-related allergies as a result of exposure to small mammalian animals (i.e., guinea pigs, hamsters, mice, rabbits, and rats) in veterinary and animal research settings where high exposures to animal allergens can be expected. Persons at risk of exposure include animal caretakers, researchers, veterinarians, veterinary technicians, students, and anyone else having contact with animals, their bedding, or their bodily fluids or feces. Risk industries include breeding facilities, pharmaceutical industries, and academic and non-academic research institutions [12]. Allergic conditions, primarily laboratory animal allergy (LAA), historically afflicted up to 20% of a highly trained and skilled workforce [13] with significant health and economic consequences for workers, their families, employing institutions, and the wider scientific research fraternity. While LAA is universally recognized as a significant occupational health problem, unfortunately, formal health, and safety advice on the issue only exists in some countries.

16.7.1 What Is the Prevalence of Laboratory Animal Allergy?

The prevalence of allergic diseases among animal care staff has been well documented; however, few studies have investigated allergic diseases among veterinary staff [14]. In the absence of specific prevention strategies, the prevalence of LAA in exposed populations in the first years of animal work varies between 5 and 44%, depending on the diagnostic methods (questionnaire or laboratory testing) used [15, 16]. Historical data suggest that 15% of laboratory animal workers develop IgE sensitization and 10% clinically apparent disease, including LAA and occupational asthma [13].

In a Canadian survey, 39% of respondents developed allergies during their veterinary career, with hair and dander from companion animals as the most common trigger [17].

16.7.2 Which Laboratory Animal Allergens Are Most Common?

Laboratory animal allergens are characterized by animal species and include proteins found in dander, feces, hair, saliva, serum, and urine. As for

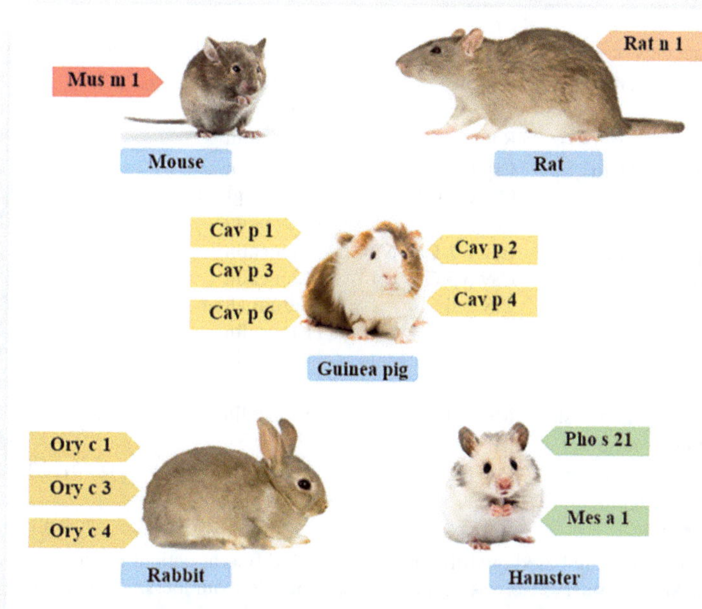

Fig. 16.5 Major allergens found in common small laboratory animals such as mice, rats, hamsters, guinea pigs, and rabbits

most mammalian inhalant allergens, there are major (Fig. 16.5) and minor allergens. Several specific allergens have been isolated from mice (Mus m 1 and Mus m 2, albumin), rats (Rat n 1a and Rat n 1b, albumin, α2μ-globulin), guinea pigs (Cav p 1 and Cav p 2), hamsters (Mes a 1 and Pho s 21), and rabbits (Ory c 1 and Ory c 4) of which the major allergens are lipocalins (Table 16.3) [18]. Rat and mouse allergies are the most prevalent probably as a consequence of the increased use of these species in animal research. However, most laboratory animal species produce allergenic proteins [18].

Nevertheless, personnel may also be exposed to other workplace allergens. This may include but is not limited to allergens in animal food (e.g., mealworm or corncob), natural rubber latex (e.g., found in gloves), molds, storage pests, mites, pollens, enzymes, antibiotics, and several sensitizing chemicals.

Mouse Allergens The major mouse allergen (*Mus musculus*, Mus m 1) is a pre-albumin and lipocalin-odorant binding protein [19] belonging to the rodent family of the major urinary proteins (MUPs) [20]. These proteins are produced hormonally in the liver and other exocrine glands, transported by blood and secreted in urine. The mouse MUPs have 15 forms detectable in urine and appear to play a complex role in chemosensory signalling among rodents. Mouse MUPs are encoded by 35 genes and their expression varies according to species, strains, and sex. The Mus m 1 allergen is carried on particles with aerodynamic diameters ranging from 0.4 to >10 μm, with the majority on particles between 3.3 and 10 μm [21]. Urine is the main source of allergenic proteins in both mice and rats [18].

Rat Allergens Similarly, the major rat allergen Rat n 1 (*Rattus norvegicus*) is a pre-albumin or variant of alpha-2μ-globulin belonging to the lipocalin group and the family of MUPs [22]. There is ~65% amino acid identity between mouse and rat MUPs; the difference is that MUPs from rats are glycosylated. Airborne Rat n 1 was detected on particles ranging from <0.5 to 20 μm, with the majority on particles greater than 8 μm. Male rat urine appears to have larger quantities of Rat n 1 than urine from females, influencing exposure risk [21].

Table 16.3 Major allergens of small laboratory animals

Animal species	Allergen	Protein family	MW (kDa)	Allergen source	Sensitization rate (%)[a]
Mouse (*Mus musculus*)	Mus m 1	Lipocalin/Urinary pre-albumin	17	Urine, Hair, Dander	66
Rat (*Rattus norvegicus*)	Rat n 1	Lipocalin	17	Urine	73–87
Rabbit (*Oryctolagus cuniculus*)	Ory c 1 Ory c 3 Ory c 4	Lipocalin Secretoglobin Lipocalin	17-18 19-21 24	Saliva, Dander Saliva, Dander Saliva	– 77 46
Guinea pig (*Cavia porcellus*)	Cav p 1 Cav p 2 Cav p 3 Cav p 4 Cav p 6	Lipocalin Lipocalin Serum albumin Lipocalin Lipocalin	20 17 18 66 18	Dander, Urine Saliva, Dander, Tears Saliva, Dander Serum Saliva	70 65 54 52 –
Golden or Syrian hamster (*Mesocricetus auratus*)	Mes a 1	Lipocalin	20-30	Saliva, Tears, Urine, Dander	–
Siberian or Djungarian hamster (*Phodopus roborovskii*)	Pho s 21 kDa†	Lipocalin	18, 21, 23	Saliva, Dander	100

[a]Sensitization rates are based on different studies with different patient groups and test systems (ELISA, immunoblot, ImmunoCAP). They served as orientation points, no absolute numbers. †Allergen listed in Allergome; this lipocalin had no cross-reactivity with common and golden hamster. MW: molecular weight

Rabbit Allergens Rabbit serum albumin, two lipocalins (Ory c 1 and Ory c 4), and a secretoglobin (Ory c 3) are described as allergens in saliva and dander of rabbits (*Oryctolagus cuniculus*) [23, 24].

Guinea pig allergens Members of the lipocalin superfamily are also relevant allergens in guinea pigs (*Cavia porcellus*) [25]. The Cav p 1 allergen was identified in hair extracts and urine and can form monomers and dimers. Similarly, Cav p 3 and 6 are also lipocalins, while Cav p 2, is a non-glycosylated lipocalin, and Cav p 4 is a serum albumin [21, 26].

Hamster Allergens The Siberian or Djungarian hamsters (*Phodopus sungorus*) are slightly easier to distinguish from the common hamsters (European: *Cricetus cricetus* and Golden: *Mesocricetus auratus*). The Golden hamster is mostly used for animal research. The male-specific submaxillary gland protein, a lipocalin expressed in a sex- and tissue-specific manner in the submaxillary and lacrimal glands, is secreted in the saliva, tears, and urine of golden hamsters (Mes a 1). While, the major allergen from the Siberian hamster, Pho s 21 kDa, is also a lipocalin secreted by the submaxillary gland [27].

16.7.3 What Are the Key Determinants of Exposure to Laboratory Animal Allergens?

Allergen levels vary in different workplaces and are dependent on numerous factors such as animal presence, type of animal model, animal hair (e.g., straight or curly), as well as facility-related factors (e.g., size and type of room, type of flooring and furnishing, cleaning frequency, and ventilation system) [28]. For example, advances in genetic manipulation have led to a shift in animal models with mice, rather than rats, being the major animal model used. However, there is currently no occupational exposure standard for LAA due to the severe health effects, the variation in the susceptibility of individuals, and the lack of method standardization to quantify allergens [15].

Workplace contamination may occur by the allergens becoming airborne or being carried on clothing and other surfaces [15]. In some facilities, animal receipt can cause significant exposure due to animals being anxious in unfamiliar environments. Other activities posing a risk of exposure include bleeding, culling, and dosing, and those involving the handling of animals outside of cages [29].

16.7.4 What Are the Risk Factors Associated with Laboratory Animal Allergy?

Several risk factors are associated with the development of LAA, including the level of exposure, job activity, duration of employment, atopy, and smoking.

1. Level of exposure: The most important risk factor for the development of an allergy to rodents is the level of exposure to laboratory animal allergens [21]. An exposure–response relationship has been shown for airborne rat urinary proteins and LAA, with higher risks of IgE sensitization and LAA at elevated exposure levels [13]. However, the relationship between allergen exposure and clinical symptoms development is complex and not linear. Jeal and colleagues [30] demonstrated that elevated exposure to rat allergens is associated with lower rates of specific IgE (sIgE) and symptoms and higher specific IgG (sIgG) and IgG4 (sIgG4) production. The risk of developing work-related chest symptoms is reduced with the dual production of sIgG4 and sIgE compared with specific IgE solely produced [30–32].
2. Job activity: Workers who work directly or indirectly with animals and their waste products (including maintenance workers and waste disposal workers) are at risk of developing LAA [15]. Regarding mice, the major mouse urinary protein, Mus m 1, is excreted mainly in urine which is aerosolized by various activities like handling the animal and bedding material [13]. Straumfors et al. [33] showed that cage emptying and cage washing gave the highest exposure, whereas animal experiments in lab/operation rooms gave the lowest exposure for mouse (Mus m 1) and rat (rat n 1) allergens. Furthermore, significantly different exposure levels were identified for various tasks implying different risks for sensitization and allergy development [33]. While guinea pigs are widely studied, minimal data currently exists on allergen exposure levels due to a lack of quantification methods [21].
3. Duration of employment: Generally, workers acquire LAA within the first three years of exposure. Initial exposure may prime the immune system to produce specific IgE antibodies to one or more animal allergens; subsequent exposure may stimulate the onset of clinical symptoms. However, there is great variation in the latency period before allergy is expressed clinically [15].
4. Atopy: A history of common environmental allergens (atopy) and animal exposure are considered important risk factors for developing allergies [15]. Atopic individuals are up to 11 times more likely to become sensitized to animal allergens than non-atopics and thus, have an increased risk of experiencing symptoms. Atopy may also influence the time course of symptoms with a median time of 2.2 years for atopics compared to 8.2 years for non-atopics. Atopics were also shown to be at a 2.2 times greater risk of developing a more severe form of the disease and at a faster rate [15]. Another study also demonstrated that workers exposed to low levels of rat allergen for a few hours per week were sufficient to sensitize atopics; however, the risk for non-atopics increased significantly with increased intensity of exposure [34]. Nevertheless, it is important to note that atopy is not a sufficiently good predictor of LAA for preplacement selection [15].
5. Apart from an atopic predisposition, smoking is considered a possible risk factor for animal

allergy development, but a definite link has not been proven [35]. In a prospective epidemiological study among university employees, individuals with a smoking history had significantly greater declines in pulmonary function compared with non-smokers [36]. According to Bush and Stave [18], the finding is an expected effect of concomitant exposure to tobacco smoke and laboratory animals. Tobacco smoke results in elevated serum IgE levels, which could predispose smokers to increased risk for LAA [37].

16.7.5 Common Symptoms and Health Outcomes of Laboratory Animal Allergen Exposure

Laboratory animal allergens can cause serious adverse health effects, which may impact workers' quality of life and affect the continuity of work with the animals. However, a chain of events is typically necessary for this to occur. After initial exposure to the allergen, some individuals develop sensitization to the agent; upon repeated exposure, sensitized individuals may develop an allergy. Continuous exposure to laboratory animal allergens may exacerbate asthma symptoms, possibly leading to reduced lung function. Once a respiratory disease is present, additional exposures can cause exacerbated respiratory symptoms.

Workers may experience symptoms such as runny nose, itchy eyes, mouth, or skin, sneezing, stuffy nose, red, watery eyes, and coughing in keeping with rhinoconjunctivitis and urticarial. Approximately 10% of allergic workers will develop more severe respiratory disease symptoms, such as asthma and upper airway hypersensitivity. In rare circumstances, allergic reactions may lead to anaphylaxis [15] with potential shock or even death [35]. Some workers with a mouse allergy may also experience symptoms when exposed to other laboratory animals such as rats, guinea pigs, hamsters, and rabbits due to cross-reactivity between the major allergens [21].

16.7.6 How to Clinically Manage Worker Symptoms?

Occupational health professionals play a critical role in identifying at-risk and affected workers early through necessary treatment, referrals, education, and recommendations to prevent debilitating illnesses [38].

The onset of allergic symptoms can be immediate or may be delayed for several hours after exposure. Delayed reactions make diagnosing the cause of the symptoms difficult and sometimes mistakenly attributed to an event that is not the actual trigger [35].

While symptom frequency and intensity can be reduced through exposure reduction, sensitized subjects who develop sensitivity to one type of laboratory animal are at increased risk of developing allergies to other small mammalian animals. Therefore, workplace management should focus on reducing exposure to a clinically insignificant level (i.e., when the affected worker is free of symptoms in the absence of treatment). This may be achieved by changes in working practices or relocation to areas away from the specific animal/s. It is recommended that individuals with LAA and occupational asthma be removed from exposure within the first year of work-related symptoms for a better prognosis. It is also essential to prevent other workers from developing occupational asthma [21]. In rare cases, will affected workers have to leave their employment if all reasonable measures, including redeployment, have been exhausted with no positive health outcome [15].

The formulation of allergy vaccines for specific immunotherapy relies on knowledge about and good characterization of the relevant allergens. However, the production of recombinant allergens from the small mammalian species is also insufficient so far [21].

16.7.7 How Is Laboratory Animal Allergy Diagnosed?

Workplace exposure to laboratory animal allergens is a risk factor for hypersensitization, allergic diseases, and asthma. The pathophysiology manifests an IgE-associated sensitization to animal proteins through direct or indirect contact with animal dander, hair, saliva, and urine allergens [14].

Clinical signs and occupational history (working in laboratory animal facilities) given by the worker often lead to a provisional allergy diagnosis. The diagnosis is contingent on the demonstration of specific antibodies to the putative allergen/s and needs to be confirmed by either in vivo (e.g., skin prick test) or in vitro tests (e.g., specific IgE) coupled with proper interpretation thereof. Workplace-related inhalant challenge tests are optional to supplement and strengthen the diagnostic workup. However, specific allergens needed for testing are not readily available [21, 35].

Skin Prick Testing Commercial allergen extracts of hair, epithelia, and/or dander from mouse, rat, rabbit, and guinea pig are often used in the diagnostic procedure. Extracts from hamsters are based on Golden or Syrian hamsters. However, sensitization to Siberian or Djungarian hamsters cannot be determined accurately due to potential cross-reactivity between the lipocalins Mes a 1 and Pho s 21 kD [21].

Specific IgE Testing Specific antibody (IgE) testing to the suspected animal allergen extracts is commonly performed. The testing is based on extracts prepared from epithelia, serum protein, and urine protein as a mixture or alone. It has to be considered that dual sensitization to rat and mouse urinary allergens reflect cross-reactive molecules rather than atopy; thus, identifying the primary sensitizer is challenging. Therefore, information from the exposure assessment and the clinical history is crucial. To date, there is insufficient evidence to advise using single recombinant molecules for in vitro diagnosis (Table 16.4).

Table 16.4 Individual or a mixture of LAA allergens for sIgE testing

No.	Animal type	Laboratory animal allergens		
		Epithelia	Serum proteins	Urine proteins
e71	Mice	•		
e76	Mice		•	
e72	Mice			•
e88	Mice	•	•	•
e73	Rat	•		
e75	Rat		•	
e74	Rat			•
e87	Rat	•	•	•
e84	Hamster	•		
e6	Guinea pig	•		
e82	Rabbit	•		
e206	Rabbit		•	
e211	Rabbit			•

Inhalant Challenge Tests On rare occasions, it may be necessary to perform a bronchoprovocation challenge with a laboratory animal allergen. When the diagnosis is in doubt, a positive test is considered the gold standard for confirming a diagnosis of occupational asthma due to laboratory animal exposure. In such instances, a lung function test (usually spirometry or peak flow rate) is performed on the worker before and after inhaling a control saline solution. The individual then gradually inhales incremental doses of the allergen followed by lung function measurements every 10–15 minute intervals after each dose. A decrease in lung function (≥20% decrease in FEV_1 or ≥25% decrease in PEFR) is indicative of a positive test. The worker's lung function may be monitored for up to 12 hours post-challenge to determine a late-phase response. Due to the risk of anaphylactic reaction, these tests should only be administered in specially equipped facilities with emergency protocols in place and supervised by experienced physicians [39].

16.7.8 What Are the Components of a Health Surveillance Programme for LAA?

Previous studies suggest that airborne exposure must be eliminated for sensitization to be prevented among most workers. This implies that even the most stringent exposure control methods may be insufficient to prevent sensitization in all workers therefore, health surveillance is required. Since atopy is a poor predictor and immunological tests to measure specific IgE add little value, it is impossible to predict who will develop work-related allergies or asthma. Therefore, preplacement testing and regular health surveillance screening may be used to gather baseline data, raise awareness of animal allergies and related symptoms, assess worker vulnerability, and provide information on the prevention of allergic diseases. Candidates with pre-existing pet allergies or LAA from previous employment and a history of asthma or anaphylaxis may not be suited to animal work [38].

Health surveillance would be informed by the workplace risk assessment or following the onset of occupational allergies from working with laboratory animals. The workplace health and safety procedures will dictate the frequency of the review but typically are performed annually. More frequent checks may be necessary for the first 2–3 years of exposure when the risk of disease is greatest. Components of a surveillance programme may include a recent medical and occupational history supported by a questionnaire, lung function tests, and specific IgE measurements as described above (Sect. 7.7) [15].

16.7.9 How Can Laboratory Animal Allergies Be Prevented?

The primary goal of animal allergy intervention or prevention strategies is to reduce airborne exposure with consideration to controlling exposure via other routes such as ingestion, skin absorption, and percutaneous injury. Exposure control should be designed to reduce both the intensity and the duration of exposure by applying the hierarchy of controls (elimination, substitution, engineering, administrative, and PPE), while it is acknowledged that elimination and substitution may not be practical. A multi-tiered approach may be required to reduce allergen exposure sufficiently for very high exposure tasks or to a clinically insignificant level (i.e., when the affected worker is free of symptoms in the absence of treatment). Careful selection of equipment, maintenance, and training in its use is fundamentally important, as misuse can compromise the safety and effectiveness of the systems [15, 40]. Those responsible for protecting their workforce in laboratory animal facilities need to comply with the appropriate regulatory authority's legislation and/or guidance [29]. The principle elements of an occupational health and safety program are shown in Table 16.5.

Adapted from NIOSH and HSE OSH programme [41, 42]

16.7.9.1 Engineering Controls

Engineering controls and architectural features are the primary defense and assist in containing allergens within the animal facility and reducing contamination in other areas [35]. Animal facilities should be designed to incorporate engineering controls where practicable to reduce potential exposure. Various engineering controls exist and should be implemented

Table 16.5 Principal elements of an occupational health and safety programme to reduce animal allergen exposure

	Programme elements
1	Implementation of a health and safety management system
2	Facility design and operations
3	Risk assessment
4	Prevention and control of exposure
	– Engineering controls (e.g., ventilation)
	– Administrative procedures (e.g., systems of work, education, and training)
	– Personal protective equipment
5	Maintenance and equipment performance testing
6	Occupational health services (e.g., health surveillance)
7	Information management networks
8	Emergency procedures
9	Program evaluation and audit

depending on the activities and risks. Some are task specific and may include humidity control systems, room and building ventilation, local ventilation systems (e.g., biosafety cabinets, fume cupboards and ventilated workstations that use down-draft or back-draft systems, vacuum systems), and building designs that enclose and separate animal use space from public and office space. In addition, automated systems to reduce ambient allergen levels are widely available. It is accepted that ventilation design may contribute to a reduction in particle counts; design features that direct allergen-contaminated air away from personnel or communal areas may effectively reduce widespread contamination throughout an animal unit. Alternatively, a one-way airflow system in animal holding rooms equipped with sliding perforated screens, behind which the cage racks and exhaust vents were situated, has effectively reduced allergen levels in the center of the room. Similarly, pressure gradients within animal units (e.g., having the animal holding rooms at negative pressure to corridors) assist in containing animal allergens in specific areas.

Lastly, cage design can further contribute to aeroallergen control. With the modernization of research facilities, individually ventilated cages (IVCs) are replacing conventional open cages but at a cost. As such, in contemporary practice, LAA is now largely preventable with the use of these IVC systems and the astute use of appropriate respiratory protection [13] informed by a workplace risk assessment. These cages are generally supplemented with other engineering control "systems" supported by local exhaust ventilation and thus may also reduce the levels of aeroallergen depending on the design, functionality, and the purpose it is intended for [43] IVCs were strong exposure-reducing predictors compared to open shelves and sliding doors which largely increased the Rat n 1 exposure in the animal rooms [33].

It should be noted that measures designed to reduce exposure to animal allergens contribute to reducing the incidence of related symptoms; however, it may not affect the incidence of those sensitized to animal allergens as previously shown [44].

16.7.9.2 Administrative Controls

Administrative controls may include limiting animal and people density within rooms; restricting access to animal areas, minimizing movement of animals and people inside and outside the facility; transporting animals in filter-top caging; appropriate work practices and procedures (e.g., rotating job assignments to limit individuals' exposure levels and duration). Another important aspect of administrative control is the occupational health and safety programme, which includes education about potential risks, preplacement, and periodic medical evaluations to recognize symptoms before chronic conditions may develop [45].

Procedural controls should be implemented to ensure that work activities are conducted to minimize aeroallergen levels and prevent transmission. Such measures may include the choice of animal depending on sex and age. Older male animals have been shown to excrete more allergens in their urine [45]. Furthermore, consideration should be given when selecting environmental enrichment or bedding material as litter type may influence the airborne dissemination of allergens. Administrative controls should also be applied to the cleaning of animal units, in the handling of contaminated documents and clothing and in the disposal and handling of animal waste and litter. Minimizing the number of people exposed may be achieved by situating the facility away from non-animal workers and, further separating animal work from other work activities; or setting boundaries for "clean" and "dirty" work areas, which facilitates control of the spread of contamination [15].

16.7.9.3 Personal Protective Equipment

It may be necessary to augment engineering and administrative control measures with PPE. The correct use of personal protective equipment, general hygiene, changing routines for protective clothing, provision of information, and training is critical in reducing exposure to workers; however, its effectiveness depends on individual behavior [15]. A comprehensive workplace risk assessment needs to inform the type of PPE used. Allergen particles may be carried on clothing and be transported to offices and other public areas. Therefore, work clothes should not be taken home to be laundered. If respirators are required, they must be fit tested, worn, and maintained properly [35].

16.7.10 Summary

For the foreseeable future, animal models will remain a crucial part of clinical studies and other research. Therefore, awareness of symptoms, early diagnosis, and effective clinical and environmental management are paramount to protecting and promoting workers' health and sustaining work activities. Demonstrating causality may be challenging, therefore, it is recommended that other immunologic tests are considered depending on the exposure (e.g., sIgE and IgG for rat exposure) and if initial tests are negative.

16.8 How Do You Address Compassion Fatigue?

16.8.1 What Is Compassion Fatigue?

As shown in previous sections, physical well-being is a requirement in laboratory animal facilities: the employer has to develop an environment that is safe for all the workers, implementing processes and equipment that help to protect the worker. At the same level should be considered mental and emotional health.

Compassion Fatigue it is the cumulative physical and emotional effects of providing care. The concept was initially used for people in the care-giving professions, like nurses and counselors [46]. Compassion Fatigue was described as burnout, due to loss of the ability to cope with the chronic discomfort and stress related to the caregiver profession. The stress is overpowering and interferes with the ability of the person to function.

Later on the term was applied to all personnel involved in human and animal care. Compassion fatigue in animal-related professions is mostly considered a direct result of the impact of euthanasia in veterinary clinics, animal shelters, and research facilities. Arluke named the experience of moral stress of euthanasia as the "caring-killing paradox" [47]. However, other common occupational stressors are involved in these negative feelings, such as employee workload, long-term care of patients with diseases, and end-of-life care [48]. In animal care settings, compassion fatigue is a combination of physical, emotional, and psychological depletion, associated with working and caring for animals and their well-being in a captive environment.

Personnel (research staff, facilities staff, Animal Welfare Body, or IACUC members) deeply care for the animals they work with, developing a strong bond. Close contact with animals can create feelings of satisfaction and affection. However, they see animals also in situations of distress and pain or the bond comes to an end at the of the research. Therefore, personnel may experience emotional stress, with conflicting emotions. They may feel guilty, powerless, and without a voice. All this can translate into depression, exhaustion, and frustration. The cost of caring for others and the empathy shown for their pain is known as compassion fatigue. Compassion fatigue is not specific to the lab animal workers. Other categories such as nurses, social workers, human doctors, veterinarians, palliative care workers and caregivers can develop such exhaustion, depression, anxiety, anger, and frustration.

In research animal setting, factors that can trigger compassion fatigue are the following [49]:

- Close relationship with animals
- Higher animal stress/pain
- Desire to provide better conditions (e.g., more enrichment and more contact with social species)
- Ethical or moral dilemmas
- Humane killing methods and euthanasia
- Understaffing or lack of resources
- Poor relationships within the team, including line manager

- Poor communication: inadequate information and resources being provided to carry out their job
- Lack of training/resources on compassion fatigue
- Less social support: because of public opinion they might feel not supported by society

16.8.2 What Are the Consequences of Compassion Fatigue?

Mental health is also connected to the ability of the person to adequately perform the tasks. A mentally healthy staff member or researcher will be more concentrated, paying more attention to details that could be decisive in complex animal experiments. Stress and fatigue might lead to oversights, being less vigilant about reporting, dosing, feeding/watering, and therefore animal welfare problems. Stressed and exhausted people may also respond ineffectively to emergencies. From the management point of view, undetected and untacked compassion fatigue will translate into burnout, absenteeism, increased staff turnover, and team dysfunction.

When mental health is cared for, personnel will be more collaborative, more effective in teamwork, therefore solution solving and thinking outside the box will be triggered.

However, it should be considered that some people will find it difficult to admit having problems, perhaps seeing it as a sign of weakness or inadequacy. For this reason, it is a good practice to monitor and manage work demands and resources, especially the factors triggering Compassion Fatigue.

16.8.3 Is It Possible to Manage and Monitor Compassion Fatigue?

Usually, compassion fatigue is left out of the institutional H&S programme. It is therefore important to include it in the institutional risk assessment and provide personnel involved in Lab animals with proper training, guidance, and care because this will also have an effect on the animals.

Based on the hierarchy of control measures (Section 16.3), the strategies to minimize the risk of compassion fatigue would be:

- Elimination of the stressful event: e.g., humane killing and procedures
- Substitution: change of protocols for humane killing or other stressful procedures. Not everybody is comfortable with cervical dislocation, so by providing a choice for humane killing the staff member can choose the procedure that is creating less anxiety.
- Administrative control: counseling for workers, encouraging social support, training, restricting workers who are experiencing acute distress; support for the 3Rs with internal programs, awards, and self-treat rewards [50]; create institutional compassion fatigue resiliency programs. For inspiration, we suggest the University of Washington's Dare 2 Care Program [51] and the 3Rs Collaborative Compassion Fatigue Resiliency resources [52].
- An institutional compassion fatigue resiliency program could provide the following:
- Study endpoint notification, especially in the case of animals who have been cared for a long time. It could be a notification on behalf of the main researcher or the veterinarian, to all staff providing humane care at all levels to these animals.
- Support for staff. It is important to have somebody to talk to, whether it is a peer among animal care personnel, or a support professional (e.g., counselling provider) available at the institute. Another option could be to provide a box where personnel can leave their thought anonymously.
- Recognition of the community's contribution to animal welfare and research by organizing an annual commemoration or by having a dedication tribute/area [52, 53].
- Inclusion of Compassion fatigue and self-care strategies in the training that staff (animal-

care and researchers) completes when starting animal work.

- Improve of work environment with break-rooms with pictures of some of the animals hosted or with the possibility to provide activities of self-care; provide appreciation events (e.g., lunch of coffee breaks) and promote work well-being.
- Inclusion of Compassion Fatigue assessment in the occupational health screening performed annually on staff/animal users.

Having staff satisfied with the work they do and being able to perform their activities and talk about that in a safe environment is not a glass mountain. Measures such as the one described above can be easily put in place also in small animal facilities, thus avoiding larger problems such as absenteeism and high staff turnover, which eventually impact animal welfare.

References

1. Pacheco KA, McCammon C, Liu AH, Thorne PS, O'Neill ME, Martyny J, Newman LS, Hamman RF, Rose CS. Airborne endotoxin predicts symptoms in non-mouse-sensitized technicians and research scientists exposed to laboratory mice. Am J Respir Crit Care Med. 2003;167(7):983–90. https://doi.org/10.1164/rccm.2112062.
2. Fox JG, Otto G, Colby LA. Selected zoonoses. In: Laboratory animal medicine. Academic Press; 2015. p. 1313–70.
3. Directive 2000/54/EC of the European Parliament and of the Council of 18 September 2000 on the protection of workers from risks related to exposure to biological agents at work (seventh individual directive within the meaning of Article 16(1) of Directive 89/391/EEC)
4. https://my.absa.org/Riskgroups, Accessed on 18 August 2023
5. World Health Organization, Laboratory Biosafety Manual, fourth edition and associated monographs, 2020. ISBN 978-92-4-001131-1 (electronic version)
6. Fleming DO. Risk assessment of biological hazards. In: Fleming DO, Hunt DL, editors. Biological safety: principles and practices. Washington, DC: ASM Press; 2006. https://doi.org/10.1128/9781555815899.ch5.
7. European Commission, Communication from the Commission on the use of the Precautionary Principle, published on 02/02/2000 CELEX: 52000DC0001
8. https://www.cdc.gov/niosh/topics/hierarchy/, Accessed on 18 August 2023
9. United Nations, Globally Harmonized System of Classification and labelling of Chemicals (GHS), tenth edition, 2023.
10. https://www.ebsaweb.eu/biosafety/biosecurity-resources/guidance-documents-/-manuals, accessed on 24 July 2023.
11. Center for Disease Control and Prevention 2011. Guidelines for Biosafety Laboratory Competency MMWR 60(02);1–6
12. Zahradnik E, Raulf M. Animal allergens and their presence in the environment. Front Immunol. 2014;5:76.
13. Feary JR, Schofield SJ, Canizales J, Fitzgerald B, Potts J, Jones M, Cullinan P. Laboratory animal allergy is preventable in modern research facilities. Eur Respir J. 2019;53(6)
14. Zahradnik E, Sander I, Kleinmüller O, Lotz A, Liebers V, Janssen-Weets B, et al. Animal allergens, endotoxin, and β-(1,3)-Glucan in small animal practices: exposure levels at work and in homes of veterinary staff. Ann Work Exposur Health. 2021:1–14.
15. Gordon S, Preece R. Prevention of laboratory animal allergy. Occup Med. 2003;53(6):371–7.
16. Aoyama K, Ueda A, Manda F, Matsushita T, Ueda T, Yamauchi C. Allergy to laboratory animals: an epidemiological study. Br J Ind Med. 1992;49:41–7.
17. Epp T, Waldner C. Occupational health hazards in veterinary medicine: zoonoses and other biological hazards. Can Vet J. 2012;53:144–50.
18. Bush RK, Stave GM. Laboratory animal allergy: an update. ILAR J. 2003;44(1):28–37.
19. Lorusso JR, Moffat S, Ohman JLJ. Immunologic and biochemical properties of the major mouse urinary allergen (Mus m 1). J Allergy Clin Immunol. 1986;78:928–37.
20. Cavaggioni A, Mucignat-Caretta C. Major urinary proteins, alpha(2U)-globulins and aphrodisin. Biochim Biophys Acta. 2000;1482:218–28.
21. Matricardi PM, Kleine-Tebbe J, Hoffmann HJ, Valenta R, Hilger C, Hofmaier S, et al. EAACI molecular allergology user's guide. Pediatr Allergy Immunol. 2016;27(suppl 23):1–250.
22. Bayard C, Holmquist L, Vesterberg O. Purification and identification of allergenic alpha (2u)-globulin species of rat urine. Biochim Biophys Acta. 1996;1290:129–34.
23. Hentges F, Leonard C, Arumugam K, Hilger C. Immune responses to inhalant Mammalian allergens. Front Immunol. 2014;5:234.
24. Willerton L, Mason HJ. The development of methods to measure exposure to a major rabbit allergen (Ory c 1). AIMS Public Health. 2018;5(2):99–110.
25. Hilger C, Kuehn A, Hentges F. Animal lipocalin allergens. Curr Allergy Asthma Rep. 2012;12:438–47.
26. Swiontek K, Kler S, Lehners C, Ollert M, Hentges F, Hilger C. Component-resolved diagnosis using guinea-pig allergens elucidates allergen sensitization

profiles in allergy to furry animals. Clin Exp Allergy. 2021;51(6):829–35.
27. Torres JA, de las Heras M, Maroto AS, Vivanco F, Sastre J, Pastor-Vargas C. Molecular and immunological characterization of the first allergenic lipocalin in hamster: the major allergen from Siberian hamster (Phodopus sungorus). J Biol Chem. 2014;289:23382–8.
28. Zahradnik E, Raulf M. Animal allergens and their presence in the environment. Front Immunol. 2014;5(76)
29. Howard J, Mason HJ, Willerton L. Airborne exposure to laboratory animal allergens. AIMS Allergy Immunol. 2017;1(2):78–88.
30. Jeal H, Draper A, Harris J, Taylor AN, Cullinan P, Jones M. Modified Th2 responses at high-dose exposures to allergen: using an occupational model. Am J Respir Crit Care Med. 2006;174:21–5.
31. Jones M, Jeal H. IgG4 antibodies against rodents in laboratory animal workers. Allergy. 2011;66:1249.
32. Jones M, Jeal H, Schofield S. Rat-specific IgG and IgG_4 antibodies associated with inhibition of IgE-allergen complex binding in laboratory animal workers 619–23. Occup Environ Med. 2014;71:619–23.
33. Straumfors A, Eduard W, Andresen K, Sjaastad AK. Predictors for increased and reduced rat and mouse allergen exposure in laboratory animal facilities. Ann Work Exposur Health. 2018;62(8):953–65.
34. Heederik D, Venables KM, Malmberg P. Exposure–response relationship for work-related sensitization in workers exposed to rat urinary allergens: results from a pooled study. J Allergy Clin Immunol. 1999;103:678–84.
35. Figler N. Laboratory animal allergies: overview of causation and prevention. Lab Animal. 2004;33(10):25–7.
36. Fuortes LJ, Weih L, Pomrehn P, Thorne PS, Jones M, Burmeister L, et al. Prospective epidemiologic evaluation of laboratory animal allergy among university employees. Am J Ind Med. 1997;32:665–9.
37. Bush RK, Stave GM. Laboratory animal allergy: an update. ILAR J. 2003;44(1):28–51.
38. Acton D, Linda McCauley L. Laboratory animal allergy: an occupational hazard. AAOHN J. 2007;55(6)
39. Bush RK. Assessment and treatment of laboratory animal allergy. ILAR J. 2001;42(1):55–64.
40. Filon FL, Drusian A, Mauro M, Negro C. Laboratory animal allergy reduction from 2001 to 2016: an intervention study. Respir Med. 2018;136:71–6.
41. NIOSH. National Institute for Occupational Safety and Health. NIOSH Alert: Preventing Asthma in Animal Handlers, Publication No. 97-116. 1998.
42. HSE. Health & Safety Executive. Control of Laboratory Animal Allergy, Guidance Note EH76. London: HSE Books; 2002.
43. Renstrom A, Bjoring G, Hoglund AU. Evaluation of individually ventilated cage systems for laboratory rodents: occupational health aspects. Lab Anim. 2001;35:42–50.
44. Botham PA, Lamb CT, Teasdale EL, Bonner SM, Tomenson JA. Allergy to laboratory animals: a follow-up study of its incidence and of the influence of atopy and pre-existing sensitization on its development. Occup Environ Med. 1995;52:129–33.
45. Gordon S, Tee RD, Newman Taylor AJ. Analysis of rat urine proteins and allergens by sodium dodecyl sulfate–polyacrylamide gel electrophoresis and immunoblotting. J Allergy Clin Immunol. 1993;92:298–305.
46. Joinson C. Coping with compassion fatigue. Nursing. 1992;22:116–21. https://doi.org/10.1097/00152193-199204000-00035.
47. Arluke A. Managing emotions in an animal shelter. In: Manning A, Serpell J, editors. Animals and human society: changing perspectives. New York: Routledge; 1994. p. 145–65.
48. Scotney RL, McLaughlin D, Keates HL. A systematic review of the effects of euthanasia and occupational stress in personnel working with animals in animal shelters, veterinary clinics, and biomedical research facilities. J Am Veterin Med Assoc. 2015;247:1121–30. https://doi.org/10.2460/javma.247.10.1121.
49. LaFollette MR, Riley MC, Cloutier S, Brady CM, O'Haire ME, Gaskill BN. Laboratory animal welfare meets human welfare: a cross-sectional study of professional quality of life, including compassion fatigue in laboratory animal personnel. Front. Vet. Sci. 2020;7:114. https://doi.org/10.3389/fvets.2020.00114.
50. Kerton A, Tremoleda JL. Emotional challenges in our work with laboratory animals: tools that support caring for others and yourself. Animal Technol Welfare. 2021;20(1)
51. https://sites.uw.edu/d2c/, accessed on 18 July 2023
52. https://www.na3rsc.org/compassion-fatigue/institutional-resources/, accessed on 18 July 2023
53. Iliff SA. An additional "R": Remembering the animals. ILAR J. 2002;43(1):38–47.

17 Emergency and Disaster Plans

Gabi Itter and Thierry Decelle

Abstract

The value of disaster planning and preparedness was one of the global lessons learned from the recent COVID-19 pandemic. As other than biohazard disasters can occur like natural or technological ones, the ones based on human errors, criminal activities, and other threats, inclusion of all risks is key when issuing a disaster plan. It should be adapted to the location, research activities, and animals housed and supported by specific training and preparedness to ensure rapid recovery. There are various organizations and regulatory bodies that require disaster plans when animals are used for research with different levels of expectations, such as the European Directive 2010/63/EU, the [1], the World Organization for Animal Health, The NRC Guide 2011, and others. Disaster and contingency plans should be reviewed and updated periodically to reflect any changes in the facility, staff, or local regulations, and any previous experiences. This ensures that the plan remains relevant and effective. As there is a lot to reflect upon while generating "your" disaster plan, this chapter should assist you with recommendations to take into consideration when issuing or reviewing your current plans.

Keywords

Disaster · Contingency plan · Animal facility · Emergency · Pandemic

17.1 What Is a Disaster and What Type of Disasters Can Occur in an Animal Facility?

A disaster is a sudden and severe event that causes great damage or hardship to people, property, reputation, and the environment or can damage animals directly. It often leads to significant loss of life, injury, destruction of infrastructure, and business disruption. As this may impact animal welfare it is of utmost importance to be prepared by having a disaster plan. Disasters may be caused by natural events, technological failures, biological contamination (people, animal, and environment) like the recent COVID-19 Pandemic [2], and from human origins.

Disaster plans need to identify potential hazards, specific to the research institution. Below are some examples of disasters:

– Natural disasters such as flooding, storm, tornado, earthquake, and fire, need consideration

G. Itter (✉)
Sanofi-Aventis, Frankfurt, Germany
e-mail: Gabi.Itter@sanofi.com

T. Decelle
DCL Solutions, Paris, France
e-mail: thierry@DCL-solutions.com

J. Guillén, V. Galligioni (eds.), *Practical Management of Research Animal Care and Use Programs*, Laboratory Animal Science and Medicine 3, https://doi.org/10.1007/978-3-031-65414-5_17

of likelihoodness depending on the geographic locale [3]. Flooding needs to be considered when the area is prone to have flooding, most recent examples are the flooding in Germany's Ahr Region in 2021, with catastrophic consequences, but also happened in other areas like the superstorm Sandy, in New York, 2021 where Laboratory mice were sacrificed, what was hardly criticized in the press (Reuters, 7th Jan [4])

- Technological and premise disasters such as critical equipment failures, structural disruptions, or acts of vandalism within the facility that may also cause harm to the animals or personnel should be included. Planning for power outages is essential as it can disrupt environmental control systems, affect animal welfare due to the loss of ventilation and temperature regulation, and compromise the overall functionality of the facility, including biosecurity. In the twenty-first century, disasters like cyberattacks and energy breakdowns are to be taken into consideration as they could impact laboratory animal facilities, operations, and staff security as well.
- Human exposure disasters should also be included in the disaster plan. Biohazard-related disasters in facilities that deal with infectious agents or work with biohazardous materials can occur, so, therefore, the plan should include measures for potential outbreaks or accidental releases to protect people, animals, and the environment. It should address quarantine procedures, infection control measures, diagnostic methods, clear instructions, and internal communication. The most recent pandemic has shown great impact on personnel and animal facilities evidencing the need to anticipate a similar situation to ensure contingency not only for housing and care of the animals, but also for personnel. Other exposure should be considered as laboratories often handle hazardous chemicals, and spills or leaks can pose serious risks to the personnel and the environment. Plans should include procedures for containing, mitigating, and cleaning up any spills or leaks to minimize harm. Other hazards are stored in laboratories, like flammable materials, which could have devastating consequences in case of fire. Fire prevention measures, evacuation plans, and fire suppression systems should be outlined to ensure the safety of all within the facility and the protection of the assets.
- Disease outbreak represents a disaster for research and breeding centers as it can be deleterious for the whole research program; it requires rapid response to prevent the contamination of all the colonies. Preventative measures should be in place to control microbiological barriers, but the research and care staff should be trained to take the appropriate measures from the beginning of an outbreak. In the case of zoonotic agents, additional measures with involvement of Occupational Health and Safety (OHS) department are required.
- Other threats that need to be included are criminal activities such as personnel harassment and assault, facility break-ins, arson, and vandalism as they could occur to institutions working with and housing laboratory animals. Criminal activities, like undercover investigation, may remain, even silent during long time periods as a threat that needs to be watched. When animal activists have entered animal facilities, there is a high risk for personnel security, and for animals being released into the wild. In the event of animal escape or release, plans should be developed to safely capture or recapture the animals without causing harm or spreading any potential diseases. Apart from the financial impact and the impact on mental health of personnel an adverse event like this could cause a major institutional reputation damage due to video footage and misleading press releases.

Potential hazards are specific to the institution and therefore a disaster plan can never be generic. Every research institution should develop its own list of hazards and assess the likelihood. For example, research laboratories may require specific protocols for handling hazardous substances or managing specialized equipment during emergencies. The specific plans and protocols will vary based on the location, nature of the research conducted, species housed, and overall risk assessment for each facility.

Therefore, disaster and contingency plans should be reviewed and updated periodically to reflect any changes in the facility, staff, or local regulations (types of risks, likelihood, severity). This ensures that the plan remains relevant and effective.

17.2 What Are the Key Elements of a Disaster Plan to Define General Actions?

The plan should define the actions necessary to prevent and manage staff and animal injuries, and to ensure rapid recovery. Knowledge of the geographic locale may provide guidance as to the probability of a particular type of disaster and is required to detail mitigation and remediation plans.

Guidance on how to develop and maintain a disaster plan is given by several Institutions, such as FEMA [5], so-called the "General Emergency Preparedness Plan." In the United States (US), the Animal and Plant Health Inspection Service (APHIS USDA) issued a final rule on December 31, 2012, to establish regulations under which research facilities and dealers, exhibitors, intermediate handlers, and carriers must meet certain requirements for contingency planning and training of personnel been updated [6].

The OHS Department should be included in the preparation of the disaster to ensure that human life is guaranteed before others. *The mitigation and remediation plan should be aligned with the business continuity plan of the site.* However, specific to animal facilities, the disaster plan should also describe actions to ensure animals can be secured, receive the appropriate care, or are humanely euthanized.

Regarding animals, the plan should define the *actions necessary to provide daily care and to prevent and manage animal pain, distress, and deaths*. If possible, the plan should describe how the facility will preserve animals that are critical for research activities or are irreplaceable. Actions to be taken in case of lack of care, distress, and pain should describe when and how animals will be relocated or humanely euthanized [7]. A system should be in place to maintain accurate records of all animals in the facility, including their identification, health status, and any special needs they may have.

Clear and detailed instructions should be provided on *how to safely evacuate animals from the facility* in case of an emergency. This includes ensuring the availability of proper transportation and establishing escape routes. This may involve establishing partnerships with other facilities or setting up temporary shelters. Guidelines for when it is safe to return animals to the facility after an evacuation or emergency should be part of the plans.

Proper *communication between all stakeholders* (details in item k, next section) should be established, ensuring that all staff members are aware of their roles and responsibilities in case of a disaster. This includes establishing communication methods between team members, veterinarians, scientists, local authorities, site direction, and other relevant stakeholders.

The plan should have outlined the list and quantity of *husbandry supplies and resources that should be readily available* in case of an emergency. This includes food, water, medications, first aid kits, housing material, and access to any other essential items and backup equipment needed to care for animals. The plan should address procedures and equipment for ensuring the continued care and well-being of animals. As an example, Fig. 17.1 illustrates a decision tree approach to ensure business continuity.

Regular *training sessions and drills* should be conducted to educate staff members on their roles and responsibilities during emergencies. This helps ensure everyone knows how to respond effectively and efficiently and that the remediation plan is realistic. The recent pandemic has shown that cross-training of animal teams is important to ensure the routine husbandry and care of animals is guaranteed if key staff is ill or under quarantine.

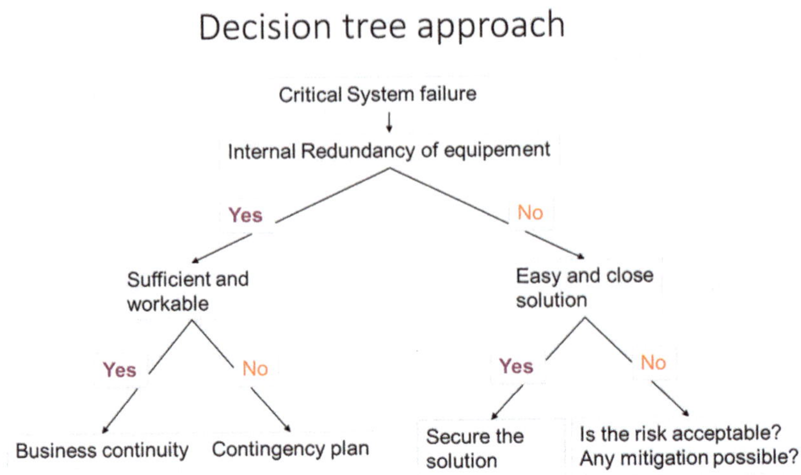

Fig. 17.1 Decision tree approach for critical system failures

17.3 What Particular Actions Should Be Considered in the Disaster Plan?

17.3.1 What Happens If There Is a Need to Close Down a Site?

The access to site may be limited or the site may be closed down and only crucial tasks will be continued, for instance, in order to facilitate interventions of civil security in case of natural disaster, to reduce the risk of spreading infections, or to react to a possible curfew or a breakdown of public transportation.

For such an event, the management of the animal facilities needs to take rapid decisions together with the researchers and the customers: What tasks will be continued, how many animals will be kept, and what staff needs to be present at work? The number of animals will determine how much supply needs to be in storage. In the USA, the Guide for the Care and Use of Laboratory Animals [8] states that it is important to consider both the priorities for triaging animal populations and the institutional needs and resources, whereas the transposition of European legislation into national laws does not clearly indicate that a critical situation does allow the euthanasia of the animals [9], so this must be carefully considered beforehand.

For those employees who will stay at home, the need for outside access to the company's Information Technology (IT) network should be granted and, if not already existing, provisions need to be made for short-term installation of lines and equipment.

17.3.2 What Are the Products That Need to be Considered for Storage?

The list of products, which are critical for the care of animals are diet, water, bedding, basic veterinary intervention drugs, including euthanasia products, and materials, respiratory protection (e.g., masks), disposable garments, and disinfectants. Other products may be considered on a case-by-case basis as it varies depending on the research subject of the institution. Other products such as enrichment, clean cages, and bottles may be optional. The list of products and materials should be reviewed by the husbandry team to be as comprehensive as possible.

17.3.3 How Materials Need to Be Stored?

It has to be decided whether storage of material is to be established and how much, and storage space is ensured to cover the time of a possible shortage situation. Expiration dates of extra materials should be managed. If the decision is not to have storage of products, a detailed plan for rapid supply should be in place, and its operationalization should be checked. Immediate orders in case of disaster or at the first announcement of a disaster, e.g., major weather event could be challenging on short notice. If needed, anticipating temporary storage space in case of short notice is an option.

17.3.4 What Needs to be Done in Case of Stored Material Is Not Enough or Headcount Is Not Available?

On the first sign of an approaching disaster, management should be asked to prioritize care, studies, and research activities. The prioritization criteria should be defined with the research teams as early as possible and be part of the general disaster plan. The prioritization criteria need to be updated on an agreed interval, with arbitrage of the top management if necessary. This also could prevent difficult discussions and disagreements with study directors over study priorities during a disaster. Communication between the management, the staff, and the scientists might be limited. Using a prioritization list for ongoing studies and research projects, the animal facility management can react in an agile manner by autonomously stopping the studies with the least priority and allocating tasks to the staff present on site.

17.3.5 What Alternatives Apart from Study and Research Prioritization Exist?

During the last pandemic, some staff members were sick or unable to leave their houses, regardless of how urged they were needed or whether they possessed special skills. The remaining staff needed to take over crucial tasks by decreasing the level of care for a limited period of time, by limiting the introduction of new animals or stopping the breeding. If not sufficient, option to depopulate the animal facility should be considered.

The priority is to limit the delivery and birth of new animals until the full recovery. Then, the decisions need to be taken about minimal care without jeopardizing the welfare of animals. In order to replace absent staff, as many people as possible need to be cross-trained for specific procedures. When depopulation (euthanasia) is required, it can be assumed that studies in one research department might get a higher priority than others. This is why it is important to agree upon prioritization criteria prior to any occurrence of disaster. On sites with both, researchers and animal facility operations, research staff could be shifted to animal facility operations—when the number of staff there is dropping below the critical line. However, in order to have this option available it is a prerequisite that research staff has been trained for daily care of animals.

17.3.6 Are There Any Key People and Companies Outside That Need to Be Involved?

Efforts must be made to preserve the minimal care for animal welfare, ongoing research projects, ensure minimal disruption, and act for a rapid recovery and business continuity. Ensuring the availability of essential support services such as power, water, and medical supplies is critical. This may involve backup power systems, storage of samples or data in secure locations, and contingency plans for continuing experiments remotely or in alternative facilities. Developing contingency plans for situations where these services may become compromised is necessary. In addition to technical services, other site departments may be involved: purchasing, OHS, IT staff, Communication, Public Affairs… Animal breeders could be also informed to stop any delivery of animals and adjust the breeding whenever possible.

17.3.7 What Is Important to Consider Concerning the Animal Food Supplier?

In respect with the amount of food stored and the expected food consumption, and the estimated duration of the crisis, it is important to inform animal food suppliers that an order for animal feed and special diets will come on a short notice. The suppliers need to be prepared to hold the capacity and raw materials to produce and deliver the amount within a short period. It requires active discussion between the animal facility management and the supplier. The animal facility management needs to avoid any food waste by adjusting the diet amount and to make sure to hold enough adequate storage for the required amount.

If sufficient storage space is available at a site, keeping a permanent stock of feed with a first-in-first-out process should be considered.

17.3.8 What Is Important to Consider Concerning the Animal Suppliers?

When facing a disaster, or if possible by anticipation, the beginning of new studies will presumably be delayed until the event is over. During the crisis, fewer animals will be used and supplied by the breeders. Breeders need to be aware of the crisis situation as early as possible, to adjust the breeding plan. They should be encouraged to have their own plan to preserve lines of genetically modified animals or other invaluable animals for you. In addition, due to the disaster affecting your business, transport conditions may be affected.

17.3.9 What Is Important to Consider Concerning Genetically Modified and Other Important Research Animals?

In case of disaster, transgenic breeding activity should be prioritized, as these are often unique rodent models. Regular cryoconservation of lines should be considered to secure valuable animal models. In case of unanticipated disruptive events, relocation can be considered. However, options for relocation should have been assessed upfront by the staff and detailed in the disaster plan.

Likewise, of as importance is to secure large animals such as non human primates and other large species. In case of disaster, the operational constraints for those species require furthering the preparedness plan and ensuring that the actions to be taken are realistic, as relocation and other logistical aspects for some species may be more complicated.

17.3.10 What Are Other Essential Key Activities That Need to Be Considered?

17.3.10.1 Plan for Reduction of Quality in Husbandry

Animal Facility Management needs to list the current activities and the ones that could be reduced or abandoned if the number of staff drops to the point where the usual quality of husbandry cannot be maintained anymore, e.g., reduced frequency of cage changes. In case of decreased standards, welfare should be monitored closely. It should be decided when to reduce quality or when to stop the next study with the least priority. It may be necessary to obtain the consent or approval of the site's internal Oversight Body (OB), but at least, the OB needs to be informed of measures.

17.3.10.2 Communications

A list of key staff with office, home, and mobile numbers has already been generated and should be kept updated. Animal Facility Management should get access to the communication list of their customers/researchers and any internal or external relevant staff (institutional official/site head, maintenance, OHS staff, OB, security, communication, etc.) in case of a disaster to ensure communication on the alignment of priorities. Establishing effective communication channels both within the institution and with external emergency response agencies is crucial. The institution should have reliable means of communication to coordinate responses and seek assistance if required.

17.3.10.3 Inter-site Transfer of Activities

Different sites of the animal program might be affected differently by the disaster at a given time. Animal Facility Management could consider the transfer of studies from affected to non-affected sites. Management should discuss under what conditions a study could be transferred, what a shipment could include and what kind of equipment is needed for shipment without jeopardizing the health of animals and the outcomes of studies. All simple in theory, the operationalization of animal transfer is challenging and raises many questions. All those operational aspects need to be included in the disaster plan in order to get an effective solution in case of disaster.

17.3.11 What Are the Key People, and How They Should Be Organized?

It is recommended to set up a Site Disaster Committee that should include at a minimum the Institutional Official/License Holder/Site Head (IO), Designated Veterinarian or equivalent Attending Veterinarian (DV, AV), Clinical Veterinarian(s), Facility/operations Manager, Medical Doctor and OHS representatives, relevant study directors (PIs), Quality Assurance (QS) if GLP (Good Laboratory Practices) or GMP (Good Manufacturing Practices) apply, and members of the OB. Other key functions could be included on a case-by-case basis: communication, public affairs, internal security, civil security, representatives of the local community, etc.

The site disaster committee should oversee the elaboration of the disaster plan and its periodic update, the training and mock exercise, and the initiation of the remediation plan in case of disaster. The colony manager or veterinarian responsible for the animals should be a key member of the appropriate committee at the institution, an "official responder" in the institution, and a participant in the response to a disaster [7].

In case of disaster, the committee should have defined its remits:

(1) The Chair of the committee (e.g., the IO) should activate the remediation plan.
(2) This Committee should meet as often as needed and maintain active communication with all internal and external stakeholders (care staff, scientists, suppliers, etc.). If needed a spokesperson will be appointed.
(3) The Committee should perform an in-depth analysis of the situation: type of disaster, impact and potential duration; research activities and priorities; animal number and species; inventory of material and equipment; and availability of the care staff.
(4) The Committee should align on the needs or changes in regard to the storage of animal housing materials and disposables, study prioritization, cross training, confinement, and quarantine in alignment with OHS, outsourcing of studies, transportation of animals, animal orders, and breeding needs.
(5) If husbandry and study support are affected, conservative measures should be taken in the following order:
    a. Manage Facility and studies with cross-trained personnel.
    b. Reduce housing (no delivery, stop of the breeding, early termination of some studies, etc.) and husbandry to the minimum required (to facilitate a correct study execution of running studies).
    c. Study termination, and euthanasia of animals.
(6) When the disaster situation is considered as managed, the Committee should issue a summary and value the experiences to update the disaster plan.

17.3.12 If Euthanasia Needs to Be Applied Which Ethical Considerations Are Important?

If euthanasia cannot be avoided, respective laws and regulations have to be applied. However, depending on the country and local animal welfare laws and other regulations, a disaster situation is not a justification for euthanasia. The same rules apply to animal suppliers and contract research organizations (CROs). The Guide for the Care and Use of Laboratory Animals takes into consideration both the priorities for triaging animal populations and the institutional needs and resources (NRC, 2011—*Page 35, Disaster Planning and Emergency Preparedness*). Whenever possible, the OB should be consulted before any decision and informed about effective euthanasia. Setting upfront criteria for triaging animal populations approved by the OB facilitates rapid decision. If animals need to be euthanized it should be taken into consideration, if animals are in study, to apply an earlier time point for necropsies to gain the maximum information out of the study. It should also be considered if re-homing of the animals is an option.

17.3.13 How to Ensure That Local Regulations Are All Applied?

It must be ensured that all regulations are applied during a disaster in a laboratory animal facility. Therefore, it is needed to familiarize with local regulations. Collaboration with local authorities should be initiated as early as possible. Sharing the disaster plan details in advance could be considered helpful, for example, by establishing and maintaining a good working relationship with relevant local authorities, such as veterinary inspectors, emergency management services, and animal welfare organizations. Collaborating with these entities will ensure that the plan is updated on any changes to local regulations and guidance can be sought in case of a disaster. Regular inspections and audits of the laboratory animal facility will help to ensure compliance with local regulations. This includes checking the emergency equipment, infrastructure, and ensuring that all protocols are being followed. Seeking professional advice may be needed if there are uncertainties about any specific local regulations or their application during a disaster, including experts in the field, like internal or external lawyers and respective authorities. Training of the staff with regular practice emergency response exercises is essential. In addition, to ensure that staff is well-prepared and aware of the local regulations, this will help identify any gaps in the emergency response plan and allow for adjustments and improvements.

In case of disaster, it is important to maintain accurate documentation and keep detailed records of all laboratory animal operations, including animal welfare protocols, rationale of decisions related to animals, permits, and local regulatory requirements.

17.4 What Is the Difference Between a Disaster Plan, a Mitigation Risk Plan, and a Remediation Plan

A Disaster Plan is primarily proactive and focused on disaster identification and preparedness measures. This includes risk identification, emergency management, and disaster recovery strategies (Fig. 17.2). For each risk, the likelihood and the severity should be assessed and weighed against the current level of control. The aim of the Mitigation Risk Plan is to decrease the likelihood of the risk and/or the impact of an adverse event on the business and to increase the level of control. The level of control depends on the type of risk: surveillance and monitoring system, practicality of operational options, and effective network of professionals, etc. For high-priority disasters and risks that cannot be mitigated, the Remediation Plan is a list of actions and decisions to ensure business continuity, i.e., rapid recovery with a minimum of damages to the organization.

Disaster Plan constitutes a comprehensive framework for managing a wide range of unforeseen events and various types of disruptions [10]. Mitigation and Remediation Plans are a subset of a Disaster Plan to 1/ reduce the probability and impact of a risk, 2/ ensure rapid recovery and business sustainability.

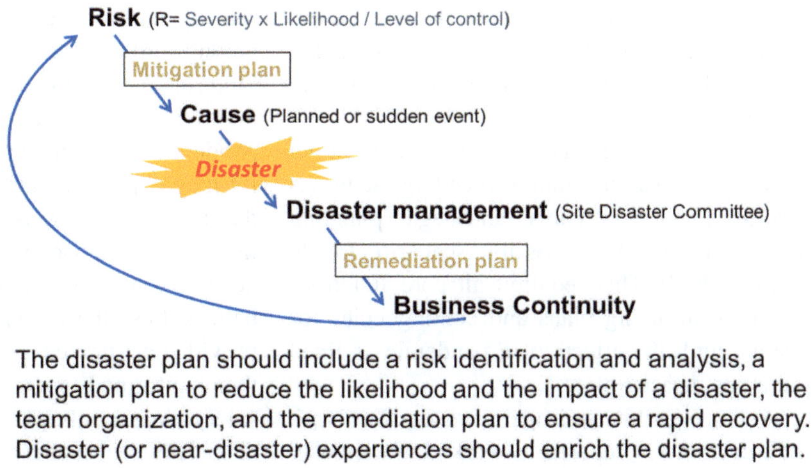

Fig. 17.2 Risk Mitigation Planning: The disaster plan should include a risk identification and analysis, a mitigation plan to reduce the likelihood and the impact of a disaster, the team organization, and the remediation plan to ensure a rapid recovery. Disaster (or near-disaster) experiences should enrich the disaster plan

17.5 Are There Any Regulations and Laws Requiring Disaster Planning and Contingency Measures?

There are various organizations and regulatory bodies that require disaster plans when animals are used for research. The European Union requires prevention measures and rapid interventions when animals are used for research. Specifically, Directive 63/2010/EU on the protection of animals used for scientific purposes does not require a formal disaster plan and contingency measures to ensure the welfare and safety of animals in research settings. However, the care for the animals should be provided on a daily basis, with rapid intervention of veterinarians; the heating, ventilation, and air conditioning (HVAC) system should have an alarm system to facilitate rapid management of any environmental anomalies [9].

In the USA, there are various organizations that require disaster plans when animals are used for research. The National Institutes of Health recommends that all institutions conducting research involving animals have a disaster plan in place [1]. This includes guidelines for emergency situations such as natural disasters, power failures, and other unforeseen events. The Office of Laboratory Animal Welfare (OLAW), as part of the NIH, provides assurance to various funding agencies that the institutions conducting animal research are following the Public Health Service (PHS) Policy on Humane Care and Use of Laboratory Animals [11]. Institutional Animal Care and Use Committees (IACUC) are responsible for overseeing animal research at the institutional level. They are responsible for establishing disaster plans as part of their animal care and use program.

Even this is not a legal requirement, but animal programs seeking for AAALAC accreditation must have a disaster plan as instructed in the Guide for the Care and Use of Laboratory Animals [8] as animal facilities may be subject to unexpected conditions that result in the catastrophic failure of critical systems or significant personnel absenteeism, or other unexpected events that severely compromise ongoing animal care and well-being [12].

There are other laws and regulations that require disaster plans, e.g., WOAH Terrestrial Code. Especially when working under GMP or GLP regulations, as set in OECD Guidelines. Working under or in hazardous containment facilities requires it as well [13].

17.6 What Is the Most Recent Example of a Disaster?

In 2020, the World Health Organization issued a "Pandemic Alert" after the outbreak of coronavirus disease (COVID-19) that was first reported from Wuhan, China, on December 31, 2019. The

COVID-19 pandemic, caused by the novel coronavirus SARS-CoV-2, quickly spread globally, resulting in a major health crisis and an ongoing pandemic.

As a result of this alert institutions executing in vivo studies or animal breeding activities formed "Pandemic Teams" and began planning and preparations for a possible scenario already in early 2020. This required all core functions including initiating plans and contingencies for dealing with the effects of a pandemic as lined out in the disaster plan.

Animal facility management together with their customers prepared to work autonomously as far as possible under conditions of a reduced workforce and diminishing supply of consumables for the time of the pandemic. At a certain point of an approaching pandemic, site management may decide to close down the site and reduce all work to that which is absolutely crucial for long-term success. Studies may be completely stopped and only prioritized studies may be continued. As not all countries are affected at the same time when operating in different regions or time zones, this allows a bit more flexibility in global institutions.

Nowadays, we are in the lessons learned phase after the pandemic, which will improve disaster planning massively. However, at the onset of the pandemic, nobody could predict impact and outcome and there was a lot of uncertainty. However, this pandemic has shown the importance of "living disaster plans" [14].

17.7 Lessons Learned During the Recent COVID-19 Pandemic?

Preparedness and Contingency Planning including communication and training are key. It is essential to inform facility staff about the proper safety measures and protocols required during a disaster, especially during a pandemic. This includes practices such as wearing personal protective equipment, hand hygiene, and social distancing. Clear communication channels and regular training sessions can help minimize the risk of exposure and transmission of the virus among staff members. Laboratory animals play a vital role in scientific research, and it is crucial to maintain their health and well-being during a pandemic. Personnel in a laboratory animal facility may experience increased stress and anxiety due to several reasons such as fear of infection, increased workload, or uncertainty about the situation. Regular communication and training can help address these concerns, boost morale, and provide reassurance to staff members by keeping them informed about the facility's response, safety measures in place, and any support available. However, concerns and stress of personal need to be followed up and measures to ensure social and psychological wellbeing need to be established. The pandemic emphasized the importance of prioritizing health and safety measures for both researchers and animals.

Supply disruption has valued existing stocks and ensured adequate supplies of all needed consumables and equipment for housing, husbandry, and studies.

The pandemic accelerated the adoption of remote collaboration tools and highlighted the benefits of data sharing among research institutions. Animal research institutes should explore and invest in technologies that enable remote collaboration, data sharing, and virtual conferences. This been respected by human resources, and allows been flexible with rules of applying work time and conditions [15].

Not only disasters like the COVID-19 pandemic raise ethical questions regarding the use of animals in research. Institutes should continuously evaluate and refine their ethical frameworks to ensure that animal welfare is prioritized while balancing the need for scientific advancement. This includes exploring alternative research methods and promoting the principles of the 3Rs (Replacement, Reduction, and Refinement) established.

17.8 Helpful Links?

AALAS Homepage; Disaster Preparedness (aalas.org)

NIH Homepage: Disaster Planning and Response Resources | OLAW (nih.gov)

References

1. National Institutes of Health (NIH). U. S. Department of Health and Human Services; Intramural Research Program Animal Program Disaster Plan Overview Final Version – 11/17; 2022.
2. Petervary N, Pullium JK. Research continuity in responsible animal research. ILAR J. 2019;60(1):74–85.
3. Ballard MD, Smith SM, Johnson HF, Range F. Crisis Management Planning. Disaster Recov J Winter. 1999:49–51.
4. Reuters, Nov 7, 2012, 12:29 AM EST, |Updated Jan 7, 2013]. New York University Faces Growing Criticism After Superstorm Sandy Kills Lab Mice at Medical Research Center, Criticism Over Death of Mice At NYU, Major Loss for Research.
5. Federal Emergency Management Agency. FEMA Developing and maintaining emergency operations plans. Comprehensive preparedness guide (CPG) 101 Version 2.0., Published November 2010. 2018. Accessed February 1st
6. USDA, Animal and Plant Health Inspection Service. Federal Register, National Archives 12th March; 2021.
7. Vogelweid CM. Developing emergency management plans for university laboratory animal programs and facilities. Contemp Top Lab Anim Sci. 1998;37:52–6.
8. National Research Council (NRC). The guide for the Care and Use of Laboratory Animals. Disaster Plan, Disaster Planning and Emergency preparedness. 2011. p. 35.
9. European Parliament and Council. Directive 2010/63/EU, 22 September, on the protection of animals used for scientific purposes; 2010.
10. Miller G. Science and the public: animal extremists get personal. Science. 2007;318:1856–8.
11. US Department of Health and Human Services. Public Health Service Policy on Humane Care and Use of Laboratory Animals. 2015. NIH Publication No. 15-8013.
12. Bayne KA. Disaster planning and management: a practicum. ILAR J. 2010;51(2):101–3.
13. Roble G, Pullium J, Hester T, Harvey S. Disaster planning for animals in hazardous agent containment units. ILAR J. 2018;59(2):195–202. https://doi.org/10.1093/ilar/ily022.
14. Fisher D, Heymann D. Q&A: the novel coronavirus outbreak causing COVID-19. BMC Med. 2020;18(1):57.
15. World Health Organization. COVID-19 Strategic Preparedness and Response Plan (SPRP 2021). WHO REFERENCE NUMBER: WHO-WHE-2021.02

Implementing Quality Systems in the Management of the Animal Care and Use Program

18

Javier Guillén, Rony Kalman, Sara Wells, Mark Gardiner, and Thomas Steckler

Abstract

The laboratory animal science community is moving toward increasing the quality of their work. There are two main reasons for that: first, the objective of improving the care and use of the animals to ensure animal well-being; and second, the general trend by animal researchers toward enhancing the quality, reproducibility, and translatability of the research outcome. Therefore, animal care and use program managers are more and more involved, by personal and/or institutional commitment, in the implementation of quality practices in all animal program areas. In addition to internal quality measures, that may or may not be imposed by regulations, there are several external quality systems that can, and have been traditionally applied, to animal care and use programs. The practical aspects of the implementation of the three most common quality systems in the animal research environment (AAALAC International, GLP, and ISO) are described.

Keywords

Quality system · Animal research · AAALAC · GLP · ISO

J. Guillén (✉)
AAALAC International, Pamplona, Spain
e-mail: jguillen@aaalac.org

R. Kalman
The Hebrew University of Jerusalem, Jerusalem, Israel

S. Wells · M. Gardiner
Mary Lyon Centre, MRC Harwell, Didcot, UK

T. Steckler
Janssen Pharmaceutica NV, Beerse, Belgium

18.1 Quality Systems in Animal Care and Use Programs

18.1.1 What Is a Quality System?

A Quality System (QS) is a collection of organizational processes defined in policies, standard operational procedures, work instructions, protocols, guidelines, or other documents.

It has the aim to meet an organization's internal and/or external requirements and expectations.

18.1.2 What Are the Quality Systems Applicable for an Animal Program?

The initial action of anyone wanting to introduce a new quality system is an assessment of the added value and the advantage one wants to achieve for an organization.

J. Guillén, V. Galligioni (eds.), *Practical Management of Research Animal Care and Use Programs*, Laboratory Animal Science and Medicine 3, https://doi.org/10.1007/978-3-031-65414-5_18

Internal requirements are defined by the organization itself. In case of an animal care and use program, these could be internal rules set by program management, responsible veterinarian, Oversight Body (e.g., Animal Welfare Body, Ethics Committee, Institutional Animal Care, and Use Committee), and/or users of the animal services.

External requirements relevant to an animal care and use program can be set by, for example, the government competent authorities and applicable legislation, voluntary organizations such as AAALAC International (AAALAC) (www.aaalac.org), the International Organization for Standardization (ISO; https://www.iso.org/home.html), the Enhancing Quality in Preclinical Data (EQIPD; https://go-eqipd.org/) project, or regulators for the Good Laboratory Practice (GLP) regulations from OECD Principles of Good Laboratory Practice (GLP) and Compliance Monitoring [1], the Food and Drug Administration (FDA; https://www.fda.gov/) in the United States (US) or the European Medicines Agency (EMA; https://www.ema.europa.eu/) in the European Union (EU).

If the focus of your quality management system is animal care and use (institutional policies and responsibilities, animal housing and management, veterinary care, and facilities) then the internationally recognized AAALAC program would apply.

However, if your organization is looking more toward efficacy and efficiencies in the delivery of services or products then a broader, more generic system such as ISO 9001:2015 standards [2] could be considered. Quality standards such as this aim to meet customer satisfaction through continuous evaluation of the processes and systems in place. Animal facilities also involve animal care regimes as one of these processes. Customers in this instance could be any stakeholder within your organization that you provide a service or product to.

There are a number of other quality systems and guidelines that may be relevant for animal care and use program, such as, e.g., Good Manufacturing Practice (GMP) [3, 4] for feed produced and delivered or for veterinary drugs; Enhancing Quality in Preclinical Data (EQIPD: https://go-eqipd.org/) [5]; several FELASA guidelines such as those for health monitoring or genotyping [6]; and AVMA guidelines for euthanasia [7], but for the purpose of this chapter we will focus on AAALAC, ISO, and GLP, which have been already recognized as the most common QS applied in the animal research environment [8].

Whatever decision you take on which type of quality management systems you may pursue, an assessment of how these standards are recognized and respected internationally is also very important.

18.1.3 What Are the Differences and Commonalities Between the Most Commonly Implemented Systems?

A summary of differences and commonalities between the most common systems implemented in animal care and use programs is presented in Table 18.1. Important to note, while some systems have very well-defined scope and applicability (AAALAC, GLP), others (like ISO or internal systems) may be applied at the institutional level or exclusively in the animal unit, which will have implications for the role of the animal program manager in implementing a quality system.

18.1.4 Can Different Quality Systems Coexist in Our Animal Program?

The short answer is yes, different QS can coexist in an animal program. In fact, this is the norm rather than the exception. For example, animal facilities must comply with their national legal requirements and this is overseen by the government in most countries. This really represents nothing else than a QS. In addition to these basic legal requirements on quality, the unit may have any of the other QSs in place. Institutions can have AAALAC accreditation, which is more focused on animal welfare and/

Table 18.1 Differences and commonalities between most commonly implemented systems

	AAALAC	GLP	ISO	Institutional systems	
				Internal quality system	Compliance with ethical/legal legislation
Applicability	All kinds of animal research and breeder institutions	Institutions performing safety-regulated studies	Any kind of institution	Own institution	Own animal care and use program
Voluntary vs. Mandatory	Voluntary	Mandatory for certain safety-regulated studies	Voluntary	Voluntary	Mandatory
Accrediting/ Certifying Body	Independent organization	Government Body	National approved agencies	No external	Government
Inspectors/site visitors' specialty	Independent Lab animal professionals	Variable, government inspectors	Organization of processes	Internal quality personnel	Government
Main focus	Animal care and use program	Preclinical studies[a]	Organization of processes and customer satisfaction	Organization of processes	Animal welfare
Institutional Quality Assurance Unit	Not needed	Needed	Needed	Not needed, but usually present	Not needed
International recognition	Animal Research community/ Funding agencies/Potential collaborators	Regulatory Agencies/ Private Sector[c]	Commercial/Potential collaborators	Potential collaborators	Potential collaborators
Confidentiality	Very high	Very high	Very high	Internal	Depends on legislation
Support from upper management	Needed	Needed	Needed	Needed	Needed
Role of animal program team[b]	Principal role in the implementation	Support of the process	Support of the process unless applied in animal unit exclusively (principal role)	Support of the process unless applied in animal unit exclusively (principal role)	Principal role in implementation

[a]Reference elements
[b]Manager, veterinarians, technicians, etc.
[c]Purchase of a service (e.g., CRO)

or can hold GLP (Good Laboratory Practice) to comply with regulatory requirements, and/or they may be ISO certified (mostly ISO 9001).

But why should different QS coexist? Animal facilities may have two or three of these QSs established because there will be approaches unique for each QS (see Question 18.1.3 on similarities/differences). Institutions may see value in running different QSs, either because they need to comply with regulatory requirements or because they voluntarily wish to improve their way of working. Naturally, there are also overlapping aspects among the different QSs, but those usually do not conflict with each other. Rather, having experience with one QS facilitates the implementation of another QS, although the workload to establish a new QS can be substantial and should not be underestimated.

18.1.5 What Are the Challenges and Opportunities When Developing and Implementing a Quality System?

There are a number of challenges and opportunities when implementing a QS, for example:

Challenges:

- Buy in from all staff, including senior management and researchers, agreeing that developing and maintaining the QS provides value and the best use of resources.
- Engagement of animal care personnel is needed as they will be first-in-line in the implementation.
- Likely, information from different departments needs to be assembled and someone should have an overarching view to bring all information together.
- Time will be required to identify and evaluate all processes.
- Time will also be required to develop documentation, whether this means new standard operating procedures (SOPs), process maps, training, and/or competency records.
- Resources will be required, including manpower and time commitment, to start up and maintain the QS, in addition to the direct application fees that a QS may have.
- A decision must be taken on which QS provides the best value; for example, for an animal care program AAALAC may provide more value than a process-based system looking at preventive measures and continuous improvement such as ISO9001:2015.
- Maintaining requirements of the QS and a need to meet the standards required, e.g., via annual reports that may have to be provided to an external organization or external audits that may have to be hosted.

Opportunities:

- You are probably already carrying out many of the QS practices anyway and following the QS provides further confidence in the high standards already in place.
- Challenge some long-term established practices and evaluate your processes against best practices and current legislation and compliance.
- In the case of GLP, market the ability to perform regulated studies.
- To evaluate the efficiency and effectiveness of already established and new procedures.
- Gaining confidence that processes are being carried out and meet the current institution QS and industry standards, as well as in how this is implemented.
- Get engaged in a continuous improvement process.
- Establish a better research environment for the research community at the institution.
- Foster team building.
- Motivate animal care staff by bringing them together to discuss QS and explain the key role they play within the organization. Pride in the workplace once the QS implementation has been achieved, all people working in the animal facility can feel they have contributed to the achievement and be recognized by the institution.

- Provide confidence to stakeholders including clients, researchers, and regulatory authority that processes are being managed well and are in line with independent national and international standards.
- Implementing a QS (especially AAALAC) can demonstrate to the public the institutional commitment to animal welfare.

18.2 Elements and Implementation of a Quality System in Practice

18.2.1 What Are the Basic Practical Elements of a Quality System?

The implementation of a QS entails putting order in and defining all the activities that have to be performed, ensuring the personnel who perform the activities understand their role in the program and have the necessary competence to perform them, and ensuring the tools used to perform the activities are fit for purpose. To achieve this, a certain amount of documentation, variable in extent and level of confidentiality across the quality systems, is needed. Basic elements to consider are:

- Standard Operating Procedures (SOPs). The SOPs are written instructions on how a process or procedure is performed. They serve to define and standardize the way the activities are performed. They should be clear, concise, and easily available, and ideally should be detailed in a way that a new person could perform every task following the respective SOP.
- Personnel management. Responsibilities and reporting lines of personnel involved should be clear, known by everybody, and documented (i.e., organizational chart, job descriptions and updated curriculum vitae (CV)).
- Training and competency assessment. Standards for how staff are trained and how competency is assessed and reassessed as appropriate.
- Equipment and facilities management. Equipment and facilities used are expected to be under a maintenance program appropriate for the specific characteristics and use (see more in the specific question on equipment and facilities below).
- Self-evaluation and continuous improvement. Once a quality system is implemented, it requires an active mechanism to self-evaluate the progress of the implementation. This self-evaluation, which can be conducted via internal audits, should also focus on continuous improvement, since the quality standards will evolve over time.
- External evaluation. The quality principles may be implemented by an institution without external help, and tailored to the institutional needs as an internal quality system. However, external independent evaluation is needed to obtain official recognition of the implementation of the most widely recognized quality systems, through inspections, audits, or site visits performed by the certifying/accrediting bodies.
- Quality Assurance Unit (QAU). Although not obligatory in all systems (e.g., AAALAC), a QAU with personnel specifically qualified will be necessary for the more "formal" quality systems, especially the GLP, that involve a higher level of documentation and coordination with other areas of the institution.
- Documentation management. How documents are reviewed, managed, changed, disseminated, and archived. The administrative work is one critical aspect to consider when considering the implementation of a quality system.

18.2.2 What Program Topics Does the Quality System (QS) Need to Cover?

A QS can cover many topics but will be based on the commitment and the decision made by an establishment on what QS to implement. This will also be heavily influenced by the standards of the QS which they are going to follow (i.e., whether this is to acquire certification or accreditation or as a guide to implementing their own in-house system).

These are Questions about the topics to consider when developing a QS:

- How are you going to meet the needs of the stakeholders and ensure assurance to all statutory and regulatory requirements?
- What is the purpose of the work and the strategic direction that may affect its ability to achieve the QS?
- What are the organizations objectives, risks, and opportunities, how have these been considered and how are they being addressed?
- Within an organizational structure, who are the key representatives and what are their responsibilities? How will they deliver the resources required for the implementation, maintenance, and continual improvement of the QS?
- How does the institutional management demonstrate leadership and commitment to the QS?
- Does the type of research being carried out require a specific QS to meet client requirements or is this covered by local rules and regulations?
- How is training and competency delivered and assessed?
- Within Health and Safety, what are the programs for identifying hazards, managing risk, and the maintenance of occupational health and safety of personnel?
- How are the animal facilities' environment controls managed and maintained?
- What housing and management is specific to each of the species held?
- How can an effective veterinary care program be implemented during all phases of animal care and use?
- What types of records are kept to demonstrate all aspects of the QS are in place and being managed?
- What systems are in place to allow an open culture for reporting and managing welfare concerns?
- How does the ethical review process, through the work by the Oversight Body (e.g., AWB, Ethics Committee, IACUC, and relation with the competent authority), comply with legal requirements including harm benefit analysis and the 3Rs, and be effective?
- What type of management system is in place for crisis management planning and implementation?
- How is security and plant maintenance managed and what systems are in place to deal quickly with breakdowns that may affect animal welfare or legislative requirements?
- How is performance monitored, evaluated, analyzed and evaluated, and how are opportunities for improvement identified and managed?

18.2.3 What SOPs Are More Important to Consider?

The most important factor to consider when embarking on SOP writing is to be clear about the requirements, what process are you describing and whether it is likely to be misinterpreted if you do not include a detailed procedure to follow. Moreover, it is important to include evidence of processes that may be required during audits of the quality management system, including calibration and training records.

For many animal facilities the most important SOPs are:

- Husbandry SOPs providing instructions about the care of animals, including, for example, SOPs for animal management such as acquisition, acclimatization, housing, feeding, sexing and breeding, euthanasia, as well as sanitization practices.
- Training and competency of animal care and research staff.
- Environmental SOPs outlining the process for recording temperature, humidity, noise, lighting, and the systems for alerting and remedying issues of non-compliance with expected environmental conditions.
- SOPs for the most common experimental procedures (e.g., blood sampling) providing details on how research experiments are car-

ried out, such as procedures authorized under national legislation, including those involving anesthesia, analgesia, and euthanasia techniques. This may include data management, animal welfare, and outline the scientific requirements.
- Facility Management SOPs for the calibration and servicing of equipment will provide evidence for the quality system audits and that suitable controls are being maintained for safety and collecting experimental data.

18.2.4 How Is Training/Competence of Personnel to Be Addressed Under a Quality System?

Ensuring trained and competent staff is key to a QS and providing suitable and sufficient evidence of this will be required within any internal or external audit process.

Key questions to consider are:

- Are staff in all functions following a training program? These may include animal care staff, veterinarians, researchers, Animal Welfare Officers, and Oversight Body members.
- The scope and type of training required to carry out a task/process and attain the standards required. This could range from reading a document, online training, taught courses, or individual practical one-to-one training.
- Is the person carrying out the training the most suitable and experienced person to deliver the training? Do they have an understanding of the process in enough depth to answer questions and provide additional support if further training is required?
- How is competency going to be assessed? For example, a written assessment, observational assessment, or a combination of all of these methods?
- Is the individual assessing competency independent enough to the person carrying out the training so that they can do this in a standard, non-biased way? Do they understand the level of competency required to sign an individual off as competent?
- How often does competency need to be reassessed?
- What training documents are needed? This could be a whole range of different formats including SOPs, competency documents, and observation recordings.
- Is the training program in compliance with applicable legal requirements?

All training and competency records are required to be in a format that can provide assurance to any internal or external auditor that the training has been undertaken and competency has been assessed including all dates this occurred.

18.2.5 How Are Equipment and Facilities Management (e.g., Calibration/Verification/Maintenance) to Be Addressed Under a Quality System?

Equipment and facility management are essential to produce accurate and consistent research data and reduce unwanted effects on animals, thus are an integral part of any laboratory animal operation and are vital for both maintaining animal welfare as well as data quality assurance.

Equipment may require verification (which ensures correct operation according to its stated operating specifications), and/or calibration (which ensures measurement accuracy compared to a known standard) and/or validation (which ensures that a system satisfies the stated functional intent of the system).

Key points to consider are:

- Type of equipment related to animal use.
- Level of management required (calibration/verification/validation). For example, under GLP, full validation may be required for certain types of equipment (e.g., software), whereas it may not be required under other QS (e.g., AAALAC).
- Frequency of use.
- Competence of responsible personnel.
- Records of management activities.

Most common equipment and facilities on which to perform some of these activities will include:

- Heating, ventilation and air conditioning (HVAC) system, including environmental conditions (temperature and relative humidity) and air pressure difference between areas.
- Lighting system (intensity levels, on/off).
- Watering system (microbiological monitoring, decontamination systems).
- Sterilization equipment.
- Cage washing equipment.
- Anesthesia equipment.
- Health and safety equipment (e.g., eye wash stations and safety hoods).
- Housing systems (e.g., ventilated racks).
- Surfaces of animal facility.
- Laboratory research equipment (e.g., balances): this will apply at least to the equipment directly involved in animal procedures. When applying a QS that covers the entire laboratory work, and not only the animal use (i.e., GLP and ISO), these processes will be implemented also for the equipment of the entire laboratory, and the entire facility.

All records are required to be in a format that can provide assurance to any internal or external auditor that the procedures have taken place, including all dates this occurred. In many cases, this may involve the use of stickers directly applied on equipment.

18.2.6 What Level of Documentation Is Necessary?

Most external QS have specific standards that outline the documentation required for assistance and evidence that you have reached the QS standards. Such documentation can also serve for any kind of audit. With an internal based QS, the decision on the amount of documentation and the duration of archiving can be made by that individual establishment, whereas external QS may have specific requirements.

In general, most of the documentation will refer to:

- Standard operating procedures/work instructions
- Personnel (training, competence)
- Husbandry and veterinary records
- Oversight Body meeting minutes
- Equipment/facilities (calibration/verification/maintenance)
- Occupational health and safety

It is important to ensure that the documentation being kept reflects actual practices and the requirements of the QS in place. For example, if work is being carried out using equipment that needs to be calibrated, the documentation should show evidence that this is being carried out. Or if you have a system in place for training staff and assessing competence, it should demonstrate that this is being carried out.

The records can be in any format but would need to be accessible, archived where necessary and disposed of securely once the archive period has been reached.

18.2.7 Why Consider a Quality System for an Animal Care and Use Program?

The objective of a QS is to satisfy the needs or requirements of stakeholders, either internal and/or external. The stakeholders can include:

- The institutional management.
- The research community.
- The competent authority (regulatory agency).
- The buyer of a product (e.g., animals) or service (e.g., studies) offered by the institution.
- The institutional Oversight Body (EC/IACUC/AWB…).
- External collaborators.
- Funding agencies.
- The public.
- Publishers.

With an animal care and use program it is an expectation from all stakeholders that:

1. Refined animal husbandry and welfare is an integral part of scientific programs.
2. The establishment is carrying out current best practices according to established procedures.
3. All animal use has undergone an effective ethical review and required authorization.
4. Staff are highly trained and competent.
5. A culture of care is implemented throughout the establishment.

A QS during initial discussion, implementation, and maintenance assists an establishment to reflect on the five areas highlighted above and to look for continuous improvement. This is essential to demonstrate to stakeholders and auditors/inspectors that you have a robust animal care and use program in place.

18.2.8 How Can We Use What We Already Have in Our Program Relating to Quality, Such as the Oversight Body (EC/AWB/IACUC)?

A good place to start when deciding to implement a QS is to highlight what is already available within the establishment, especially controls and processes required to cover any legal obligations. These will help develop a foundation to build your quality program and identify areas that need additional information and or processes to be put into place.

The *legal requirements* an animal care and use program must adhere to will also be—to different levels of detail—evaluated by agencies such as AAALAC, GLP, and ISO.

Also, a functional institutional Oversight Body is a legal requirement in many countries including the European Union member states, the UK, and the USA. The *roles of an institutional Oversight Body* such as oversight and evaluation of the animal care and use programs are key contributors to a QS and usually cover aspects such as:

- The establishment of animal welfare policies towards a culture of care.
- The inclusion of the 3Rs in programs of work.
- The review of standard operational procedures/work instructions.
- The review of animal research projects.
- The periodic review of the animal program and facilities.
- Additional activities such as retrospective assessments of projects and advising on rehoming schemes.

Additional useful, quality-related guidance can be obtained from documents such as implemented legislation (e.g., Directive 2010/63/EU in the European Union) [9] or other guidance documents such as the Guide for the Care and Use of Laboratory Animals [10] and FELASA recommendations [7].

Thus, a functional institutional Oversight Body and adherence to legal and guiding documents will cover at least part of the animal care and use requirements of the three external quality systems mentioned above.

The external quality systems, in particular, the accreditation process of AAALAC, in return will ensure the proper implementation of the processes mentioned in the guidance documents, including those to be executed by the institutional Oversight Body. They thus facilitate the management of the requirements imposed by legislation and recognized standards, and address additional quality aspects relevant to an animal program.

There is a close interrelationship between the legally mandated infrastructure of an animal facility and the requirements of the external QS. But importantly, the already existing infrastructure imposed by legal requirements can be used to implement and manage the quality requirements of AAALAC, GLP and ISO.

In essence, there are already a lot of good practices and processes being carried out within animal facilities that can be utilized directly into a QS. The real challenge when adding current practices in a QS is in auditing the processes regularly and looking for continuous improvements.

18.3 Institutional and Personal Responsibilities

18.3.1 Where Can the Initiative to Implement a Quality System Come from Within the Institution?

There is not only one potential source within the institution to promote a QS.

A QS is very often implemented to protect the brand, organization processes, and the customers' interest. In these cases, the normal process would be coming from institutional management. This situation can happen for all applicable quality systems and has the practical advantage of management making the necessary resources available, which can have a positive impact on the animal program.

When the reason for the implementation is compliance with legal requirements (i.e., Ethical regulatory bodies such as AWBs or IACUCs, GLP for regulated studies), or customer requirements, the process is also normally the same.

However, when the intention is focused more on reducing concerns about the reproducibility and translatability of animal studies and/or assuring animal welfare and the 3Rs, the initial interest may come from other institutional representatives, such as veterinarians, investigators (i.e., internal customers), and/or animal program responsible persons. This case is usually more related to AAALAC, ISO, or EQIPD. When this occurs, the success will depend on if/how/when the interested parties convince top management to dedicate the resources needed. Not easy, but not impossible.

18.3.2 Does the Type of Institution Make a Difference in the Type of Quality System and Way of Implementation?

Yes, it does. Whereas all institutions must have, to some extent, some kind of internal QS due to compliance with legal requirements and their own commitment to quality, the nature of the institution, type of research, and relation with external customers make a difference when considering the more standard systems such as AAALAC, GLP, or ISO.

Institutions performing regulated preclinical research will implement GLP as a legal requirement. This is more common in the field of contract research organizations (CRO) where this type of work is mostly conducted, but GLP will have to be implemented in any type of institution conducting regulated preclinical research, for example, in pharmaceutical companies and, albeit with less frequency, in academic institutions.

Institutions dealing with external customers may be interested in ISO to offer evidence of consistency of the product or service. This is more typical in breeders and CROs. However, when other types of institutions want to consider their own researchers as customers, they can also consider ISO, which may also be seen in academic and other institutions. However, due to the lack of specialization of this scheme on animal research, the implementation of ISO in animal facilities outside the commercial environment is low.

AAALAC can be implemented in all kinds of institutions, and in fact this is what happens in practice. In addition to the particular commitment to improving the animal care and use program that any institution may have, it offers a visible label of promoting animal welfare, which can be used to gain confidence of customers (e.g., in CROs and breeders), the public (all institutions), and collaborators (academia, pharmaceutical companies, biotechs, etc.).

It is important to note that the cited QSs are not exclusive, and certain types of institutions implement more than one, or even the three of them together. For example, there are institutions, including a number of CROs, which perform regulated research and must have GLP as a legal need, implemented ISO to focus on the consistency of their processes, and AAALAC to cover better animal welfare, care, and use aspects.

18.3.3 Who Are the Key Institutional Players to Get Engaged in the Implementation Project?

A QS may cover many areas within an establishment, some of which will require specialist knowledge outside of the normal routine working processes, e.g., calibration of temperature and humidity sensors in ductwork will require maintenance service input.

The main point to consider in any change or implementation project is what individual roles need to be involved to ensure success and this will normally include representatives of:

- Senior institutional management, with authority and resources.
- Quality Assurance Unit, as appropriate.
- Research staff.
- Technical and procedural services staff.
- Animal facility manager.
- Animal care staff.
- Veterinary staff.
- Human Resources.
- Health and Safety.
- Maintenance Service.

Input from other professionals related to areas such as security, information technology, or laboratory services may also be needed.

The main point to consider is who should lead and coordinate all the above players. Sufficient authority and backup should be given by management to the project leader responsible for the implementation of the QS.

18.3.4 What Are the Obligations for Researchers Under a Quality System in the Animal Care and Use Program?

Researchers must be engaged in the implementation of the QS in the animal program from the beginning, as they will have to follow the QS requirements. Researchers will have to be involved in any QS, but their level of involvement may differ depending on the QS. For example, their involvement will be higher under GLP, because the research process is the main protagonist (with the Study Director as main responsible), whereas under AAALAC, the main focus is on the animal care and the research involvement is less. Aspects of the researcher's involvement in the QS may include:

- Coordination with the responsible person for the implementation of the QS (e.g., quality assurance unit and facility manager) to define the requirements for researchers.
- Provision of personnel documentation and definition of responsibilities and reporting lines, job descriptions, and training. Common to all QS.
- Preparation of experimental SOPs. Absolutely necessary under GLP for all experimental procedures. Some experimental SOPs can be necessary for other systems too, especially when they are generally used (e.g., blood sampling).
- Keeping detailed records related to research activities with animals and following their clinical signs and welfare status.
- Participation in inspections/audits/site visits. Absolutely necessary under GLP. In other QS, there may be a variable level of interaction with researchers during the onsite assessment to describe certain research processes. For those participating in the institutional Oversight Body (IACUC/EC, AWB, etc.) activities, they may be asked to describe their

role in the oversight and ethical review processes.
- Compliance with institutional health and safety policies relating to animal use. For example, AAALAC thoroughly evaluates the occupational health and safety program, which must apply to all staff relating to animal care and use, including researchers.

To better engage researchers and ensure their effective involvement, it is advisable to explain the QS and the benefits they receive as early as possible and invite them to actively participate during the implementation process. Their perception may also be different depending on the necessity of the QS: whereas they must implement GLP to perform certain types of studies, ISO and AAALAC are voluntary, which may limit their engagement.

18.3.5 What Is the Process of Applying for a Quality System?

After deciding which of the QS you would like to establish, initiating the process within your organization, getting the appropriate approvals, and identifying your key people for the process, you should make contact with the organizations that will accompany you through the process and assist you in achieving the desired quality system.

ISO application: ISO certification is issued by certification/registration bodies that are independent of ISO. The task will be to identify the certification body in the region/country, which will walk you through the standards, documentation to be provided, and the audit process. A list of certification bodies by country can be found at: https://iaf.nu/en/home/

AAALAC application: There is single application process for any institution around the world, accessible at: https://www.aaalac.org/accreditation-program/apply-for-accreditation/. In summary, the applicant must submit an application form and a description of the animal care and use program using the Program Description (PD) template freely available on the website. There is the standard PD, a European version of the PD, and a Thai version. It is also very important to read carefully the instructions on how to complete the PD. In addition to the main office in the USA, AAALAC has a European office that can help applicants from Europe, Latin America, Africa, and the Middle East, and an office in Thailand for the entire Asia Pacific area.

GLP application: GLP certification is issued by national government GLP compliance programs which are in place to ensure compliance with GLP by the institutions that conduct the tests. Furthermore, the signing of Mutual Recognition Agreements (MRA) on data ensures that the results of these tests are recognized by other countries. The applicant has to contact the government office (in some countries this may be at the regional level) responsible for this certification, who will coordinate with the institution the submission of documentation and inspection procedure. Links to National Web Sites on Good Laboratory Practice can be found at: https://www.oecd.org/chemicalsafety/testing/linkstonationalwebsitesongoodlaboratorypractice.htm

18.3.6 Have Quality Systems Regulatory Implications?

Out of the QS reviewed in this chapter, only GLP has direct regulatory implications. Certain safety and efficacy studies have to be performed following GLP requirements as defined by regulators. Details of regulations vary across geographical regions (for example, based on EMA in the European Union or FDA in the USA) [11, 12]. Certification of GLP requirements is performed by inspectors from the applicable government authorities, at regional or national level. The results of the studies are officially informed and registered as part, for example, of the preclinical development of medicinal products.

AAALAC and ISO represent voluntary systems with no direct regulatory implications. However, it can be argued that AAALAC may have an indirect impact on certain activities. For example, it can facilitate the application process for funding by government agencies (such as the NIH in the USA). Also, it is mentioned as a risk-mitigating factor in the working document for guidance on inspections and enforcement to fulfil the requirements under Articles 34 and 60 of Directive 2010/63/EU [7] when evaluating the risk and deciding on the frequency of inspections of institutions by competent authorities in the European Union [13].

18.3.7 Is a Quality Assurance Unit Needed for the Implementation of a Quality System?

A Quality Assurance Unit can be defined as a group of people in a QS that is focused on providing confidence that all quality requirements will be fulfilled both internally and externally. Assurance relates to how a process is performed.

Overall a QAU provides evidence-based confidence to management, regulators, and other stakeholders. It evidences that high-quality work is being carried out in an organization and that the organization addresses key areas such as best practices and evaluation of essential metrics to identify continued delivery and engagement in quality. By addressing different units of assurance you are in effect building up and maintaining a QS. For example, when assessing competency, the quality assurance units would encompass areas such as training of the learner and trainer, documents used for training and assessment, examples of assessment criteria, retraining, user feedback, and record keeping of all relevant stages.

Under ISO and GLP, the work and auditing of a QAU is a necessary part of the quality standards in place, not only for the internal implementation but also to prepare the external audit/inspection by the respective certification bodies. However, a QAU may not be necessary if the QS has no external certification criteria (i.e., internal systems), or the level of documentation can be managed by the animal care and use management (i.e., AAALAC). Although not required in all cases, developing an auditing QAU would in essence help to ensure no area had been missed and help to identify strengths, weaknesses, threats, and opportunities within the system.

18.3.8 What Is the Time Commitment Needed for the Implementation of a Quality System?

The time commitment required for a quality system is dependent on the resources available and whether a QS is going to be implemented in its entirety or parts of an already defined standard used as a reference for improvement. When considering a QS you need to think about the following time constraints:

- Commitment from senior staff as there are needs to be top management buy-in to discuss scope, mission statements, and organizational objectives.
- Processes already in place, changes required, and potential hurdles to change.
- Time requirements by others that need to be involved.
- Frequency of group meetings needed to develop the QS and the best use of resources to be productive at each meeting.
- Evaluation and auditing of how items are calibrated and records maintained.
- Development of process maps and/or standard operating procedures to highlight and standards to maintain.
- Development of training programs and assessing both training and competency.
- Audit of the QS system once in place.
- Ongoing time commitments in establishment of a quality culture framework and maintaining it.

In summary, implementing a QS requires a significant time investment (from several months to a few years) that has to be considered in the initial planning.

18.3.9 What Are the Financial Costs of Implementing a Quality System?

There are two types of financial costs associated to the QS:

(a) The costs associated with the organization (e.g., staffing) and potential necessary updates in the animal program (e.g., facility or equipment improvements) to get ready for the implementation. This cost can be very variable and will be inversely related to the initial baseline quality of the animal program. The size and complexity of the program will be a significant factor in the final cost. It is important to note that this cost will significantly be higher than the official fees of the applicable certification process described below, because it will include costs associated with requirements to continuously train people, assure documentation is up-to-date, procedures being compliant with requirements imposed by the QS, run internal audits/assessments, prepare external audits, etc.
(b) The fees charged by the external body responsible for the administration/auditing/certification/accreditation processes:

    ISO9001:2015: This is dependent on the quality organization chosen to certificate your program; however, on average a surveillance audit costs in the range of 1000–2000 € per day. The number of site visits will be dependent on the size and complexity of the organization. The average would be one to two visits per year for general auditing purposes with a full recertification visit lasting 2–3 days every 3 years.

    AAALAC International: There is an application fee and an annual fee to be paid once the program is accredited. The fees are associated to the size of the program, and can be seen at: https://www.aaalac.org/accreditation-program/fees-and-deadlines/ Most of the application fees are in the range of 5000–10,000 €, with an annual fee in the lower range.

    GLP: The daily cost for the certification audit may vary across countries and regulatory bodies. In the European context, it can be estimated in the range of 1000–4000 per day or complete process. As with ISO, the final sum may depend on the complexity of the research unit.

18.3.10 How Is the Quality System to Be Maintained in Time?

Active maintenance of a QS is important to ensure the QS remains functional, fit for purpose, and includes the latest updates and information. This will require time and effort from a team that should be committed to investing in this process. The responsible person(s) for the implementation of the QS should plan and identify all the resources required to maintain the QS, which may be substantial (including finances), e.g., to implement improvements that were identified during the last external inspection, audit or AAALAC site visit. It will ensure that good practices are maintained, ongoing processes (including documents such as SOPs), and existing competences (including training needs and resources) are reviewed and adjusted as required, and new developments in the field are taken into consideration. This is a continuous improvement process and a large part of any QS.

A culture of quality needs to be maintained or even strengthened to keep people engaged, not to lose momentum, and ensure the continuous process is in place to be ready for the requirements of each QS visiting/auditing/inspection procedure. Any important changes in the animal care and use program must be dealt with appropriately and, in case of an AAALAC-accredited organization, should be reported to AAALAC annually. The program description should be revised as needed in preparation for the next AAALAC visit (the process is repeated every 3 years). With other external QS, auditing requirements may vary (e.g., audits performed annually, semi-annually, or ad hoc). Time and effort needed for these activities should not be underestimated, although proper planning with clearly defined responsibilities and timelines will help. Similar efforts should be considered for the maintenance of other QS. A cost-benefit analysis will be useful to better understand whether the benefits that come from the QS justify the investments made into the maintenance of the system or whether an internal system would work, limiting the need to meet an external standard and audit requirements.

18.3.11 How to Ensure and Demonstrate the Value of the Quality System?

Efforts toward quality management not only demonstrate effective and controlled operational systems and processes to external stakeholders but can be invaluable in developing and monitoring progress within your own institution. This is particularly important in areas such as welfare, training, and data management.

External users of services, especially those who are aspiring to reach standards set by regulatory bodies or who are seeking funding and additional resources, may frequently quote the QS of the facility they have or planning to use.

Requesting regular feedback from researchers working within an accredited facility will give an indication of the impact of the QS on the success of services delivered. This also aids continuous improvement and provides feedback to staff on the value they make toward the establishment.

For internal purposes that include staff, welfare, and research, the value of a QS is not limited to times around a periodic audit, but in a sustained effort to meet the standards throughout the year, every year. Regular reviews, meetings of teams, and internal efforts will ensure that changes, and issues which arise between official audits are identified at early stages and corrected appropriately. Monitoring metrics of the QS can be vital in demonstrating the effectiveness and therefore the value of the quality-driven efforts. This information can also be used for root cause analysis to delve deeply into processes to identify more robust systems, if necessary. These can include:

- Registers tracking incidents of non-compliance and subsequent corrective actions.
- Improvement in data accuracy, transparency, traceability, and appropriate data storage.
- Appropriate and fit-for-purpose documentation of processes (including up-to-date SOPs and effective risk assessments).
- Help with the timely and accurate delivery of projects.

Prospective implementation of a QS will help to avoid errors from the start and continuous evaluation of the measurements described above will enable a retrospective assessment of improvements and give a tangible readout of value and service improvements.

The QS should become part of the culture of an establishment where all systems and processes are constantly evaluated and questioning of the effectiveness and efficiency becomes a normal part of any review process. This is not carried out alone by institutional management but by those carrying out the processes to provide additional value and ownership that leads to highly motivated staff.

References

1. OECD series on principles of good laboratory practice (GLP) and compliance monitoring. 1998. https://www.oecd.org/officialdocuments/publicdisplaydocumentpdf/?cote=env/mc/chem(98)17&doclanguage=en
2. ISO 9001:2015 Quality management systems—Requirements. 2021. https://www.iso.org/standard/62085.html
3. European Medicines Agency. Good manufacturing practice. 2010. https://www.ema.europa.eu/en/human-regulatory/research-development/compliance/good-manufacturing-practice
4. Food and Drug Administration. 2021. https://www.fda.gov/drugs/pharmaceutical-quality-resources/current-good-manufacturing-practice-cgmp-regulations
5. Bespalov A, Bernard R, Gilis A, et al. Introduction to the EQIPD quality system. eLife. 2021;2021(10): e63294. https://doi.org/10.7554/eLife.63294.
6. FELASA guidelines and recommendations. https://felasa.eu/working-groups/guidelines
7. American Medical Veterinary Association. 2020. https://www.avma.org/sites/default/files/2020-01/2020-Euthanasia-Final-1-17-20.pdf

8. Guillén J, Medina CL, Denais-Lalieve DG. Assessment of animal care and use programs. In: Hau J, Schapiro SJ, editors. Handbook of laboratory animal science. Essential principles and practices. 4th ed. London: CRC; 2021.
9. The European Parliament and the Council of the European Union. Directive 2010/63/EU of the European Parliament and of the Council of 22 September 2010 on the protection of animals used for scientific purposes. Off J Eur Union. 2010;L 276/33–79.
10. National Research Council, National Academy of Sciences. Guide for the care and use of laboratory animals. Washington: National Academy Press; 2011.
11. European Medicines Agency. Good laboratory practice compliance. https://www.ema.europa.eu/en/human-regulatory/research-development/compliance/good-laboratory-practice-compliance
12. Food and Drug Administration. CFR—Code of Federal Regulations Title 21. https://www.accessdata.fda.gov/scripts/cdrh/cfdocs/cfcfr/CFRSearch.cfm?CFRPart=58
13. National Competent Authorities for the implementation of Directive 2010/63/EU on the protection of animals used for scientific purposes. 2014. A working document on Inspections and Enforcement to fulfil the requirements under the Directive. Available at: https://ec.europa.eu/environment/chemicals/lab_animals/pdf/endorsed_inspection-enforcement.pdf

Inter-institutional Collaborations 19

Joachim Coenen, Thomas Steckler, and William W. King

Abstract

There are many sound reasons for initiating an inter-institutional collaboration, such as additional or complementary scientific expertise, knowledge, labor, technical capabilities, and financial resources. This is why multi-institutional projects have gained increasing popularity in recent years. For some studies, these collaborations may be initiated and terminated rather spontaneously and without significant repercussions. However, when animal subjects are involved, numerous implications, caveats, and consequences must be considered, not only to cultivate favorable outcomes but also to avoid subsequent problems, including animal welfare and regulatory issues. This chapter defines and describes inter-institutional collaborations, which parties could be involved, how partnerships are created, what details need to be considered, and why a written mutual agreement of understanding (or equivalent document) is important. Regulatory implications, roles and responsibilities, animal ownership, sourcing, and financial aspects are also discussed. While success is always anticipated, this chapter also clarifies legal and animal welfare considerations in cases when collaborations must be terminated prematurely.

Keywords

Collaborations · Animal welfare · Responsibilities

19.1 Definitions and General Concepts

19.1.1 What Is an Inter-institutional Collaboration?

An Inter-Institutional Collaboration (IIC) occurs when members of any two or more organizations or establishments initiate a cooperative effort toward a common product or goal. In research, this frequently occurs when two or more individuals or teams engage to address a scientific question based on their specific experience, abilities, interest, or access to research tools of otherwise limited availability.

In animal use-based scenarios, such cooperative arrangements can range from a simple sharing of a unique genetically modified mouse strain from a neighboring university to a complex,

J. Coenen (✉)
Merck KGaA, Darmstadt, Germany
e-mail: joachim.coenen@merckgroup.com

T. Steckler
Janssen Pharmaceutica NV, Beerse, Belgium

W. W. King
University of Michigan, Ann Arbor, MI, USA

J. Guillén, V. Galligioni (eds.), *Practical Management of Research Animal Care and Use Programs*, Laboratory Animal Science and Medicine 3, https://doi.org/10.1007/978-3-031-65414-5_19

international, multi-institutional endeavor to identify innovative approaches to developing therapeutics to a specific disease. Examples of the inspiration for potential collaborations are potentially limitless:

- A research scientist with a need for a specialized imaging device learns that a unit is available at a nearby research institution or university.
- Two researchers from different institutions learn from each other's work during a scientific society meeting and wish to develop a collaborative effort that may involve complementary experiments at each other's laboratories.
- A sponsor wishes to outsource various components of a widely scoped project to experts in separate institutions.
- Two companies decide to jointly develop a therapeutic agent, involving the use of a Contract Research Organization (CRO) and/or an academic institution.

Each of these cases represents a collective approach to a scientific challenge that may have many potential legal ramifications and other complications that must be considered before the actual collaboration starts.

In fact, modern pundits strongly advocate for scientific collaboration and team science [1–4]. The sharing of expertise, knowledge, and increasingly specialized and expensive equipment provides essential opportunities for scientific exploration in a progressively complex research environment. However, as this chapter will examine, careful consideration of common challenges associated with sharing of information and resources is prudent.

This chapter will focus primarily on animal welfare and regulatory implications of IIC. As with any scientific partnership, there are many additional considerations associated with such matters as intellectual property, authorship and publication rights, data sharing and ownership, conflicts of interest, and other contractual obligations. Such details are discussed only briefly in this chapter; however, a general understanding and acknowledgment of the business-like aspects of IIC may prove useful.

For the purposes of this chapter, an academic institution is a university, college, academy, school, or other institution of higher learning with research and/or educational missions. The term "industry" represents a private or publicly traded company that includes, in entirety or in part, research and development within its scope and mission, such as a pharmaceutical company, CRO, or medical device company.

Examples provided in this chapter will primarily incorporate perspectives of Europe and the United States; readers are encouraged to explore the implications discussed based on their regional and national regulatory environment.

19.1.2 What Are the Types of Inter-institutional Collaborations?

Inter-institutional collaborations can come in various forms and may have many facets. Partnerships can involve academic partners such as universities or governmental (research) institutions, and partners from industry, e.g., large pharmaceutical companies, smaller biotechnology companies, or CROs. Collaborations may involve various combinations of these parties, with academic/academic, industry/industry, and academic/industry likely being the most common. The type and nature of the collaboration may also vary, as described below.

The intricacies of a collaboration, including contractual complexity, usually increase with the number of partners participating. An example of a large collaborative effort between academia and industry is the European Innovative Medicines Initiative (IMI; [5]), which funds big consortia within not only large pharmaceutical companies and academic institutions, but also biotechnology companies, CROs, learned societies, and others.

Collaborations can be characterized as:

- *Cooperating*, where each party does part of the work, for example, two academic laboratories from two institutions contributing mutually to a project.
- *Enabling*, where the involvement of one party may be limited, e.g., to providing resources, expertise, and advice, or access to a genetically modified mouse line, exclusive assay, animal model or method, but without active involvement.
- *Contracting*, where one party outsources work, with the contractor providing a fee-for-service product; examples may include establishing a breeding colony or generating and surrendering data from a specific set of experiments.

A special case of enabling collaboration is investigator-initiated work, where one party, mostly academic, requests resources from the other, often industry, partner to enable its own study, for example, free access to a drug or a device.

A collaboration can be *precompetitive* or *competitive* in nature, which should be defined in a contractual agreement between the collaborators. In a precompetitive collaboration, parties work together on a shared question or problem presenting no competitive advantage for any, i.e., the outcome from the collaboration is shared as well. An example of a precompetitive collaboration would be the IMI consortia mentioned above. In a competitive collaboration, the potential for scientific or financial advantage is sustained for those involved. Specific examples of competitive collaborations include *outsourcing agreements*, where ownership of results generated by a contracted laboratory would be retained by the study sponsor; *joint ventures*, often involving the creation of a new business entity by two partnering institutions; and *licensing efforts*, such as the in-licensing of an animal model, assay, or method by one institution that is patent-protected and owned by another institution.

19.1.3 Will My Staff and I Be Able to Conduct Animal Experiments at My Collaborator's Institution (and Vice Versa)?

Ultimately, collaborators are likely able to conduct research at each other's institutions. After all, an IIC is intended to be a mutually beneficial relationship that combines expertise and/or other assets of the individual partners. However, there are certain requirements to ensure an effective, efficient, compliant, and seamless collaboration that involves scientists and staff conducting work at a partnering institution. Three primary considerations, which should be addressed well in advance to ensure safe and legal conduct of animal experiments, include:

1. *Institutional requirements*

   Contingent on location, type of institution, and individual requirements, there may be a number of logistical and administrative considerations:
   (a) General onboarding activities, such as facility orientation, physical access and security requirements, and work hours.
   (b) Training, such as institutional animal care and use expectations, specific biomethodology, occupational health and safety, and physical and information security.
   (c) Insurance needs, such as workers compensation and liability.
   (d) Licenses, e.g., personal license granted by the UK Secretary of State [6] or other national competent authorities.
2. *Regulatory requirements*

   National regulations (e.g., the US Animal Welfare Act [7], German Animal Welfare Act [8]), the UK Home Office's guidance, "Animal Testing and Research: Personal Licence Process" [6], and international legislation or guidance (e.g., EU Directive 2010/63 [9], *Guide for the Care and Use of Laboratory Animals* (the Guide; [10]) may dictate licensing and specific training. If it is intended that scientists from both or all parties are to perform animal activities, it is mandatory to closely review these requirements, undergo necessary certification, and apply for required licenses and/or approvals as necessary. There are many other regulatory implications for IIC, as described throughout the remainder of this chapter.

3. *Contractual agreements*

   Satisfying legal and regulatory requirements is imperative. Furthermore, it is highly recommended to create (a) written agreement(s) detailing all aspects of the collaboration, as described below.

19.1.4 Who Establishes an IIC?

Initial discussions regarding scientific partnerships are usually launched among specific researchers. But as the rest of this chapter will illustrate, there are numerous other stakeholders involved in an IIC that must be engaged to address considerations not normally involved in performing animal-based research by employees at their home institution.

From a practical standpoint, animal facility management must verify that the vivarium and other research areas provide the infrastructure needed and, if applicable, facilitate the logistical aspects of animal transport. Facility management may also be asked to assist the scientists in reviewing husbandry and physical plant standards. Although uncommon, some collaborations encourage or require as much consistency as possible across locations, e.g., environmental control, water quality, sanitation practices, feed, and bedding. Both or all parties should be involved in decision-making and identifying acceptable exceptions. The attending or designated veterinarians at each site must oversee animal health and well-being during transit, housing, and use, including protection of animal biosecurity.

The pertinent animal welfare oversight body (OB), such as the Animal Welfare Body, Ethics Committee, Institutional Animal Care and Use Committee (IACUC; which will be referred to as IACUC/OB in this text), and other institutional regulatory authorities (such as biological safety, chemical hygiene, and/or environmental health, as applicable), usually must review and approve all projects and procedures conducted within their own institutions. In addition, the committees should also understand the relationships between the investigators and how the procedures conducted at various locations support the overall goals of the study and impact individual animal welfare. Quality management teams at each institution, if applicable, may also require engagement.

Personnel or offices associated with procurement and finance will often be involved in the acquisition of animals and research-related materials, establishment of institutional accounts, and the oversight and transfer of funding. Information technology may be involved in projects requiring significant data exchange. In many institutions, legal counsel and technology transfer offices are responsible for ensuring that each site's interests are preserved and that research products are appropriately distributed in accordance with established agreements. In certain circumstances, in particular in industry, executive management approval may be required as well.

In some instances, the sponsoring agency may also dictate certain requirements. An example involves the funding by the US Public Health Service (PHS) of a scientist whose home institution does not otherwise have a centralized animal care and use program with requisite oversight components. This situation requires partnering with another institution that maintains an "Assurance of Compliance with the PHS Policy on the Humane Care and Use of Laboratory Animals" with the PHS Office of Laboratory Animal Welfare (OLAW). In these cases, an "Interinstitutional Assurance" is created by the awardee and endorsed by the assured institution, which verifies that the hosting institution assumes regulatory responsibility for appropriate study conduct [11].

19.1.5 What Are the Operational Aspects of IIC?

There are numerous functional elements to consider when organizing an IIC. Partners should agree in advance on the work schedule, including resources needed and timelines. Determining the distribution of workload, i.e., who will be responsible for performing specific aspects of the study, will optimize planning and avoid unnecessary and unpleasant surprises. Collaborators need to identify the origin of required resources such as animals, equipment, labor, consumables, and reagents, especially if some must be acquired from a third-party or supplier. For resources that are not readily available, decisions regarding the financial sources will be needed. This is of particular importance when third-party grant funding is used to support IIC, to not only abide by the conditions of the grant award but also to ensure fair distribution of the budget allocation within the partnership.

An agreement should also be reached among the partners on the proposed rigor to be applied (for example, whether and how experiments should be randomized, blinded, and to what level they should be powered; how outliers are defined; or whether a study is considered exploratory or confirmatory), the expected quality of the animal care and use program (see also Sect. 19.1.4), the degree of harmonization/standardization that may be required across sites, and on the type/method and duration of record retention.

Data and other research product dispositions are especially important for many collaborations. Partners should agree on the level of confidentiality required, i.e., what information can and cannot be shared with others. Intellectual property discussions will determine ownership of data, inventions, and potential patents. Other products or outcomes also require decisions, such as responsibility for presentations, publications, and authorship. Finally, the liabilities associated with the violation of any of these principles should be outlined.

As scientific projects do not always progress as expected, agreements should also include contingency plans discussing the need for repeating failed studies or experiments with indecisive results and their subsequent financial, personnel, and resource obligations. Conversely, there must be alignment in the initiation of additional or supplemental studies. Waning scientific enthusiasm or changing focus may occasionally lead to conduct of studies that are not in the best interest of all partners. Given the involvement of live animals, this may present significant ethical and animal welfare challenges when considering study termination and potential animal euthanasia.

19.1.6 Why Is a Written Agreement/Contract Required?

Especially given the myriad of details requiring active decision-making described above, and acknowledging that parties have overlapping but distinct interests, it is essential to establish expectations in writing. Collaborations are spawned from common scientific interests combined with complementing expertise, resources, and capacities; a partnership is considered a "win-win" situation. Without clear assurances, however, such feelings can dissipate rapidly. Most importantly, regulatory responsibilities must be considered based on local laws and responsibilities.

A proper written agreement in advance amongst all parties involved will facilitate the success of the collaboration. At a minimum, documentation of the above discussions could be in the form of informal meeting minutes. More formal records are advisable, including memoranda of understanding (MOU) or contractually binding agreements, depending on the nature and complexity of the IIC [10].

Table 19.1 outlines recommended components of written agreements involving animal use in IIC.

19.1.7 Why Should I Perform a Risk/Benefit Analysis Before Commencing a Partnership?

As in any endeavor, there are a number of benefits involved in an IIC that should be balanced

Table 19.1 Recommended components of written agreements involving animal use in IIC

1. General administration		
Financial agreements and animal-related costs	Responsibility for • Procurement • Housing (per diem charge?) • Responsibility for costs for animal care and procedures applied (daily charges?)	
Intellectual property	Ownership of intellectual property, data sharing, conflicts of interest, other contractual obligations, how to protect intellectual property	
Access rights	• List of roles/representatives/individuals allowed to enter the facility • List of activities these roles/representatives/individuals are allowed to perform • Relationships between investigators (supervision of study personnel, final decision-making authority)	Could also be defined or referenced in the IACUC/OB-approved study protocol
Institutional requirements	General onboarding activities, training, insurance needs, licenses	
Associated departments	For example, • Procurement • Finance • Legal • Technology Transfer	
Funding sources	• Associated reporting requirements/updates/final reports and responsibility • Associated costs	Necessary assurances, e.g., inter-institutional assurance
Operational aspects	• Work schedules • Workload balance • Financial responsibilities • Operational responsibilities (e.g., equipment, labor, consumables, and reagents)	
Study objective and experimental design	Randomization, blinding, statistical rigor, definition of outliers, expected quality of the animal care and use program, degree of harmonization/standardization	
Definition of milestones and completion date	There should also be a mechanism in place to report delays or concerns (e.g., safety, efficacy, formulation, physicochemical properties, and galenic issues)	
Data security	Including data transfer and cyber security	
Authorship/publications	• Responsibilities for presentations and publications • Definition of authorship • Approval process • Conflict of interest	

(continued)

Table 19.1 (continued)

2. Legal, regulatory, and compliance		
Regulatory environment	Laws, directives, and regulations to be followed	• The approval process differs from country to country • Involvement of ethics committees and competent authorities may apply • Transport of animals may require specific permits • If procedures are performed at several locations/institutions, more than one competent authority may have to approve the project
Regulatory requirements	Required licenses (establishment, project, personal), certificates, and approvals	
3. Animal care and use		
Roles and Responsibilities	• Institutional Official(s) • Oversight Body(-ies) • Attending Veterinarian(s) • Sponsor(s) • Principal Investigators(s) • Animal Facility Manager(s)	For all roles it is important to define institutional expectations, how the final decision is made in their respective areas of responsibilities and by which partner(s)
Definition of the decision-making process	Definition of the roles of the partners in the project, their participation in the design, planning, and conduct of the study, access to resources, utilization of study outcomes	
Animal ownership	Definition Transfer of ownership in case of termination of collaboration, closure of business, or disagreement	Potential legal and ethical implications
Sourcing	Animals, supplies, and equipment	Restrictions due to international regulations (e.g., CITES)
Contractual agreements	Further aspects of collaboration • Animal facility infrastructure/equipment • Animal transport • Review of husbandry and physical plant standards • Veterinary oversight • Environmental control • Supplies (e.g., feed and bedding) • Sanitary requirements (hygiene)	Includes housing standards
Organizational responsibilities/ relationships	• IACUC/OB • Other institutional regulatory bodies (e.g., biological safety chemical hygiene, environmental health)	
Adverse event reporting	Definition of adverse events, to whom they need to be addressed to, who needs to report, who decides on consequences and CAPAs	

(continued)

Table 19.1 (continued)

Contingency plans	Decision on repetition of studies or experiments with decisive results, subsequent financial, personnel, and resource obligations. Relocation of collaborating partners.	
Termination of collaboration, project, and/or study	• Definition of financial consequences • Ethical and animal welfare consequences, legal consequences, disposition (e.g., euthanasia, rehoming, (re-) use in other studies/projects) • Definition and financial consequences for early termination	
Relocation of collaborating partners or PIs	• Identification of the new roles and responsibilities • Requirement of new licenses	
Closure of business/ disagreement without scientific and/or animal welfare justification	• Contingency assurance of the animal study • Animal and data ownership • Potential legal and ethical implications • Withdrawal of animals • Financial fall back position	
Animal transport	• Frequency • Method • Costs	In addition, impact of frequent transport on animal welfare and study results should be considered
4. Quality control and assurance		
Quality management and audits	• Assurance of ethical standards and legal requirements • Quality of the animal care and use program • Accreditations or certifications of the animal care and use program (e.g., AAALAC International) • Quality standards to be adhered to (e.g., GLP and ISO) • Additional procedures to be adhered to (e.g., ARRIVE, PREPARE, and EQIPD)	
Audits	• Frequency • Personnel involved • Associated costs/financial responsibility • Format • Outcome/consequences	

against potential risks. Benefits should clearly outweigh the risks to make a collaboration viable. Questions one may wish to ask before engaging in an IIC could include the following:

- Will I/my institution gain additional knowledge; develop greater expertise, experience, and skills; and/or establish new or more valuable networks?
- Will the data generated be more robust or of higher quality?
- Will there be greater scientific efficiency due to cost-sharing and/or increased access to existing infrastructure?
- Will the potential for sharing of new ideas lead to greater innovation ("thinking outside of the box")?

- Is there a possibility to enhance the impact of the work due to the collaboration?
- Is there a potential for higher reputation and credibility?

Even with affirmative responses to any/all of these questions, the potential benefits should be weighed against potential negative side effects, such as:

- Will I/my institution experience an unacceptable loss of autonomy due to the collaboration?
- Will I/my institution face unmanageable conflicts of interest?
- Will the collaboration result in an unacceptable drain of resources?
- Will there be unsurmountable logistical challenges?
- Is there a potential for a negative impact on my or my institution's reputation if the collaboration proves unsuccessful or animal-welfare-related questions are raised?

As in most aspects of scientific endeavors, the conduct of collaborative studies is rarely routine or outcomes predetermined. An acceptable balance must be decided on a case-by-case basis given the risk/benefit threshold that the individuals and institutions are willing to accept.

19.1.8 Are There Special Considerations for IIC Involving Partners from Academic Institutions and Commercial Organizations?

When considering an IIC, it is important to consider and acknowledge cultural and organizational differences, and potential differences in goals and objectives between collaborating institutions, especially when partnerships between academic and commercial institutions are to be established.

In general, research in industry is applied, deadline-driven, and more standardized to ensure comparability of data over time. Industrial research has the goal to support business objectives and often aims at developing a clinical product (e.g., a drug or device). In this environment, individual animal experiments are part of a larger scheme and should enable decisions on continuing project development, based on whether or not the product has the desired properties (e.g., in terms of efficacy, pharmacokinetics, safety, and tolerability). Furthermore, failure to recognize and report concerns, such as safety, efficacy, or others (e.g., formulation, physicochemical properties, or galenic issues), may be costly or result in litigation. This requires more control and oversight, both internally and externally (e.g., from regulators), and has a bearing on the animal care and use programs, which should ensure standardized and stable processes in terms of animal source and availability, health status, housing, husbandry, etc.

Working in academic research in general means more research freedom, flexibility, and autonomy, with the primary research goal of gaining knowledge and disseminating new findings. Obviously, quality standards in academic animal facilities should be high as well, but this environment allows and requires a more adjustable approach to support the potentially more diverse and dynamic research ventures.

Collaboration partners should be aware of these differences and acknowledge their strengths and limitations to establish expectations and avoid disappointment.

19.1.9 As a Member of a Large Organization, Are There Special Considerations for Partnering with a Colleague at a Small Institution?

Larger organizations, including multi-national commercial or pharmaceutical companies, may choose to collaborate with smaller institutions that offer special talents or capabilities. In these situations, especially if the IIC involves shared regulatory or legal responsibilities, bigger companies may at least perceive a higher degree of risk from any impropriety that may occur associated with the study. For one thing, the broader footprint of the larger company dictates more public scrutiny. As stated by American humorist and writer Will Rogers, "It takes a lifetime to build a good reputation, but you can lose it in a minute."

Furthermore, many animal welfare regulations and accrediting bodies authorize institutions, not individual principal investigators. A case of serious non-compliance emanating from a single laboratory employing external collaborators risks the accreditation and regulatory status of the entire institution. Large organizations may therefore be more averse to such risk when considering an IIC, unless the perceived benefit is considerable.

19.1.10 As a Smaller Partner, What Do I Have to Consider When I Collaborate with a Large Organization?

It is also advantageous for the smaller partner to ensure that expectations are clearly defined. Often, the smaller partner provides very specific expertise or owns specialized equipment desired by the larger partner. However, smaller organizations may depend upon infrastructure available at larger institutions, such as electronic data handling, a wider array of scientific capabilities, and information security. This may tempt a larger partner to take the lead in the collaboration and to consider the smaller party as a secondary or junior partner.

Consequently, the smaller partner must confirm their role in the project, including their participation in the design, planning, and conduct of the study; access to resources such as the animal facilities; and utilization of study outcomes. This also underscores the importance of a written agreement to protect the independent expertise of the smaller partner.

19.2 Regulatory Roles and Responsibilities

19.2.1 What Are the General Considerations and Legal Implications When Initiating an IIC?

As this section will elucidate, there are important legal, ethical, and logistic considerations when initiating an IIC involving animals with respect to local, national, and international regulations. The specific prerequisites for executing animal experiments in the countries of each of the institutions participating in a collaboration must be taken into consideration. For example, in member states of the European Union, this is driven by the Directive 2010/63 [9], and in the United States, the Animal Welfare Regulations [7] and Public Health Service Policy on Humane Care and Use of Laboratory Animals [12], which relies on the *Guide* [10], determine what can and must be done. The legal ramifications in other countries involved likely differ and must be considered. If an institution is accredited by AAALAC International, the *Guide* also applies.

The application of regulations begins during the planning stages of the collaboration (see Sect. 19.1.3). Ethical considerations include the rules and expectations of the participating IACUC/OBs and/or governmental competent authorities (as applicable), as well as the relevant local and national animal welfare regulations. This is especially true when animal transfer and transportation are involved. Of course, ethical approval must be obtained prior to the conduct of any animal experiment, and most often prior to any animal shipment. It is best for the IACUC/OB from the institute from where animals originate to have a general understanding of their fate at the collaborating institution, and vice versa. In general, the IACUC/OBs from both the shipping and the receiving institutions should authorize animal transfer. In addition, and as applicable, competent authorities must be involved in the authorization and oversight process. Physical relocation of animals in research is highly regulated and involves many logistical issues; these and other considerations impacting animal shipping are discussed in Sect. 19.3.4 and Chap. 5.

19.2.2 Which Institution Maintains the Authority for IACUC/OB Oversight for Animals Involved in IIC; Is It Simply the Body from the Institution Housing the Animals?

In general, the IACUC/OB of the institution housing the animals is responsible for their health and welfare. If animals are transferred to multiple sites, oversight changes with the transfer. In some countries (e.g., all EU member states), in addition to local animal welfare bodies, independent ethics committees and/or Competent Authorities must approve study projects. In case animals are transferred, all respective authorities must approve the study protocol if manipulations are applied at multiple sites (e.g., project-specific surgery at one location and nuclear magnetic resonance imaging at another; note that this may not apply to commercially available surgical models such as catheterized animals). In these cases, it is crucial to consider all applicable legislation in detail to be compliant with all legislation and specific local expectations.

In the United Kingdom, it is important to ensure that all relevant licenses (establishment, project, and personal licenses) cover all aspects of the programs involved, that license holders for the respective animal sites are identified, and that these licenses cover all aspects of the project [6]. Similar requirements apply in many other countries, for example, within the European Union.

In the United States, each institution has an overarching responsibility to ensure appropriate review, approval, and oversight of research involving animals. Additional complexity emerges when institutions must oversee research that is occurring at or otherwise involves multiple institutions. In these situations, the division of responsibilities between and among institutions must be clear and involved parties should share a common understanding. This is particularly relevant as animal regulations differ by funding agency and individual institutional policies may also vary. Both the National Institutes of Health Office of Laboratory Animal Welfare [12] and the United States Department of Agriculture [7] require an IACUC to review the care and use of animals in research and determine whether proposed research projects are in accordance with federal policy, regardless of whether the work occurs at one or multiple institutions.

19.2.3 Do PIs at Each of the Collaborating Institutions Need IACUC/OB Approval?

Here again, national legislation must be considered first. Principal Investigators at each of the collaborating institutions require approval by the responsible IACUC/OB or Competent Authority unless specified otherwise in legislation.

Unless defined otherwise, there is no expectation that both/all IACUC/OBs must review and approve the entire collaborative project, including all experiments and animal procedures that will be performed elsewhere, as long as there is a written agreement designating each individual IACUC/OB oversight authority for actions occurring at their institution. Seeking means of avoiding review by multiple IACUC/OBs, when allowed by regulations, is recommended to preclude the potential for conflicting oversight expectations. However, especially in cases where animals are transported or when procedures are performed at multiple locations, most IACUC/OBs will expect at least a summary of procedures conducted remotely that could be expected to have an impact on animal welfare. Once again, the need for a reciprocal understanding and commitment to assigning oversight responsibility highlights the importance of a written agreement with an understanding of local regulations or institutional policy.

In some instances where two institutions may collaborate frequently, a Master Reciprocal Institutional Agreement for Animal Care and Use (Master IACUC Agreement; [13]) may be useful. Such documents codify the overarching, as opposed to project-specific, responsibilities for animal oversight and care between institutions with the goal of facilitating research yet reducing redundant regulatory oversight efforts.

19.2.4 What If the Collaboration Is Limited to Use of Specialized Equipment at a Colleague's Institution? Are There Reduced Expectations for Pilot Studies?

Once again, the responsibilities depend on the national regulations applicable to each institution, and potentially the funding agency, even for pilot studies using a minimum number of animals. As mentioned above, when animals are transported between institutions, the IACUC/OB at each collaborating institution should maintain some understanding of animal use at each location, even if that use is restricted to use of specialized equipment. This remains true regardless of the number of animals involved or the duration of their stay.

In cases where animals are transported to another institution solely for use with a specialized laboratory/equipment/procedure, the originating institution that owns the animals must understand the use of the facility providing the specialized equipment/procedure(s) in the context of the overall study. The procedures must be adequately described so that the approving IACUC/OB understands their need and potential impact on the animals for which it is responsible. For most circumstances, primary regulatory responsibility is retained by the originating institution and follows animal ownership. If regulations dictate that the IACUC/OB extend their oversight to the collaborating site, a written agreement is especially useful to outline each stakeholder's expectations.

If use of a specialized imaging equipment, for example, by outside collaborators becomes routine, some hosting institutions may agree to a blanket approval with minimal to no experiment-to-experiment oversight of animals owned by another institution and that are on-site for brief periods of time. In this scenario, the laboratory with specialized equipment or services functions as a contracted service provider with a reduced need for regulatory oversight. Nonetheless, the prudent IACUC/OB will still require enough information from the scientists operating the contracted space to determine any potential risks to institutionally owned animals using the facility or housed nearby. As mentioned above, in addition, authorizations from respective competent authorities may also apply.

19.2.5 What Happens If IACUC/OBs or Facility Management at Collaborating Organizations Have Different Institutional Expectations or Regulatory Requirements?

At some stage of a collaboration, differences in opinion may be inevitable. Should this occur, there are three possible outcomes: (1) compromise (i.e., a willingness by both parties to concede to a "middle ground" or an agreement that the different parties involved can continue to adhere to their respective standards), (2) adoption of the more stringent criteria by all parties involved, or (3) acceptance of the inability to pursue those specific parts of the collaboration where disagreements cannot be settled. However, termination of an ongoing study solely because the parties involved cannot find a compromise may cause ethical problems (see next question). Where a compromise is sought, animal program representatives may need to be involved to evaluate whether a compromise is acceptable and to advise on minimum required standards of animal care and use.

As was addressed in previous questions, this situation should best be prevented, or at least controlled, by a written agreement in advance that clearly delineates roles and responsibilities, study objectives, and the processes to be employed to reach outcomes (see Sect. 19.1.6). However, even with the best intentions of the parties involved, unforeseen situations may occur that violate the expectations of at least one collaborating partner and that require remediation to avoid unfortunate outcomes such as unacceptable data variability or invalid data, legal or reputational issues, or ethically unacceptable conditions. Again, written agreements should contain clauses that define the collaborators' options should such a situation occur, which in the worst-case scenario could be a termination of the collaboration.

Written agreements can also serve to help avoid late surprises triggered by unacceptable differences in animal care and use standards across institutions, especially if located in different countries that may have diverse legal animal welfare requirements and a different culture of care. As discussed in the last section, agreements should address the methods of animal procurement, transportation, and minimal expectations regarding health status, veterinary care, husbandry practices, and ethical review to harmonize processes as much as is feasible. Clearly, it is not realistic to expect complete alignment of processes across institutions; e.g., it may not be reasonable to expect an institution to acquire a new individually ventilated caging system for a limited rodent study if existing rodent husbandry practices meet regulatory requirements and are not expected to impact study outcomes. However, if institutions cannot reach a consensus on acceptable standards, either from irreconcilable differences deemed unacceptable by one IACUC/OB or untenable by facility management, then the viability of collaboration must be questioned and it may be advisable not to engage.

19.2.6 What Happens If One Collaboration Partner Relocates, Closes Business, or Other Unforeseen Circumstances Impact Pre-study Agreements?

Relocation of a PI's laboratory is always fraught with challenges; this will be compounded when an existing IIC is involved. Particularly when moving across national borders, it is critical that national legislation and regulatory expectations are resolved prior to recommencing any animal work. A properly executed and thorough written agreement will provide invaluable assistance by providing a framework for negotiation with the PI's new institution. This document will identify the roles and responsibilities of the individual parties and their regulatory requirements based on the national legislation, such as a need for a personal license for each person conducting animal procedures, a project license for the program of work, and an establishment license for the study location. All licenses (personal, project, and establishment) must be obtained prior to reinitiation of the study, which involves both IACUC/OB and/or Competent Authority(ies), as applicable.

A contingency plan should include the option to complete the study if one partner closes business or otherwise can no longer participate. Animal and data ownership should be defined in the written plan.

It is also important that the contingencies following a termination of the partnership are defined in the written agreement. Collaborating institutions must be aware of the potential legal and ethical implications of a premature termination of an animal study. Euthanasia of animals assigned to a study prematurely terminated for reasons such as collaborator relocation or disagreement without scientific and/or animal welfare justification would be ethically unacceptable and potentially legally questionable. The ownership of existing data and the options available for ultimate disposition of study animals may present considerable ethical and financial challenges.

19.3 Animal Ownership and Animal Resources

19.3.1 Why Is Defining Animal "Ownership" Important?

Determining which institution retains ownership of animals associated with an IIC has animal welfare, regulatory, and legal ramifications. The implications may be complex and not straightforward; therefore, it is imperative that such discussions are fully explored and defined in writing prior to commencing animal-based work. Advance determination of animal ownership may be especially important when scarce or especially valuable (both ethically and financially) resources have to be considered, such as non-human primates or genetically modified mice, or for potentially sensitive decisions such as initiating veterinary intercession, ultimate animal disposition, or euthanasia. Note that although the definition of ownership is vital, it must not interfere with clinical decisions or other interventions as authorized by the protocol; written agreements should include language that prevents a partner from retrospectively requesting compensation for veterinary or animal welfare-related activities.

Different regulatory bodies place various weights on animal ownership, ranging from ignoring to emphasizing it:

1. Most regulatory agencies in Europe and the United States focus responsibility for animal welfare on the site providing direct care and use regardless of ownership.
2. Some regulatory agencies that are associated with funding, e.g., the US Public Health Service National Institutes of Health Office of Laboratory Animal Welfare [12], may extend oversight only to those animals purchased and housed with the award provided.
3. Others, such as the US Department of Agriculture [7], acknowledge a shared responsibility between both parties regardless of which institution legally owns the animals—the hosting institution providing animal housing and veterinary care as well as the parent institution involved in study rationale and design [14]. Likewise, the UK Association of Medical Research Charities [15] requires that researchers and local ethics committees satisfy themselves of adherence to welfare standards consistent with the principles of UK legislation (e.g., the Animals [Scientific Procedures] Act 1986; [16]) when collaborating with other partners.
4. Animal ownership is of particular importance to accreditation by AAALAC International. AAALAC's Rules of Accreditation stipulate that the use of all animals owned by the accredited unit be incorporated into the association's review [17]. This includes not only animals housed at the institution during their initial and triennial site visit, but also animals that are located elsewhere. In essence, this extends the "accredited program" to the location where the animals are housed and/or used, including all the programmatic aspects that impact the animals in question, such as husbandry and environment, veterinary care, ethical oversight body review and approval, and occupational health and safety for individuals working with the animals [18]. Relationships are simplified when the hosting institution maintains its own accreditation, because the program will be reviewed during its initial and triennial site visit; however, if the hosting site is not accredited, the parent institution is expected to provide direct oversight and must make special arrangements with AAALAC to include the hosting site during its evaluation [14]. For institutions that contract animal care or use, and for which the contractor is considered the animals' owner, accreditation does not extend. Thus, some institutions insist that ownership is transferred to eliminate risk to their accreditation status should deficiencies be identified in the hosting unit.

Discussions regarding the legal implications of animal ownership are often based on intellectual property laws. During negotiations regarding information sharing, retaining ownership of animals involved in studies may be seen as an opportunity to ensure retention of the data obtained from them [14]. However, transfer of ownership can be outlined independent of data management, and likely fosters a better understanding of the responsibilities of the institution housing the animals in question.

For these reasons, transfer of animal ownership is recommended, when possible, to simplify legal and oversight responsibilities. Regardless, all parties have a stake in the animal welfare aspects of a collaboration. Institutional reputation may still be at risk should animal welfare be compromised during a study associated with a collaboration, despite relinquished animal ownership [19]. Thus, a written agreement clearly delineating animal ownership, roles, and responsibilities to assure appropriate animal care and use is highly recommended.

19.3.2 What Should Be Considered When Sourcing Animals from Vendors for Multi-site Studies?

A number of points must be carefully considered when ordering animals from commercial suppliers as part of an IIC, especially when the work is to be conducted in different parts of the world with different time zones and different legal requirements. A principal agreement should be reached regarding the species, strain, sex, and age of the animals to be used, and a number of additional important questions should be addressed:

- Can my facility or the facility of my partners accommodate certain species?
- Is the source of animals qualified (acceptable to all partner institutions)?
- Will all partners expected to house animals be legally allowed to import this species? For example, it may be allowed to use wild-caught non-human primates in some countries, but not in others.
- Is strain or sub-strain important? For example, it may well be relevant for certain types of studies whether C57/BL6J or C57/BL6N mice are tested, and just agreeing on C57/BL6 mice may not be sufficient [20, 21].
- Will the study use males, females, or both, and what would be the logistics required to keep and use both sexes? Outcomes of experiments may well differ, depending on sex of the animals being tested.
- At what age should animals be tested? Again, this can affect experimental outcomes, but can also become a logistical issue as availability of animals at a certain age may be limited, or difficult or even impossible to transport, e.g., preweaning. The age of the animals also greatly influences their size, which must also be considered.
- How many animals should each institution acquire and test?
- Is there sufficient holding capacity at each institution?
- Should animals have a certain health status and are there any exclusion criteria? First, health status may directly affect the outcome of the planned studies; second, it may also limit whether an institution is willing to accept animals into its animal facility due to exclusion of certain microorganisms. Institutions may also differ in quarantine requirements, which should be taken into consideration when planning the collaboration.
- To what environmental conditions have the animals been exposed? Housing and husbandry history of the animals ordered should also be taken into consideration, especially if not from the same supplier, as this may well differ at source of origin and again could affect the data.
- What is the animals' current location? Depending on availability and sourcing strategy, animals may also have substantially different distances to travel, potentially resulting in different time zones between place of origin and test facility. This in turn may result in the need for lengthy acclimation periods, well above the minimum acclimation period that may be imposed by an animal facility, in order to normalize the circadian rhythm of the animals.

Potential remediation strategies may include ordering all animals used in an IIC from the same supplier, as this increases the likelihood that genetic background, breeding methods, housing, and husbandry conditions are comparable, even if breeding facilities are located in different countries. However, there may be subtle differences due to different regulatory requirements in those countries or animals may not be available from all sites. To avoid this issue, animals could all be ordered from the same breeding facility. However, this has to be balanced against potentially large differences in transport requirements and transit time, the associated need for appropriate acclimation, and potentially higher costs. What is best should be decided case-by-case and will depend on animal sources available, requirements imposed by the animal facilities, and demands of the experiments.

Clearly, animals originating from different vendors for multi-site studies, or animals originating from the same vendor but without consideration of different acclimation needs for collaborating sites that are in different time zones, may not only increase the variability of the data, but may also negatively impact the ability to replicate experiments. On the other hand, if properly controlled, use of different animal sources could increase heterogenization, and hence increase external validity by making results more generalizable to the population.

19.3.3 Who Is Responsible for Paying for Animal Acquisition and per Diem Charges?

To ensure the success of projects using animals, it is essential to define the following financial aspects:

- Who is responsible for the ownership of the animals (sponsorship)?
- Who is responsible for purchasing/acquisition of the animals (payments for animals)?
- Who is responsible for the animal care and the procedures applied to the animals (daily charges)?

While there are no right or wrong responses to these questions, responsibility for budgetary concerns must be assigned and documented in the written agreement. What needs to be considered, however, is that the origin (source) of the budget carries certain implications. Depending on legislation and regulations, responsibility for the animals may follow the origin of the money. Sponsors should be aware of this implication and the responsibility this entails prior to signing a written agreement.

In general, partnerships are formed to generate the ideal combination of scientific excellence and financial background or opportunity. Depending on their expertise, partners may be equally focused on both funding and experimental conduct; alternatively, some collaborations rely on one partner concentrating on financial sponsorship and the other(s) on completing the experimental work. When projects are successful, and proceed with the anticipated pace and direction, partners will continue to share the same objectives. However, if tensions arise, agreements, including the financial aspects of those agreements, may be challenged. In extreme cases, a party may wish to relocate animals or withhold data in response to an impression that financial obligations are not being fulfilled. Once again, details on conflict resolution within written agreements become critical at these moments. While agreements cannot predict all eventualities, these aspects and potential financial fallback positions must be considered (see also Sects. 19.1.6 and 19.2.5).

19.3.4 What Should Be Considered When Transporting Animals Between Institutions?

There is a considerable body of knowledge identifying the impact of transportation and distress on laboratory animals. Therefore, any plans for animal relocation must be made thoughtfully and carefully with the principal aim of minimizing transit time and duplicating the environmental conditions of housing as much as possible. The *Guide* notes that oversight of transportation is a key component of a veterinary care program [10]. There are a number of additional texts and manuscripts that provide overviews of the subject in great detail, including those by the Laboratory Animal Science Association [22], ILAR [23], National Academies of Science, Engineering, and Medicine [24], Animal Transport Association [25], and the International Air Transport Association [26]. Primary considerations include regulations impacting relocation and transportation (e.g., [27–29]), transportation method and route, required documentation, environmental conditions, enclosures and space, access to food and water, appropriate facilities for receipt, health assessment, and acclimation periods (see also Chap. 5).

Note that there are numerous legal and regulatory factors that must be considered when even considering animal transfer. Animal transportation relies on high-quality shipping services with appropriately trained personnel that can ensure appropriate spatial, thermal, nutritional, and social requirements. Other factors include addressing biosafety standards, e.g., shipment of genetically modified animals, ensuring appropriate monitoring during transport, and implementing appropriate emergency procedures if required. There are limitations to transporting certain species, for example, legal restrictions on relocating species covered by the Convention on International Trade in Endangered Species (CITES) [30]. Local or regional laws may prohibit importation of certain species. Violation of applicable regulations can lead to serious liabilities and complications with customs. To ensure a seamless transfer and arrival of the animals, cooperation with all involved governmental authorities is vital.

The willingness of the receiving institution to accept a shipment is often driven by the health status of the animals and capacity of the facility to house them; this usually falls under the authority of both the animal facility management and the Attending Veterinarian. Ideally, acceptable health status is pre-defined in a quality document or written agreement. Animal ownership must also be predetermined, as was described in Sect. 19.3.1.

Lastly, there are a number of logistical items requiring attention. For example, the receiving animal facility must be aware of animal transport plans and be prepared to receive the animals. Shipment schedules should avoid the risk of arrival on weekends or holidays. Depending on the length of transport, sufficient nutrition and hydration should be provided. Shipping should occur in secure transport containers, fulfilling the animal welfare and biosafety requirements mentioned above, exposure of the animals to extreme temperatures during the transport must be avoided. Finally, all required documents should be duly completed to avoid unnecessary delays during transport, especially international customs.

19.4 Qualification (Auditing)

19.4.1 Why Is It Important to Qualify the Partner Facility?

Qualification is the process of ensuring that parties in a collaboration adhere to common expectations and standards. In the context of IIC involving animals, qualification of a partnering facility allows an assurance of the status of the animal care and use program of that partner.

There are at least three important reasons for doing so:

1. Alignment and adherence to *ethical standards and legal requirements* must be ensured. For example, a collaborator should not use methods or equipment that would not be approved by one's own IACUC/OB or that would violate local and/or international standards, e.g., with respect to minimum housing space requirements.
2. It is important to confirm that relevant aspects of the animal care and use programs of collaborators are *sufficiently consistent* to enable the generation of robust and comparable data. Some aspects are likely covered in the study protocol, while other factors, for example, how animals are handled by animal care technicians (method and frequency of cage-changing or other disturbance) or under what environmental conditions animals are kept (housing temperature, humidity, noise, light intensity, etc.), are less likely to be addressed in the study protocol yet could dramatically affect experimental data. But even if relevant animal care and use program details are included in the study protocol, it may be advisable to monitor the study conduct to ensure that the protocol is followed and that deviations are recorded and timely reported

among the collaborating partners. For example, do all animals indeed receive the enrichment that is specified in the protocol? Are non-aversive handling methods applied consistenly to all animals? Are there any singly housed animals, even though the protocol dictates social housing? Note there may be logical reasons why study animals must be single housed (e.g., aggression), but were the other partners informed about this change or process?
3. If a collaborator does not adhere to acceptable animal care and use standards, this may backfire on the *reputation* of one's own institution if the public becomes aware of the collaboration. Thus, there is a sound rationale for why it is useful to check and ensure that partners in a collaboration adhere to common expectations and avoid late surprises.

Qualifications can take different forms, ranging from informal teleconferences to agree on common practices, shared self-assessments, detailed questionnaires, to full site visit assessments, or combinations thereof. What would work best should be decided case-by-case and likely depends on the perceived risks associated with the IIC.

19.4.2 What Are Important Factors to Be Considered to Ensure that High Quality, Robust, Repeatable, and Coherent Data Are Obtained at the Collaborators?

A high-quality animal care and use program is essential for high-quality studies and subsequently high-quality results. The *Guide* [10], in combination with national and international legislation, forms its basis and AAALAC accreditation provides evidence. However, there are many more aspects required to conduct a sound and well-planned animal study, to generate robust and repeatable data, and finally to write a concise, transparent, and thorough manuscript that provides reviewers and readers all information needed "to scrutinize the research adequately, evaluate its methodological rigor, and reproduce the methods or findings" [31].

Quality aspects must be considered in planning, conducting, writing, and/or reviewing an animal experiment. For each step of an experiment, there are a number of references to assist in these efforts.

- For planning and designing experiments, the PREPARE (Planning Research and Experimental Procedures on Animals: Recommendations for Excellence; [32]) guidelines provide an extensive set of recommendations. Although primarily designed as a reporting tool, the ARRIVE (Animal Research: Reporting of In Vivo Experiments; [31, 33]) guidelines also provide excellent references for planning.
- Post-approval monitoring (PAM) is a program that monitors active projects to confirm that the research is being conducted as approved, thus ensuring compliance with the federal regulations, policies, and guidelines that govern the protection of study participants [10]. The level of formality and intensity of PAM should be tailored to institutional size and complexity, and in all cases should support a culture of care focusing on the animals' well-being [34]. Both OLAW and the USDA require the IACUC to review the animal care and use program, including inspection of all animal care and use facilities, every 6 months [7, 12].
- The European Quality in Preclinical Data (EQIPD) quality system is designed for non-clinical biomedical studies, aiming to provide "simple and sustainable solutions that facilitate improvements in data quality without impacting innovation and freedom of research" [35].
- As mentioned above, the ARRIVE guidelines provide a checklist of recommendations to improve the reporting of research involving animals—maximizing the quality and reliability of published research, and enabling others to better scrutinize, evaluate, and reproduce it [31, 33].

Chapter 18, "Quality," discusses these topics, detailing aspects that should be included and examples of quality systems.

19.4.3 Does Institutional Accreditation or Certification Preclude the Need for Qualification/Audit?

Collaborating with institutions maintaining accreditation by AAALAC, International, provides a valuable means of ensuring overall animal care and use program excellence. Other quality management certifications, such as those outlined in Chap. 18, "Quality," can also furnish some assurance of appropriate oversight and general study conduct. Such programs may also be viewed to mitigate risk and may facilitate qualification, especially if partners are willing to share relevant documents. A review of other available programmatic assessments, such as regulatory inspection reports, may also reveal institutional weaknesses, or a lack thereof. While it may be tempting to rely on such third-party assessments, none of these provide the intricate details needed to verify adherence to expectations among collaborators. Accreditation and positive regulatory reviews illustrate adherence to acceptable guidance; however, there are likely study- or collaborator-specific expectations that far exceed minimally acceptable standards. Furthermore, many practices that ensure appropriate project execution, such as data handling and scientific recordkeeping, are generally exempt from regulatory and accreditation reviews.

Given the relatively limited nature of regulatory and accreditation reviews and the likelihood of a range of attention to protocol details, a study-specific, bilateral review for verifying alignment with the expectations established by the partnership is strongly recommended.

19.4.4 How Should an Audit Be Performed?

If it is decided to conduct an audit as a means of qualification, it should be performed with mutual respect and the understanding that information provided by the auditee will be treated confidentially. It can be conceptualized as a process with the following steps:

1. *Planning*: First, prioritize where and how to audit. This is often risk-based; regardless, the audit scope should be defined.
2. *Preparation*: Auditees should be notified about the plans to audit, and auditors should familiarize themselves with applicable laws and regulations and, if required, complete additional training (e.g., how to enter a biocontainment facility). The hosting animal facility will usually provide the information needed regarding personal health (e.g., vaccination, tuberculosis testing, and respiratory fitness) and training requirements, as well as any other expectations such as additional animal facility access precautions, mutually agreeable dates and agendas, and other documentation. Some animal facilities may agree to forward pertinent documents in advance; some prefer the auditor to review documents while on-site. For an on-site visit, travel and accommodations should be arranged.
3. *Opening meeting*: During the opening meeting, which can be virtual or face-to-face while on-site, the auditors introduce themselves, as well as the scope of the audit. In most instances, the auditees will also use the opportunity to provide some information about the animal facility and the animal care and use program.
4. *Conduct*: In many instances, conduct consists of document review and facility tours. Both can be independent of each other (e.g., the document review could be conducted virtually, while the tour would be while the auditor is on-site).

5. *Exit briefing*: At the end of a site visit, it is good practice to arrange a short meeting with the auditees to discuss preliminary observations. This also allows the auditees to ask additional questions or to provide further clarification. Some time may be needed prior to the exit briefing for note review and preparation of any findings. This is more relevant if more than one auditor is involved in aligning any observations made by the auditors. Usually, this is done in a closed meeting without the auditees being present.
6. *Reporting*: A report should be written, documenting all observations, and distributed to relevant parties. Most auditees will appreciate a copy of the report. Both recommendations and concerns should be included and, if possible, the severity of any findings graded as this prioritizes follow-up actions.
7. *CAPA and CAPA follow-up*: Some issues require a so-called CAPA (corrective action/preventive action). Auditors and auditees should agree on a CAPA plan and timelines to address the CAPA. The auditor should follow up to ensure progress, effective implementation, and timely closure of the CAPA. Again, this should be documented in a report.

References

1. Bennett LM, Gadlin H, Marchand C. Collaboration and team science field guide. 2nd ed. NIH Publication No. 18-7660. Center for Research Strategy, National Cancer Institute, National Institutes of Health; 2018.
2. Didegah F, Thelwall M. Which factors help authors produce the highest impact research? Collaboration, journal and document properties. J Inform. 2013;7(4):861–73.
3. Joos S, Nettelbeck DM, Reil-Held A, Engelmann K, Moosmann A, Eggert A, Hiddemann W, Krause M, Peters C, Schuler M, Schulze-Osthoff K, Serve H, Wick W, Puchta J, Baumann M. German Cancer Consortium (DKTK)—A national consortium for translational cancer research. Mol Oncol. 2019;13(3):535–42.
4. Varner M, Logan J, Bjorklund T, Whitfield J, Reed P, Lesher L, Sikalis A, Brown B, Drollinger S, Larrabee K, Thompson K, Clark E, Workman M, Boi L. Process improvement for interinstitutional research contracting. Clin Transl Sci. 2015;8(4):334–40.
5. Innovative Medicines Initiative (IMI). 2022. https://www.imi.europa.eu/about-imi. Last accessed 05/12/2022.
6. UK Home Office. Animal testing and research: guidance for the regulated community. 2022. https://www.gov.uk/guidance/research-and-testing-using-animals. Last accessed 05/12/2022.
7. U.S. Department of Agriculture. Animal Welfare Act and Regulations. 2022. https://www.nal.usda.gov/legacy/awic/animal-welfare-act. Last accessed 05/12/2022.
8. Administration of Justice. Animal Welfare Act. 2021. TierSchG—Tierschutzgesetz. https://www.gesetze--im-internet.de/tierschg/BJNR012770972.html. Last accessed 05/12/2022.
9. European Parliament and the Council of the European Union. Directive 2010/63/EU of the European Parliament and of the Council of 22 September 2010 on the protection of animals used for scientific purposes. Off J Eur Union. 2010;L276/33–79.
10. Institute for Laboratory Animal Research, Committee for the Update of the Guide for the Care and Use of Laboratory Animals, National Research Council. Guide for the care and use of laboratory animals. 8th ed. Washington, DC: National Academies Press; 2011.
11. Office of Laboratory Animal Welfare, National Institutes of Health. Interinstitutional assurance. Bethesda, MD: OLAW; 2020. https://olaw.nih.gov/resources/documents/interinstitutional-assurance.htm. Last accessed 05/12/2022.
12. Office of Laboratory Animal Welfare, National Institutes of Health. Public health service policy on humane care and use of laboratory animals. Bethesda, MD: OLAW; 2002.
13. Holthaus K, Goldberg D, Connelly C, Corning B, Nascimento C, Witte E, Bierer BE. Facilitating collaborative animal research: The development and implementation of a master reciprocal institutional agreement for animal care and use. J Clin Transl Sci. 2020;4:96–101.
14. AAALAC International. Who's responsible for offsite animals? AAALAC Connect Newsl. 2003;2003(Spring):6–11.
15. Association of Medical Research Charities. Responsibility in the use of animals in bioscience research: Expectations of the major research councils and charitable funding bodies. 2017. https://bbsrc.ukri.org/documents/animals-in-bioscience-research-pdf/. Last accessed 05/12/2022.
16. UK Home Office. Animals (Scientific Procedures) Act of 1986. 2022. https://www.legislation.gov.uk/ukpga/1986/14/contents. Last accessed 05/12/2022.
17. AAALAC International. Rules of accreditation. 2022. https://www.aaalac.org/accreditation-program/rules-of-accreditation/. Last accessed 05/12/2022.

18. AAALAC International. Frequently asked question: animals included in the AAALAC International accredited 'unit.' 2022. https://www.aaalac.org/accreditation-program/faqs/. Last accessed 05/12/2022.
19. Bayne K, Turner PV. Animal welfare standards and international collaborations. ILAR J. 2019;60(1):86–94.
20. Aredo B, Zhang K, Chen X, Wang CX, Li T, Ufret-Vincenty RL. Differences in the distribution, phenotype and gene expression of subretinal microglia/macrophages in C57BL/6N (Crb1 rd8/rd8) versus C57BL6/J (Crb1 wt/wt) mice. J Neuroinflamm. 2015;12:6.
21. Fergusson G, Éthier M, Guévremont M, Chrétien C, Attané C, Joly E, Fioramonti X, Prentki M, Poitout V, Alquier T. Defective insulin secretory response to intravenous glucose in C57Bl/6J compared to C57Bl/6N mice. Mol Metabol. 2014;3:848–54.
22. Swallow J, Anderson D, Buckwell AC, Harris T, Hawkins P, Kirkwood J, Lomas M, Meacham S, Peters A, Prescott M, Owen S, Quest R, Sutcliffe R, Thompson K, Transport Working Group, Laboratory Animal Science Association (LASA). Guidance on the transport of laboratory animals. Lab Anim. 2005;39(1):1–39.
23. Institute for Laboratory Animal Research, Committee on Guidelines for the Humane Transportation of Laboratory Animals, National Research Council. Guidelines for the humane transportation of research animals. Washington, DC: National Academies Press; 2006.
24. National Academies of Sciences, Engineering, and Medicine. Transportation of laboratory animals: proceedings of a workshop. Washington, DC: National Academies Press; 2017.
25. Animal Transport Association. 2022. https://www.animaltransportationassociation.org/. Last accessed 05/12/2022.
26. International Air Transport Association. Live animal regulations (LAR), 47th ed. 2022. https://www.iata.org/en/publications/store/live-animals-regulations/. Last accessed 05/12/2022.
27. Council of Europe. Council Regulation (EC) No 1/2005 of 22 December 2004 on the protection of animals during transport and related operations and amending Directives 64/432/EEC and 93/119/EC and Regulation (EC) No 1255/97. 2019. https://eur-lex.europa.eu/legal-content/EN/TXT/?uri=celex%3A32005R0001. Last accessed 05/12/2022.
28. Council of Europe. European Convention for the Protection of Animals during International Transport (Revised) ETS No. 193. 2006. https://www.coe.int/en/web/conventions/full-list/-/conventions/treaty/193. Last accessed 05/12/2022.
29. U.S. Department of Agriculture. Import and export: animal and animal products. 2020. https://www.aphis.usda.gov/aphis/ourfocus/importexport/animal-import-and-export. Last accessed 05/12/2022.
30. Convention on International Trade in Endangered Species. 2022. https://cites.org/eng. Last accessed 05/12/2022.
31. Percie du Sert N, Hurst V, Ahluwalia A, Alam S, Avey MT, Baker M, Browne WJ, Clark A, Cuthill IC, Dirnagl U, Emerson M, Garner P, Holgate ST, Howells DW, Karp NA, Lazic SE, Lidster K, MacCallum CJ, Macleod M, Pearl EJ, Petersen O, Rawle F, Peynolds P, Rooney K, Sena ES, Silberberg SD, Steckler T, Würbel H. The ARRIVE guidelines 2.0: Updated guidelines for reporting animal research. PLoS Biol. 2020;18(7):e3000410.
32. Smith AJ, Clutton RE, Lilley E, Hansen KEA, Brattelid T. PREPARE: Guidelines for planning animal research and testing. Lab Anim. 2018;52(2):135–41.
33. Percie du Sert N, Ahluwalia A, Alam S, Avey MT, Baker M, Browne WJ, Clark A, Cuthill IC, Dirnagl U, Emerson M, Garner P, Holgate ST, Howells DW, Hurst V, Karp NA, Lazic SE, Lidster K, MacCallum CJ, Macleod M, Pearl EJ, Petersen OH, Rawle F, Reynolds P, Rooney K, Sena ES, Silberberg SD, Steckler T, Würbel H. Reporting animal research: Explanation and elaboration for the ARRIVE guidelines 2.0. PLoS Biol. 2020;18(7):e3000411.
34. Klein HJ, Bayne KA. Establishing a culture of care, conscience, and responsibility: Addressing the improvement of scientific discovery and animal welfare through science-based performance standards. ILAR J. 2007;48:3–1.
35. Bespalov A, Bernard R, Gilis A, Gerlach B, Guillen J, Castagne V, Lefevre IA, Ducrey F, Monk L, Bongiovanni S, Altevogt B, Arroyo-Araujo M, Bikovski L, De Bruin M, CastanosVelez E, Dityatev A, Emmerich C, Fares R, Ferland-Beckham C, Froger-Colleaux C, Gailus-Durner V, Hölter SM, Hofmann M, Kabitzke P, Kas MJ, Kurreck C, Moser P, Pietraszek M, Popik P, Potschka H, Prado Montes de Oca E, Restivo L, Riedel G, Ritskes-Hoitinga M, Samardzic J, Schunn M, Stöger C, Voikar V, Vollert J, Wever K, Wuyts K, Macleod M, Dirnagl U, Steckler T. Introduction to the EQIPD quality system. eLife. 2021;10:e63294. https://doi.org/10.7554/eLife.63294.

Transparency: External Communication

20

Bob Tolliday and Kirk Leech

Abstract

Opponents of the use of animals in research are well-funded, organised, and co-ordinated. They promote a message to the public and policymakers that animal research is unethical, unnecessary, and old fashioned (EARA. EARA executive director speech at SECAL conference. 'Hearts and minds' approach needed to talk about animal research, EARA tells Spanish scientists. Available at: https://www.eara.eu/post/hearts-and-minds-approach-needed-to-talk-about-research-eara-tells-spanish-scientists, 2021). Allowing these claims therefore allows for a one-sided narrative to go unchallenged—essentially that animals in scientific research is torture, with no societal benefit. This has a severe impact on biomedical research and scientific understanding and consequently on the prospect of new life-saving treatments for currently incurable diseases.

To counter this narrative, public confidence in biomedical research relies on the scientific community embracing an open and transparent approach as part of an ongoing dialogue about why and how animals are used in scientific, medical, and veterinary research and the enduring benefits of this.

In recent years, there has been a cultural change taking place, prompted by the European Animal Research Association (EARA) (EARA website. Available at: https://www.eara.eu, 2023) founded in 2014, its members and other advocacy associations around the world that support the use of animals in research. The chapter seeks to empower animal care professionals and research institutions with the tools needed to develop a proactive communications strategy on animal research, with the aim of promoting a balanced and informed debate throughout society. Based on this guidance, this chapter includes a step-by-step guide to developing a communications strategy, and advice on how to handle those crisis situations that will inevitably occur.

Keywords

Animal care professionals · Veterinarians · Biomedical research · Proactive communications · Transparency · Animal research

B. Tolliday · K. Leech (✉)
European Animal Research Association (EARA), London, UK
e-mail: btolliday@eara.eu; kleech@eara.eu

J. Guillén, V. Galligioni (eds.), *Practical Management of Research Animal Care and Use Programs*, Laboratory Animal Science and Medicine 3, https://doi.org/10.1007/978-3-031-65414-5_20

20.1 What Does the European Public Think About the Use of Animals in Research?

In recent years, unfortunately there has been no pan-European polling on public attitudes to the use of animals for scientific purposes to indicate public opinion trends. The last polling, the Eurobarometer poll on Science and Technology [1], tool place back in 2010 and found that European citizens' opinion of the necessity of using animals in research was divided: specifically, only 44% of interviewees agreed that scientists should be allowed to experiment on animals like dogs and monkeys—even when it leads to improvements in human health—and 37% disagreed. When asked the same about animals like mice, 66% of respondents were supportive and 18% were not.

That divide in public opinion was in large part caused by an imbalance in the information available to the public about animal research—because in general access to information from opponents of animal research is more readily available than from the scientific community [2]. Historically groups that oppose animal research have also increasingly gained ground in Europe [3], influencing decision makers and public opinion. Therefore, leaving the claims of these groups unchallenged and/or censoring communications has made the life sciences sector appear as if it has something to hide.

One interesting, but much smaller scale poll was carried out by Understanding Animal Research [4] in 2020, during the COVID-19 pandemic. The findings were that almost three-quarters of people in the UK (73%) think that it is acceptable for scientists to develop tests, treatments, or vaccines for COVID-19 using animals, such as mice, dogs, or monkeys, if it is the only way this research can be done. However, and significantly, many people in the poll felt conflicted and remained uncomfortable with the idea of animal research, 'I can accept animal research, but that doesn't mean that I like it', was the prevailing view.

Although for many years, researchers and research institutions have sometimes faced invidious campaigning by those opposed to the use of animals in research, since 2010, animal research extremism and unlawful activity have declined dramatically [5]. Animal research opponents currently prefer to use a successful potpourri of lawful campaigning methods that include political lobbying, public relations campaigns, social media activity, and also non-violent demonstrations and reputational challenges. Significant political challenges and lobbying have come through motions in the European Parliament in 2021 [6], and the European Citizens' Initiative (ECI) *Save Cruelty Free Cosmetics*, in 2023 [7].

Added to this, the reluctance of the European scientific community to openly make the case for animal research to the public has exacerbated an already difficult situation. Institutional websites are one of the places the public is most likely to look for answers and where explanatory information should logically be kept. However, in the most recent series of studies on the website content of close to 1000 biomedical institutions in the European Union [2], under half were assessed as having a clearly recognisable public-facing statement acknowledging their use of animals, with some of the larger countries, such as France and Italy, with under a third of their biomedical institutions with this basic information for the public.

The general lack of proactive communications from research institutions has meant the general public and patients find it hard to find website content, or any other materials, that support animal research. The study of EU-based websites also found an absence of statistics on animal use, images/videos of research animals or animal facilities, or case studies to highlight how animals were used in research studies. Even when the content exists on an institutional website there is often no easy way to find it either through searches or navigation from a website homepage.

To counter the threat of these campaigns, many in the scientific community, alongside EARA, are increasingly committed to speaking openly about the use of animals for scientific purposes 8]. The belief is that by providing regular, fact-based, proactive communications there will be an improvement in an institution's reputation and provide it with the opportunity to promote its work and engage in a public dialogue.

Now, more than ever, is the time for institutions to develop a more proactive and open approach to their communications on animal research. There are many good stories and examples, outlined in this chapter, that show how the scientific community has moved from an essentially passive and heads-down approach to public engagement, to a more proactive one thanks to proactive communications. Animal care professionals have a significant part to play in this approach.

20.2 Why Should Institutions Adopt a Proactive Approach to Communications on the Use of Animals in Scientific Research?

The need to foster open and transparent communication with the general public, about the benefits to society of using animals in biomedical research, has been one of the life sciences' key priorities over the last decade. Public perceptions and ethical concerns [9] about the use of animals have often clouded the significance of their contribution and fostered a conservative approach to engaging with the public by research institutions.

Instead of being forced to react to anti-animal research campaigns, a proactive communications strategy, involving key staff, allows an institution to develop well thought out communications about animal research at its own pace. Openness about animal research gives organisations an advantage over those opposed to animal research, as well as showing the public that they are willing to engage openly on the topic [10].

In fact, the European Commission has for some time encouraged a public mandate for openness and transparency. In its response to the previous ECI *Stop Vivisection* in 2015 [11], the Commission made a direct call for the scientific community to proactively engage in the dialogue on animal research and developments in this area [12] and this is also enshrined in the EU Directive 2010/63 on the use of animals for scientific purposes [13].

With cultural change on openness growing across Europe and networks spreading no institution needs feel isolated in publicly communicating about the role of animals in research. Initiatives, such as the eight Transparency Agreements on Animal Research [14] (in Belgium, France, Germany, Netherlands, Portugal, Spain, Switzerland, and the UK), have more than 500 signatory institutions [15]—there are also agreements in Australia and New Zealand. Each signatory institution commits to transparency regarding its animal research and pledges to uphold its commitment to be transparent about communication on the when, how, and why animals are used in research, ensuring comprehensive disclosure to both the media and the public regarding research conditions, and outcomes. The signatories also actively engage in initiatives fostering broader societal awareness of animal research, whilst committing to an annual progress report to share their experiences.

Social media campaigns such as *Be Open About Animal Research Day* (#BOARD) [16] and *Biomedical Research Awareness Day* (BRAD) [17] have shown that proactive communication both helps remove the air of secrecy that surrounds animal research and fosters a balanced public dialogue. BOARD and BRAD are both annual events, that take place in person and on social media, that give animal care staff, vets, researchers, and communicators a platform to speak publicly about their work with animals and to give inspiration to others in the biomedical community to do likewise.

20.3 How Should Research Institutions Develop a Proactive Approach to Communicating Their Use of Animals in Scientific Research?

The aim of any animal research communications strategy is to generate long-term support for the fundamental role of animal models in scientific research and their benefits to society and hopefully to minimise the effectiveness of any shock tactics used by activists. Ultimately, it means engaging with the public and media. You are likely to need a higher level of internal support and reassurance within your organisation to embark on this kind of proactive communication activity, as working with the media will undoubtedly raise your profile.

Here, we provide a step-by-step guide for any institution to put in place a robust communications strategy for the use of animals for scientific purposes. Adopting these measures will inevitably require cultural change as part of a long-term communications strategy. First, the focus should be on internal communications.

20.4 Why Are Internal Communications on Animal Research Important as the First Step in External Communications?

Before you can begin working on any proactive communications strategy, a vital first step is to obtain internal support for openness on animal research. However, achieving institutional openness on animal research can be a slow process and is also about building trust between the communicators and the different staff groups, including animal care professionals.

Why do you need to focus on internal communications?

- It will raise awareness of your animal research communications strategy across your institution and gain top-level approval of communication messages.
- A carefully planned internal communications strategy can build the support and confidence of scientific and management staff. It can also boost the morale of those involved in research, especially those in animal facilities, as they begin to understand how being open is better than remaining secretive. It will also help address the concerns of staff members who are not directly involved in the animal research at your institution.
- It can also help keep staff and other stakeholders up-to-date with developments regarding animal research, openness, and any counter-activity from opponents of animal research.

20.5 What Internal Structures Are Needed for an Effective Communications Strategy?

It is essential to involve the entire institution in your communications strategy, and not restrict it solely to the department(s) dealing with biomedical research. This will ensure a more consistent approach is followed in the event of adverse publicity about your institution, or should your organisation be the focus of a reputational campaign led by activists?

To gain commitment for a new institutional communication strategy, the proposals will need to be approved by the most senior management team of your research institution. Setting up an Animal Research Expert Committee will be key to develop and coordinate the communications strategy concerning the use of animals. Ideally, this committee will have a broad reach involving key animal care professionals.

The committee should include the animal facility manager, one or more senior researchers, representatives from the communications department, the head of biomedical services, the central administration, the Establishment Licence Holder/Responsible Person, a senior veterinarian if not already included in the representatives mentioned here and possibly, a representative of the institution's animal research ethics committee.

The Expert Committee should meet and assess the institute's current stand on communicating its use of animals in scientific research and where the institute wants to be in 1 year from now in terms of progress. The Committee should then outline the steps it intends to take over the next 12 months to meet that target.

The Committee should meet at regular intervals to discuss progress on its communications plan. Communication channels within the

Committee should be actively maintained to update its members on developments, actions, and issues of interest including media coverage and events. Leading members of the Expert Committee should be fully aware of the crisis response plan and there should be at least two spokespeople identified—media training for the spokespeople would also be extremely valuable. Media training sources are available from some advocacy organisations [18], and can be used to train specific categories of personnel. For example, the European Society of Laboratory Animals (ESLAV) provided media training to its members [19].

20.6 How Do You Improve Understanding of the Use of Animals in Research Within Your Institution?

Beyond your organisation's internal decision makers, a large proportion of the people working or studying at your institution will not be directly involved with any animal research. Making them aware of the animal research and welfare standards, the legislation that regulates animal procedures and projects in which animal research plays a part will help staff and students understand the context and need for animal research at your institution.

Make sure that members of staff, who feel nervous about proactive communication, have an opportunity to voice their concerns. Attempts to engage on the issue of animal research can often generate resistance in different sections of an institution. This also reflects on the issues related to the culture of care [20] within an institution, which places good communication to the fore and where members of staff that have any concerns regarding the use or care of animals should be encouraged to raise the matter.

Using existing channels of communication is a good way to start discussing animal research at your institution. Seek to place articles in the institute newsletter, the annual report or, in case of academic institutions, in the alumni blog. It is not necessary to focus solely on animal experimentation—mentioning the use of animals in your regular communications about the research work at your institution is also extremely useful. The role of animal care professionals in animal welfare is an obvious starting point for any such article.

Animal care professionals and scientists are proud of their work and their efforts to improve animal welfare, advance scientific knowledge, and search for effective drugs and treatments. Institutions should therefore encourage them to give talks to researchers, students, other staff, and alumni groups, or at established lecture series, open days, summer schools, or local community forums to showcase how and why animals are used in research and what the benefits will be and also help address any concerns before your institution embarks on a wider proactive communications strategy.

One illustrative example of this comes from the body responsible for animal welfare (ORBEA) of the faculty of sciences at the University of Lisbon, who welcomed high school students and showed them around the animal facilities. The visit was filmed which then had the added benefit of highlighting the university's efforts towards open communication to a wider audience [21].

There may also be public engagement opportunities with other stakeholders, or public bodies to which an institution already has contacts, such as local schools, or residents' associations, or at suitable venues such as patient forums or other community groups [22]. In addition, you could encourage staff to spend a day or more with your communications team to understand the work that they do and likewise for the communications staff to become familiar with the work of facilities and lab staff and researchers. In addition, most life sciences students will understand the value of animal research and they may be willing to participate in student debates and roundtables to explain why they stand on the side of animal research. Workshop courses, on communication in animal research, can be a useful way to inform and encourage greater participation by students [23].

20.7 What Are the Key Steps That Lead to Improved Internal Communications?

Before any communication strategy can be implemented there needs to be a period of discussion with facility managers/directors about how they can help the communication department. A strong partnership at management level and continuous assessment of the progress being made is an important part of the process. An efficient internal communications strategy should follow these steps:

1. Select an institutional contact person for animal research issues. This person should preferably be a member of your Animal Research Expert Committee.
2. Front-line staff at your institution cannot be expected to have all the answers at their fingertips, but they should know where to go for information and what the policies are. It is good practice to have prepared information ready in order to respond to common enquiries.
3. Inform all staff—not just those who work in biological sciences, but employees across the entire organisation—about the animal research carried out at your institution. This should include developing materials that explain in non-technical terms the work of animal staff, how there is continuous progress in improving animal welfare and the principles of the 3Rs, with practical examples of how these are being implemented.
4. Make sure that everyone involved in developing or implementing the communications strategy has visited an animal lab and understands the rationale for animal research. Staff lab visits can also be good practice in preparation for visits by the media etc. Key animal care professionals should be part of those hosting these visits.
5. Give support staff in biomedical services (receptionists, secretaries) training or information so they know how to deal with enquiries on animal research. Enquiries to the central secretariat should be forwarded to the biomedical services administrative department or your institution's approved communications contact.
6. Remind all departments that use animals for research to regularly update any news (a new project licence, any unexpected event, any media mention) or developments to the Animal Research Expert Committee. By doing so, you can make any necessary preparations for publicity surrounding new investments or research programmes, new buildings, changes in experimental procedures, new project licence applications, or high-profile appointments or announcements.
7. Identify an institutional point of contact, preferably a security, or facilities management representative, to liaise with your local police force should a problem arise. Ensure that this person keeps the police up to date with any activity from opponents to animal research, no matter how insignificant it might seem. A deputy should be appointed and should be kept aware of the latest issues for when the designated police liaison officer is out of office.
8. Set some targets. Decide what progress on communications you would like your institution to have made in 6 months and in a year's time.

20.8 What Are the Steps Needed to Develop an External Communications Strategy for the Use of Animals in Scientific Research?

20.8.1 Identify External Target Audiences

Without a clear understanding of the different audiences that you want to influence and inform, your institution will not be able to design an effective strategy to target them. Different target groups engage through different communications channels and your institution will inevitably require different methods and different key messages in order to engage with them. Generally, speaking, these target audiences can be categorised as:

1. Local community
2. Media/opinion formers
3. Professional bodies
4. Legislators and regulators
5. Activist group opponents

Local Community Local stakeholders are potentially a receptive audience who will be interested to learn about the research at your institution and the role of animal studies within that research. If your institution is a major employer in the area those in the local community could know employees personally and may have concerns, but are likely to give a fair hearing to the institution on animal research issues. Local people could also be an important ally if your institution is targeted by protesters and may be willing to make a public case for animal research themselves.

The goal of local community engagement is not aggressive propaganda, but rather regular, low-key reminders of the institution's activities, especially when they benefit the community (for instance, a bioscience spin-off that will boost employment and bring revenue to a community). This 'drip-drip' feed of information serves to keep your institution on the community's radar, and allows you to influence at least some of the information the community receives about your institution. Consider outreach work such as leaflets, open days, and public presentations.

Engaging with schools is especially important since teachers across Europe are inundated with materials from groups opposed to animal research. Even when they want to address the issue, they might not have adequate information that supports their views on the use of animals in medical and scientific research. Persuade your institute staff to talk at local schools. Animal care professionals and animal technicians often give a very positive impression to school children because they can talk about how they care for the animals themselves. Use existing forums like institutional open days, science fairs or schools' road shows to communicate with local school students [21].

Opinion Formers These are defined as people who can shape the perception of animal research and your institution's reputation, such as journalists and local influencers. Making opinion formers aware of the important role of animals in biomedical research will help make the case for animal research in both the public and political spheres.

Opinion formers often need to very quickly gain an understanding of the main facts, figures, and issues about a controversial issue, such as animal research, so offer to meet them face-to-face for a briefing. For instance, highlight the relevance of animal research at your institution, and the guidelines regulating animal research and welfare in Europe, your country, and your institution.

Professional Bodies There is strength in numbers, so professional associations, research funders, industry partners, and other research institutes are some of the professional bodies that can offer support and guidance. It is useful to make them aware of the research that you conduct and to build contacts within them. If your institution then comes under pressure, the way that you handle any crisis can help build your institution's reputation and the perception of its competence. It is also useful to discuss with colleagues in other institutions any openness methods they have used and found successful, or unsuccessful.

Legislators and Regulators Politicians, including those at the local, regional and national level will also be important audiences to influence and inform about the benefits of using animals in biomedical research. Local politicians could be particularly useful supporters if the institution comes under criticism, as it is possible the media might look to them for comment. Provide their offices with the sort of general information provided to the public and offer invitations to tour your research facilities and meet with senior staff. If possible, relationships should be built with regulators as well.

An example of this was the visit of a prominent French MP, who had chaired hearings on animal research and alternatives, to the University of Strasbourg, in conjunction with CNRS, Inserm, and Gircor, the French advocacy organisation. He heard presentations on animal research, spoke with scientists, and visited the animal facilities. Similarly, a German MEP was invited on a fact-finding visit to the Centre for Stroke and Dementia Research at the Ludwig Maximilian University of Munich. Over a 3-h visit, she met with researchers and technicians, delving into discussions about strokes, Alzheimer's disease, the role of animal research, and a tour of the animal facilities [24, 25].

Opponents Engaging with local groups that are critical of different aspects of animal research can be constructive even if minds are not changed on either side. When first engaging with these organisations, try to find out whether they are open-minded and prepared to enter the constructive discussion. If they ask you to provide a speaker for a debate about animal experimentation, we suggest you do so—provided they have received sufficient training for such an event. This will avoid being perceived as trying to hide your use of animals, which can be met with disdain even by supportive groups. You should also ask if a speaker from a national pro-research organisation can also attend, as they are likely to have a good overview of the debate.

20.9 How Do You Develop Your Key External Communication Messages?

After identifying your communications goals and target audiences you can begin developing your key messages to help achieve these. It is important to keep the messages simple and to the point. The tone of this messaging should be that your institution is willing to engage in open discussion on the issue of animal research.

- It is helpful to prepare a Frequently Asked Questions (FAQ) document or factsheets (see the section on website communication) addressing major concerns, so that you can supply opinion formers with a handy overview in case of time-pressured requests. Animal care professionals have a keen role to play in ensuring that these messages include evidence of animal welfare regulations.

Information packs tailored to different audiences can be distributed to prospective students or employees, decision makers, journalists, or funders. Multinational pharmaceutical company, Sanofi, has produced a factsheet for all its staff and available on its website, which sets out its commitments to high standards of animal protection and welfare, its progress towards replacement of animals and the other 3R principles, all within the context of the continuing importance of animal use for biomedical studies [26].

The messages should be at the forefront of any document or statement that is produced by your institution. The themes of your messaging are likely to include, the high standards of animal welfare and the strict regulation at both national and EU levels and reference to the medical and research breakthroughs which have involved animal research. The principles of replacement, refinement, and reduction (the 3Rs) guide research in the EU. This means that every effort is made to improve animal welfare, minimise the use of animals and adopt alternative methods.

Emphasise the ethical dimension of animal research, that it is done when there is no alternative and with animal welfare at the forefront. You might include quotes from your institution's animal care professionals or animal technicians about how they maintain a culture of care and how they promote good animal welfare standards. A good example of this comes from the Lyon Neuroscience Research Center, France, which has a website interview with the designated veterinarian, describing her career and her responsibilities [27].

The key messages need specific supporting facts and figures, examples, anecdotes, pictures, film etc. Photographs of good-quality housing for the animals look particularly impressive (see the section on website communication). This is important because the media tends to run with pictures from activist NGOs, even in balanced stories, due to a lack of pictures/footage of contemporary facilities. Be aware that key facts and statistics can take some time to collect, verify, and sign off and will always need to be dated.

20.10 What Approach Should Be Taken to Develop an External Communications Plan and What Resources Are Needed?

1. Mention the species of animal used in research when publicising biomedical breakthroughs and advances in press releases and information packs. The animals that are used are rarely the main story, but if one has been used, mention it.
2. Ensure that all the documents you produce include a short version of your institutes' animal research statement with a link back to the full document.
3. Banners and leaflets at public engagement events and open days are a good way of reaching out to the local community. The informal atmosphere and direct contact between the audience and researchers are an opportunity to discuss animal research within its larger scientific and societal context.
4. Infographics are a visually interesting tool to present a quick overview of complex information. Depending on the topic, this type of graphic is particularly suitable for use in schools, in briefings for politicians, and for use on social media. EARA has produced a series of features that explain why different species of animals are used in biomedical research and has used infographics and videos to illustrate various points [28].
5. When justifying the use of animals in your research, it is better to put forward the benefits of animal research rather than counter the arguments used by the opponents of animal research.
6. Explain some of your institution's research and why it is carried out (see the section below on website communication). Put this into context by also mentioning some of your non-animal work, or the work to replace or reduce the use of animals at the institution. Openness means acknowledging that research means harm to animals as well as benefits to humans (and animals). Showing the steps taken to reduce these harms will show the care taken by your staff and help reinforce the message that, by law, animals are only used where there are no other options. Hearing directly from researchers about how and why they use animals in their research can give the public insights into why animal research is necessary. It is important to be as open as possible and the institution's position statement can be used as the basis for a response.

A good example of public outreach was given by staff from the Institute of Biomedicine Seville, in Spain, and the Gulbenkian Institute of Science and the Institute of Molecular Medicine, in Portugal, who took part in the annual European Researchers Night. This showcased the impact of researchers' work on people's daily lives and inspired the interest of young people in science and research careers [29]. Consider publishing an annual report or executive summary about animal research at your institution—Imperial College London produces an annual report on animal research, which contains numerous pictures of animals in research settings and shows how biomedical studies using animals are an important part of their institution's groundbreaking work [30]. An annual review could include the yearly figures provided to regulatory authorities, a number of case studies of the research at your institution that involves animals, 3Rs initiatives, or other relevant information that might avoid time-consuming Freedom of Information requests. The best statistical information will include a breakdown of the number of animals by species and the purpose of the research.

20.11 What Plans Should Be Made for Organised Animal Facility Visits?

Inviting small groups (politicians, journalists, school pupils, or staff who do not work directly with animals) into an animal research facility allows you to engage directly with target groups and is the most direct way of putting openness into practice. A laboratory tour allows visitors to meet animal technicians and directly experience the welfare standards at your institution. A laboratory tour does not guarantee that the visitors leave your facility being entirely supportive of animal research, but it does allow for a more informed debate in future.

- Be sure to notify anyone in advance who will be present in the facilities at the time of the tour. Some staff might wish to avoid being in an animal house if certain visitors are being shown around.
- Make sure that staff have given their consent if photographs are going to be taken.
- Ensure that there are no notices, or signs that might provoke questions that the institution does not want to discuss.
- If you want to show biosecurity/biosafety environments, consider installing cameras in the room that link to monitors outside.
- Consider inviting the media to visit following any major redevelopment or expansion of your research facilities. Anticipate any questions that a journalist might ask and prepare them in writing as well in more detail. If you are asked a question you were not prepared for, just tell the journalist that you will reply as soon as possible by email. There is no guarantee that a news report is without criticism, but any responsible reporting will include your key messages about the work you conduct.
- To reach a larger audience remotely, one way is to create a virtual lab tour via a web link. These are interactive tours where the visitor can click to enter different parts of the facility, with information points available to give additional information. This sort of demonstration of openness is usually much appreciated by the media and the public, and ends some of the mystery about what goes on at laboratories [31, 32].

20.12 What Role Can an Institute's Website Play in Improving Communications and Public Understanding?

Most European countries, and also the USA, have some form of freedom of information (FOI) legislation. This allows members of the general public to request information held by their government; in many cases, this type of legislation also applies to publicly funded bodies, including research institutions. Groups opposed to animal research sometimes make use of FOI legislation to request data on animal use at public research institutions. If your institution has an FOI officer, make sure you consult them before acting on the request. A good way to prevent these time-consuming FOI requests is therefore to ensure that the information is already available to the public.

Developing effective web pages and a social media plan are key elements for any research institution. Your institution's website is likely to be the first point of contact with many of your key audiences and it is essential that it contains an easily accessible and prominent section on animal research. The best animal research webpages should include the following sections:

- A recognisable public-facing statement on the use of animals.
- Statistics on animal research and the species used at your institution.
- Case studies that highlight the role of animal studies.
- Images and videos of research animals and animal facilities.
- Frequently Asked Questions (FAQs), or other additional information on the 3Rs and alternative non-animal methods, and/or external links to further information.

Position Statement Providing a statement on your website shows that you are open about animal research. It lets the public and your supporters know why you support such research. It is also an opportunity to explain the high standards of animal welfare that this research must meet.

This should be a collaborative process, between the communication department and the senior management staff. There are numerous examples of good statements available, either from your national Transparency Agreement, or from national advocacy organisations, or EARA. Once these have been assessed and a template agreed, we would recommend the first draft is written by the designated vet, facility manager, or director, ready for circulation and comment.

Aim to make your statement the first piece of information available for anyone interested in looking for information about animal research at your institution. A statement can pre-empt questions from the public or media; provide the basis for replying to news stories; reassure its audiences about the importance of animal research; and show researchers that the institution is proud of the important work it does.

More detailed information on animal welfare, housing, and environment can help get across your institution's commitment to the refinement of animal research and the minimising of animal suffering. However, the statement needs to be non-technical and easy to understand for a general reader. It does not need to go into the details of compliance with various national or international regulations on animal welfare or staff training, which can be mentioned in other sections of the website content. You should be prepared to update any facts or statistics used in the statement each year. Here are some elements of a good position statement:

- Explain why animal research is necessary and its benefits [33–35].
- Animal research has been key to medical progress.
- Research into debilitating diseases still involves animal studies.
- In certain aspects of fundamental and applied research, animal studies play a vital role.
- Explain, in overview, that the use of animals in research is only allowed when the potential benefits outweigh the expected harm and provide links to the laws and regulations that govern animal research in the EU, such as Directive 2010/63/EU on the protection of animals used for scientific purposes, whilst staff, laboratories, and animal housing have to adhere to strict criteria.
- Animals can only be used for a limited number of research purposes.
- Animal testing of cosmetics is no longer permitted in the EU.

Animal Use Statistics Publishing annual animal research statistics on your website will give an accurate overview of the species and numbers of animals used at your institution [36, 37]. It shows that you have a clear intention to be open and transparent and can pre-empt opponents of animal research from targeting your institution with time-consuming Freedom of Information requests. Good statistical information will include a breakdown of the number of animals by species and research purpose. Further information giving the details on why different species are used is also a clear demonstration of openness [38, 39].

Case Studies In a case study, you can make the narrative about animal research at your institution more tangible, and place it into context. It should contain the sort of content that you would be pleased to see featured in a newspaper article. A case study can explain how and why animals were used in a piece of research and connect the research back to the larger scientific, clinical, or societal impact. This should include case studies about innovation and progress in the 3Rs principles and the development of viable alternative non-animal methods, as well as examples of good animal welfare practices within animal studies.

- Consider case studies on animal research used to study diseases and also research to advance fundamental knowledge, as these are two separate aspects of animal testing.

- If you are looking at fundamental research, it may still be useful to mention any future disease research which could benefit from this research.
- Include the impact of any disease being studied, such as the symptoms and number of people affected.
- Include why animals were necessary to investigate the scientific questions being addressed. Why was the specific species involved chosen?
- Address any specific steps taken by the researchers to reduce animal use or alleviate possible suffering.
- Include information about the ethical review the research underwent before it could go ahead and how it is regulated.
- For the most impact see if you can, work with charities or other patient groups to provide a patient perspective and how the treatments developed, thanks to animal research, have helped them personally.

Images and Video These are a powerful way of providing an accurate representation of the research environment at your institution. A handful of pictures, or a short video [38–40], including an interview with researchers, can do more to dispel many common misconceptions about the conditions and treatment of animals in laboratories than a paragraph of text. Images might be of enclosures, animals, or procedures.

Remember that most members of the public are unfamiliar with lab equipment, so a short caption would be useful, for instance, stating that individually ventilated cages can protect animals from external diseases. It is useful to allow the easy reuse of your image, such as by creating an image library, as it increases the chances they will be used instead of another image found by a journalist on the internet (many of these are not representative of modern animal research) [40–42].

FAQs and Additional Information FAQs can help directly address some of the more common questions you are asked both by journalists and the public. These answers can also be helpful for dealing with questions that come through social media. It is better not to use negative phrasing (e.g. 'we don't conduct research on primates'). It can be seen as an implied criticism of those institutions that conduct certain types of research and could cause problems if your areas of research change in the future [43, 44].

The 3Rs are pretty much unknown outside of the scientific community, so use your website to explain what they mean. This also presents an opportunity for staff to demonstrate their commitment, through a culture of care, to the proactive implementation of good experimental design, good care, and the 3Rs. You could reference some or all of the following [45, 46]:

- High animal welfare and a culture of care supports good science.
- The 3Rs are guiding principles in animal research.
- How are the 3Rs applied in practice?
- The EU Directive enshrines the 3Rs into EU law, and has been implemented into national law.

20.13 Should Social Media Be Used as Part of Our Communications Strategy?

Social media is an important way to engage directly with those who are interested in your institution and the research that it carries out without the filter of the media. The public may also ask questions about your institution's research through your social media platforms. The most likely platforms for this interaction are X formerly known as Twitter, LinkedIn, and Facebook [16, 47, 48]. Consider scheduling recurring posts, such as those about the benefits of animal research to society, and include links to your institution's animal research webpages.

Presenting what happens inside an animal facility, or explaining the work of animal technicians can be a powerful way to present an open and understandable message about the use of animals in research. The Netherlands Cancer Institute has produced a video detailing its work, with staff speaking plainly and directly to the public in a very engaging way [49]. Of course, not everyone is comfortable talking to the camera and anything produced for social media should be developed in conjunction with the communications department.

20.14 How Should You Respond to Comments Made on Social Media?

Questions and comments on social media can come in a great many forms. It is useful to outline a strategy to help you decide when and how to answer questions, and when wider action is required to deal with the questions. Answer questions about the animal research at your institution in a brief and polite manner. Your key messages will help answer social media questions and comments quickly and consistently. Space is limited on social media so include helpful links to your own web resources (or via hashtags # on X) or those of other bodies where relevant, to refer to more detailed information. Providing an email address for people to contact you directly can be effective in moving the discussion offline.

Avoid getting stuck in lengthy conversations. When answering people's questions, you are not trying to convince them of the value of animal research. The aim of your institution's social media engagement is to set out your institution's official position and the reasons for supporting animal research, so the user can make up their own mind.

In the case of abusive comments, it is often unhelpful to engage with the content of the comment itself. You can choose to reply with a standard sentence referring to your web statement or to ignore this type of reaction. However, in the interest of an open and balanced debate, we would advise not to delete negative comments unless they clearly break community guidelines or if they are part of a large-scale campaign clogging up your page—you are also likely to find that supportive users will stick up for your institution. Deleting or blocking comments can be seen as censorship, but is sometimes necessary when they are abusive or are personal attacks on those involved in animal research at your institution. If there are clear threats or incitement in a comment then you should immediately report it to your institution's security staff and the police.

20.15 How Should You Prepare for a Crisis Communications Situation?

As we have outlined committing your institution to a proactive communications strategy will mean preparing materials and messages in advance and ensuring that there is a good understanding of the arguments in favour of animal research amongst senior management and those research staff involved on a day-to-day basis with animals. However, often the first time your systems will be truly tested is when your institution has to respond to media enquiries, possibly following allegations made by animal research opponents. These are the likely crisis scenarios that you may have to deal with and which may be of interest to the media:

- Animal activist groups publicising the fact that animal research is taking place at your institution with statistics on the number and/or species used. This information may have been acquired through a Freedom of Information request or by scouring published scientific papers.
- A protest outside your facilities, organised by an activist group. These may start in response to details of specific studies, the planned open-

ing of a new or expanded research facility, or national or international 'days of action' by animal activists.
- Undercover infiltration of your facilities by one or more individuals—often by someone working as a technician for many months previously—which might include photos and video footage. These are less likely, but are something to be aware of.
- Spill over protests from demonstrations against other targets, such as commercial companies which your institution may have commercial links with.
- Articles or letters published in newspapers, magazines, and websites where private or public institutions are named and criticised for their research using animals.
- Online petitions or high-volume phone/mail campaigns that target individuals at an institution, criticising animal research.

The aim of these techniques is probably to make an emotive attack on your institution for conducting 'cruel' or 'unnecessary' research, or citing evidence of mistreatment, either maliciously or based on misunderstandings about the nature of the experiments. Without a crisis plan, there is a danger that your institution will fail to deal effectively at an early stage with the allegations leading to damaging articles in the press before a counter-argument has been made.

The basic rules of preparation for crisis communications are:

- React appropriately and recognise the level of risk to the reputation of the institution—not all attacks require the full mobilisation of your communications resources—you do not want to highlight a story or event that has little credibility or media impact.
- Ensure that internal staff are ready to react at short notice, both through media training and by maintaining out-of-hours contact details. It is better to keep your response team as small as possible. Set up a WhatsApp group, to include the most important internal contacts, for use during a crisis.
- Contact your networks and institutions that have experienced similar situations and certainly ask for advice from professionals (e.g., from EARA) in a crisis.

20.16 What Actions Should Be Taken to Handle Protesters Outside Animal Facilities?

Whilst a couple of tweets probably do not suggest the beginning of a campaign, a new Facebook page aimed at criticising/stopping an institution's animal research could well be. Similarly, a student group requesting information about your institution's research is better seen as an opportunity to engage with the student population, than as a campaign that needs to be contained. If such a group emerges it can be a good opportunity to engage with them—for instance, through laboratory visits or a talk from a scientist or animal welfare technician.

If your institution is targeted a brief should be sent, as soon as possible, to senior management. As they may not be familiar with any animal activist groups involved or their tactics, providing some of the guidance contained in this document may be helpful. Animal rights extremism is at a historical low, but many senior managers remember a time when extremism was a more present risk.

Activists have a democratic right to protest. Such protests are almost always entirely peaceful and within the law. If you hear of an upcoming protest, your institution's security staff should be able to advise on any security implications. The protest limitations should be provided in writing to the protesters, and a message should be sent to staff asking them not to engage with any protesters, reminding them that both police and activists may be filming.

As protesters are likely to have tipped off local journalists (or student journalists at a university), a prepared statement can be helpful in case of any media interest. The statement should note the importance of the research that the institution carries out, and how it fulfils its commitment to ethical practice, animal welfare, and the 3Rs. If the protest is about a new facility make sure to explain what diseases the research will be trying to find treatments for. The box below shows a real-life scenario of a response to a crisis situation.

Response by the Max Delbrück Center, Berlin (MDC) to a Protest Outside Their Facility

MDC was the target of a campaign Ärzte gegen Tierversuche (ÄgTV; 'physicians against animal experimentation') when one of its scientists was awarded the so-called 'Heart of Stone' for the 'worst animal experiment 2017' The research they targeted was a study of naked mole rats which sought to protect the heart and brain of human patients after infarction and stroke, by studying how these animals survive in oxygen-starved conditions.

The activists announced that they would present this prize together with supporters and media representatives on the MDC campus. MDC decided to welcome these visitors to the campus and show that the centre was willing to enter into a fact-based discussion and that it stood behind its scientists. An email was sent out to all staff explaining what was happening by Martin Lohse, CEO of MDC and asking them to show solidarity with the targeted colleague and meet with the protesters. Staff were also asked to point out any unusual activity to reception or security.

Mr Lohse said: 'We accept manifestations against our views and our opinions, and we are willing to enter into a dialogue. Our key messages are: We stand up for our researchers and we and our institution are not willing to accept this generalising denunciation. We do not have a heart of stone and we are willing to discuss with members of ÄgTV and to listen to their criticism. But we demand a respectful discourse'.

A small group of activist protesters was then met by 120 MDC staff with leaflets stating 'Let us talk', and asking the activists to discuss the issues in a proper dialogue.

A robust justification of the research and the benefits of animal research was put on the MDC website, which also included the centre's commitment to the 3Rs. Other links included a Q&A about the research and why it was done and write-up on the study and fuller details on why research is conducted at MDC.

https://www.mdc-berlin.de/de/news/press/kein-herz-aus-stein

20.17 What Actions Should Be Taken If There Has Been Undercover Filling at an Animal Facility?

Animal activist groups have set aside large amounts of money for 'investigations', and over the last few years there have been a number of high-profile infiltrations of labs. Developing a process for communicating with the media—and for supporting staff in the event of allegations being made—can significantly reduce the negative impacts of an infiltration.

The best defence against an infiltration is to be as open as possible. Invite journalists in to see your laboratories, preferably before any story goes to print. Contact the affected scientists to get first-hand information on the aims, potential benefits and welfare considerations of the research, and relay this information to the journalist.

You should also immediately contact organisations such as your national advocacy organisation, or EARA, and/or your national lab animal science association (if existing) for additional support. You will also need to go through the specific allegations made by the activists one by one to establish the facts. This will form the basis of any response then put forward by your institution. Be aware that an infiltration can have a profound effect on staff wellbeing and trust. Try to keep your staff updated with the latest information.

Response by the Vrije Universiteit Brussel (VUB), Belgium to Secret Filming in Their Institution

In November 2016, animal activists GAIA published a hidden camera video of the housing and euthanising of research animals at VUB, accusing it of animal suffering and breaches of the law. Two days later, in one reaction to the news, students and staff were evacuated from the VUB campuses following bomb threats. The university also temporarily suspended all its animal testing following a request of state secretary Bianca Debaets, Brussels State Secretary.

VUB immediately launched an internal investigation, to verify whether the documented situations and actions were in line with the legislation and its ethical guidelines, and to see how and where existing internal procedures on animal welfare could be tightened. As a result the university then took measures in the fields of animal wellbeing, administration, infrastructure, and scientific research. New structural controls were put in place allowing outsiders to audit and oversee the laboratories and an academic lead was appointed to co-ordinate the working of the testing facilities, in close collaboration with the Ethical Commission Animal Testing and the Animal Welfare Body. The entire upgrade of the 40-year-old facilities cost around 100,000 euros.

These measures meant that VUB and Ms. Debaets reached an agreement on the resumption of animal testing. Now every 2 months VUB reports to the state secretary on the proceedings at the animal testing unit, under the supervision of an inspector-veterinarian. In the future, VUB wants to commit even more too animal wellbeing. In the investment plan of the university 13.8 m euros was been earmarked for a new animal testing unit. The new animal testing facility will meet international criteria for animal wellbeing. Construction should be finished by 2018–2019. 'With those changes, we explicitly aim to push the boundaries of housing and general care of lab animals', added vice rector for research policy, Karin Vanderkerken.

20.18 What Actions Should Be Taken If There Is a Petition or Campaign Against Animal Research at an Institution?

The main frustration with an online petition [50] is that often it can send an email to a number of very busy staff members every time someone signs it. Since the wording of the emails is often identical, it may be advisable to set up an email rule to manage these emails. It is not necessary to reply to every email given the very low effort required to send them (many petition websites will not even check an email address is real before sending the email)—perhaps just those that have been personalised or from recognised opinion formers. It is important to alert (but not alarm) anyone who may be affected by these mass communications so they can take steps to minimise the disruption it may cause.

20.19 How Should Critical Articles About an Institution Be Handled?

In theory, if your institution has a policy of openness this should mean that there are no surprises in store from revelations about the number of animals used in research, or the types of research being conducted. Problems may arise if statistics have been revealed that have not been made publicly available previously as this may be seen as an example of the institution's secretiveness. Otherwise, any arguments put forward in the media articles should be refuted at the earliest opportunity.

20.20 Chapter Summary

20.20.1 What Are the Main Points for Developing a Long-Term Communications Strategy?

The aim of any animal research communications strategy is to generate long-term support, both from external audiences and those within your institution, for the fundamental role of animal models in scientific research.

- Before you can begin working on any proactive communications strategy, a vital first step is to obtain internal support for openness on animal research.
- Set some targets. Decide what progress on communications you would like your institution to have made in 6 months and in a year's time.
- It is essential to involve the entire organisation in your communications strategy, and not restrict it to the department(s) dealing with external audiences. Mention the use of animals in research as a normal part of your information about research at your institution.
- Setting up an Animal Research Expert Committee can be helpful as you design and co-ordinate the communications strategy. Ideally, this committee will have a broad reach and not be limited to researchers.
- Without a clear understanding of the different external audiences that you want to influence and inform your institution will not be able to design an effective strategy and the key messages with which to target them.
- Key messages will always need specific supporting facts and figures, examples, anecdotes, pictures, film etc.

20.20.2 What Are the Main Points for Developing Effective Web Pages and Social Media?

- The best animal research webpages will include a position statement; frequently asked questions; statistics on animal research at your institution; case studies; images and videos.
- The aim of your institution's social media engagement is to set out your institution's official position, rather than to win an argument on the pros and cons of animal research.
- Consider scheduling recurring posts, such as those about the benefits of animal research to society, and include links to your institution's animal research web pages.

20.20.3 What Are the Main Points for Handling Crisis Communications?

A good crisis plan is more likely to succeed if materials and messages have been prepared in advance and it is worth testing out your plan with a mock scenario.

- React appropriately and recognise the level of risk to the reputation of the institution of any particular adverse publicity [51].
- Be prepared and ensure that the relevant internal staff are aware of how to react at short notice.
- Have a preliminary statement ready and signed off. This will contain information on your institution, the type of research conducted the standards you adhere to, and the benefits of animal research.
- Conduct a debrief on the actions and responses of your institution once a crisis has passed. Build also on the relationships with the journalists who covered the story.

References

1. European Commission. Eurobarometer—science and technology. 2010. pp. 60–64. Available at: https://europa.eu/eurobarometer/surveys/detail/806.
2. EARA. EARA Study of EU-based websites. 2024. A new study of the websites of biomedical research bodies across the EU, by EARA, to assess how openly they discuss their research using animals, reveals that an increasing number of institutions are meeting this objective - in particular, institutions that are signatories of national Transparency Agreements on animal research. Available at: https://www.eara.eu/post/transparency-agreements-on-animal-research-set-the-benchmark-for-openness-earawebsite-study-2024
3. Intergroup for Animal Welfare. 2023. Available at: https://www.animalwelfareintergroup.eu.
4. Understanding Animal Research (UAR). Attitudes to animal research under Covid-19. 2020. Available at: https://www.understandinganimalresearch.org.uk/application/files/2016/5226/6731/attitudes_to_animal_research_under_covid-19_final.pdf.
5. Animal Rights Extremism. A global information service about animal rights extremism. Available at: http://www.animalrightsextremism.info.
6. European Parliament. MEPs demand EU action plan to end the use of animals in research and testing. 2021. Available at: https://www.europarl.europa.eu/news/en/press-room/20210910IPR11926/meps-demand-eu-action-plan-to-end-the-use-of-animals-in-research-and-testing?mc_cid=15a90a2c89&mc_eid=UNIQID.
7. European Citizens Initiative (ECI). Save cruelty free cosmetics—commit to a Europe without animal testing. 2023. Available at: https://citizens-initiative.europa.eu/save-cruelty-free-cosmetics-commit-europe-without-animal-testing_en#:~:text=The%20%27Save%20Cruelty%20Free%20Cosmetics,1%2C217%2C916verified%20statements%20of%20support.
8. UAR. UAR conference 2024. Openness in animal research: a conference to celebrate a decade of the concordat. Available at: https://www.understandinganimalresearch.org.uk/news/openness-in-animal-research-a-conference-to-celebrate-a-decade-of-the-concordat.
9. RSPCA Science Group. Welfare and severity assessment. 2023. Available at: https://science.rspca.org.uk/-/welfare-and-severity-assessment.
10. Current Biology. Dutch scientists highlight the need for animal research during Covid-19. 2020. Available at: https://www.sciencedirect.com/science/article/pii/S0960982220311842?via%3Dihub&mc_cid=5d59e09e3a&mc_eid=[UNIQID]#
11. European Citizens' Initiative (ECI). Stop vivisection. 2015. Available at: https://citizens-initiative.europa.eu/initiatives/details/2012/000007/stop-vivisection_en.
12. European Commission. Commission replies to 'stop vivisection' ECI. 2015. Available at: https://ec.europa.eu/commission/presscorner/detail/en/IP_15_5094
13. European Commission. Directive EU/2010/63. 2010. Available at: https://environment.ec.europa.eu/topics/chemicals/animals-science_en.
14. EARA. Transparency Agreements on Animal Research. Signatories agree to a series of commitments on openness and transparency about animal research. 2023. Available at: https://www.eara.eu/transparency-agreements.
15. EARA. 500 biomedical institutions in Europe have signed a National Transparency Agreement. 2023. Available at: https://www.eara.eu/post/500-biomedical-institutions-have-signed-a-national-transparency-agreement.
16. EARA. #BOARD24 - The fourth edition of Be Open About Animal Research Day (#BOARD24), EARA's global, 24-hour social media campaign, that celebrates examples of openness in animal research with the public, took place on 3 May, 2024. It had a record 220 partner institutions pledging their support from 48 countries across six continents (Europe, North America, South America, Oceania, Asia and Africa). 94 institutions produced materials for the campaign, which included statements, videos, events, infographics, articles and case studies. Available at: https://www.eara.eu/board24
17. Biomedical Research Awareness Day (BRAD). 2023. Available at: https://www.bradglobal.org.
18. EARA. EARA media training. EARA Media Training workshops equip researchers and communication professionals with essential tools to effectively communicate animal research, covering the significance of transparency, providing media communication tips, and offering crisis management advice, all focusing on enhancing public engagement. 2024. Available at: https://www.eara.eu/media-training. League of European Research Universities (LERU). Good practice in communicating animal research at universities. Developing an open and transparent approach to animal research within a university can help increase the awareness of the public about animal research. This short note provides a guide for universities how this could be achieved. It suggests how universities could improve their internal and external communications, gives several examples of good practice in developing webpages and gives links to European and national associations which can give further advice on this sensitive issue. 2021. Available at: https://www.leru.org/publications/good-practice-in-communicating-animal-research-at-universities
19. European Society of Laboratory Animal Veterinarians (ESLAV). Online media training for veterinarians. Media training designed to ensure veterinarians involved in animal research have the necessary tools to communicate the need for the use of

animals. 2023. Available at: https://www.eslav.org/online-media-training-for-veterinarians.
20. Manchester Hive—Manchester University Press. Culturing care in animal research. 2024. https://www.manchesterhive.com/display/9781526165770/9781526165770.00014.xml#9781526165770.00014
21. Faculty of Sciences of the University of Lisbon. Open day ORBEA. 2023. Available at: https://www.youtube.com/watch?v=OM8tXPUQGWg.
22. EARA. EARA Patient Discovery. EARA is currently leading a project called Patient Discovery, engaging patient associations and connecting patients and caretakers with researchers doing research relative to their disease, with adapted talks and visits to the laboratories and research facilities, including where animals are housed. Participants then volunteer for further media training so they can become advocates for the use of animals in biomedical research. 2023. Available at: https://www.eara.eu/post/eara-patient-discovery-project-launched.
23. LERU. Communication workshop for students. Researchers from LERU member universities took part in a science communication workshop on animal research, entitled From Emotion to Communication: What can we Learn?. The event was co-organised with the University of Heidelberg. 2022. Available at: https://www.leru.org/news/young-researchers-learn-to-better-communicate-about-animal-research
24. Gircor. French MP visits research center. Visit of a French MEP to the University of Strasbourg, in conjunction with CNRS, Inserm, and Gircor, which included animal facilities. 2022. Available at: https://www.gircor.fr/transparence-cedric-villani-visite-deux-animaleries-de-recherche-a-strasbourg/
25. EARA. German MEP laboratory animal fact-finding visit. Visit of a German MEP to the Ludwig Maximilian University of Munich (LMU), which included animal facilities. 2022. Available at: https://www.eara.eu/post/german-mep-laboratory-animal-fact-finding-visit.
26. Sanofi. Animal protection. 2022. Available at: https://www.sanofi.com/assets/dotcom/content-app/documents/Animal-Protection.pdf.
27. Lyon Neurosciences Research Centre. Commitment to animals and research—profile of designated veterinarian. 2023. Available at: https://www.crnl.fr/en/actualite/commitment-animals-and-research-profile?language=en.
28. EARA. Feature article: Why are animals used in brain research?. 2023. Available at: https://www.eara.eu/why-are-animals-used-in-brain-research.
29. Institute of Biomedicine Seville, in Spain, and the Gulbenkian Institute of Science and the Institute of Molecular Medicine in Portugal. Meeting the public at Researchers' Night. European Researchers Night in 2023 which showcased the impact of researchers' work on people's daily lives and inspire the interest of young people in science and research careers. 2023. Available at: https://www.eara.eu/post/meeting-the-public-at-researchers-night.
30. Imperial College London. Animal research report 2020–2021. 2022. Available at: https://www.imperial.ac.uk/media/imperial-college/research-and-innovation/public/animal-research/21_06_Annual-Report_Animal-Research_digital_SP_TP.pdf.
31. MRC Harwell Institute. 360° laboratory animal tours. 2023. Available at: https://labanimaltour.org/harwell.
32. University of Lübeck. 360° tour of the animal facility. 2023. Available at: https://vr-tour.gth.uni-luebeck.de/.
33. Max Planck Institute of Molecular Cell Biology and Genetics (MPI-CBG). Animal studies in basic research. 2023. Available at: https://www.mpi-cbg.de/research/animals-in-research/animal-research-in-basic-research.
34. Inotiv. Animal welfare statement. 2023. Available at: https://www.inotivco.com/animal-welfare-statement.
35. University of Zurich. Research involving animals and animal welfare. The statement leads to other links with further information. 2023. Available at: https://www.uzh.ch/cmsssl/en/researchinnovation/ethics/animals.html.
36. Merck. Animal research statement. The statement begins with a welfare statement, but includes other important information, including statistics on animal use. 2023. Available at: https://www.merckgroup.com/en/cr-report/2018/business-ethics/animal-welfare.html.
37. AstraZeneca. Animals in research. A comprehensive statement that includes statistics on animal use. 2023. Available at: https://www.astrazeneca.com/sustainability/ethics-and-transparency/animals-in-research.html.
38. Institute of Functional Genomics of Lyon (IGFL). Animal models. Further information on each species of animal used. 2023. Available at: https://igfl.ens-lyon.fr/offres-et-technologies/modeles-animaux.
39. German Rheumatism Research Centre Berlin (DRFZ). Animal experiments at the DRFZ. The statement also includes details on the severity of experiments. 2023. Available at: https://www.drfz.de/en/ueber-uns/tierversuche-am-drfz.
40. Charité Berlin. Charité 3R—Replace | Reduce | Refine. Images of animals and lab staff. 2023. Available at: https://charite3r.charite.de.
41. Novo Nordisk. Responsible use of animals. Numerous videos of animal housing for different species. 2023. Available at: https://www.novonordisk.com/science-and-technology/bioethics/animal-ethics.html.
42. Spanish Society of Science for Laboratory Animals (SECAL). Spanish researchers answer difficult questions—video. A video where scientists and caretakers answer frequently asked questions about animal research. 2021. Available at: https://secal.es/video-la-experimentacion-animal-da-vida/
43. Helmholtz Munich. Animal research. A statement that includes FAQs. 2023. Available at:

https://www.helmholtz-munich.de/en/about-us/understanding-animal-experiments-initative.
44. Biomedical Primate Research Centre. Questions & answers. Detailed answers to a range of questions. 2023. Available at: https://www.bprc.nl/en/questions-answers-bprc.
45. University of Antwerp. Wetgeving. Further example of a public-facing statement on animal research. 2023. Available at: https://www.uantwerpen.be/nl/projecten/dierproeven/wetgeving.
46. GSK. Use of animals. A very clearly set out statement on animal research with lots of detail on the 3Rs. 2023. Available at: https://www.gsk.com/en-gb/responsibility/ethical-standards/use-of-animals/.
47. EARA X/formerly Twitter. Social media on EU animal research annual statistics. Infographics produced by EARA to publicise the publication of the EU annual statistical report on animal use for scientific purposes. 2023. Available at: https://twitter.com/hashtag/EUAnimalStats?src=hashtag_click.
48. EARA. EARA's #TransparencyThursday. Transparency Thursdays give voice to researchers to talk about their research in an informal manner and how animals play such an important part in it. 2021. Available at: https://www.eara.eu/post/transparencythursday.
49. Netherlands Cancer Institute (YouTube). How research is conducted at the Netherlands Cancer Institute. Behind the scenes at the research facility with staff explaining the work they do directly to the camera. 2023. Available at: https://www.youtube.com/watch?v=cMFXcvM-lUQ&t=146s
50. Speaking of Research. Animal Justice Project misleading public over Swedish malaria study. 2016. Available at: https://speakingofresearch.com/2016/03/23/animal-justice-project-misleading-public-over-swedish-malaria-study/.
51. Le Soir. Belgian researchers respond to misinformation about animal testing. Open letter by researchers from Université Libre de Bruxelles, UC Louvain, University of Liège, University of Mons and University of Namur, responding to misinformation about the use of animal experiments on Belgian channel RTBF. 2019. Available at: https://www.lesoir.be/125453/article/2017-11-21/lexperimentation-animale-une-pratique-medicalement-et-ethiquement-tres-encadree

21 Analyzing Our Organization and Strategizing to Grow or Survive. A Case Scenario

Aurora Brønstad

Abstract

Strategy is the field of topics about the best hypothesis about relationships, causalities, and how things are connected, and which is important as a roadmap under changed and uncertain conditions. This chapter gives an overview of different response patterns to changes, what an organization is in relation to its surroundings, and how different systems essential for the organization are integrated. The relational interactions with the organization come into play under changing conditions. Adaptions will be necessary, and the strategic roadmap will be helpful in balancing formal and informal mechanisms, rational and emotional factors that are not under hierarchical the control of organization. Such understanding is necessary to arrive at the favored condition. A scenario at the end of the chapter will exemplify the theories.

Keywords

Strategy · Change management · Organizational relationships

A. Brønstad (✉)
Department of Clinical Medicine, University of Bergen, Bergen, Norway
e-mail: aurora.bronstad@uib.no

21.1 What Is Strategy and Why Is It Important?

Many important decisions are based on limited information and uncertainty about the outcome.

There is always unpredictability about the future and there might be a need to adjust assumptions about internal and external circumstances. Strategy is the field of topics about making the best hypothesis about relationships, causalities, and how things are connected. A strategy may be a roadmap to either success or survival under changed conditions. Most organizations aim to safely arrive at the preferred place or in a preferred condition. A popular way of saying this is "you need to understand the map and the surroundings - not only the highway." It is important to understand the surroundings—the external factors—as well as your "engine"—the internal factors to arrive safely and timely at the target.

21.2 How to Respond to Changes?

There are different ways to respond to changes, as disregard, ridicule, adaptation, and actions to take control of the process.

Disregard and ridicule, and maybe also resistance [1], maybe humane responses to changes or threats; however, the outcome of this approach is likely not very beneficial and may, in the end, lead to a disaster. Resistance includes both emotional

J. Guillén, V. Galligioni (eds.), *Practical Management of Research Animal Care and Use Programs*, Laboratory Animal Science and Medicine 3, https://doi.org/10.1007/978-3-031-65414-5_21

and political components and ranges from indifference to active or even aggressive resistance [2].

Adaption is necessary to survive as things are changing, though the outcome might not be the optimal or the favored one. This is a reactive response to change. Changes do happen because the organizations have to adapt [1]. All organizations go through some level of adaption through their lifetime [3].

Taking control best reflects a strategical approach to changes, where the relevant actors analyze the conditions, grab the steering wheel, maneuver with control, and use their influence to reduce risks and lead a process in a favorable direction. This will be a proactive response to the understanding of internal and external factors that either offer opportunities for growth or avoid a disaster for the organization [1]. Making a disaster plan for how to secure animals and scientific activities is an example of taking control of worst-case scenario [4].

In this chapter, the models will be introduced for analyzing internal and external factors that are relevant and important for decisions about the future. Such models are helpful to get a better overview, or "helicopter perspective" of the situation, and avoid the risk of taking short-term decisions and solving "nearby" problems. It is important to understand how changes might influence us, as it is necessary for how we decide to cope in the best way. A scenario at the end of this chapter will exemplify the theory.

There is uncertainty about what future scenarios will be—so I see it pointless to be descriptive of solutions as they likely do not fit or are not relevant for other cases.

The aim of this chapter is to present and illustrate tools that can be useful in a strategic approach to change. But first, how can we describe an organization and its relationship to the surroundings as well as internal constitution?

21.3 What Is an Organization?

An organization is a group of people working to achieve certain goals and objectives. The activity in the organization is characterized by a high level of formalized rules and procedures. The work tasks are shared and coordinated between individuals and groups in the organization. An organization does not exist in a vacuum—independent of the rest of the world. Ideally, the organization stays in a symbiotic relationship with its stakeholders.

An organization has legitimacy as long as the stakeholders perceive benefits from the input resources they bring to the organization. The organization and its stakeholders are dependent on each other by providing resources to customers, employees, and owners (input), and the organization provides benefits back to the stakeholders. In this way, the organization exists in a relationship with the surrounding world (Fig. 21.1).

Organizations are like organic systems, and the organizational culture is influenced and characterized by elements like social values, norms, behavior, and perceptions of reality. When these are established in the organization, and almost getting the feel of being taken for granted, we say that they are "institutionalized" [5].

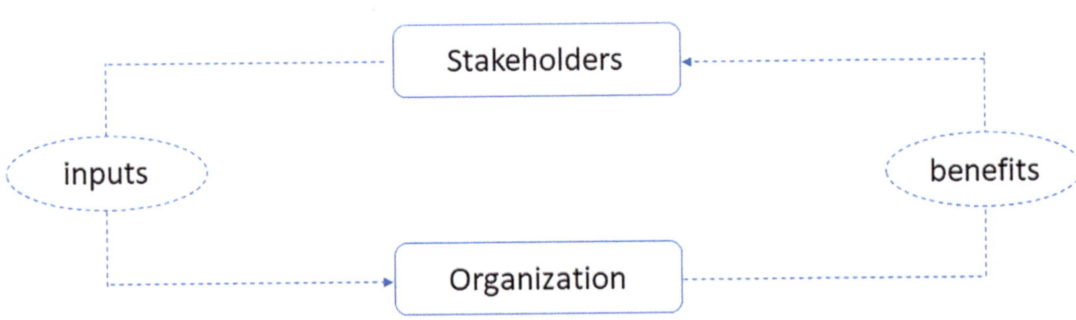

Fig. 21.1 How stakeholder inputs to the organization are transformed to benefits for the stakeholders

21.4 What Is the "Technical Environment" and Why Is It Important?

It is important to gain knowledge about and understanding of the technical environment for the organization's effectiveness. In general, the "technical environment" includes all matters outside the organization's boundaries of hierarchical control, but they are still important for the organization to maintain production of goods and services [6]. The technical environment includes the political system that determines important framework conditions for the organization and the economic systems that define rules for economic activity and possibilities for financing activities [6]. Further, the technical environment includes labor market and the availability of qualified workers at a reasonable cost, and last but not least customers of whatever the organization provides or produces [6].

Technological opportunities, or the opportunities at institutional level, define abilities to transform input factors (money, material, support, etc.) into values, benefits, or profits for customers. Competence in the use of technologies to achieve the best, favorable result is an important component of the machinery.

All these factors have an impact on the organization's ability to achieve its missions and goals and are linked directly to the organization's transformation system which is necessary for the production of goods and services.

21.5 What Is the "Institutional Environment" and Why Is It Important?

While the technical environment is important for the efficiency of the institution, the institutional environment is important for the organization's legitimacy [6]. The behavior of the organization must be in harmony with the general norms and expectations of the society [7]. The use of animals in research raises ethical issues and the general public is concerned on how animals are used and for what purposes [8, 9]. Compliance with rules and regulations is a minimum requirement for legal legitimacy of an animal research organization [7]. Regulations for animal studies, like harmonization with the common European directive [10], define the baseline for what is legally acceptable. Lack of compliance with rules and regulations damages the reputation of the organization and harms research fields that are dependent on the use of animals. Consumers' power may finally harm the organization if consumers perceive that animal studies are not performed in an ethical, responsible manner.

> Legitimacy is a generalized perception or assumption that the actions of an entity are desirable, proper, or appropriate within some socially constructed system of norms, values, beliefs, and definitions [11].

Legitimacy is a value of its own, independent of the effectiveness of the organization [7].

Adaption by institutionalizing is important for an organization, both for survival as well as reducing potential conflicts. For example, by not violating laws and regulations for animal research, as well as meeting society's norms on how to treat research animals in a humane way. Such adaptations are important for the legitimacy of the organization.

Cultural artifacts provide information about values in the organizational culture [12]. Demonstrating 3R compliance [13], adherence to the concept of culture of care, including appropriate attitudes, behavior, mindsets and mutual respect [14], and participation in voluntary accreditation programs like AAALAC International [15], reflect ways of demonstrating social responsibility in accordance with current expectations, values, and norms proving normative legitimacy for the organization [7].

While legal compliance with animal research regulations provides a formal license to operate (so the organization will not be legally punished, have to pay penalty fees or have representatives go to jail), demonstrating harmony with society's norms and expectations on how to treat animals are necessary for smooth operations without recurring conflicts. Recurring conflicts drain energy and resources from the organization and harm effectiveness of core activities.

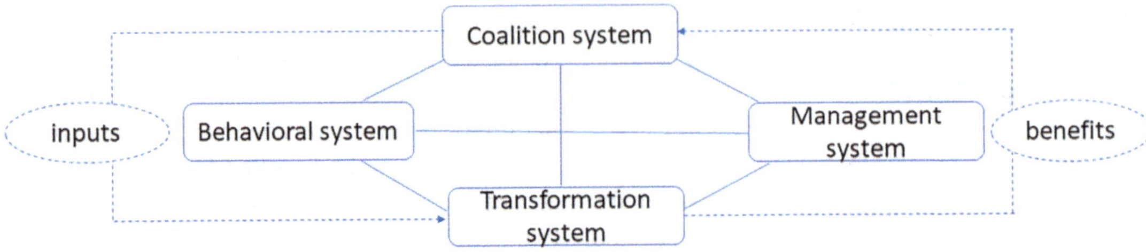

Fig. 21.2 An integrated model showing how critical components of an organization are interrelated and how inputs and outputs as profit for the stakeholders may be modulated by the different components

21.6 How Can We Map and Understand Relevant Components?—and How Do These Factors Influence Each Other?

To be sustainable, any organization must show they are effective in producing values or benefits—for their owners or society in general. If the input-reward balance turns out to be negative, stakeholders may withdraw their contributions and support that constitute the basis of existence for an organization.

Tor Busch and Jan Ole Vanebo together with Eirik Johnsen, developed a generic, integrated model for how internal and external components were influencing the effectiveness and operational capacity of an organization [16]. Such a model does represent a simplification, but still gives an overview of important interaction of components influencing any organization. Such understanding is valuable for strategy and decision-making under changing circumstances. It is also important for growth, success, or survival of the organization. The components of the model will be explained, and it will be exemplified how they may impact an animal research organization (Fig. 21.2).

21.7 What Is the "Coalition System"?

A coalition system represents actors in an environment who have common interests vis-à-vis an organization within a defined area. The coalition system represents stakeholders, meaning organizations or groups that have an interest in the existence, presence, continuation, and function of an organization. The coalition system gives inputs to the organization in the form of resources or support and achieves benefits or profits back from the organization. And usually, what they achieve back is regarded as more valuable (better, more beneficial, or profitable) than generating that same or similar value on their own. The stakeholders perceive the benefits as "good value for money."

So, stakeholders, such as customers, employees, and owners, contribute to a reward relationship with the organization through contracts with the organization. For example, the life science industry is interested in basic preclinical research, as this is a source of new knowledge that might have commercial potential as new treatments or other products. Industry can make contracts with academia on specific research projects where they see a commercial possibility, or they do so to demonstrate social responsibility—without any other obligations—for financing any kind of research. Patient organizations are interested in how industry can provide us with better treatments, but also the industry is dependent on consumers, willing to pay for their products. Lawmakers and similar bodies are an important component of the coalition system as they define borders of operation for the organizations. For example, the European Medicines Agency (EMA) contributes to protection of public and animal health in European Union (EU) Member States by ensuring that all medicines available on the EU market are safe, effective, and of high quality—which is also of interest to consumers.

21.8 What Is the Transformation System?

The transformation system is the "machinery" of the organization and includes all human, physical, and financial resources necessary for the organization to create value for the stakeholders. The transformation system is the fundament for continuation of existence. Typical components are physical plants, facilities and equipment, methodologies, procedures, and routines, and, not least, competence by employees, as abilities, knowledge, and skills. Competent animal care staff and competent veterinarians are an important part of the transformation system for animal research activities, and a high level of competence is desired for any organization providing services.

All these are input factors in the transformation system that convert them to values and benefits for customers like new treatment, raw materials for production, knowledge, smarter solutions, new technology, and innovations. This happens through value-creation processes in the transformation system. Important to notice is the fact that humans are a part of the transformation system. The employees' work satisfaction, perception of the meaning of their tasks, and fair work conditions will influence the performance of the organization. The internal environment is important for the organization's effectiveness and smooth operation through the transformation system.

21.9 What Is the Management System?

The management system is highly formalized through a hierarchy and an organizational map. The management system has two main functions: negotiations with the stakeholders and contract fulfillment vis-à-vis the stakeholders [17]. The management system defines roles and responsibilities for different work tasks—that influence the behavior of the employees. Further, the management system must regularly adjust ambitions and objectives to the organizations' resources based on changes in the environment. This is a challenge because adaptations may be costly, unaffordable, and in the worst case threatening the fundament of existence of the organization in its current form. Management has been defined as the power and initiative to participate in a binding, goal- or objective-defining, problem-solving, and language-developing behavior [17]. That means to define the target the organization is aiming for, what the organization needs to reach the target, and what is the common language to use, so that everyone in the organization understands and supports the direction.

Management behavior can be described as defining objectives and allocating resources necessary to achieve them. Creating a common language that resonates among the people is also an important function of management behavior. Communicating objectives and openness on the resources is important for the people in the organization, as those people in the end will be the "machinery" responsible for the deliveries.

Defining the organization structure, that is how activities are managed and coordinated and how decision-making authority is assigned are important tasks of the management system [17]. The need for coordination starts when individuals or groups perform special tasks that other groups are dependent on for their function.

Formally, job descriptions define tasks, authority, and responsibilities. Specialized functions are very much related to competence. Whether a work task is standardized following a formal job description (for example, Standard Operation Procedures, SOPs) or there is a need for professional case-by-case judgement, should be reflected in the job description. Freedom to take own decisions independent of formal procedures is important for job satisfaction for many professionals. If not, there is a risk of bureaucratic inefficiency, as well as loss of job satisfaction. The management must balance needs for control, high efficacy, and good legitimacy. An organization often mirrors the existing coalition and the organization structure is there to direct the behavior of the people, and reduce the risk of people behaving according to self-interest at the cost of the organizations' interest [17].

21.10 What Is the Behavioral System?

The interest in organizational behavior as a key to success very much stems from studies of American successful companies [18]. Motivated employees engaged in meaningful activities, positive feedback, and a feeling of connection to the organization are important factors to success [18]. Advocates of the importance of organizational behavior and the behavioral system say that this is just as important as formal structures [19], and research on organizations has shown that organizational culture is important for actual behavior [18].

The people in the organization make their footprint by informal structures. Organizational culture includes interpersonal relations or relationships, roles, values, norms, attitudes, and not at least "perceptions of reality" and how things are connected [12]. Organizational culture has a significant impact on how the organization presents itself and how well it performs, and has close connections to both the coalition and the transformation systems [19].

A functional perspective of organizational culture is described as an "instinct to survive."

The organizational culture is necessary for survival and development to preserve important functions is a result of a long process [12, 19]. So, we behave and act the way we believe is the best to remain in the business and for job security, and people in the organization adapt to these beliefs.

This way of behavior is learned and taken for granted, and seldom questioned if this is the best way to behave. This way behavioral patterns are conserved within a group of people. It may include behavior on how people interact and new members of the organization must learn this way of behavior.

Schein (1987) defined organizational culture as a response to demands from the environment [12]. According to Schein [12], organizational culture represents a pattern of basic assumptions that are taken for granted. The pattern of basic assumptions is created or developed by a social group as they experience mastering their problems. This strategy works appropriately to be regarded as "true" and is learned to new members of the group as the right way to think, understand, and feel concerning problem solving [12]. This way, the culture becomes a fundament for behavior. The organizational culture is formed by external adaptation to the surroundings as well as internal integration within the group or organization. For animal research fostering, a culture of care [14] (see also Chap. 6) is an example focusing on the concern for the welfare of other sentient beings, as the research animals as well as the people in this industry.

A culture is informal and cannot be changed just by decision—as organizational culture is anchored in basic assumptions about right and wrong among the individual people. The management can try to *foster* a certain culture anchored in values they would like to be recognized with—but it is difficult to enforce a certain culture, especially if there are cognitive dissonance or conflicts with people's core values, beliefs, or desires on what is regarded as true and suitable for problem solving. For example, if the management expresses that the organization shall be characterized by a "culture of care" [14], however, in priorities in practice—this is not the case (See Chap. 6 on Culture of Care).

While rules and regulations can be changed overnight, it takes a long time to change the culture in the organization. However, demands, limitations, and opportunities in the surroundings may have an impact and modify the culture.

From a rational perspective, the organizational culture is an instrument to create a well-functioning organization [19]. The benefit of a common value platform that direct employees' behavior is important versus the stakeholders for continued support [19]. For example establishing a 3R-reward, can be a rational attempt and a symbol of acknowledgement of employees efforts to fulfill the core values of the principle by Russel and Burch [20] or a culture of care that the organizations like to be identified with.

In the rational perspective, organizations emphasize a common culture and subcultures within the organization are regarded as less desirable [19].

Organizational culture can also be understood from a symbolic perspective as a pattern of symbols or expressions that are communicated by members of the organization. 3Rs-rewards may be a typical symbolic ritual or tradition and an incentive to stimulate more focus on the animals' intrinsic value as well as the animals right to the best possible welfare. The culture is created through social interactions that connect people and nurture a common identity [19].

Argyris and Shön distinguish between expressed values and used values [21]. Used values are the behavior we actually perform. The behavior does not have to correspond with what we say we are doing, the expressed behavior [21]. There is not always a correspondence between what is expressed and actual behavior [22]. An organization can claim that they have implemented the 3Rs, but this is not necessarily reflected in changes in behavior or prioritized when important decisions are made.

21.11 What Have We Learned So Far?

So far, we have learned about the components in the model of an organization and how the components are in relation to each other. Changes in one of them may very likely have influence on the others, and this is of strategic importance to understand. Demands for effectiveness may come in conflict with legitimacy demands if the welfare of humans, animals, or environment is compromised. Loss of legitimacy may undermine the basis of existence of your organization if support from the coalition system comes to an end. Employees who perceive conflicts with their core values and professional pride and make efforts to deliver with a high level of professional standards may lose motivation and momentum with the cost of work performance.

21.12 Analysis of a Scenario: What If There Will Be a Total Ban of Animal Studies?

Case: A very popular politician has announced in his program that he will ban all animal studies if he is elected as president. Opinion polls show that its very like that he will win.

You are the manager of a preclinical research unit housing rodents, pigs and zebrafish. Your site has a long record of success with researchers publishing in highly rated journals, winning prizes and contributing to innovations and significant progress in translational medicine. Your company receives generous private and public funding and there is a strategic plan to invest millions in expansion for the next 25 years. You are a part of the project team to realize this ambition.

How do you respond to potential change in the political environment?

Despite initiatives to ban animal research, animals are still (January 2024) needed for medical progress when alternative methods do not exist. How should the company deal with the scenario—how should they proceed with their strategy and expansion plan?

A careless response can be to just ignore the prognosis from the opinion poll, have faith in the long history of success, the support from the public and the private companies and continue the expansion plan as if nothing happened. Ridiculing the politician saying things like "It's stupid – we will always need animals", "only stupid, uneducated people propose such things", or "just wait until he becomes seriously ill and need treatment" may sustaining the narrative of historical merits and assumption of invulnerability. However, this might not be enough to convince the majority eligible to vote and politics is just as much about feelings than facts.

The adaptation position will be a wait and see and take necessary adjustments along the road as they come. This might sound like a safe and sound approach, not worrying about things that may never happen. It may be a risk to take regarding the expansion plan and the significant investments. Also, the employer's job security might be at stake. If not a significant threat to the organization—it might not be optimal either.

To behave as an actor, taking the steering wheel, trying to control the potential threat, it might be sensible to use some strategic tool to better understand the external factors that might influence the outcome.

It is not only this politician that want to end animal research. There are groups and organizations demanding EU to make an action plan to end the use of animals in research and testing, as, for example, the "Stop Vivisection" European Citizens' Initiative in 2012 [23] and the "Save cruelty-free cosmetics – Commit to a Europe without animal testing" of 2023 [24].

Important components of your coalition system include medical and life science research institutions, pharmaceutical companies, and patient organizations. Representatives from your supplier chain of goods for animals may also be influenced by the alarming signal of the opinion polls and statements from this politician. An analysis of the interests of the coalition system may be valuable.

Your transformation system has been rigged for animal studies, spare parts, and maintenance service may be unavailable, physical equipment may be too specialized in its current form for other purposes and those investments may be lost. The human resource base and collective competence in your company may possibly be transformed to fit into other industries or services. The behavioral system may be affected both by the threat of losing jobs and by the dissonance between what was assumed to be a responsible, important industry—now becomes illegal. The organization's culture will impact perception of the new reality, how people behave and perceive support when a potential threat appears. The management system must take the correct action to limit damage to the organization. Personally, you have already used efforts in the investment and expansion plan, which now seems to be in danger.

To get a better overview of the scenario, a PESTEL analysis might be helpful. PESTEL stands for *p*olitical, *e*conomic, *s*ocietal, *t*echnological, *e*nvironmental, and *l*egal and is a tool to systematically evaluate factors that may have an impact on an outcome.

21.13 What Can a PESTEL Analysis Tell?

An example of a PESTEL analysis on this scenario of banning animal use in preclinical studies can look like as described in Table 21.1.

Politics is not mainly based on scientific facts or rational choices, but to a large extent on feelings, moods, and trends in society. An important alliance for you in the coalition system is the research community. Recent years "fake news" and "alternative facts" have entered discussion causing confusion of what is facts and what is

Table 21.1 Example of a PESTEL analysis

P—political	• Named politicians will ban animal use in preclinical research • Politicians define laws and regulations • Politics is not based on scientific or rational choices needs, but also on feelings, moods, and trends in society
E—economic	• Running animal facilities is costly, demands high-quality buildings, specially trained and competent staff
S—Society	• There is a "vegan"/vegetarian movement in society. Not only for animal welfare reasons but also for our own health and the sustainability of the environment. European Citizens' Initiative for Vegan meals was already been proposed in 2022 [25] • Several surveys among lay people reflect a concern for research animals and a position that they should be replaced by other methods, the number of animals used should be minimized and animals should not suffer. These values can be recognized as the 3Rs [20]
T—Technology	• There are some "non-animal" alternatives like organoids, data-simulations, and other in vitro models • However, technology has not yet been able to replace all animal studies • Automatization may reduce some labor costs for manual work—however, they demand large investments
E—Environment	• Energy costly running animal houses, use of chemical for disinfectants Sanitation and sterilization equipment that is energy consuming
L—Legal	• If total ban is not going to happen, there is still an aspiration to limit animal use reflected in 3Rs explicitly mentioned in the EU Directive [10]

faults. Researchers must be better at communicating, in a fact-based manner, why animal studies are still important for medical progress in certain fields. Regarding economy and saving costs—the plan for big investments should be considered—and maybe include opportunities for flexibility, especially if new, more cost-saving non-animal models technology seems to be evolving and new better methods are emerging. The vegan trend may be anchored in an animal rights position [26], but is also motivated by health concerns and the sustainability of the environment. For the legitimacy of your organization and support with the public, it will be important to communicate a shared concern for unsolved health issues, as well as communicating how the 3Rs are implemented in all activities involving animals in order to improve animal welfare.

Looking at this PESTEL analysis, there is more than just this politician talking against expansion of animal studies. And you might wonder why animal studies have not been replaced a long time ago for several other reasons? We might raise the hypothetical question if animal research was never invented—based on this analysis—it would maybe never be started? There are many explanations why using animals for research was established as a tool, and those decisions were made in another context and under other conditions than today.

21.14 What Can a SWOT Analysis Tell?

The outcome of this PESTEL analysis did not show the most optimistic result for this scenario. It could be useful to do a complementary SWOT analysis, standing for *s*trength, *w*eaknesses, *o*pportunities, and *t*hreats—as this is an analysis includes potential upsides (Table 21.2).

It is important to include all elements of the model in the SWOT analysis (Table 21.3).

The existing coalition system may be a strength; however, changes might open doors for opportunities to build a new and even better coalition. The management should try to identify strengths in their transformation system, like, for example, competent staff, that is able to transform their skills into new directions. A very specialized, little flexible technology may be a weakness when circumstances are changing. A solid organizational culture will be a strength in the behavioral system with loyal employees who will do their best to support the management. Competent management is essential to build and nurture a strong organizational culture with loyal employees. On the other hand, poor management will be harmful to the organization under changing and difficult conditions.

Table 21.2 Generic model of components of a SWOT analysis

	Helpful	Harmful
Internal origin	Strength	Weaknesses
External origin	Opportunities	Threats

Table 21.3 Integrating components of the Coalition system in a SWOT analysis

	Helpful	Harmful
Internal origin	Strength – In the Coalition system – In the Transformation system – In the Behavioral system – In the Management system	Weaknesses – In the Coalition system – In the Transformation system – In the Behavioral system – In the Management system
External origin	Opportunities – in the Coalition system – in the Transformation system – in the Behavioral system – in the Management system	Threats – in the Coalition system – in the Transformation system – in the Behavioral system – in the Management system

21.15 What Can We Learn from This Chapter?

Important decisions about the future are based on limited information and there is always uncertainty about the outcome. Strategy, the field about making the best hypothesis about how things are connected and to make the best roadmap to navigate under changed, unknown circumstances, depends on a good understanding of internal and external components and how they are in play with each other.

An ignorant attitude or passive adaptation to warned changes will in most cases not lead to a favorable outcome. Taking an active approach and gaining knowledge for a more complete understanding of factors that are in play provides information that can reduce the risk of harm to the organization and increase the opportunity of a favorable outcome.

References

1. Jacobsen DI. Endringsprosesser - tid, oversettelse og motstand. In: Jacobsen DI, editor. Organisasjonsendringer og endringsledelse. Bergen: Fagbokforlaget; 2004. p. 137–80.
2. Nadler DA. The effective management of organizational change. In: Lorsch JW, editor. Handbook of organizational behavior. Englewood Cliffs, NJ: Prentice-Hall; 1987.
3. Diamond MA. Resistance to change: a psychoanalytic critique of Argyris and Schon's contribution to organization theory and intervention. J Manage Stud. 1986;23(5):543.
4. Garber JC, et al. Animal care and use program. In: Academies TN, editor. Guide for the care and use of laboratory animals. 8th ed. Committee for the Update of the Guide for the Care and Use of Laboratory Animals; National Research Council: National Academies Press; 2010. p. 11–40.
5. Selznick P. Foundations of the theory of organization. Am Sociol Rev. 1948;13(1):25–35.
6. Vanebo JO, Busch T. Tekniske omgivelser. In: Organisasjon og Ledelse: Et integrert perspektiv. Oslo, Norway: Universitetsforlaget AS; 2003. p. 56–85.
7. Vanebo JO, Busch T. Institusjonelle omgivelser. In: Organisasjon og Ledelse: Et integrert perspektiv. Oslo, Norway: Universitetsforlaget AS; 2003. p. 88–108.
8. SwedishResearchCouncil, Public opinion in Sweden on the use of animals research. 2008.
9. Lund TB, et al. Painful dilemmas: a study of the way the public's assessment of animal research balances costs to animals against human benefits. Public Underst Sci. 2014;23(4):428–44.
10. European Commission. Directive 2010/63/EU of the European Parliament anf of the council of 22 September 2010 on the protection of animals used for scientific purposes. European Commission; 2010.
11. Suchman MC. Managing legitimacy: strategic and institutional approaches. Acad Manage Rev. 1995;20(3):571–610.
12. Schein EH. Organizational culture and leadership, The Jossey-Bass business & management series, vol. XVI. 3rd ed. San Francisco, CA: Jossey-Bass; 2004. p. 437s.
13. Brønstad A, Berg A-GT. 3R Culture, compliance and consequences. Lab Anim. 2011;40(1):22–6.
14. Bertelsen T, Hawkins P. In: Sørensen DB, Pedersen A, Bailey RE, editors. A culture of care, in animal-centric care and management: enhancing refinement in biomedical research. CRC Press; 2020.
15. AAALAC International. Private, nonprofit organization that promotes the humane treatment of animals in science through voluntary accreditation and assessment programs]. 2023. Available from: https://www.aaalac.org/about/what-is-aaalac/
16. Vanebo JO, Busch T, editors. Organisasjon og Ledelse: Et integrert perspektiv. 5th ed. Oslo, Norway: Universitetsforlaget AS; 2003. p. 447.
17. Vanebo JO, Busch T. Organisasjonsstruktur. In: Vanebo JO, Busch T, editors. Organisasjon og Ledelse : Et integrert perspektiv. Oslo, Norway: Universitetsforlaget AS; 2003. p. 143–86.
18. Peters T, Waterman RH. In search of excellence: lessons from America's best-run companies. New York: Harper & Row; 1982.
19. Vanebo JO, Busch T. Organisasjonskultur. In: Vanebo JO, Busch T, editors. Organisasjon og Ledelse: Et integrert perspektiv. Oslo, Norway: Universitetsforlaget AS; 2003. p. 187–218.
20. Russell WMS, Burch RL. The principles of humane experimental technique. London: Methuen; 1959. p. 238s.
21. Argyris C, Schön DA. Organizational learning / a theory of action perspective, vol. VII. Reading, MA: Addison-Wesley; 1978. p. 344s.
22. Haukelid K. Theories of (safety) culture revisited - an anthropological approach. Saf Sci. 2008;46:413–26.
23. European Commission. European Citizens' Initiative "Stop Vivisection". Brussel, Belgium: 2012.
24. European Commission. Save cruelty-free cosmetics – commit to a Europe without animal testing. Brussel, Belgium: 2023.
25. European Citizens' Initiative for VEGAN MEAL. 2022 [cited 2023 July 13]; Available from: https://europa.eu/citizens-initiative/initiatives/details/2022/000009_en
26. Regan T, editor. The case for animal rights. Updated with a new preface. Berkeley, CA: University of California Press; 2004.

MIX
Papier aus verantwortungsvollen Quellen
Paper from responsible sources
FSC® C105338

If you have any concerns about our products,
you can contact us on
ProductSafety@springernature.com

In case Publisher is established outside the EU,
the EU authorized representative is:
Springer Nature Customer Service Center GmbH
Europaplatz 3, 69115 Heidelberg, Germany

Printed by Libri Plureos GmbH
in Hamburg, Germany